DIABETES IN
CARDIOVASCULAR
DISEASE

A Companion to Braunwald's Heart Disease

DIABETES IN CARDIOVASCULAR DISEASE

A Companion to Braunwald's Heart Disease

Darren K. McGuire, MD, MHSc, FAHA, FACC
Professor of Internal Medicine
Dallas Heart Ball Chair for Research on Heart Disease in Women
Director, Parkland Hospital and Health System Cardiology Clinics
University of Texas Southwestern Medical Center
Dallas, Texas

Nikolaus Marx, MD, FAHA
Professor of Medicine/Cardiology
Head of Department of Internal Medicine I
University Hospital Aachen
Aachen, Germany

ELSEVIER
SAUNDERS

1600 John F. Kennedy Blvd.
Ste 1800
Philadelphia, PA 19103-2899

DIABETES IN CARDIOVASCULAR DISEASE: A COMPANION TO BRAUNWALD'S HEART DISEASE   ISBN: 978-1-4557-5418-2

Library of Congress Cataloging-in-Publication Data

Diabetes in cardiovascular disease: a companion to Braunwald's heart disease / [edited by] Darren K. McGuire, Nikolaus Marx.
       p.; cm.
   Complemented by: Braunwald's heart disease / edited by Robert O. Bonow ... [et al.]. 9th ed. 2012.
   Includes bibliographical references and index.
   ISBN 978-1-4557-5418-2 (hardcover: alk. paper)
   I. McGuire, Darren K., editor. II. Marx, Nikolaus (Professor of medicine/cardiology), editor. III. Braunwald's heart disease.
Complemented by (work):
   [DNLM: 1. Cardiovascular Diseases–complications. 2. Diabetes Complications. 3. Diabetes Mellitus–physiopathology.
4. Diabetes Mellitus–therapy. 5. Risk Factors. WG 120]
   RC681
   616.1'2–dc23
                                        2014012925

Executive Content Strategist: Dolores Meloni
Content Development Specialist: Angela Rufino
Publishing Services Manager: Anne Altepeter
Project Manager: Cindy Thoms
Design Manager: Steven Stave
Illustrations Manager: Lesley Frazier

Printed in China

Last digit is the print number: 9 8 7 6 5 4 3 2 1

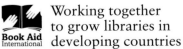

To my wife, Julia, and our children, Emma and Jack, for their support, encouragement, and sacrifices for the time and effort required to develop this book. Thanks to each of you for keeping me focused on what is really most important, always.

To the patients around the world afflicted with diabetes, with hopes of an increasingly bright future.

Darren K. McGuire

To Nicole, and to my children, Nadine, Julian, and Florian, for their remarkable support through this endeavor.

In memory of my father Hans-Albert.

Nikolaus Marx

Contributors

David Aguilar, MD
Assistant Professor of Medicine
Internal Medicine and Cardiology
Baylor College of Medicine
Houston, Texas

Sylvie A. Ahn, MD
Division of Cardiology
Cliniques Universitaires – St-Luc
Pôle de Recherche Cardiovasculaire
Institut de Recherche Expérimentale et Clinique (IREC)
Université Catholique de Louvain
Brussels, Belgium

Pavan K. Battiprolu, PhD
Departments of Internal Medicine, Cardiology, and
    Metabolic Disorders
University of Texas Southwestern Medical Center
Dallas, Texas

Joshua A. Beckman, MD, MS
Associate Professor of Medicine
Harvard Medical School
Director, Cardiovascular Fellowship Program
Cardiovascular Division
Brigham and Women's Hospital
Boston, Massachusetts

Deepak L. Bhatt, MD, MPH
Executive Director of Interventional Cardiovascular
    Programs
Brigham and Women's Hospital Heart and Vascular Center
Senior Physician
Brigham and Women's Hospital
Senior Investigator
TIMI Study Group
Boston, Massachusetts

Petter Bjornstad, MD
Department of Pediatrics
Children's Hospital Colorado
University of Colorado School of Medicine
Aurora, Colorado

Jonathan D. Brown, MD
Instructor
Harvard Medical School
Cardiovascular Division
Brigham and Women's Hospital
Boston, Massachusetts

Melanie J. Davies, MD, PhD
Diabetes Research Centre
College of Medicine
Biological Sciences and Psychology
University of Leicester
Leicester, United Kingdom

Robert H. Eckel, MD
Professor of Medicine
University of Colorado Anschutz Medical Campus
Aurora, Colorado

Leonard E. Egede, MD, MS
Professor of Medicine
Health Equity and Rural Outreach Innovation Center
Ralph H. Johnson Department of Veterans Affairs Medical
    Center
Center for Health Disparities Research, Division of General
    Internal Medicine
Medical University of South Carolina
Charleston, South Carolina

Frank Joachim Erbguth, MD, PhD
Professor of Neurology
Department of Neurology
Nuremberg Municipal Academic Hospital
Nuremberg, Germany

Jason S. Fish, MD, MSHS
Director of Ambulatory Quality and Optimization
Assistant Professor
Internal Medicine
University of Texas Southwestern Medical Center
Dallas, Texas

B. Miles Fisher, MD, MB ChB
Consultant Physician
Glasgow Royal Infirmary
Honorary Professor
University of Glasgow
Glasgow, Scotland

Barry A. Franklin, PhD
Director
Preventive Cardiology and Cardiac Rehabilitation
William Beaumont Hospital
Royal Oak, Michigan
Professor of Internal Medicine
Oakland University
William Beaumont School of Medicine
Rochester, Michigan

Baptist Gallwitz, MD
Deputy Head of Department
Department of Medicine IV (Endocrinology, Diabetology,
     Angiology, Nephrology, and Clinical Chemistry)
Eberhard Karls University Tübingen
Tübingen, Germany

Baris Gencer, MD
Fellow
Interventional Cardiology Unit
Cardiology Division
University Hospital
Geneva, Switzerland

Anselm K. Gitt, MD, FESC
Herzzentrum Ludwigshafen
Medizinische Klinik B, Kardiologie
Stiftung Institut für Herzinfarktforschung Ludwigshafen
Ludwigshafen, Germany

Colin Greaves, PhD
Senior Research Fellow
University of Exeter Medical School
University of Exeter
Exeter, Devon, United Kingdom

Hans Ulrich Häring, MD, PhD
Head of Department
Department of Medicine IV (Endocrinology, Diabetology,
     Angiology, Nephrology, and Clinical Chemistry)
Eberhard Karls University Tübingen
Tübingen, Germany

Markolf Hanefeld, MD, PhD
Professor
Study Centre Professor Hanefeld
University Hospital
Carl Gustav Carus Technical University
Dresden, Germany

**Michel P. Hermans, MD, PhD, DipNatSci, DipEarthSci,
DipGeogEnv, PGCert(SocSc)**
Professor
Endocrinology and Nutrition
Cliniques Universitaires Saint-Luc
Brussels, Belgium

Adrian F. Hernandez, MD, MHS
Director, Outcomes Research
Duke Clinical Research Institute
Associate Professor of Medicine
Cardiology
Duke University School of Medicine
Durham, North Carolina

Joseph A. Hill, MD, PhD
Departments of Internal Medicine (Cardiology) and
     Molecular Biology
Division of Cardiology
University of Texas Southwestern Medical Center
Dallas, Texas

Kelly J. Hunt, PhD
Health Equity and Rural Outreach Innovation Center
Ralph H. Johnson Department of Veterans Affairs
     Medical Center
Center for Health Disparities Research,
     Division of General Internal Medicine
Department of Public Health Sciences
Medical University of South Carolina
Charleston, South Carolina

Silvio E. Inzucchi, MD
Professor
Internal Medicine (Endocrinology)
Yale University School of Medicine
Clinical Chief, Endocrinology
Director, Yale Diabetes Center
Yale-New Haven Hospital
New Haven, Connecticut

Stefan K. James, MD, PhD
Department of Medical Sciences
Uppsala Clinical Research Center
Uppsala University
Uppsala, Sweden

Tracy R. Juliao, PhD, LP, NCC
Director of Psychology
Weight Control Center
William Beaumont Hospital
Royal Oak, Michigan
Assistant Professor
Oakland University
William Beaumont School of Medicine
Rochester, Michigan

Wolfgang Koenig, MD, FRCP, FESC, FACC, FAHA
Professor of Medicine and Cardiology
Department of Internal Medicine II – Cardiology
University of Ulm Medical Center
Ulm, Germany

Frank D. Kolodgie, MD
CVPath Institute
Gaithersburg, Maryland

Mikhail Kosiborod, MD
Professor of Medicine
St. Luke's Mid America Heart Institute
University of Missouri – Kansas City
Kansas City, Missouri

Elena Ladich, MD
Chief, Cardiovascular Pathology
CVPath Institute
Gaithersburg, Maryland

Harold L. Lazar, MD
Professor of Cardiothoracic Surgery
Department of Cardiothoracic Surgery
Boston Medical Center
Boston, Massachusetts

Kasia J. Lipska, MD, MHS
Instructor in Medicine
Section of Endocrinology
Department of Medicine Yale School of Medicine
New Haven, Connecticut

Cheryl P. Lynch, MD, MPH
Physician-Investigator
Health Equity and Rural Outreach Innovation Center
Ralph H. Johnson, Department of Veterans Affairs Medical
    Center
Assistant Professor of Medicine
Center for Health Disparities Research, Division of General
    Internal Medicine
Medical University of South Carolina
Charleston, South Carolina

David M. Maahs, MD, PhD
Assistant Professor of Pediatrics
Barbara Davis Center for Diabetes
Department of Medicine
Aurora, Colorado

John J.V. McMurray, MSc(Hons), MB ChB(Hons), MD,
FESC, FACC, FAHA
British Heart Foundation Cardiovascular Research Centre
University of Glasgow
Glasgow, Scotland

Wendy M. Miller, MD
Director
Nutrition and Preventive Medicine
William Beaumont Hospital
Royal Oak, Michigan
Professor of Internal Medicine
Oakland University
William Beaumont School of Medicine
Rochester, Michigan

Masataka Nakano, MD
CVPath Institute
Gaithersburg, Maryland

K.M. Venkat Narayan, MD
Hubert Department of Global Health
Rollins School of Public Health
Emory University
Atlanta, Georgia

Franz-Josef Neumann, MD
Professor
Cardiology and Angiology II
University Heart Center Freiburg – Bad Krozingen
Bad Krozingen, Germany

Michelle L. O'Donoghue, MD, MPH
TIMI Study Group
Cardiovascular Division
Brigham and Women's Hospital
Boston, Massachusetts

Fumiyuki Otsuka, MD
CVPath Institute
Gaithersburg, Maryland

Anushka A. Patel, MBBS, SM, PhD, FRACP
Professor
Sydney Medical School
Chief Scientist
The George Institute for Global Health
Cardiologist
Royal Prince Alfred Hospital
Sydney, Australia

Mark C. Petrie, MD
Scottish National Advanced Heart Failure Service
Golden Jubilee National Hospital
Clydebank
Glasgow Royal Infirmary
Glasgow, Scotland

Frank Pistrosch, MD
Study Centre Professor Hanefeld
University Hospital
Carl Gustav Carus Technical University
Dresden, Germany

Jorge Plutzky, MD
Director
Vascular Disease Prevention Program
Co-Director, Preventive Cardiology
Brigham and Women's Hospital
Associate Professor
Harvard Medical School
Boston, Massachusetts

Paul Poirier, MD, PhD, FRCPC, FACC, FAHA
Chief, Cardiac Prevention and Rehabilitation
Cardiology
Institut Universitaire de Cardiologie et de Pneumologie de
    Québec
Professor
Faculty of Pharmacy
Laval University
Quebec City, Quebec, Canada

Ravichandran Ramasamy, PhD
Diabetes Research Program
Division of Endocrinology
Department of Medicine
New York University School of Medicine
New York, New York

Marian J. Rewers, MD, PhD
Barbara Davis Center for Diabetes
University of Colorado School of Medicine
Aurora, Colorado

Marco Roffi, MD
Associate Professor
Vice-Chairman of Cardiology
Director
Interventional Cardiology Unit
University Hospital
Geneva, Switzerland

CONTRIBUTORS

Michel F. Rousseau, MD, PhD, FACC, FAHA
Professor, Division of Cardiology
Cliniques Universitaires Saint-Luc
Pôle de Recherche Cardiovasculaire
Institut de Recherche Expérimentale et Clinique (IREC)
Université Catholique de Louvain
Brussels, Belgium

Kenichi Sakakura, MD
CVPath Institute
Gaithersburg, Maryland

Frank Schaper, MD
Study Centre Professor Hanefeld
University Hospital
Carl Gustav Carus Technical University
Dresden, Germany

Ann Marie Schmidt, MD
Diabetes Research Program
Division of Endocrinology
Department of Medicine
New York University School of Medicine
New York, New York

Peter E.H. Schwarz, MD, PhD, MBA
Professor
Department for Prevention and Care of Diabetes
Medical Clinic III
University Hospital
Carl Gustav Carus Technical University
Dresden, Germany

Paul Valensi, MD
Professor
Endocrinology Diabetology Nutrition
Jean Verdier Hospital
Bondy, France

Renu Virmani, MD
Medical Director, President
CVPath Institute
Gaithersburg, Maryland

Lars Wallentin, MD, PhD
Department of Medical Sciences
Uppsala Clinical Research Center
Uppsala University
Uppsala, Sweden

Zhao V. Wang, PhD
Department of Internal Medicine (Cardiology)
University of Texas Southwestern Medical Center
Dallas, Texas

Mary Beth Weber, MPH, PhD
Assistant Professor
Hubert Department of Global Health
Rollins School of Public Health
Emory University
Atlanta, Georgia

Neil J. Wimmer, MD
Fellow in Cardiovascular Medicine
Division of Cardiovascular Medicine
Brigham and Women's Hospital
Boston, Massachusetts

Yee Weng Wong, MD
Advanced Heart Failure and Cardiac Transplant Unit
The Prince Charles Hospital
Chermside, Queensland, Australia

Shi Fang Yan, MD
Diabetes Research Program
Division of Endocrinology
Department of Medicine
New York University School of Medicine
New York, New York

Thomas Yates, PhD
Diabetes Research Centre
College of Medicine
Biological Sciences and Psychology
University of Leicester
Leicester, United Kingdom

Barak Zafrir, MD
Cardiovascular Division
Department of Medicine
Brigham and Women's Hospital
Harvard Medical School
Boston, Massachusetts

Foreword

Science often takes great strides when two fields intersect and when each contributes its special knowledge, expertise, and technology to create a powerful hybrid. An example is astrophysics, in which principles of physics are applied to astronomical observations. Such intersections abound in biomedical science. For example, the relatively new field of pharmacogenetics combines the expertise of the founding sciences – pharmacology and genetics – to provide an understanding of the (sometimes enormous) differences in the response of individual patients to identical doses of drugs, and this has advanced the field of personalized medicine. In cardiology, an understanding of the electrical properties of cardiac cells and clinical arrhythmology has been combined to form the important new subspecialty of clinical electrophysiology.

The substantial increase in caloric intake and reduction in physical activity throughout the world have resulted in a pandemic of obesity that, in turn, has led to an enormous increase in the incidence of type 2 diabetes mellitus. It is widely appreciated that diabetes accelerates atherogenesis, and along with hypertension and dyslipidemia, is a cardinal risk factor for atherosclerotic disease of coronary, carotid, and other systemic arteries. Therefore, cardiologists must learn how to assess and manage diabetes in patients with this diagnosis and clinical evidence of atherosclerotic disease in the same manner in which they have become accustomed to managing hypertension and hyperlipidemia. Similarly, diabetologists (or endocrinologists) must learn how to prevent and recognize atherosclerotic complications that are responsible for the most frequent cause of death or serious illness of their patients with diabetes. As a consequence, these two specialties – cardiology and diabetology– are now "joined at the hip."

We are pleased to welcome *Diabetes in Cardiovascular Disease* as a new companion to *Braunwald's Heart Disease*. It has succeeded in placing into a single text much of what is known about the effects of diabetes on cardiovascular disease. The book is eminently readable, thorough but not encyclopedic. Part I presents the epidemiology, pathophysiology, and management of diabetes and of the metabolic syndrome. Part II focuses on the pathobiology of diabetic atherosclerosis, as well as the risk and epidemiology of this condition. The management of chronic coronary heart disease in diabetic patients is complex and is described in Part III. It involves lifestyle interventions and management of glucose, blood pressure, lipids, and anti-platelet drugs, as well as coronary revascularization. Part IV presents similar considerations for acute coronary syndromes, while Part V focuses on the special features of heart failure in patients with diabetes. Last – but certainly not least important – Part VI deals with diabetes-accelerated atherosclerosis in other vascular beds, including the peripheral and the cerebrovascular arteries, as well as autonomic neuropathy.

The 60 authors, ably led by the talented editors, Drs. McGuire and Marx, are international authorities who have provided excellent and up-to-date information in this rapidly expanding field, which is positioned at the intersection of these two specialties. The optimum care of patients with diabetes now requires a team approach involving both diabetologists and cardiologists (as well as nephrologists, neurologists, and ophthalmologists). It is likely that, if the incidence of diabetic cardiovascular disease continues to mushroom, it may become necessary to create a new subspecialty, *Diabetocardiology*, and this book would be an excellent text to prepare physicians for this important, emerging field.

Eugene Braunwald

Douglas L. Mann

Douglas P. Zipes

Peter Libby

Robert O. Bonow

Preface

Over the past several decades, obesity and diabetes mellitus have become an increasing problem that constitutes a global epidemic, representing one of the most important chronic disease conditions in the world with critically important public health implications. Patients with diabetes exhibit an increased propensity to develop myriad cardiovascular diseases; its key sequelae are myocardial infarction, heart failure, stroke, and cardiovascular death. Over this same time period, the cardiology community has increasingly recognized the adverse cardiovascular prognosis of patients with diabetes, with increasing understanding of the heterogeneity of efficacy of available medical and interventional strategies by diabetes status and a notable unmet clinical need to mitigate the incremental "residual" cardiovascular risk associated with diabetes. Based on these observations and resultant evolution of regulatory requirements for diabetes drug development around the world, it is only within the past few years that the cardiovascular effects and safety of glucose-lowering therapies have begun to undergo rigorous assessment in large-scale randomized cardiovascular outcome trials focusing specifically on patients with diabetes. Thus the field of cardiovascular disease in diabetes has gained momentum over the past years, resulting in joint activities and guidelines from cardiology and diabetes associations around the world, requiring and fostering a truly interdisciplinary collaborative research and clinical partnership among cardiologists, endocrinologists, primary care providers, nutritionists, exercise physiologists, pharmacists, and diabetes educators—reflected in the diverse authorship of chapters in this textbook.

The first edition of *Diabetes in Cardiovascular Disease: A Companion to Braunwald's Heart Disease* includes 31 chapters that address the spectrum of topics relevant to the nexus of diabetes and cardiovascular disease. These chapters cover the epidemiology, pathophysiologic and genetic underpinnings, clinical presentation and consequences, and diagnostic and therapeutic approaches for prevention and treatment of high-risk diabetes patients, and review systems approaches to apply such interventions. Each of the chapters is written by international leaders in their respective fields, and for us it has been a true pleasure and honor to work with such a fabulous group of experts. They are our colleagues, collaborators, and friends and represent the remarkable interdisciplinary collaborative spirit bridging our specialties and advancing the field of science and health care for the betterment of our patients.

We believe that this book will be an invaluable resource for cardiologists, diabetologists, and all other health care providers taking care of patients with diabetes and cardiovascular disease.

We thank our many friends, our colleagues, and the experts from around the world who contributed to this book. Without their expertise and contribution the text could not have been completed.

Acknowledgments

We offer our heartfelt gratitude to those who have supported the development of this textbook. First, to Professors Braunwald and Libby, who had the confidence to allow us to edit an addition to the family of texts with the internationally revered imprimatur of *Braunwald's Heart Disease*. Second, to our colleagues and friends around the world who accepted our invitation to author chapters and delivered such excellent content that most commonly exceeded our highest expectations. Finally, to the editorial staff at Elsevier who so ably assisted and facilitated the development of this book at every step of the way: Dolores Meloni, Angela Rufino, and Cindy Thoms. To each of you, thank you.

Contents

xviii

CONTENTS

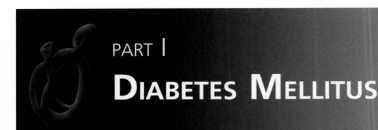

PART I

DIABETES MELLITUS

1

Definition and Epidemiology of Type 2 Diabetes Mellitus

Mary Beth Weber and K.M. Venkat Narayan

Worldwide, diabetes has reached epidemic proportions. Although diabetes encompasses a range of disorders (e.g., type 1 diabetes mellitus [T1DM], type 2 diabetes mellitus [T2DM], gestational diabetes mellitus, drug- or chemical-induced diabetes [from, for example, some second-generation antipsychotic drugs[1] and some anti–human immunodeficiency virus [HIV] drugs, as well as exposure to combination antiretroviral therapy[2]]), most cases of diabetes—approximately 90% to 95%—are T2DM (hereafter referred to simply as *diabetes*). Diabetes affects multiple systems of the body and can result in serious and debilitating complications, particularly when an individual has poor glucose control. In this chapter, we provide an overview of diabetes and its complications, describe the global burden of diabetes, discuss the causal underpinnings of diabetes, and conclude with a discussion of the future of diabetes research and prevention.

TYPE 2 DIABETES—DEFINITIONS AND OUTCOMES

Glucose intolerance ranges from impaired glucose tolerance (IGT) and impaired fasting glucose (together termed *prediabetes*, a precursor to and risk factor for diabetes) to diabetes. The diagnostic criteria for prediabetes and diabetes are shown in **Table 1-1**. Traditionally, diabetes is diagnosed by fasting plasma glucose (FPG) measurements and/or a 2-hour, 75-g oral glucose tolerance test (considered the gold standard for diagnosis of diabetes). In 2009, an international expert committee (including the American Diabetes Association [ADA], the International Diabetes Federation [IDF], and the European Association for the Study of Diabetes) recommended the use of glycosylated hemoglobin A1c (HbA1c) for diabetes diagnosis.[3]

Diabetes can result in severe morbidity and increased mortality as a result of secondary complications, which affect multiple body systems, including the cardiovascular system (cerebrovascular disease and coronary heart disease), renal system (nephropathy), eyes (retinopathy), peripheral nervous system (neuropathy), and limbs (foot ulcers, peripheral vascular disease, amputations).[6-8] For a more thorough discussion of these diabetes complications, see Chapters 7, 19, 23, 27, and 28.[6-8] Diabetes is also associated with other hitherto underappreciated complications, namely, infections, liver and digestive diseases, falls and mental illness, lung diseases, some cancers, and cognitive decline.[9] Individuals with diabetes also are at an increased risk for other conditions including erectile dysfunction, tuberculosis, sleep apnea, and periodontal disease,[6,10-12] and this population reports a lower quality of life than other groups.[13] Furthermore, individuals with diabetes have an increased risk of death from conditions ranging from cardiovascular diseases and kidney failure to infections, mental disorders, and liver disease.[9] Because of the severity of the conditions associated with diabetes, diabetes is associated with an attenuated lifespan.[14]

Diabetes-related complications are not infrequent, and they affect public health systems worldwide (**Fig. 1-1**). Diabetic retinopathy is the leading cause of blindness in adults in developed countries.[6,7] An audit of the United Kingdom's National Health System's data showed additional risk for complications caused by diabetes: compared with the general population, people with diabetes were 64.9% more likely to be admitted to a hospital with heart failure, 48.0% more likely to have a myocardial infarction (MI), 331% more likely to have an amputation below the ankle, 210% more likely to have an above-ankle amputation, 24.9% more likely to have a stroke, and 139% more likely to require renal replacement therapy.[15] In the United States, diabetes is the leading cause of nontraumatic amputations of the lower limbs, blindness, and kidney failure.[16]

Diabetes is an economically costly disease. Diabetes and its complications lead to increases in work-place

TABLE 1-1 American Diabetes Association Diagnostic Criteria for Diabetes and Prediabetes

		DIAGNOSTIC TEST		
		Fasting Plasma Glucose	OGTT*	HbA1c
Type 2 diabetes		≥126 mg/dL (7.0 mmol/L)	≥200 mg/dL (11.1 mmol/L)	≥6.5%
Prediabetes	Impaired fasting glucose†	100-125 mg/dL (5.6-6.9 mmol/L)		5.7-6.4%
	Impaired glucose tolerance		140-199 mg/dL (7.8-11.0 mmol/L)	

OGTT = Oral glucose tolerance test.
*Two-hour, 75-g oral glucose tolerance test.
†The World Health Organization (WHO) defines impaired fasting glucose with a narrower range: 110-125 mg/dL (6.1-6.9 mmol/L).[5]
Data from American Diabetes Association: Standards of medical care in diabetes—2014, *Diabetes Care* 37(Suppl 1):S14-S80, 2014.[4]

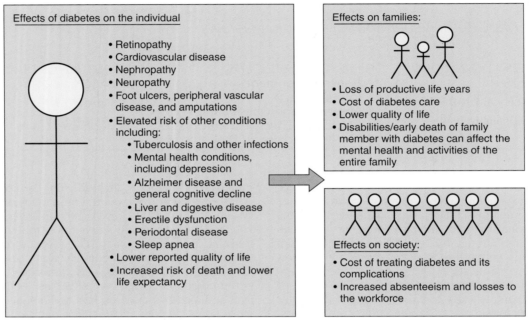

FIGURE 1-1 Secondary complications of diabetes. The effects of diabetes go beyond those on the individual—secondary complications in multiple systems of the body and increased risk of serious diseases and earlier death. Families and society as a whole are negatively affected by diabetes and its complications.

absenteeism and loss of productive life-years.[14,17] In the United States the cost of diabetes was estimated to be $245 billion dollars in 2012. This includes $176 billon dollars in direct medical costs (medications, office visits, hospitalizations, emergency care) and $69 billion in indirect medical costs (unemployment, absenteeism, and reduced productivity resulting from diabetes, and the loss to the workforce because of premature mortality associated with diabetes).[18] The costs to individuals with diabetes is also great; U.S. men and women with diagnosed diabetes have medical expenditures that are 2.3 times higher than they would have if the individual did not have diabetes.[18] In low- and middle-income countries (LMICs), the economic ramifications of diabetes can be even worse than in high-income countries such as the United States. A study conducted in India reported that few patients had health insurance, instead relying on personal savings, loans, mortgages, and property sales to pay for medical bills associated with diabetes care[19]; in this situation, the high costs of routine diabetes care and treatment of diabetes-related complications are enough to put even comfortable, middle-class Indian families into poverty.

Given the strong evidence that treatment of multiple risk factors simultaneously in patients with diabetes improves outcomes,[20,21] expert groups recommend that patients with diabetes undergo regular preventative examinations (e.g., foot and eye examinations, measures of urine protein) and manage risk factors associated with diabetes-related complications (e.g., manage blood pressure [BP], plasma lipids, and blood glucose; eliminate tobacco use; undergo treatment of albuminuria with angiotensin-converting enzyme [ACE] inhibitor or angiotensin receptor blocker [ARB] medications; do regular exercise; be referred to a dietician).[18,22,23] Unfortunately, achievement of diabetes care targets is suboptimal. In the United States, even though there have been improvements in process of care and intermediate outcomes, two fifths of patients with diabetes have poor control of low-density lipoprotein (LDL) cholesterol, one fifth have poor glycemic control, and one third have poor BP control.[22] Data collected during a 5-year observational study in Asia, Eastern Europe, Latin America, the Middle East, and Africa show that the situation is worse in LMICs; among 9901 patients with diabetes, 36% had never had an HbA1c measurement, 11% to 36% had not been screened for secondary complications in the previous 2 years, and only 3.6% had achieved optimal LDL, BP, and HbA1c targets.[24]

GLOBAL BURDEN OF DIABETES

The burden of noncommunicable diseases (NCDs), such as diabetes, is growing worldwide, and these diseases and conditions already contribute to most mortality and morbidity worldwide. Globally, we are witnessing a major shift from communicable and undernutrition-related diseases to NCDs in adulthood.[25–27] Disability-adjusted life years (DALYs) from NCDs increased 25% between 1990 and 2010, whereas those resulting from communicable diseases and maternal, neonatal, and nutrition-deficiency disorders decreased by 26.5% in the same time period. A large proportion of the increase in the burdens of NCDs is driven by population growth and ageing, yet almost half of the increase in DALYs from NCDs between 1990 and 2010 resulted from factors other than population growth and ageing.[26]

Among NCDs, the growth of diabetes appears to be especially dramatic and worrisome. As a cause of death, diabetes has advanced in ranking from 15 in 1990 to 9 in 2010.[25] High blood glucose and associated cardiometabolic risk factors (e.g., physical inactivity, overweight and obesity, low fruit and vegetable intake) are now consistently among the top 10 risk factors for mortality globally, and across high-, middle-, and low-income countries alike.[28,29] Furthermore, high blood glucose, high body mass index (BMI), diets low in fruits and vegetables, diets low in whole grains, and physical inactivity and low physical activity were among the leading risk factors for DALYs globally in 2010, and they ranked high as risk factors for DALYs in all regions of the world.[26] Overall, over the past two decades, there has been a steady and disturbing increase in mean BMI and mean FPG globally, and this trend is affecting almost all countries of the world, barring a few exceptions, with the rate of increase most acute among developing countries undergoing industrial transformation in their economies.[30,31] In contrast, mean BP and mean total cholesterol levels have decreased globally, largely driven by decreases in high-income countries, although their levels have increased in many developing countries.[32,33]

These changes in BMI and glucose levels have translated into increases in prevalence of diabetes worldwide. The number of people with diabetes is increasing in every country of the world (**Table 1-2**), although prevalence estimates are conservative given that in 50% to 80% of those with the disease it remains undetected.[34] According to the latest IDF Diabetes Atlas, at least 382 million people worldwide had diabetes in 2013, 80% of whom lived in LMICs. By 2035 the number of people with diabetes will rise to 592 million,[34] although the growth may be greater given the overall population trends of increasing weight, aging, and urbanization.[35]

Although there are differences in diabetes risk by ethnicity (e.g., Native Americans, Hispanics, Blacks, and Asians in the United States have higher risks than non-Hispanic whites; Indians in the United Kingdom have higher risks than their Caucasian counterparts; Indians have higher risks than Chinese and Malays in Singapore),[36–38] it is generally true that the rise in diabetes prevalence is affecting all ethnic groups.[34] Similarly, both genders are affected by the increasing prevalence of diabetes.[34] As a consequence, on a global level the number of people with diabetes is projected to increase between 2013 and 2035 in every continent (+109% increase in Africa; +96% in the Middle East and North Africa; +71% in South-East Asia; +60% in South and Central America; +46% in the Western Pacific; +37% in North America and the Caribbean; and +22% in Europe; see **Table 1-2**).[34]

The steepest growth in the number of people with diabetes is occurring in LMICs. In fact, 7 of the top 10 countries worldwide in terms of number of people with diabetes are already LMICs, and by 2030 only 1 of the top 10 countries will be other than an LMIC (**Table 1-3**).[34] The number of adults with diabetes in LMICs is expected to increase at a pace that far exceeds that of developing countries (69% increase in developing countries compared with a 20% increase in developed countries by 2030).[39] In terms of diabetes prevalence, the top 10 countries or territories of the world are the Tokelau (37.5%), Federated States of Micronesia (35%), Marshall Islands (34.9%), Kiribati (28.8%), Cook Island (25.7%), Vanuatu (24%), Saudi Arabia (24%), Nauru (23.3%), Kuwait (23.1%), and Qatar (22.9%).[34]

Although the burden of diabetes is already staggering, two additional patterns are a cause for further concern. First, the number of young people with diabetes is high and increasing. The highest numbers of people with diabetes worldwide are in the economically productive age group of 40 to 59 years, and half the people who die from diabetes are under the age of 60 years—a pattern of major concern to global economic productivity and development, the health and economic costs of the disease itself notwithstanding.[34,40] In 2011 there were an estimated 490,100 children aged 0 to 14 years with T1DM worldwide, and an estimated

TABLE 1-2 Numbers of People with Diabetes (in Millions), 2013 and 2035, Globally[1]

REGION	2013	2035	INCREASE
Africa	19.8	41.4	109%
Middle East and North Africa	34.6	67.9	96%
South-East Asia	72.1	123	71%
South and Central America	24.1	38.5	60%
Western Pacific	138.2	201.8	46%
North America and Caribbean	36.7	50.4	37%
Europe	56.3	68.9	22%
World	381.8	591.9	55%

Data from International Diabetes Foundation (IDF): IDF Diabetes Atlas, Sixth Edition. Brussels, Belgium: International Diabetes Federation; 2013.

TABLE 1-3 Countries with the Highest Number of People with Diabetes (20-79 years), 2013 and 2035[1]

COUNTRY	2013 (MILLIONS)	COUNTRY	2035 (MILLIONS)
China	98.4	China	142.7
India	65.1	India	109.0
United States	24.4	United States	29.7
Brazil	11.9	Brazil	19.2
Russian Federation	10.9	Mexico	15.7
Mexico	8.7	Indonesia	14.1
Indonesia	8.5	Egypt	13.1
Germany	7.6	Pakistan	12.48
Egypt	7.5	Turkey	11.8
Japan	7.2	Russian Federation	11.2

Data from International Diabetes Foundation (IDF): IDF Diabetes Atlas, Sixth Edition. Brussels, Belgium: International Diabetes Federation; 2013.

778,000 new cases of T1DM were being diagnosed each year, representing a 3.0% increase in annual incidence. Furthermore, there has been an increase in occurrence of T2DM, traditionally believed to be a disease of adults, at younger ages.[41] There is uncertainty about the actual prevalence and incidence of youth-onset diabetes, because data are limited; however, reports suggest that T2DM may account for 10% to 30% of all youth-onset diabetes patients and that certain ethnic groups (e.g., Native Americans, Asian Indians) may be at especially high risk.[42] The best-characterized data available are from the SEARCH for Diabetes in Youth study, a multicenter investigation in the United States. The SEARCH study has reported a physician-diagnosed T2DM prevalence of 0.01/1000 among 0 to 9 year olds, and among 10 to 19 year olds the prevalence ranged from 1.74/1000 in American Indians to 0.19/1000 in non-Hispanic whites.[43]

Second, whereas the growth of diabetes was largely believed to have been an urban phenomenon, a recent systematic review of diabetes in rural parts of LMICs indicates that the diabetes epidemic is rapidly spreading through rural areas across the world. The pooled prevalence of rural diabetes among LMICs was estimated to be 5.6%, and moreover, it had quintupled in a 25-year time period.[44] Although the IDF projects a 47% rise in the number of people with diabetes globally by 2030,[34] these rural data suggest that the rise may be even higher because an estimated 55% of LMIC populations worldwide live in rural areas.[44]

CAUSAL UNDERPINNINGS OF DIABETES

Diabetes results from poor insulin resistance paired with insufficient insulin secretion (**Fig. 1-2**). Under normal

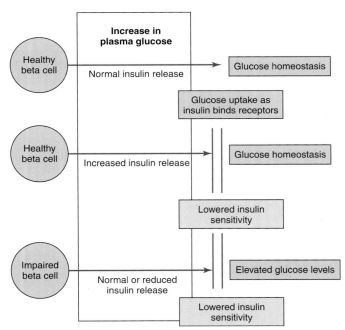

FIGURE 1-2 Beta cell response in a healthy individual compared with an individual with impaired beta cells. In a healthy individual, the beta cells are able to compensate for decreases in insulin sensitivity (because of, for example, physical inactivity or weight gain) by increasing insulin production and release, thereby maintaining glucose homeostasis in the blood. In an individual with beta cell dysfunction, however, beta cells are not able to increase insulin production sufficiently to overcome insulin resistance, resulting in sustained hyperglycemia. In the long term, this sustained elevation in blood glucose can lead to the development of prediabetes and diabetes.

metabolic conditions, pancreatic beta cells can compensate for decreases in insulin sensitivity (because of, for example, increasing age, weight gain, or physical inactivity) by producing more insulin,[45] thereby maintaining glucose homeostasis and avoiding the progression from normal glucose tolerance to prediabetes and diabetes. However, when the beta cells are impaired (because of, for example, genetic predisposition or overuse[46,47]), they are unable to adjust production of insulin to respond to increased glucose levels or decreased insulin action, leading to a hyperglycemic state. Over time, frequent or consistent hyperglycemic states will result in loss in the number of beta cells (in individuals with prediabetes, beta cell mass is about 60% of normal; it is about 40% of normal in individuals with T2DM[48]) and their functional capacity,[45,48–50] making it more and more difficult for the body to maintain glucose homeostasis unassisted.

Genes, Epigenetics, and Gene-Environment Interactions

The development of diabetes and its precursors, insulin resistance and beta cell dysfunction, is caused by a confluence of factors, both genetic and environmental. (For more information on the causal factors of insulin resistance, see Chapter 2.) Although insulin resistance increases with age, this is most likely the result of age-related weight gain and loss of physical activity; among nonobese, fit individuals, older people are not insulin resistant compared with younger individuals.[47] Inheritance of diabetes is polygenic, and the associated gene variants act together to confer risk[51]; however, the risk conferred by most known gene variants associated with diabetes is small[52] (the exception to this is the transcription factor 7–like 2 gene *[TCF7L2]*, a transcription factor involved in the Wnt signaling pathway[53,54]). It is likely that genes alone will not lead to diabetes in most people, although lack of underlying genetic risk may explain why many at-risk (e.g., overweight) people never develop diabetes.[55]

Family history is a strong, independent risk factor for diabetes; individuals having two parents with diabetes report a significantly higher rate of diabetes than individuals having no family history (16.7 vs. 1.8 cases of diabetes per 1000 person-years).[56] Family history as a risk factor reflects not only genetic inheritance, but also shared lifestyles and environments among families and the effects of the environment on previous generations.[57–60] Nutritional or metabolic factors can lead to temporal changes to genetic factors (so called "metabolic imprinting"), which can persist throughout life.[42,61–63] The "thrifty phenotype hypothesis" describes how maternal undernutrition (as occurs during famine or in less severe food or nutrient shortages) changes the intrauterine environment, resulting in fetal adaptations that can affect the child throughout life.[64–67] Infants born to mothers with diabetes have an increased risk of glucose intolerance, independent of genetic inheritance.[68]

The interaction of genes and environment in diabetes risk occurs throughout life and is well illustrated by considering the Pima Indians, a Native American population living in the southwest United States and Mexico. Pima Indians living in Mexico are more physically active (mean physical activity of 27.4 hr/wk) and less obese (13.2% prevalence of obesity) than Pima Indians living on a reservation in Arizona (7.6 hr/wk of physical activity and 69.3% obese). Although both populations share the same elevated genetic risk for diabetes, the prevalence of diabetes is much higher among U.S. Pima Indians (37.5%, the highest of any race-ethnic group in the United States) than among Pima Indians residing in Mexico (8.0%).[69] A similar pattern can be seen in populations with low genetic diabetes risk. Japanese Americans tend to weigh more than their Japanese counterparts and consume a significantly greater percentage of daily calories from animal protein[70]; the prevalence of diabetes is approximately fourfold higher among second-generation Japanese-Americans than among native Japanese.[71]

Overweight and Obesity and Associated Lifestyle Behaviors

Diabetes risk is strongly associated with excess body weight[72-75]; with each one unit increase in BMI, diabetes risk increases by 12%.[76] Overweight and obesity increase diabetes risk by increasing liver and skeletal muscle insulin resistance.[77-82] How body fat is distributed, particularly abdominal adiposity, contributes to diabetes risk, independent of BMI.[77,83-85] Visceral fat, as an active endocrine organ, can lead to the development of insulin resistance and increased glucose intolerance,[86-89] through the release and accumulation of free fatty acids, cytokines, and other "toxic messengers" that impair the ability of insulin to limit glucose production in the liver and promote glucose disposal in the muscle tissue.[77-82,90]

Conversely, reducing body weight and increasing exercise counter the effects of obesity on hyperglycemia and reduce the risk for developing diabetes.[91-93] Depending on gender, baseline BMI, and age, a 10% weight loss reduces diabetes risk by 0.5% to 1.7%.[94] Exercise acts directly on glucose intolerance by enhancing insulin sensitivity[95] and improving glucose uptake,[96,97] and indirectly by decreasing concentrations of fatty acid metabolites, thereby improving insulin resistance.[78,98] Exercise also helps prevent diabetes by promoting healthy body weight. Even short-term interventions that increase moderate-intensity exercise reduce risk factors for diabetes[95,99,100] and cardiovascular disease.[101-104]

Excessive caloric intake as well as poor diet quality (e.g., low intake of dietary fiber, whole grain cereals, and low-glycemic carbohydrates or high intake of saturated and trans fats) increase the risk of cardiometabolic diseases such as diabetes.[81,105-107] On the other hand, following a healthy diet improves insulin action and reduces hepatic glucose production, thereby countering the effects of obesity on hyperglycemia.[79] A review of the data on obesity interventions concludes that low-fat diets with exercise or behavioral therapy result in prevention of diabetes and improved glycemic control.[73] Both the DASH diet (Dietary Approaches to Stop Hypertension; a low-fat, high-fiber diet rich in vegetables, fruit, and low-fat dairy products)[108] and a Mediterranean-style diet (high intake of vegetables, beans, fruits, nuts, fish, and olive oils with a low consumption of meat, high-fat dairy products, and processed foods) supplemented with extra virgin olive oil or mixed nuts[109] are associated with reduction in diabetes risk. Similarly, a healthy diet pattern (low-fat dairy, whole grains, fruits and vegetables, and moderate alcohol) significantly reduces diabetes risk (hazard ratio 0.71; 95% confidence interval [CI] 0.51-0.98) compared with several other diet patterns and reduces the 15-year risk of diabetes and death from a coronary event or nonfatal MI compared with the unhealthy diet pattern (full-fat dairy products, refined grains, processed meat, and fried foods).[110]

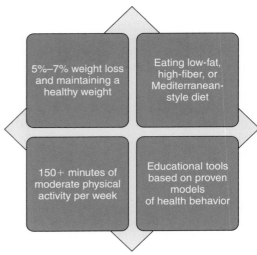

FIGURE 1-3 Behaviors associated with reduction of diabetes risk. Evidence from cohort trials and randomized studies has shown that several factors are important for successfully preventing diabetes in high-risk individuals. (1) Reaching and maintaining a healthy weight: In randomized trials a weight loss of 5% to 7% was sufficient to effect a substantial reduction in diabetes incidence. (2) Reduction in calorie intake and following a healthy diet: Both low-fat, high-fiber diets and Mediterranean-style diets have been shown to reduce diabetes risk. (3) Participation in at least 150 min/wk of moderate-level physical activity. (4) Education tools based on the science of behavior change: Diabetes prevention requires lifestyle modifications that many people find difficult to make and sustain. Health care providers should provide educational tools that are based on proven models of behavior change.

There is strong evidence from randomized controlled trials[111] that diabetes can be prevented, or at least delayed, through lifestyle education programs, programs that seek to change behaviors to improve the diets, physical activity patterns, and often body weights of participants (**Fig. 1-3**). The first randomized trial assessing lifestyle education as a tool for diabetes prevention was the Da Qing IGT and Diabetes Study.[112] In this trial, 33 health clinics in Da Qing, China were randomized to provide patients who had IGT ($N = 577$) education on (1) standard diabetes prevention (control); (2) dietary improvements; (3) increasing daily exercise; or (4) improving diet and increasing physical activity. Individuals in the intervention groups all showed statistically significant improvements in diabetes risk; compared with the control arm, participants in the diet, exercise, and diet-plus-exercise groups had reductions in diabetes incidence of 31%, 46%, and 42%, respectively.[112] After 20 years of follow-up, the cumulative incidence of diabetes, after adjustment for age and clustering by clinic, was 43% lower in the intervention group (all intervention arms combined) compared with the control group.[113] The risk reduction was slightly attenuated over time, which may reflect changing behaviors of study participants or age-related weight gain or decreased activity. Alternatively, lifestyle interventions might only be able to delay diabetes (as opposed to preventing it entirely),[114] possibly because of an inability of lifestyle interventions to reverse damage to beta cell function[115] or because age-related increases in insulin resistance paired with underlying beta cell defects may counteract the improvements in insulin resistance provided by lifestyle change.

Two other trials, the Finnish Diabetes Prevention Study (DPS) and the U.S. Diabetes Prevention Program (DPP), both showed a 58% reduction in diabetes risk in participants in lifestyle programs compared with controls.[116,117] Participants in the DPS ($N = 522$ overweight adults with IGT) were provided one-on-one counseling to help them reach study goals: (1) a 5% weight loss; (2) an increase in physical activity to 30 min/day; (3) a reduction in total fat intake to less than 30% of total energy; (4) a reduction in saturated fat intake to less than 10% of total energy; and (5) an increase in dietary fiber to at least 15 g/1000 kcal. The reduction in relative risk of diabetes was lower, but still significant at 7 years follow-up (risk reduction 36%).[118] Even participants who reached only one study goal (e.g., only increased physical activity) showed improvements compared with controls; regardless of which goals were reached, the incidence of diabetes per 100 person-years was 8.4, 7.1, 5.5, 5.8, and 2.0 for participants reaching 0, 1, 2, 3, and 4 or 5 of the study goals, respectively.[118]

The DPP was the largest trial of lifestyle intervention for diabetes prevention. The study included 3234 overweight adults with IGT and elevated FPG (90 to 125 mg/dL) at 27 sites randomized to control (standard advice on lifestyle change for diabetes prevention), metformin (a glucose-lowering drug at 850 mg twice per day), or an individualized lifestyle education program (a fourth study arm testing the pharmaceutical agent troglitazone for diabetes prevention was discontinued because of potential liver toxicity of the drug). Lifestyle coaches met with lifestyle arm participants weekly for 16 sessions and monthly for eight sessions and trained participants on the behaviors and skills needed to reach the study goals of a 7% weight loss and increase in moderate-level physical activity to at least 150 min/wk. As mentioned previously, the participants in the intervention arm showed a 58% reduction in diabetes incidence compared with controls, significantly greater than the 31% risk reduction seen in the metformin arm. These results were consistent across genders and racial or ethnic groups. All age groups benefited, with oldest participants showing the greatest reduction in diabetes incidence (71% for ages 60 years or greater compared with 48% for participants aged 24 to 44 years).[116] The increased improvements among older participants were likely a result of the effects of increased exercise and weight loss overcoming age-related insulin resistance.[119] The lifestyle program was also effective in overweight and obese individuals, although those with the lowest BMIs (22 to 30 kg/m^2) had greater reductions in diabetes risk than those with BMIs of 35 kg/m^2 or greater (65% reduction in diabetes incidence compared with controls versus 51%, respectively).[116] Finally, lifestyle interventions overcame genetic susceptibility to diabetes,[116,120] with lifestyle essentially negating baseline genetic risk.

In addition to reducing risk of diabetes, lifestyle interventions have been shown to improve other markers of disease. Lifestyle participants show significant improvements in markers of inflammation, plasma lipid levels, aerobic capacity, BP, whole body insulin sensitivity, and insulin response.[79,115,121–124] Lifestyle interventions have been shown to be cost-effective for preventing diabetes.[125–127] Based on the findings of the studies described previously and other similar trials, expert organizations such as the ADA[4] and the IDF[128] recommend lifestyle changes (e.g., increased physical activity, weight loss) for diabetes prevention.

Other Risk Factors for Diabetes

Although increasing obesity and changes in diet and activity patterns can explain much of the recent increase in the number of people with diabetes, they cannot account for all of it.

This has resulted in an increase in the number of researchers investigating so-called "nontraditional risk factors" for diabetes. For example, sleep, active smoking, and exposure to environmental contaminants have been hypothesized to increase risk of diabetes.

Several studies have correlated sleep debt with diabetes. In one study, the prevalences of diabetes and IGT were significantly greater in individuals sleeping either 5 or fewer or 6 hr/night.[129] Similar results were seen in an analysis of the Nurses' Health Study, a large cohort of 70,026 women: women sleeping less than 5 hr/night had a relative risk of diabetes of 1.57 (95% CI 1.28-1.92).[130] Compared with the same individuals in a fully rested situation, forced sleep deprivation of 4 hr/night for six nights was associated with lower glucose tolerance (glucose clearance after injection was 40% slower, glucose effectiveness was 30% lower, and active insulin response to glucose was 30% lower).[131] Sleep may increase diabetes risk through direct disturbances of glucose metabolism, but also through increasing obesity and obesity-associated insulin resistance (sleep deprivation is associated with upregulation of hormones associated with increased appetite, can provide more time to eat, and may decrease energy expenditure).[132] On the other end of the sleep spectrum, long sleeps (sleeping 9 or more hr/day) have also been significantly associated with diabetes and IGT.[129,130] The explanation for the association between long sleep and diabetes risk elevation is unclear.

There is strong evidence that individuals with diabetes who smoke have higher rates of both microvascular and macrovascular disease than smokers without diabetes.[133,134] Furthermore, some studies have suggested a possible relationship between smoking and insulin resistance and diabetes.[133] A meta-analysis of studies assessing this relationship reported a pooled relative risk for diabetes among smokers of 1.44 (95% CI 1.31-1.58) compared with nonsmokers. In addition, there is evidence of a dose response effect, with heavy smokers having a higher risk of diabetes than lighter smokers (relative risk 1.61 and 1.29, respectively) and former smokers (relative risk 1.23).[135] Further research is needed to determine if the association between smoking and diabetes is causal and to elucidate possible mechanisms of the association.

Recently an expert workshop was convened to summarize and evaluate evidence on the contribution of environmental chemicals to the current epidemics of diabetes and obesity. This group reported that there was sufficient evidence of an association between some environmental contaminants (e.g., arsenic in high-exposure areas, certain persistent organic pollutants, bisphenol A [BPA], some pesticides) and diabetes, but further research is needed to show causality. On the other hand, the evidence for the role of certain toxins, particularly in utero exposure to nicotine via maternal smoking, in causing obesity in humans is stronger.[136] By increasing obesity in the population, these exposures could indirectly increase diabetes incidence.

THE FUTURE OF DIABETES RESEARCH

Translating successful lifestyle intervention programs, such as the DPP and the DPS, for high-risk communities is a promising way to address the high and rising prevalence of diabetes. In public health, translational research attempts to apply proven clinical programs and public health interventions to the broader community.[137–141] Translational research using the curricula developed for the DPS and the DPP is underway. These studies have shown promising results, with participants displaying weight loss and, in some studies, reductions in BP, FPG, plasma lipids, or diabetes risk.[142–147]

To help ensure success of the program, translational research projects should include components shared by the most effective lifestyle programs (see **Fig. 1-3**). One important component of effective diabetes prevention programs is weight loss goals for overweight participants. In the DPP, decreases in measures of adiposity (specifically, weight, BMI, and waist circumference in men and women and waist-to-hip ratio and subcutaneous and visceral fat in men) were significant predictors of diabetes risk reduction,[91] and weight loss was determined to be the most important factor in reducing diabetes risk.[148] Successful diabetes prevention programs also promote increased physical activity, most often recommending moderate physical activity for at least 150 min/wk.[91–93,112] Diabetic Prevention Study participants who increased moderate to vigorous physical activity the most had a 63% to 65% reduction in diabetes incidence compared with other study participants.[92] In addition, following a healthy, well-balanced diet that is low in fat (<30% of total calories from fat and <10% of calories from saturated fat) and high in fiber is an important component of diabetes prevention programs. The diet recommended in the DPS (a low-fat, high-fiber diet) was associated with reduced diabetes risk and had a dose-dependent effect on sustained weight loss.[149] Successful diabetes prevention programs use proven health behavior theories (e.g., the Health Beliefs model[150] or Prochaska's Stages of Change model[151]) to design behavior change curriculums. Certain skills are required to successfully implement and maintain lifestyle behavior changes. For example, individuals need to be able to identify barriers to behavior change and ways to overcome these barriers[152]; increasing social support for lifestyle changes has been shown to be an effective tool for improving outcomes in weight loss and physical activity programs[153–155]; and in the DPP, physical activity was significantly and positively associated with exercise self-efficacy.[156] Finally, in LMIC settings where the need for effective diabetes prevention programs is greatest, community-based interventions (e.g., within families and at schools, community centers, or clinics) should include culturally tailored information, promote community ownership of the program, and be designed to be cost-effective and simple to sustain and disseminate.

For the scope of the diabetes problem to be addressed, future research is needed. Although lifestyle programs are effective at reducing diabetes risk, they are unable to completely prevent the condition; after 10 or more years of follow-up, 40% to 70% of lifestyle participants still progress to diabetes, despite weight loss and/or behavior modification during the trial, indicating that lifestyle change alone may not be sufficient to prevent diabetes.[113,118,157] Also, despite a pronounced effect on peripheral insulin resistance,[79,122] lifestyle improvements may have limited effects on beta cell dysfunction.[158] Current and future research on behavior change and the psychosocial determinants of weight gain or loss, diet choices, and other lifestyle behaviors can be used to strengthen lifestyle programs. In addition, other interventions, perhaps including pharmaceutical therapies, are required to address the gaps in prevention. Better surveillance data are needed in LMIC settings, where

available data indicate that most diabetes cases occur. Also, researchers are only beginning to understand the role of casual factors in different populations, and differences in how diabetes develops in different groups need to be studied (e.g., beta cell dysfunction may play a more important role than insulin resistance in the development of diabetes in Asian Indian populations[159]). Finally, there is a need to address the growing problems of poor nutrition, sedentary lifestyles, and expanding body sizes in all regions of the world, and research is required to identify effective policies, programs, and interventions to address these problems on the broader level (i.e., in cities, states, and countries).

SUMMARY

Diabetes is a serious public health problem with serious secondary complications. The global burden of diabetes is large and growing, affecting populations in every region of the world. The largest burden of diabetes occurs is in LMICs, settings with limited resources and, often, the dual public health burden of chronic and communicable diseases. Diabetes is caused by a confluence of factors, both genetic and environmental. Lifestyle behaviors, particularly physical inactivity and high-calorie, low-fiber diets, and resulting adiposity, worsen beta cell function and insulin sensitivity, resulting in a progression from normal glucose tolerance to prediabetes and diabetes in at-risk individuals. There is strong evidence from randomized controlled trials that diabetes can be prevented, or at least delayed, through lifestyle change programs; lifestyle interventions with intensive participant engagement (e.g., weekly classes) have been shown to reduce diabetes incidence by 30% to 60% in individuals with IGT or combined IGT-Impaired Fasting Glucose compared with low or no intervention. To address this epidemic, future research is needed to better understand how diabetes affects different populations and how to effectively translate, disseminate, and sustain proven diabetes prevention programs in communities around the world.

References

1. Consensus development conference on antipsychotic drugs and obesity and diabetes. *Diabetes Care* 27:596–601, 2004.
2. De Wit S, Sabin CA, Weber R, et al: Incidence and risk factors for new-onset diabetes in HIV-infected patients: the Data Collection on Adverse Events of Anti-HIV Drugs (D:A:D) study. *Diabetes Care* 31:1224–1229, 2008.
3. International Expert Committee report on the role of the A1C assay in the diagnosis of diabetes. *Diabetes Care* 32:1327–1334, 2009.
4. American Diabetes Association: Standards of medical care in diabetes–2014. *Diabetes Care* 37 (Suppl 1):S14–S80, 2014.
5. The World Health Organization, International Diabetes Federation: *Definition and diagnosis of diabetes mellitus and intermediate hyperglycemia: report of a WHO/IDF consultation.* Geneva, Switzerland, 2006, World Health Organization.
6. UK Prospective Diabetes Study 6. Complications in newly diagnosed type 2 diabetic patients and their association with different clinical and biochemical risk factors. *Diabetes Res* 13:1–11, 1990.
7. Hypertension in Diabetes Study (HDS): I. Prevalence of hypertension in newly presenting type 2 diabetic patients and the association with risk factors for cardiovascular and diabetic complications. *J Hypertens* 11:309–317, 1993.
8. Stratton IM, Adler AI, Neil HA, et al: Association of glycaemia with macrovascular and microvascular complications of type 2 diabetes (UKPDS 35): prospective observational study. *BMJ* 321:405–412, 2000.
9. Seshasai SR, Kaptoge S, Thompson A, et al: Diabetes mellitus, fasting glucose, and risk of cause-specific death. *N Engl J Med* 364:829–841, 2011.
10. Loe H: Periodontal disease. The sixth complication of diabetes mellitus. *Diabetes Care* 16:329–334, 1993.
11. Babu AR, Herdegen J, Fogelfeld L, et al: Type 2 diabetes, glycemic control, and continuous positive airway pressure in obstructive sleep apnea. *Arch Intern Med* 165:447–452, 2005.
12. Jeon CY, Murray MB: Diabetes mellitus increases the risk of active tuberculosis: a systematic review of 13 observational studies. *PLoS Med* 5:e152, 2008.
13. Rubin RR, Peyrot M: Quality of life and diabetes. *Diabetes Metab Res Rev* 15:205–218, 1999.
14. Narayan KM, Boyle JP, Thompson TJ, et al: Lifetime risk for diabetes mellitus in the United States. *JAMA* 290:1884–1890, 2003.
15. National diabetes audit 2010–2011 report 2: complications and mortality. September 28, 2012, at https://catalogue.ic.nhs.uk/publications/clinical/diabetes/nati-diab-audi-10-11/nati-diab-aud-10-11-comp-and-mort-v2.pdf. Accessed in 2013.
16. Centers for Disease Control and Prevention: *National diabetes fact sheet: national estimates and general information on diabetes and prediabetes in the United States, 2011,* Atlanta, GA, 2011, U.S. Department of Health and Human Services, Centers for Disease Control and Prevention.

17. Boles M, Pelletier B, Lynch W: The relationship between health risks and work productivity. *J Occup Environ Med* 46:737–745, 2004.
18. American Diabetes Association: Economic costs of diabetes in the U.S. in 2012. *Diabetes Care* 36:1033–1046, 2013.
19. Kumpatla S, Kothandan H, Tharkar S, et al: The costs of treating long term diabetic complications in a developing country: a study from India. *J Assoc Phys India* 61:16–23, 2013.
20. Gaede P, Lund-Andersen H, Parving HH, et al: Effect of a multifactorial intervention on mortality in type 2 diabetes. *N Engl J Med* 358:580–591, 2008.
21. Gaede P, Vedel P, Larsen N, et al: Multifactorial intervention and cardiovascular disease in patients with type 2 diabetes. *N Engl J Med* 348:383–393, 2003.
22. Saaddine JB, Cadwell B, Gregg EW, et al: Improvements in diabetes processes of care and intermediate outcomes: United States, 1988–2002. *Ann Intern Med* 144:465–474, 2006.
23. Performance measurement set for adult diabetes. January 21, 2005. Accessed in 2012, at www.nyqa.org/pdf-lib/NDQIA%20Diabetes%20DomainFinal2005Measures.pdf.
24. Chan JC, Gagliardino JJ, Baik SH, et al: Multifaceted determinants for achieving glycemic control: the International Diabetes Management Practice Study (IDMPS). *Diabetes Care* 32:227–233, 2009.
25. Lozano R, Naghavi M, Foreman K, et al: Global and regional mortality from 235 causes of death for 20 age groups in 1990 and 2010: a systematic analysis for the global burden of disease study 2010. *Lancet* 380:2095–2128, 2012.
26. Murray CJ, Vos T, Lozano R, et al: Disability-adjusted life years (DALYs) for 291 diseases and injuries in 21 regions, 1990-2010: a systematic analysis for the global burden of disease study 2010. *Lancet* 380:2197–2223, 2012.
27. Vos T, Flaxman AD, Naghavi M, et al: Years lived with disability (YLDs) for 1160 sequelae of 289 diseases and injuries 1990–2010: a systematic analysis for the global burden of disease study 2010. *Lancet* 380:2163–2196, 2012.
28. *Global health risks: mortality and burden of disease attributable to selected major risks,* 2010, World Health Organization. 2010, at www.who.int/healthinfo/global_burden_disease/GlobalHealthRisks_report_full.pdf.
29. Narayan KM, Ali MK, Koplan JP: Global noncommunicable diseases—where worlds meet. *N Engl J Med* 363:1196–1198, 2010.
30. Danaei G, Finucane MM, Lu Y, et al: National, regional, and global trends in fasting plasma glucose and diabetes prevalence since 1980: systematic analysis of health examination surveys and epidemiological studies with 370 country-years and 2.7 million participants. *Lancet* 378: 31–40, 2011.
31. Finucane MM, Stevens GA, Cowan MJ, et al: National, regional, and global trends in body-mass index since 1980: systematic analysis of health examination surveys and epidemiological studies with 960 country-years and 9.1 million participants. *Lancet* 377:557–567, 2011.
32. Danaei G, Finucane MM, Lin JK, et al: National, regional, and global trends in systolic blood pressure since 1980: systematic analysis of health examination surveys and epidemiological studies with 786 country-years and 5.4 million participants. *Lancet* 377:568–577, 2011.
33. Farzadfar F, Finucane MM, Danaei G, et al: National, regional, and global trends in serum total cholesterol since 1980: systematic analysis of health examination surveys and epidemiological studies with 321 country-years and 3.0 million participants. *Lancet* 377:578–586, 2011.
34. International Diabetes Federation: *IDF diabetes atlas,* ed 6, Brussels, Belgium, 2013, International Diabetes Federation.
35. Wild S, Roglic G, Green A, et al: Global prevalence of diabetes: estimates for the year 2000 and projections for 2030. *Diabetes Care* 27:1047–1053, 2004.
36. Cowie CC, Rust KF, Byrd-Holt DD, et al: Prevalence of diabetes and impaired fasting glucose in adults in the U.S. population: National Health And Nutrition Examination Survey 1999–2002. *Diabetes Care* 29:1263–1268, 2006.
37. Mather HM, Chaturvedi N, Fuller JH: Mortality and morbidity from diabetes in South Asians and Europeans: 11-year follow-up of the Southall Diabetes Survey, London, UK. *Diabet Med* 15:53–59, 1998.
38. Tan CE, Emmanuel SC, Tan BY, et al: Prevalence of diabetes and ethnic differences in cardiovascular risk factors. The 1992 Singapore National Health Survey. *Diabetes Care* 22:241–247, 1999.
39. Shaw JE, Sicree RA, Zimmet PZ: Global estimates of the prevalence of diabetes for 2010 and 2030. *Diabetes Res Clin Pract* 87:4–14, 2010.
40. *The global competitiveness report: 2009–2010,* Geneva, 2009, World Economic Forum.
41. Shaw J: Epidemiology of childhood type 2 diabetes and obesity. *Pediatr Diabetes* 8(Suppl 9):7–15, 2007.
42. Fagot-Campagna A, Pettitt DJ, Engelgau MM, et al: Type 2 diabetes among North American children and adolescents: an epidemiologic review and a public health perspective. *J Pediatr* 136:664–672, 2000.
43. Group SfDiYS, Liese AD, D'Agostino RB Jr, , et al: The burden of diabetes mellitus among U.S. youth: prevalence estimates from the SEARCH for Diabetes in Youth Study. *Pediatrics* 118:1510–1518, 2006.
44. Hwang CK, Han PV, Zabetian A, et al: Rural diabetes prevalence quintuples over twenty-five years in low- and middle-income countries: a systematic review and meta-analysis. *Diabetes Res Clin Pract,* 2012.
45. Kahn SE, Hull RL, Utzschneider KM: Mechanisms linking obesity to insulin resistance and type 2 diabetes. *Nature* 444:840–846, 2006.
46. Weber M, Staimez L, Gilligan J, et al: *Lifestyle medicine and the treatment of glucose intolerance. Textbook of lifestyle medicine and health.* 2011, Taylor and Francis.
47. Amati F, Dube JJ, Coen PM, et al: Physical inactivity and obesity underlie the insulin resistance of aging. *Diabetes Care* 32:1547–1549, 2009.
48. Butler AE, Janson J, Bonner-Weir S, et al: Beta-cell deficit and increased beta-cell apoptosis in humans with type 2 diabetes. *Diabetes* 52:102–110, 2003.
49. Jensen CC, Cnop M, Hull RL, et al: Beta-cell function is a major contributor to oral glucose tolerance in high-risk relatives of four ethnic groups in the U.S. *Diabetes* 51:2170–2178, 2002.
50. Staimez LR, Weber MB, Ranjani H, et al: Marked reduction of β-cell function in South Asians with prediabetes [abstract]. *Diabetes* 60:A352–A397, 2011.
51. Weedon MN, McCarthy MI, Hitman G, et al: Combining information from common type 2 diabetes risk polymorphisms improves disease prediction. *PLoS Med* 3:e374, 2006.
52. Jafar-Mohammadi B, McCarthy MI: Genetics of type 2 diabetes mellitus and obesity—a review. *Ann Med* 40:1–9, 2007.
53. Weedon MN: The importance of TCF7L2. *Diabet Med* 24:1062–1066, 2007.
54. Grant SF, Thorleifsson G, Reynisdottir I, et al: Variant of transcription factor 7-like 2 (TCF7L2) gene confers risk of type 2 diabetes. *Nat Genet* 38:320–323, 2006.
55. *Diabetes myths,* 2011. www.diabetes.org/diabetes-basics/diabetes-myths/at, www.diabetes.org/diabetes-basics/diabetes-myths/.
56. Goldfine AB, Bouche C, Parker RA, et al: Insulin resistance is a poor predictor of type 2 diabetes in individuals with no family history of disease. *Proc Natl Acad Sci U S A* 100:2724–2729, 2003.
57. Hariri S, Yoon PW, Qureshi N, et al: Family history of type 2 diabetes: a population-based screening tool for prevention? *Genet Med* 8:102–108, 2006.
58. Harrison TA, Hindorff LA, Kim H, et al: Family history of diabetes as a potential public health tool. *Am J Prev Med* 24:152–159, 2003.
59. O'Rahilly S, Barroso I, Wareham NJ: Genetic factors in type 2 diabetes: the end of the beginning? *Science* 307:370–373, 2005.
60. Annis AM, Caulder MS, Cook ML, et al: Family history, diabetes, and other demographic and risk factors among participants of the National Health and Nutrition Examination Survey 1999–2002. *Prev Chronic Dis* 2:A19, 2005.
61. Barker D: In utero programming of chronic disease. *Clin Sci* 95:115–128, 1998.
62. Jonnalagadda SS, Khosla P: Nutrient intake, body composition, blood cholesterol and glucose levels among adult Asian Indians in the United States. *J Immigr Minor Health* 9:171–178, 2007.
63. Kalhan R, Puthawala K, Agarwal S, et al: Altered lipid profile, leptin, insulin, and anthropometry in offspring of South Asian immigrants in the United States. *Metabolism* 50:1197–1202, 2001.
64. Hales CN, Barker DJ: Type 2 (non-insulin-dependent) diabetes mellitus: the thrifty phenotype hypothesis. *Diabetologia* 35:595–601, 1992.
65. Li Y, Jaddoe VW, Qi L, et al: Exposure to the chinese famine in early life and the risk of metabolic syndrome in adulthood. *Diabetes Care* 34:1014–1018, 2011.
66. Huang C, Li Z, Wang M, et al: Early life exposure to the 1959–1961 Chinese famine has long-term health consequences. *J Nutr* 140:1874–1878, 2010.
67. Heijmans BT, Tobi EW, Stein AD, et al: Persistent epigenetic differences associated with prenatal exposure to famine in humans. *Proc Natl Acad Sci U S A* 105:17046–17049, 2008.
68. Yajnik CS: Fetal programming of diabetes: still so much to learn!. *Diabetes Care* 33:1146–1148, 2010.
69. Schulz LO, Bennett PH, Ravussin E, et al: Effects of traditional and western environments on prevalence of type 2 diabetes in Pima Indians in Mexico and the U.S. *Diabetes Care* 29:1866–1871, 2006.
70. Fujimoto WY, Hershon K, Kinyoun J, et al: Type II diabetes mellitus in Seattle and Tokyo. *Tohoku J Exp Med* 141(Suppl):133–139, 1983.
71. Fujimoto WY, Leonetti DL, Kinyoun JL, et al: Prevalence of diabetes mellitus and impaired glucose tolerance among second-generation Japanese-American men. *Diabetes* 36:721–729, 1987.
72. Lazar MA: How obesity causes diabetes: not a tall tale. *Science* 307:373–375, 2005.
73. Avenell A, Broom J, Brown TJ, et al: Systematic review of the long-term effects and economic consequences of treatments for obesity and implications for health improvement. *Health Technol Assess* 8:1–182, 2004.
74. Thompson D, Edelsberg J, Colditz GA, et al: Lifetime health and economic consequences of obesity. *Arch Intern Med* 159:2177–2183, 1999.
75. Narayan KMV, Boyle JP, Thompson TJ, et al: Effect of body mass index on lifetime risk for diabetes mellitus in the United States. *Diabetes Care,* 2007.
76. Ford ES, Williamson DF, Liu S: Weight change and diabetes incidence: findings from a national cohort of US adults. *Am J Epidemiol* 146:214–222, 1997.
77. Report of the expert committee on the diagnosis and classification of diabetes mellitus. *Diabetes Care* 26(Suppl 1):S5–S20, 2003.
78. Samuel VT, Petersen KF, Shulman GI: Lipid-induced insulin resistance: unravelling the mechanism. *Lancet* 375:2267–2277, 2010.
79. Uusitupa M, Lindi V, Louheranta A, et al: Long-term improvement in insulin sensitivity by changing lifestyles of people with impaired glucose tolerance: 4-year results from the Finnish Diabetes Prevention Study. *Diabetes* 52:2532–2538, 2003.
80. Bogardus C, Lillioja S, Mott DM, et al: Relationship between degree of obesity and in vivo insulin action in man. *Am J Physiol* 248:E286–E291, 1985.
81. Uusitupa M: Lifestyles matter in the prevention of type 2 diabetes. *Diabetes Care* 25:1650–1651, 2002.
82. Sullivan PW, Morrato EH, Ghushchyan V, et al: Obesity, inactivity, and the prevalence of diabetes and diabetes-related cardiovascular comorbidities in the U.S., 2000–2002. *Diabetes Care* 28:1599–1603, 2005.
83. Boffetta P, McLerran D, Chen Y, et al: Body mass index and diabetes in Asia: a cross-sectional pooled analysis of 900,000 individuals in the Asia cohort consortium. *PLoS One* 6:e19930, 2011.
84. Kissebah AH, Vydelingum N, Murray R, et al: Relation of body fat distribution to metabolic complications of obesity. *J Clin Endocrinol Metab* 54:254–260, 1982.
85. Balkau B, Deanfield JE, Despres JP, et al: International Day for the Evaluation of Abdominal Obesity (IDEA): a study of waist circumference, cardiovascular disease, and diabetes mellitus in 168,000 primary care patients in 63 countries. *Circulation* 116:1942–1951, 2007.
86. Boyko EJ, Fujimoto WY, Leonetti DL, et al: Visceral adiposity and risk of type 2 diabetes: a prospective study among Japanese Americans. *Diabetes Care* 23:465–471, 2000.
87. Indulekha K, Anjana RM, Surendar J, et al: Association of visceral and subcutaneous fat with glucose intolerance, insulin resistance, adipocytokines and inflammatory markers in Asian Indians (CURES-113). *Clin Biochem* 44:281–287, 2011.
88. Shah A, Hernandez A, Mathur D, et al: Adipokines and body fat composition in South Asians: results of the Metabolic Syndrome and Atherosclerosis in South Asians Living in America (MASALA) study. *Int J Obes (Lond),* 2011.
89. Montague CT, O'Rahilly S: The perils of portliness: causes and consequences of visceral adiposity. *Diabetes* 49:883–888, 2000.
90. Furukawa S, Fujita T, Shimabukuro M, et al: Increased oxidative stress in obesity and its impact on metabolic syndrome. *J Clin Invest* 114:1752–1761, 2004.
91. Fujimoto WY, Jablonski KA, Bray GA, et al: Body size and shape changes and the risk of diabetes in the diabetes prevention program. *Diabetes* 56:1680–1685, 2007.
92. Laaksonen DE, Lindstrom J, Lakka TA, et al: Physical activity in the prevention of type 2 diabetes: the Finnish Diabetes Prevention Study. *Diabetes* 54:158–165, 2005.
93. Roumen C, Blaak EE, Corpeleijn E: Lifestyle intervention for prevention of diabetes: determinants of success for future implementation. *Nutr Rev* 67:132–146, 2009.
94. Oster G, Thompson D, Edelsberg J, et al: Lifetime health and economic benefits of weight loss among obese persons. *Am J Public Health* 89:1536–1542, 1999.
95. Eriksson J, Tuominen J, Valle T, et al: Aerobic endurance exercise or circuit-type resistance training for individuals with impaired glucose tolerance? *Horm Metab Res* 30:37–41, 1998.
96. Lund S, Holman GD, Schmitz O, et al: Contraction stimulates translocation of glucose transporter GLUT4 in skeletal muscle through a mechanism distinct from that of insulin. *Proc Natl Acad Sci U S A* 92:5817–5821, 1995.
97. Shepherd PR, Kahn BB: Glucose transporters and insulin action–implications for insulin resistance and diabetes mellitus. *N Engl J Med* 341:248–257, 1999.
98. Schenk S, Horowitz JF: Acute exercise increases triglyceride synthesis in skeletal muscle and prevents fatty acid-induced insulin resistance. *J Clin Invest* 117:1690–1698, 2007.
99. Swartz AM, Strath SJ, Bassett DR, et al: Increasing daily walking improves glucose tolerance in overweight women. *Prev Med* 37:356–362, 2003.
100. Yamanouchi K, Shinozaki T, Chikada K, et al: Daily walking combined with diet therapy is a useful means for obese NIDDM patients not only to reduce body weight but also to improve insulin sensitivity. [comment]. *Diabetes Care* 18:775–778, 1995.
101. Miyatake N, Nishikawa H, Morishita A, et al: Daily walking reduces visceral adipose tissue areas and improves insulin resistance in Japanese obese subjects. *Diabetes Res Clin Pract* 58:101–107, 2002.
102. Lee IM, Rexrode KM, Cook NR, et al: Physical activity and coronary heart disease in women: is "no pain, no gain" passe? [comment]. *JAMA* 285:1447–1454, 2001.
103. Maeda K, Ohta T, Kawamura T, et al: Effect of body weight reduction on blood pressure and biochemical data. *Nihon Koshu Eisei Zasshi* 42:534–541, 1995.
104. Ohta T, Kawamura T, Hatano K, et al: Effects of exercise on coronary risk factors in obese, middle-aged subjects. *Jpn Circ J* 54:1459–1464, 1990.

105. Hu FB, Sacks F, Willett WC: Dietary fats and prevention of cardiovascular disease. Patient compliance should have been considered. *BMJ* 323:1001–1002, 2001.

106. Hu FB: Globalization of diabetes: the role of diet, lifestyle, and genes. *Diabetes Care* 34:1249–1257, 2011.

107. Vessby B, Uusitupa M, Hermansen K, et al: Substituting dietary saturated for monounsaturated fat impairs insulin sensitivity in healthy men and women: the KANWU study. *Diabetologia* 44:312–319, 2001.

108. Liese AD, Nichols M, Sun X, et al: Adherence to the DASH Diet is inversely associated with incidence of type 2 diabetes: the insulin resistance atherosclerosis study. *Diabetes Care* 32:1434–1436, 2009.

109. Salas-Salvado J, Bullo M, Babio N, et al: Reduction in the incidence of type 2 diabetes with the Mediterranean diet: results of the PREDIMED-Reus nutrition intervention randomized trial. *Diabetes Care* 34:14–19, 2011.

110. Brunner EJ, Mosdol A, Witte DR, et al: Dietary patterns and 15-y risks of major coronary events, diabetes, and mortality. *Am J Clin Nutr* 87:1414–1421, 2008.

111. Crandall JP, Knowler WC, Kahn SE, et al: The prevention of type 2 diabetes. *Nat Clin Pract Endocrinol Metab* 4:382–393, 2008.

112. Pan XR, Li GW, Hu YH, et al: Effects of diet and exercise in preventing NIDDM in people with impaired glucose tolerance. The Da Qing IGT and Diabetes Study. *Diabetes Care* 20:537–544, 1997.

113. Li G, Zhang P, Wang J, et al: The long-term effect of lifestyle interventions to prevent diabetes in the China Da Qing Diabetes Prevention Study: a 20-year follow-up study. *Lancet* 371:1783–1789, 2008.

114. Phillips LS: Comment on: Buchanan (2007) (How) can we prevent type 2 diabetes? Diabetes 56:1502–1507. *Diabetes* 56:e19, 2007.

115. Carr DB, Utzschneider KM, Boyko EJ, et al: A reduced-fat diet and aerobic exercise in Japanese Americans with impaired glucose tolerance decreases intra-abdominal fat and improves insulin sensitivity but not beta-cell function. *Diabetes* 54:340–347, 2005.

116. Knowler WC, Barrett-Connor E, Fowler SE, et al: Reduction in the incidence of type 2 diabetes with lifestyle intervention or metformin. *N Engl J Med* 346:393–403, 2002.

117. Lindstrom J, Louheranta A, Mannelin M, et al: The Finnish Diabetes Prevention Study (DPS): Lifestyle intervention and 3-year results on diet and physical activity. *Diabetes Care* 26: 3230–3236, 2003.

118. Lindstrom J, Ilanne-Parikka P, Peltonen M, et al: Sustained reduction in the incidence of type 2 diabetes by lifestyle intervention: follow-up of the Finnish Diabetes Prevention Study. *Lancet* 368:1673–1679, 2006.

119. Wahl PW, Savage PJ, Psaty BM, et al: Diabetes in older adults: comparison of 1997 American Diabetes Association classification of diabetes mellitus with 1985 WHO classification. *Lancet* 352:1012–1015, 1998.

120. Ramachandran A, Snehalatha C, Mary S, et al: The Indian Diabetes Prevention Programme shows that lifestyle modification and metformin prevent type 2 diabetes in Asian Indian subjects with impaired glucose tolerance (IDPP-1). *Diabetologia* 49:289–297, 2006.

121. Payne WR, Walsh KJ, Harvey JT, et al: Effect of a low-resource-intensive lifestyle modification program incorporating gymnasium-based and home-based resistance training on type 2 diabetes risk in Australian adults. *Diabetes Care* 31:2244–2250, 2008.

122. Oldroyd JC, Unwin NC, White M, et al: Randomised controlled trial evaluating lifestyle interventions in people with impaired glucose tolerance. *Diabetes Res Clin Pract* 72:117–127, 2006.

123. Herder C, Peltonen M, Koenig W, et al: Anti-inflammatory effect of lifestyle changes in the Finnish Diabetes Prevention Study. *Diabetologia* 52:433–442, 2009.

124. Hamalainen H, Ronnemaa T, Virtanen A, et al: Improved fibrinolysis by an intensive lifestyle intervention in subjects with impaired glucose tolerance. The Finnish Diabetes Prevention Study. *Diabetologia* 48:2248–2253, 2005.

125. Lindgren P, Lindstrom J, Tuomilehto J, et al: Lifestyle intervention to prevent diabetes in men and women with impaired glucose tolerance is cost-effective. *Int J Technol Assess Health Care* 23:177–183, 2007.

126. Ramachandran A, Snehalatha C, Yamuna A, et al: Cost effectiveness of the interventions in the primary prevention of diabetes among Asian Indians: within trial results of the Indian Diabetes Prevention Programme (IDPP). *Diabetes Care*, 2007.

127. Diabetes Prevention Program Research Group: Within-trial cost-effectiveness of lifestyle intervention or metformin for the primary prevention of type 2 diabetes. *Diabetes Care* 26:2518–2523, 2003.

128. Alberti KG, Zimmet P, Shaw J: International Diabetes Federation: a consensus on type 2 diabetes prevention. *Diabet Med* 24:451–463, 2007.

129. Gottlieb DJ, Punjabi NM, Newman AB, et al: Association of sleep time with diabetes mellitus and impaired glucose tolerance. *Arch Intern Med* 165:863–867, 2005.

130. Ayas NT, White DP, Al-Delaimy WK, et al: A prospective study of self-reported sleep duration and incident diabetes in women. *Diabetes Care* 26:380–384, 2003.

131. Spiegel K, Leproult R, Van Cauter E: Impact of sleep debt on metabolic and endocrine function. *Lancet* 354:1435–1439, 1999.

132. Knutson KL, Spiegel K, Penev P, et al: The metabolic consequences of sleep deprivation. *Sleep Med Rev* 11:163–178, 2007.

133. Haire-Joshu D, Glasgow RE, Tibbs TL: Smoking and diabetes. *Diabetes Care* 22:1887–1898, 1999.

134. Haire-Joshu D, Glasgow RE, Tibbs TL: Smoking and diabetes. *Diabetes Care* 27(Suppl 1): S74–S75, 2004.

135. Willi C, Bodenmann P, Ghali WA, et al: Active smoking and the risk of type 2 diabetes: a systematic review and meta-analysis. *JAMA* 298:2654–2664, 2007.

136. Thayer KA, Heindel JJ, Bucher JR, et al: Role of environmental chemicals in diabetes and obesity: a National Toxicology Program workshop review. *Environ Health Perspect* 120:779–789, 2012.

137. Narayan KM, Gregg EW, Engelgau MM, et al: Translation research for chronic disease: the case of diabetes. *Diabetes Care* 23:1794–1798, 2000.

138. Narayan KM, Benjamin E, Gregg EW, et al: Diabetes translation research: where are we and where do we want to be? *Ann Intern Med* 140:958–963, 2004.

139. Garfield SA, Malozowski S, Chin MH, et al: Considerations for diabetes translational research in real-world settings. *Diabetes Care* 26:2670–2674, 2003.

140. Ogilvie D, Craig P, Griffin S, et al: A translational framework for public health research. *BMC Public Health* 9:116, 2009.

141. Woolf SH: The meaning of translational research and why it matters. *JAMA* 299:211–213, 2008.

142. Saaristo T, Moilanen L, Korpi-Hyovalti E, et al: Lifestyle intervention for prevention of type 2 diabetes in primary health care: one-year follow-up of the Finnish National Diabetes Prevention Program (FIN-D2D). *Diabetes Care* 33:2146–2151, 2010.

143. Ali MK, Echouffo-Tcheugui J, Williamson DF: How effective were lifestyle interventions in real-world settings that were modeled on the diabetes prevention program? *Health Aff (Millwood)* 31:67–75, 2012.

144. Boltri JM, Davis-Smith YM, Seale JP, et al: Diabetes prevention in a faith-based setting: results of translational research. *J Public Health Manag Pract* 14:29–32, 2008.

145. Ackermann RT, Finch EA, Brizendine E, et al: Translating the Diabetes Prevention Program into the community. The DEPLOY Pilot Study. *Am J Prev Med* 35:357–363, 2008.

146. Mau MK, Keawe'aimoku Kaholokula J, West MR, et al: Translating diabetes prevention into native Hawaiian and Pacific Islander communities: the PILI 'Ohana Pilot project. *Prog Community Health Partnersh* 4:7–16, 2010.

147. Harati H, Hadaegh F, Momenan AA, et al: Reduction in incidence of type 2 diabetes by lifestyle intervention in a middle eastern community. *Am J Prev Med* 38:628–636, 2010.

148. Hamman RF, Wing RR, Edelstein SL, et al: Effect of weight loss with lifestyle intervention on risk of diabetes. *Diabetes Care* 29:2102–2107, 2006.

149. Lindstrom J, Peltonen M, Eriksson JG, et al: High-fibre, low-fat diet predicts long-term weight loss and decreased type 2 diabetes risk: the Finnish Diabetes Prevention Study. *Diabetologia* 49:912–920, 2006.

150. Rosenstock IM: Why people use health services. *Milbank Mem Fund Q* 44(Suppl):94–127, 1966.

151. Prochaska JO, DiClemente CC: Stages and processes of self-change of smoking: toward an integrative model of change. *J Consult Clin Psychol* 51:390–395, 1983.

152. Gidding SS, Lichtenstein AH, Faith MS, et al: Implementing American Heart Association pediatric and adult nutrition guidelines: a scientific statement from the American Heart Association Nutrition Committee of the Council on Nutrition, Physical Activity and Metabolism, Council on Cardiovascular Disease in the Young, Council on Arteriosclerosis, Thrombosis and Vascular Biology, Council on Cardiovascular Nursing, Council on Epidemiology and Prevention, and Council for High Blood Pressure Research. *Circulation* 119:1161–1175, 2009.

153. Wing RR, Jeffery RW: Benefits of recruiting participants with friends and increasing social support for weight loss and maintenance. *J Consult Clin Psychol* 67:132–138, 1999.

154. Wallace JP, Raglin JS, Jastremski CA: Twelve month adherence of adults who joined a fitness program with a spouse vs without a spouse. *J Sports Med Phys Fitness* 35:206–213, 1995.

155. Unger JB, Johnson CA: Social relationships and physical activity in health club members. *Am J Health Promot* 9:340–343, 1995.

156. Delahanty LM, Conroy MB, Nathan DM: Psychological predictors of physical activity in the diabetes prevention program. *J Am Diet Assoc* 106:698–705, 2006.

157. Knowler WC, Fowler SE, Hamman RF, et al: 10-year follow-up of diabetes incidence and weight loss in the Diabetes Prevention Program Outcomes Study. *Lancet* 374:1677–1686, 2009.

158. Kitabchi AE, Temprosa M, Knowler WC, et al: Role of insulin secretion and sensitivity in the evolution of type 2 diabetes in the diabetes prevention program: effects of lifestyle intervention and metformin. *Diabetes* 54:2404–2414, 2005.

159. Amutha A, Ranjani H, Anjana RM, et al: Associations of β-cell function and insulin resistance with youth onset type 2 diabetes and prediabetes among Asian Indians. *Diabetes Technol Ther* 15:315–322, 2013.

2

Insulin Resistance
Pathophysiology, Molecular Mechanisms, Genetic Insights

Hans-Ulrich Häring and Baptist Gallwitz

Type 2 diabetes mellitus is a chronic disturbance of glucose metabolism without the absolute insulin deficiency that is typical for type 1 diabetes. Rather, type 2 diabetes is characterized by a reduced efficacy of insulin action in different peripheral tissues (insulin resistance) as well as a disturbance in beta cell function. These two important pathophysiologic characteristics in type 2 diabetes result in an imbalance of insulin availability and insulin demand. The clinical manifestation of the disease occurs mostly in the fourth to fifth decade of life, although alarming recent data show an increase in obesity and type 2 diabetes even in adolescents.

GENETIC FACTORS

Type 2 diabetes is a polygenetic disease with heterogeneous phenotypes and different gene-environment interactions. A high genetic predisposition for type 2 diabetes has been shown in population studies (e.g., the Pima Indians) and in family studies. First-degree relatives of type 2 diabetic patients have a significantly higher risk for type 2 diabetes than persons without a hereditary or genetic risk.[1] Twin studies revealed a much higher diabetes concordance in homozygous twins compared with heterozygous twins.[2] Although the existence of these genetic factors has been known for a considerable time, it was difficult to identify specific type 2 diabetes genes until recently, when genome-wide analyses and the human genome project led to progress in this field.[3,4]

The greatest success in type 2 diabetes genetics arose from the development and use of high-density single-nucleotide polymorphism (SNP) arrays in large case-control cohorts. Most of the gene variants could be confirmed in many ethnicities, whereas others, probably because of divergent risk allele frequencies, may have higher relevance for certain ethnic groups.[4]

Recent studies also provided evidence that SNPs associated with diabetes risk act in an additive manner to increase the diabetes risk.[4–6] Although significantly contributing to the type 2 diabetes risk, these gene-gene interactions do not yet allow a substantially better disease prediction than

clinical risk factors (e.g., body mass index [BMI], age, sex, family history of diabetes, fasting glucose level, blood pressure [BP], plasma triglycerides),[4,7–9] nor do they explain the heritability of type 2 diabetes.[4,5]

Beyond that, some of the diabetes-relevant genes are susceptible to persistent and partly inheritable epigenetic regulation—that is, DNA methylation and histone modifications—so gene-environment interactions are additional important factors that contribute to the complexity of type 2 diabetes genetics.[4,10–12]

Genome-wide association studies identified a series of type 2 diabetes risk loci that are for the most part associated with impaired pancreatic beta cell function.[3,13–43]

Although the underlying mechanisms by which common genetic variations within these loci affect beta cell function are not completely understood, risk variants may alter glucose-stimulated insulin secretion,[3,17,18,20,34–38] proinsulin conversion,[3,44–46] and incretin secretion or incretin action.[3] **Table 2-1** summarizes the most important diabetes genes and their functional roles.[4]

It has further become evident in recent studies that genetic variants in several diabetes risk genes may predict treatment outcome of glucose-lowering drugs. Response to thiazolidinedione therapy has been associated with peroxisome proliferator-activated receptor gamma (PPAR-γ) variations[3,47,48] in some but not all studies.[3,49,50] The genetic variants of the transcription factor 7-like 2 (TCF7L2, a transcription factor involved in the Wnt-signaling pathway and the most important genetic marker associated with type 2 diabetes) have been reported to influence disease severity and therapeutic control,[3,51] including lifestyle intervention,[3,52] and the response to sulfonylureas and possibly incretin-based therapies.[3,53]

INSULIN RESISTANCE

Type 2 diabetes, according to our present understanding, is a multifactorial disease characterized by insulin resistance of various degrees in different organs.[54] Insulin resistance is in most patients further accompanied by central obesity,

TABLE 2-1 Effects of Single-Nucleotide Polymorphisms (SNPs) in Confirmed Type 2 Diabetes Genes on Prediabetic Traits

GENE	LOCATION ON CHROMOSOME	TISSUE EXPRESSION (REPRODUCTIVE SYSTEM NOT INCLUDED)	VARIANTS (APPROXIMATE RISK ALLELE FREQUENCY IN EUROPEANS)	RISK ALLELE EFFECTS
ADAMTS9	3	Skeletal muscle, breast, thymus, kidney, prostate, pancreas, heart, lung, spinal cord, brain, all fetal tissues	rs4607103 (80%)	Unknown
CAPN10	2	Thymus, colon, bladder, brain, spleen, prostate, skeletal muscle, pancreas, heart, lymph node, lung, kidney	rs3792267 (70%), rs3842570 (40%), rs5030952 (90%)	Glucose-stimulated insulin secretion ↓; proinsulin conversion ↓; whole-body insulin sensitivity ↓
CDC123 \CAMK1D	10	Bone marrow, smooth muscle, kidney, prostate, colon, bladder, spleen, lung, lymph node, skin, breast, brain, liver, thymus and skin, retina, spleen, skeletal muscle, lung	rs12779790 (20%)	Insulin secretion ↓
CDKAL1	6	Bone marrow, breast, liver, spleen, prostate, retina, brain, lung, kidney, thymus, pancreas, skeletal muscle	rs7754840 (30%)	Glucose-stimulated insulin secretion ↓; proinsulin conversion ↓
CDKN2A/ CDKN2B	9	Ubiquitous; bladder, colon, lung, spleen, skin, liver, breast, skeletal muscle, prostate, kidney, brain, pancreas, adipose tissue	rs10811661 (80%)	Glucose-stimulated insulin secretion ↓
ENPP1	6	Thyroid gland, kidney, skeletal muscle, breast, liver, skin, thymus, salivary gland, brain capillaries	rs1044498/K121Q (10%)	Whole-body insulin sensitivity ↓; insulin secretion ↓
FTO	16	Brain, pancreas, skeletal muscle, prostate, retina, heart, skin, breast, lung, kidney, liver, thymus, fetal brain, fetal kidney, fetal liver	rs8050136 (40%), rs9939609 (40%)	Overall fat mass ↑; energy intake ↑; cerebrocortical insulin sensitivity ↓
HHEX	10	Thyroid gland, brain, lymph node, spleen, liver, lung, kidney, breast, pancreas, thymus, skin, prostate, fetal pancreas	rs7923837 (60%)	Glucose-stimulated insulin secretion ↓
HNF18	17	Colon, kidney, liver, thymus, retina, pancreas, prostate, lung	rs757210 (40%)	Unknown
IGF2BP2	3	Smooth muscle, colon, lung, retina, skeletal muscle, skin, kidney, thymus, fetal liver, fetal brain, pancreas	rs4402960 (30%)	Glucose-stimulated insulin secretion ↓
JAZF1	7	Lymph node, retina, pancreas, thymus, brain, skin, liver, skeletal muscle, lung, spleen, prostate	rs864745 (50%)	Insulin secretion ↓
KCNJ11	11	Pancreas, heart, pituitary gland, skeletal muscle, brain, smooth muscle	rs5219/E23K (50%)	Insulin secretion ↓; glucose-dependent; suppression of glucagon secretion ↓
KCNQ1	11	Thyroid gland, bone marrow, prostate, heart, pancreas, lung, thymus, skin, liver, kidney	rs2237892 (90%), rs151290 (80%)	Insulin secretion ↓; incretin secretion ↓
MTNR1B	11	Retina, brain, pancreas	rs10830963 (30%), rs10830962 (40%), rs4753426 (50%)	Glucose-stimulated insulin secretion ↓
NOTCH2	1	Lung, skin, thyroid gland, skeletal muscle, smooth muscle, kidney, bladder, lymph node, breast, colon, prostate, spleen, brain, thymus, heart, liver, pancreas	rs10923931 (10%)	Unknown
PPARG	3	Adipose tissue, colon, lung, kidney, breast, spleen, skin, prostate, bone marrow, brain, skeletal muscle, liver	rs1801282/P12A (80%)	Whole-body insulin sensitivity ↓; adipose tissue insulin sensitivity ↓; insulin clearance ↓
SLC30A8	8	Pancreas, kidney, lung, breast, amygdala	rs13266634/R325W (70%)	Glucose-stimulated insulin secretion ↓; proinsulin conversion ↓
TCF7L2	10	Brain, lung, bone marrow, thyroid gland, colon, pancreas, skin, breast, kidney, liver, thymus, prostate	rs7903146 (30%), rs12255372 (30%), rs7901695 (30%)	Incretin-stimulated insulin secretion ↓; proinsulin conversion ↓; whole-body insulin sensitivity ↓; hepatic insulin sensitivity ↓
THADA	2	Ubiquitous	rs7578597/T1187A (90%)	Unknown
TSPAN8/ LGR5	12	Spinal cord, colon, skeletal muscle, prostate, liver, lung, pancreas, kidney, skeletal muscle, skin, brain, spinal cord	rs7961581 (30%)	Insulin secretion ↓
WFS1	4	Ubiquitous	rs10010131 (60%)	Incretin-stimulated insulin secretion ↓

Data from Staiger H, Machicao F, Fritsche A, Häring HU: Pathomechanisms of type 2 diabetes genes, *Endocr Rev* 30:557, 2009.

arterial hypertension, dyslipidemia, and other risk factors for cardiovascular disease. The joint presence of these risk factors with or without manifest type 2 diabetes is summarized by the term "metabolic syndrome." The metabolic syndrome is a multifactorial metabolic disorder with a twofold to fourfold increased risk for cardiovascular disease (see Chapter 4).

The hormone insulin has a number of cellular effects and regulates not only glucose metabolism but also lipid and protein metabolism, as well as DNA synthesis and lipolysis (**Fig. 2-1**).[54] Any defect of these different cellular effects of insulin action can be seen as insulin resistance. In experimental medicine, the gold standard for measuring and quantifying insulin resistance is the euglycemic glucose clamp technique. This technique is too complicated and time- and personnel-consuming for everyday clinical practice; therefore a number of simpler tests for determining insulin resistance were developed. These are basically based on the assumption that a curvilinear relationship between insulin sensitivity and insulin secretion exists. In healthy patients it is possible to calculate the insulin sensitivity from the fasting plasma glucose concentration with a special formula for a hyperbolic relationship. However, this formula is not applicable for patients with a disturbance of glucose tolerance and diabetes because they show a disturbance in insulin secretion of varying degree in addition to being insulin resistant. The presently available simple tests to determine insulin resistance in patients with diabetes are based on the measurements of the fasting plasma glucose and insulin concentrations (homeostatic model assessment [HOMA])[55] or on the completion of an oral glucose tolerance test (OGTT) with measurements of plasma glucose and insulin concentrations (e.g., HOMA-IR [HOMA model for insulin resistance], insulin sensitivity index [ISI] [0,120], Matsuda index, and the Stumvoll index).[56-58] Whereas the glucose-clamp technique is a reliable method for the quantification

of insulin resistance, the previously mentioned simple tests do not allow an exact quantification for a single individual. Therefore the determination of insulin resistance with these tests in an individual clinical setting is feasible only in special situations. Frequent sources of error include, for example, the incorrect performance of the OGT that will eventually lead to wrong conclusions in determining insulin resistance. In everyday clinical practice, insulin resistance can be more easily detected with symptoms such as central obesity or other factors of the metabolic syndrome. Therapeutic decisions are mainly based on these clinically visible characteristics and will lead to recommendations of lifestyle changes, body weight reduction, and pharmacologic interventions with oral glucose-lowering drugs such as metformin. It should be mentioned that insulin resistance may vary considerably depending on the patient's level of physical fitness and activity, body weight, and overall health (e.g., acute and chronic infections, tumors). Insulin resistance is a common and important risk factor for development of type 2 diabetes and cardiovascular disease.[59-63] However, insulin resistance does not always lead to diabetes even though obesity is the most important risk factor. Only patients with a disturbance in insulin secretion or other risk factors will develop diabetes.

Insulin Signaling and Cellular Mechanisms of Insulin Resistance

Insulin effects are transmitted by insulin binding to a specific transmembrane insulin receptor. The receptor belongs to the family of tyrosine kinase receptors, like the receptors for many growth factors.[64] The active receptor is a dimer of two combined subunits. Insulin effects in the intact organism are mediated almost exclusively through the insulin receptor but can also be mediated by hybrid receptors that are formed by one subunit of the insulin receptor and

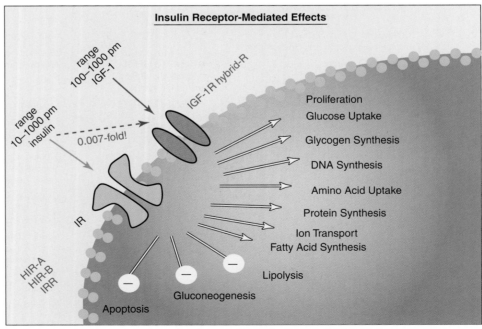

FIGURE 2-1 Insulin receptor–mediated effects. The binding of a ligand to its receptor triggers the activation of signaling pathways through effector proteins that transduce signals to several intracellular second-messenger systems, which eventually lead to biologic actions. The figure shows the insulin receptor with three different isoforms (IRR, HIR-A, and HIR-B) as well as the structurally and functionally similar receptor for insulin-like growth factor (IGF-1). The biologic actions triggered by ligand binding of insulin are depicted in a schematic manner.

another subunit of the receptor for insulin-like growth factor (IGF-1). Insulin binds with high affinity to its own receptor and with a 100 to 150 times lower affinity to the IGF-1 receptor. Therefore, insulin binding to the IGF-1 receptor does not play a notable role at physiologic insulin plasma concentrations compared with IGF-1 effects at its own receptor.[65] The affinity toward insulin–IGF-1 hybrid receptors lies between that for the insulin receptor and that for the IGF-1 receptor. The binding of insulin to its receptor leads to a cascade of cellular signals that are mostly phosphorylation and dephosphorylation events. The docking proteins IRS-1 to IRS-4 (insulin receptor substrates) have been detected as primary intracellular substrates for the postreceptor signaling. These transmit the insulin signal downstream into different cellular compartments after phosphorylation by the activated insulin receptor.[66,67] There are two distinctly different pathways in the intracellular insulin signal transmission. One pathway conveys the metabolic effects of insulin via the signaling molecules AKT/PKB; the other pathway transmits the mitogenic effects of insulin via the signaling proteins Ras/Raf/MAP kinase (**Fig. 2-2**).[54,65,67] Insulin resistance can therefore lead to a reduction of metabolic effects as well as mitogenic effects. Because redundancies and compensation mechanisms are present throughout the entire system of the intracellular signal transduction of the insulin signal, a disturbance of a single transmission element does not necessarily result in insulin resistance. Depending on the defects of the insulin signal transduction, metabolic and mitogenic effects of insulin may be affected to varying degrees.[68,69]

The Insulin Receptor, Insulin Receptor Substrates, and PKB/AKT Proteins

Numerous investigations have been carried out to investigate possible mutations in the gene for the insulin receptor in type 2 diabetes. Only very few mutations have been found that are associated with the development of insulin resistance or type 2 diabetes.[70–72] Furthermore, most studies have not shown a significant reduction in insulin receptor molecules in peripheral target tissues and organs for insulin action.[73–75] Therefore, quantitative changes in insulin receptor expression and insulin receptor mutations are not responsible for the development of insulin resistance in type 2 diabetes. It is interesting to note that a reduction in insulin receptor autophosphorylation was detected in vitro in tissues from type 2 diabetic patients in numerous former investigations.[76,77] It is hypothesized that the reduced autophosphorylation of the insulin receptor is responsible for disturbed insulin signal transduction and consequently the development of insulin resistance. The reduction in autophosphorylation and autoactivation of the insulin receptor is partially caused by modifications in the receptor molecule by an increased phosphorylation of serine residues.[78,79] The changes in insulin receptor activity are most likely secondary phenomena resulting from the metabolic changes in type 2 diabetes (e.g., hyperglycemia, dyslipidemia). Studies demonstrating normalization of the insulin receptor activity after lifestyle interventions support this hypothesis.[80–82] Only in rare patients with severe insulin resistance syndromes have insulin receptor mutations been detected that are associated with a reduced binding affinity

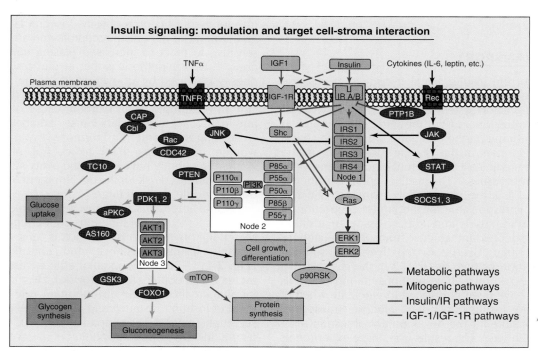

FIGURE 2-2 Insulin signaling: modulation and target cell–stroma interaction. Critical nodes form an important part of the signaling network that functions downstream of the insulin receptor (IR) and the insulin-like growth factor 1 (IGF1) receptor (IGF-1R). The important metabolic and mitogenic pathways are shown. Three important nodes in the insulin pathway are the IR and the IR substrates (IRS) 1 to 4 (node 1); the phosphatidylinositol 3-kinase (PI3K) with its several regulatory and catalytic subunits (node 2); and the three AKT/protein kinase B (PKB) isoforms (node 3). Downstream or intermediate effectors, as well as modulators, of these critical nodes include atypical protein kinase C (aPKC), AKT substrate of 160 kDa (AS160), Cas-Br-M (murine) ecotropic retroviral transforming sequence homologue (Cbl), Cbl-associated protein (CAP), cell-division cycle 42 (CDC42), extracellular signal-regulated kinase 1 and 2 (ERK1 and ERK2), forkhead box O1 (FOXO1), glycogen synthase kinase 3 (GSK3), Janus kinase (JAK), c-Jun-N-terminal kinase (JNK), mammalian target of rapamycin (mTOR), p90 ribosomal protein S6 kinase (p90RSK), phosphoinositide-dependent kinase 1 and 2 (PDK1, 2), phosphatase and tensin homologue (PTEN), protein tyrosine phosphatase-1B (PTP1B), Ras, Rac, Src-homology-2-containing protein (Shc), suppressor of cytokine signaling (SOCS), signal transducer and activator of transcription (STAT), and Ras homologue gene family, member Q (ARHQ; also called TC10). IL = Interleukin; TNF$_\alpha$ = tumor necrosis factor α; TNFR = TNF-α receptor. *(Modified from Taniguchi CM, Emanuelli B, Kahn CR: Critical nodes in signalling pathways: insights into insulin action. Nat Rev Mol Cell Biol 7:85–95, 2006.)*

of insulin to the insulin receptor or to a diminished autophosphorylation and autoactivation of the insulin receptor. These severe insulin resistance syndromes, also referred to as *type A insulin resistance,* most often lead to glucose metabolism disorders during adolescence and are often associated with acanthosis nigricans and hyperandrogenism in women.[70,78] Other very rare insulin receptor mutations involving a complete loss of function lead to severe diseases such as leprechaunism.[83]

Functional studies on the activation of the IRSs and the phosphatidylinositol 3-kinase (PI 3-kinase) that binds to the IRS were performed predominantly in muscle cells and adipocytes of patients with type 2 diabetes. These in vitro studies revealed reduced activation of IRS-1 and IRS-2 as well as reduced PI 3-kinase/PKB (PKB = protein kinase B) activity in type 2 diabetes.[68,72,84–87] Defects in the insulin signaling cascade are therefore already present in the first steps of the signal transmission in insulin resistance and type 2 diabetes. Apart from these findings, genetic polymorphisms in the genes for the IRS proteins and the PI 3-kinase/PKB/AKT complex were found in type 2 diabetes—for example, Gly972Arg for IRS-1 and Met326Iso for PI 3-kinase.[88–91] The incidence and the functional relevance of these polymorphisms is very heterogeneous in different populations. These studies suggest that the diminished activation of IRS-1, IRS-2, and PI 3-kinase/AKT in muscle cells, hepatocytes, and adipocytes may be secondary to regulatory signal changes in metabolic disturbances. It is interesting to note that a disturbance of the metabolic signal pathway via IRS/PI 3-kinase/AKT is present in insulin resistance in type 2 diabetes, whereas the mitogenic pathway of the insulin signal via MAP kinase is not affected. In summary, in insulin resistance, a reduced cellular action of insulin is found concerning the metabolic but not the mitogenic effects of insulin.[68]

GLUCOSE TRANSPORT

The activation of the insulin signal transduction cascade leads to glucose transport into the cell. The insulin effect on the glucose transport system is mediated by a translocation of glucose transporters from the intracellular pools to the plasma membrane on the one hand, and by the activation of the transporters in the plasma membrane on the other.[64,65] There are at least 12 different glucose transporter proteins in different tissues.[92] The insulin-dependent glucose transporter GLUT-4 is the most widely expressed glucose transporter and is responsible for the largest proportion of glucose transport in muscle and adipose tissue. In addition to that, glucose-dependent glucose transporters such as GLUT-1 in the brain, GLUT-2 in the liver, and sodium-dependent transporters such as GLUT-3 in the gastrointestinal tract are also known. Investigations in muscle cells and adipocytes have been performed to elucidate whether a defect in the insulin-dependent glucose transporter GLUT-4 is responsible for the development of insulin resistance in type 2 diabetes. The results from these experiments were relatively heterogeneous and revealed a reduced expression of GLUT-4 in some studies, a defect in the translocation and activation of GLUT-4 in others, as well as an unchanged GLUT-4 expression in type 2 diabetes.[86,93–96] It is interesting to note that in studies of patients with type 2 diabetes, a reduced translocation of glucose transport vesicles to the plasma membrane was found, whereas GLUT-4 expression was unchanged.[97,98] In studies investigating

possible mutations of GLUT-4 in type 2 diabetes, no functionally relevant defects were found.[99] In summary, in type 2 diabetes, a reduced capacity of insulin-dependent translocation of GLUT-4 vesicles to the plasma membrane is observed as a consequence of insulin resistance (**Fig. 2-3**).[100]

THE ROLE OF THE ADIPOCYTE AND OBESITY IN TYPE 2 DIABETES

Obesity is one of the most important predisposing factors for the development of insulin resistance and type 2 diabetes. In the past two decades, we have learned to discriminate which fat compartments contribute substantially to this development. Patients with an increased visceral (mesenteric and omental) fat mass, as well as persons with increased liver fat mass, have an increased risk for insulin resistance and type 2 diabetes.[101] This explains why measuring the waist circumference and the waist-to-hip ratio (WHR) predicts diabetes incidence more reliably than measuring the BMI. Increased subcutaneous fat depots in the hip, thigh, or gluteal region do not increase the risk for insulin resistance as long as there is no accompanying increase in visceral fat.[102] An increased subcutaneous fat accumulation around the hip and thigh is often observed in women and is termed *gynoid fat distribution,* whereas central obesity is more common in men and is termed *android fat distribution.* The causes of predominantly subcutaneous or visceral fat storage are genetic and also dependent on sex hormone concentrations and additional endocrine influences. The understanding of genetic causes for central obesity is just being unraveled, but hormones such as cortisol and androgens have already been identified as being important for the development of central obesity. Visceral fat cells express a higher number of cortisol receptors and are therefore more sensitive to react to increased plasma cortisol concentrations.[101] One hypothesis is that insulin resistance–induced obesity is caused by an overactivity of the neuroendocrine hormonal axes as well as by genetic predisposition.[101,103] One rare example of an extreme cause of central obesity and in this case a secondary cause of diabetes development is Cushing syndrome. Furthermore, hyperandrogenism in women predisposes them to central obesity.[104] These women frequently have polycystic ovary syndrome (PCOS) and an increased risk for the development of type 2 diabetes during middle age and later.

Visceral adipose tissue is now seen as an endocrine organ with respect to special functions concerning activation and secretion of numerous hormones and cytokines that mediate insulin resistance and chronic inflammation (**Fig. 2-4**).[105] Not only omental adipose tissue, but also an increased fat content in hepatocytes, muscle cells, and even intrapancreatic fat play an important role in the development of insulin resistance and even in a decrease in insulin secretion (caused by intrapancreatic fat).[4,54,63,106–109] Free fatty acids are important mediators in central obesity. Elevated free fatty acid concentrations in plasma are found in insulin resistance and in type 2 diabetes. These free fatty acids are most likely liberated by an increased lipolytic activity of the central and visceral fat depots and facilitate insulin resistance through an increased rate of fatty acid oxidation of the involved organs. Insulin and the sympathetic nervous system are important regulators of lipolysis. In central obesity, the increased sympathetic activity and a reduced

Normal

Insulin Resistant

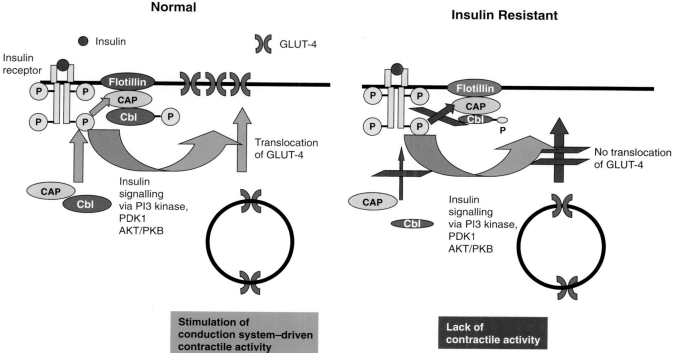

FIGURE 2-3 Differences in the regulation of GLUT-4 translocation in cardiac myocytes under normal conditions and in insulin resistance. Under normal conditions in fully differentiated cardiac myocytes (left panel), insulin stimulates the activation of the PI 3-K/PDK1/AKT signal transduction. Insulin further stimulates the phosphorylation of the proto-oncogene Cbl (Cas-Br-M [murine] ecotropic retroviral transforming sequence homologue) and its increased recruitment to a lipid raft-located complex containing flotillin and CAP (Cbl-associated protein). The joint activity of both pathways is a prerequisite for the translocation of the glucose transporter GLUT-4. In the insulin-resistant state in dedifferentiated cardiac myocytes (right panel), the stimulation of the PI 3-K/PDK1/AKT signal transduction is unchanged. Cbl, on the other hand, is reduced, and furthermore Cbl phosphorylation is impaired. As a consequence, the translocation of GLUT-4 is inhibited and the pool of available GLUT-4 is also diminished.

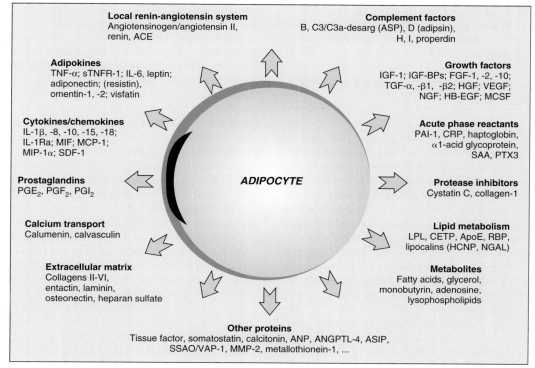

FIGURE 2-4 The adipocyte as endocrine organ. The figure shows the different hormones, cytokines, inflammatory markers, growth factors, and other transmitter molecules that are secreted by the adipocyte. These substances are involved in inflammatory processes, insulin resistance, and vascular changes. *(Modified from Staiger H, Häring HU: Adipocytokines: fat-derived humoral mediators of metabolic homeostasis,* Exp Clin Endocrinol Diabetes *113:67, 2005)*

DIABETES MELLITUS

insulin action mediate the rate of lipolysis, which results in an increase of free fatty acids.[54,62,63]

In addition to free fatty acids, numerous other factors play a role in the development of insulin resistance. In patients with insulin resistance, the insulin-sensitizing hormone adiponectin has gained much attention in the past few years, not only because circulating levels of this adipokine are markers of type 2 diabetes and an elevated risk for cardiovascular disease, but also because adiponectin is involved in the progression of these diseases.[54,110–113] Adiponectin is a protein that is synthesized and secreted by fat cells. In obese individuals, significantly reduced adiponectin plasma concentrations are observed compared with lean persons. Adiponectin is present in serum in relative high concentrations, and the serum concentrations show a negative correlation with BMI and a positive correlation with insulin resistance and even with the incidence of cardiovascular diseases.[114,115] The exogenous application of adiponectin under experimental conditions leads to an improvement in insulin sensitivity, a reduction in plasma glucose concentrations because of the activation of 5'AMP-kinase (AMP = adenosine mono-phosphate), and anti-inflammatory effects.[115–117] These effects may also be responsible for the antidiabetic and antiarteriosclerotic properties of adiponectin. Adiponectin is therefore thought to be a protective protein that is not sufficiently synthesized and secreted by adipocytes in insulin-resistant patients and patients with type 2 diabetes. Other known adipokines (e.g., leptin, resistin, retinol-binding protein, glypican-4) are currently being evaluated to determine whether they might serve as important targets for the prevention and treatment of type 2 diabetes and cardiovascular disease.[63,112,118]

Adipokines presently are the best-known "organokines", although several other classes of organokines have been identified (including myokines, lipokines, and hepatokines). Organokines are proteins exclusively or predominantly produced by and secreted from a specific tissue, but they are not simply markers of the function of their source tissue. All organokines have paracrine or endocrine actions or both (**Table 2-2**).[63,118,119]

TISSUE- AND ORGAN-SPECIFIC CONTRIBUTION TO INSULIN RESISTANCE

Muscle

The skeletal muscle plays an important role for glucose uptake. Approximately 80% of the glucose is transported into the skeletal muscle in an insulin-dependent manner. In this respect, the skeletal muscle is an important organ involved in the development of insulin resistance. This was demonstrated in glucose-clamp experiments as well as in positron emission tomography (PET)–scan investigations that showed that in insulin resistance and type 2 diabetes, insulin-dependent glucose uptake into the skeletal muscle is significantly reduced.[97,120] Ectopic fat deposition seems also to be highly important for the development of insulin resistance of skeletal muscle. Increased intramyocellular fat depositions are found in insulin resistance and type 2 diabetes.[121–124] The ectopic fat deposition creates an altered metabolic atmosphere with increased free fatty acid concentrations and increased adipokines that lead to enhanced lipid oxidation and an increase in chronic inflammation resulting in the development of insulin resistance and diminished glucose uptake into the skeletal muscle.[122] The cause for the increased intramyocellular fat deposition in insulin resistance

TABLE 2-2 Important Organokines and Mediators of Insulin Resistance and Chronic Inflammation

ORGAN	IMPORTANT ORGANOKINES	REMARKS
Adipose tissue (visceral)	Adiponectin Interleukin-6 (IL-6) Leptin Omentin-1 Omentin-2 Resistin Transforming growth factor beta (TGF-β) Tumor necrosis factor alpha (TNF-α) Visfatin	For details see also Figures 2-4 and 2-5 and the text discussion of tissue- and organ-specific contribution to insulin resistance—adipose tissue (References 54, 63, 105, 132, 134)
Liver	Angiopoietin-related protein 6 Fetuin A Fetal growth factor 21 (FGF-21) Insulin-like growth factors (IGFs) Insulin-like growth factor binding proteins (IGFBP) Selenoprotein P Sex hormone binding globulin (SHBG)	For details see also Table 2-3, Figure 2-5, and the text discussion of tissue- and organ-specific contribution to insulin resistance—liver (References 63, 108, 130, 135-147)
Muscle	Brain-derived neurotrophic factor (BDNF) Erythropoietin (EPO) Interleukin-6 (IL-6) Interleukin-15 (IL-15) Interleukin-1β (IL-1β) Tumor necrosis factor alpha (TNF-α)	For details see also the text discussion of tissue- and organ-specific contribution to insulin resistance—muscle (References 89, 97, 120-127)

and type 2 diabetes is most likely a genetic disposition. The triglyceride accumulation in skeletal muscle in obesity derives from a reduced capacity for fat oxidation. An inflexibility in regulating fat oxidation, rather than a defect in fatty acid uptake, is related to insulin resistance and type 2 diabetes.[125] On the other hand, elevated circulating free fatty serum concentrations may secondarily lead to an increase in intramyocellular triglyceride accumulation.[126–128]

The humoral crosstalk between skeletal muscle and liver seems to be of interest and importance; in animal studies, an acute increase in physical activity quickly and strongly regulates the expression of a large number of genes in the liver.[63,129]

In humans, aerobic fitness specifically regulates liver fat content, but not total or visceral obesity.[63,130] Whether myokines are involved in this important crosstalk between skeletal muscle and liver in humans needs to be further investigated and characterized.[63]

In addition to insulin-dependent glucose uptake, the transport of glucose into the skeletal muscle can also be mediated by physical activity in an insulin-independent manner. This insulin- independent glucose uptake is mainly mediated by an increase in the 5'AMP-kinase concentration with the consecutive activation of the 5'AMP-activated protein kinase (AMPK). Most data indicate that this pathway, activated by physical activity, is not altered in insulin resistance and in type 2 diabetes, in contrast to perturbations of insulin-dependent glucose transport.[131]

In this respect, interleukin 6 (IL-6) produced in the working muscle during physical activity could act as an energy sensor by activating AMP-activated kinase and enhancing glucose disposal, lipolysis, and fat oxidation.[132,133] In addition to the numerous positive effects of physical activity on all aspects of the metabolic syndrome and beyond, physical fitness and training improve glucose uptake into the skeletal muscle via the AMPK pathway.

Adipose Tissue

The role of central and visceral obesity in the development of insulin resistance was described previously. On a molecular level, the mediators secreted by the adipocytes in dependence of fat mass and fat distribution play an important role in the development of insulin resistance. In addition to the free fatty acids, adiponectin and numerous inflammatory cytokines such as tumor necrosis factor alpha (TNF-α), IL-6, and transforming growth factor beta (TGF-β) are secreted by the adipocytes. These inflammatory cytokines cause insulin resistance via an inhibition of the intracellular insulin signaling.[54,132] In addition, they lead to inflammatory processes that are frequently observed in insulin-resistant patients. The visceral fat stores therefore mediate insulin resistance and chronic inflammation, as well as arteriosclerotic development, through their secretory capacity of adipokines and cytokines.[63,134]

Liver

One of the most important physiologic functions of the liver in glucose metabolism is to make glucose available for other organs in the fasting state, especially during the night. The regulation of hepatic glucose production is mediated by the influence of insulin on gluconeogenesis. In the postprandial state, the plasma glucose concentration rises, as do the concentrations of the incretin hormones (mainly glucagon-like peptide 1 [GLP-1]) that stimulate insulin secretion. Insulin reaches the liver directly in high concentrations via the portal vein system and physiologically suppresses hepatic glucose production, which would be counterproductive in the postprandial state, when plasma glucose is elevated already.[135] Only during the fasting state with low glucose and insulin concentrations do low insulin concentrations disinhibit hepatic gluconeogenesis, leading to sufficiently high glucose concentrations in the circulation in the fasting state. In insulin resistance and type 2 diabetes, an increased hepatic glucose production is observed that is caused by a diminished hepatocyte response to insulin failing to suppress gluconeogenesis.[136] Insulin resistance of the liver is typically detected in the clinical setting through elevated fasting glucose concentration, which is caused by the increased hepatic glucose production. Different mechanisms that lead to an increased hepatic gluconeogenesis are discussed: the insensitivity of the liver toward insulin itself on the one hand, but also elevated free fatty acid concentrations, as well as hyperglucagonemia, and increased activity of phosphoenolpyruvate-carboxykinase (PEPCK), a key enzyme of gluconeogenesis.[136–138] One important trigger for insulin resistance of the liver is the fat accumulation in this organ. Different studies have shown a correlation between triglyceride content in hepatocytes and insulin resistance within the liver.[63,108,139,140] Patients with type 2 diabetes frequently also have nonalcoholic steatohepatosis (NASH) or nonalcoholic fatty liver disease (NAFLD), which are tightly correlated with insulin resistance.[63,108] Successful implementation of a lifestyle intervention may reduce liver fat mass and may improve insulin resistance.[63,108,130] The insulin-sensitizing effect of metformin and glitazones is partially explained by the reduction of the triglyceride content in the liver.[141] NAFLD is the most common liver disease and, along with the worldwide increase in prevalence of general and abdominal obesity, NAFLD has become a prevalent general health problem in many industrialized countries. NAFLD represents a continuum of liver disease from simple steatosis to NASH and cirrhosis. Up to 20% of patients with simple steatosis will develop NASH, and in a subgroup of these patients NASH can progress further to NASH with fibrosis and cirrhosis.[63,142,143] Cirrhosis is the main risk factor for development of hepatocellular carcinoma.[63,144,145] In addition, NAFLD was identified as a strong and independent predictor of type 2 diabetes and cardiovascular disease.[63,146] Thus, much effort is currently focused worldwide on precisely quantifying liver fat content in humans for predictive and therapeutic purposes.[63,143] However, this endeavor might not be sufficient to completely understand the pathophysiology of NAFLD.

During conditions of a positive energy balance, subcutaneous and visceral adipose tissues expand in a manner that is predominantly genetically determined. Subcutaneous obesity is not strongly associated with metabolic diseases, whereas visceral obesity is a strong predictor of these diseases. Increased availability of fatty acids (resulting from increased lipolysis), increased subclinical inflammation, and dysregulation of adipokine production and release are thought to promote insulin resistance, atherosclerosis, and beta cell dysfunction. Accumulation of lipids in the liver is also largely genetically determined, and two distinct phenotypes have been identified. When hepatic detoxification processes are active, storage of lipids in the liver is not associated with metabolic diseases. By contrast, when lipotoxicity is present, hepatic glucose production increases and lipids are released, with an atherogenic profile. Dysregulated hepatokine production also contributes to the development of metabolic diseases. The important heptokines are listed in **Table 2-3**, and **Figure 2-5** shows a schematic diagram of the

TABLE 2-3 Function of Important Hepatokines In Vitro and In Vivo

| Hepatokine | EFFECTS | |
	In Vitro or Animal Studies	In Humans
Angiopoietin-related protein 6	Energy expenditure ↑ Obesity ↓ NAFLD ↓ Insulin resistance ↓	Insulin resistance ↑
Fetuin A	Obesity ↔/↑ Insulin resistance ↑ Subclinical inflammation ↑	Obesity ↔ NAFLD ↑ Insulin resistance ↑ Subclinical inflammation ↑ T2DM ↑ CVD ↑
FGF 21	Energy expenditure ↑ Insulin resistance ↓ Beta cell survival ↑	Obesity ↑ NAFLD ↑ Insulin resistance ↑
IGFs and IGFBPs	Insulin resistance ↔/↑/↓	Insulin resistance ↑/↓
Selenoprotein P	Insulin resistance ↑	Insulin resistance ↑ Subclinical inflammation ↑
Sex hormone-binding globulin	Sex hormone bioavailability ↑ Sex hormone signaling ↑	Obesity ↓ NAFLD ↓ Insulin resistance ↓ Subclinical inflammation ↓ T2DM ↓ Cardiovascular disease ↓

CVD = Cardiovascular disease; T2DM = type 2 diabetes mellitus.
Data from Stefan N, Häring HU: The role of hepatokines in metabolism, *Nat Rev Endocrinol* 9:144, 2013.

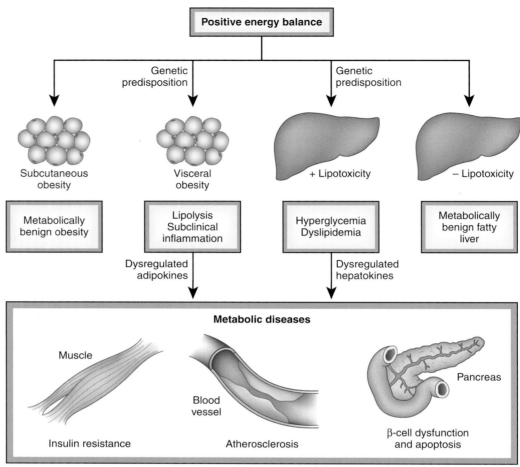

FIGURE 2-5 Novel roles of liver and adipose tissue in the development of metabolic diseases. During conditions of a positive energy balance, subcutaneous and visceral adipose tissues expand in a manner that is predominantly genetically determined. Subcutaneous obesity is not strongly associated with metabolic diseases, whereas visceral obesity is a strong predictor of these diseases. Increased availability of fatty acids (resulting from increased lipolysis), increased subclinical inflammation, and dysregulation of adipokine production and release are thought to promote insulin resistance, atherosclerosis, and beta cell dysfunction. Accumulation of lipids in the liver is also largely genetically determined, and two distinct phenotypes have been identified. When hepatic detoxification processes are active, storage of lipids in the liver is not associated with metabolic diseases. By contrast, when lipotoxicity is present, hepatic glucose production increases and lipids are released, with an atherogenic profile. Dysregulated hepatokine production also contributes to the development of metabolic diseases. *(Modified from Stefan N, Häring HU: The role of hepatokines in metabolism,* Nat Rev Endocrinol *9:144, 2013.)*

putative roles of liver and adipose tissue in the development of metabolic diseases.[63]

The glycoprotein fetuin-A is an important hepatokine. It is a natural inhibitor of the insulin-stimulated insulin receptor tyrosine kinase and induces insulin resistance in rodents. In humans, circulating fetuin-A levels are positively associated with fat accumulation in the liver, insulin resistance, the metabolic syndrome, and type 2 diabetes mellitus. In addition to inducing insulin resistance, fetuin-A is involved in subclinical inflammation and correlates positively with high-sensitive C-reactive protein (hsCRP) levels in humans. It also induces cytokine expression in human monocytes and reduces the expression of the atheroprotective adipokine adiponectin in animals. Taken together, fetuin-A may represent a pathway linking fatty liver with cardiovascular events by inducing insulin resistance and inflammation. Indeed, an investigation in the cohort of the EPIC study (European Prospective Investigation into Cancer and Nutrition; EPIC-Potsdam) revealed a link between high plasma fetuin-A levels and an increased risk of myocardial infarction (MI) and ischemic stroke. High fetuin-A plasma concentrations led to a threefold to fourfold increased risk for MI and ischemic stroke.[147]

Brain

During the past years an increasingly important role of the brain in the development of insulin resistance and obesity has been found. The brain is not only an important organ for glucose disposal, but has recently also been recognized as an insulin-sensitive organ. Insulin receptors are expressed in brain tissue.[148] A high degree of insulin sensitivity of the human brain facilitates loss of body weight and body fat during a lifestyle intervention.[149]

Furthermore, insulin has important functions in regulating satiety signals and energy expenditure within the central nervous system and therefore has an influence on the development of obesity.[150] Intracerebroventricular application of insulin promotes satiety in experimental models in animals and human studies. Neutralizing insulin effects in the brain in animal experiments leads to hyperphagia and obesity[151] and to a reduced peripheral action of insulin in the liver.[152] The results of these experiments point to insulin effects in the brain that most likely lead to a neurotransmitter response that has an influence on hepatic glucose production. The brain is therefore an important central regulator for peripheral insulin action in the liver.

BETA CELL DYSFUNCTION IN TYPE 2 DIABETES

The Role of Insulin Secretion and the Beta Cell in Type 2 Diabetes

Disturbed beta cell function and a loss of beta cell mass of the pancreatic islets play important pathogenetic roles in the development and progression of type 2 diabetes. Regarding the beta cell, a loss of insulin secretion and defects in the early phase of insulin secretion are important in the pathogenesis of type 2 diabetes. As diabetes progresses, a loss of beta cell mass is also observed. In addition, a disturbance in glucagon secretion from the pancreatic alpha cells in the islet with hyperglucagonemia also contributes to the disorder of glucose metabolism. Although insulin resistance is relatively stable in the course of type 2 diabetes, the defects in beta cell function and the loss of beta cell mass are responsible for the progressive nature of the disease.

Pulsatility

Insulin secretion is regulated through a complex interplay of glucose, hormones, incretins, amino acids, and neuronal signals, among other factors. Physiologic insulin secretion follows a pulsatile pattern; in healthy individuals, every 5 to 10 minutes insulin is secreted in a pulse.[153–155] These short-lasting insulin pulses add up to an insulin secretion profile that is repeated every 80 to 150 minutes. The pulsatile secretion of insulin is significantly more effective in lowering plasma glucose concentrations than continuous secretion.[156] Patients with type 2 diabetes already show defective pulsatile insulin secretion even before the clinical manifestation of their diabetes. This defect is characterized by a reduction in pulse frequency as well as lower amplitudes of the insulin pulses. These disturbances can be observed in glucose-dependent as well as glucose-independent fashion.[138,157,158] Insulin secreted from the beta cells reaches the liver via the portal system in the described pulsatile manner. It is degraded by approximately 60% in the liver and not distributed in the same pulsatile fashion into the systemic circulation. As a consequence of the defective pulsatile insulin secretion, hepatic glucose production is elevated.[159,160]

Glucose-Dependent Insulin Secretion

The insulin secretion response after glucose administration in healthy individuals has a typical biphasic pattern, with an immediate insulin secretion peak approximately 3 to 5 minutes after an intravenous glucose bolus and approximately 20 minutes after oral glucose administration, which lasts for around 10 minutes. This acute or first phase of insulin secretion is followed by a second phase with a slower and more sustained elevation of plasma insulin concentrations.

The duration of the second phase of insulin secretion is dependent on the elevation of plasma glucose. The first phase of insulin secretion results from liberation of insulin from the fast recruitable secretory vesicles that are close to the plasma membrane of the beta cell. The second phase of insulin secretion is recruited from a less readily recruitable reserve pool of insulin vesicles. This reserve pool comprises newly synthesized insulin vesicles and so-called "storage vesicles" and is located further away from the outside cell membrane of the beta cell.[161–164] In type 2 diabetes as well as in the prediabetic state of impaired glucose tolerance (see **Table 2-4** for classification),[165] a significantly reduced or even absent first phase of insulin secretion is observed after a glucose stimulus.[166–168] This defect in the first phase of insulin secretion especially has an impact on the postprandial glucose concentrations.[169] Several mechanisms have been reported to cause the defect in the first phase of insulin secretion: chronic hyperglycemia, elevated free fatty acid plasma concentrations, and a reduction in beta cell mass.[170] Some studies indicate that the first phase of insulin secretion can be restored by normalizing glucose metabolism.[171] In addition to the described changes of the first phase of insulin secretion, the second phase is also changed in type 2 diabetes. Because of persistent hyperglycemia, the second phase of insulin secretion is often prolonged and more pronounced compared with the second phase in healthy individuals.[166] There is a reciprocal nonlinear hyperbolic relationship between insulin secretion and insulin resistance. Insulin secretion can therefore be evaluated only with respect to the amount of peripheral insulin resistance. In insulin-resistant patients with type 2 diabetes, elevated plasma insulin concentrations may be observed compared with healthy controls, but these may be inappropriately low in relation to the degree of insulin resistance or to the elevation of plasma glucose concentrations during chronic hyperglycemia and may not be sufficient to normalize the plasma glucose. The insulin secretion in type 2 diabetes is therefore insufficient and often inadequate to cover the actual demand for glucose normalization. In addition to the disturbed insulin secretion, a defect in glucagon secretion is found in type 2 diabetes. Usually, an inappropriately high glucagon secretion is observed that mediates increased hepatic glucose production.[172] This hyperglucagonemia is partially caused by the lack of the tonic inhibition of glucagon secretion by insulin and the beta cell activity.[159,160,173]

Proinsulin-to-Insulin Ratio

In addition to the described defects in insulin secretion kinetics, in type 2 diabetes a change in the proinsulin-to-insulin ratio is observed that is characterized by a higher proinsulin secretion.[174] In the secretory granules of the beta cell,

TABLE 2-4 Classification and Detection of Type 2 Diabetes and Prediabetic States with a Standardized Oral Glucose Tolerance Test (OGTT, 75 g Glucose)

TIME POINT OF GLUCOSE MEASUREMENT	NORMOGLYCEMIA	IMPAIRED FASTING GLUCOSE (IFG)	IMPAIRED GLUCOSE TOLERANCE (IGT)	TYPE 2 DIABETES
Fasting (0 minutes)	<100 mg/dL <5.6 mmol/L	100-125 mg/dL 5.6-6.9 mmol/L		≥126 mg/dL ≥7.0 mmol/L
2 hours postglucose	<140 mg/dL <7.8 mmol/L		140-199 mg/dL 7.8-11.0 mmol/L	≥200 mg/dL ≥11.1 mmol/L

Glucose measured in venous plasma.
Data from American Diabetes Association: Diagnosis and classification of diabetes mellitus, *Diabetes Care* 36(Suppl 1):S67, 2013.

insulin and C peptide are formed by the enzymatic cleavage of proinsulin. In healthy individuals, approximately 2.5% of immunoreactive insulin originates from proinsulin or intermediate split products of proinsulin; in patients with type 2 diabetes, this proportion is much higher and amounts to approximately 8%. This finding indicates a defective or incomplete processing of proinsulin in type 2 diabetes.[175,176] It is interesting to note that in healthy individuals the proinsulin-to-insulin ratio is also dependent on the degree of peripheral insulin resistance and on the fasting plasma glucose concentration. The proinsulin proportions vary from minimally 8% under normoglycemic conditions to approximately 30% under overt hyperglycemia with glucose concentrations of 15 mmol/L.[177] It is hypothesized that chronic hyperglycemia is a continuous stimulatory impulse for insulin granules. Because of this chronic hypersecretion, matured insulin granules are depleted and immature insulin granules with a higher proportion of proinsulin prevail.[178] In addition, other mechanisms of defects in insulin biosynthesis that are not primarily dependent on hyperglycemia are discussed as being responsible for the increased proinsulin secretion in type 2 diabetes. Because proinsulin has only a very low insulin-like biologic activity, a further reduction of insulin action for insulin- sensitive organs results from the change in the proinsulin-to-insulin ratio. The increased proinsulin secretion is further seen as a marker for beta cell stress and as a predictor for diabetes development.[175,176]

Incretin Hormones and Type 2 Diabetes

The so-called "incretin effect" describes the phenomenon by which orally ingested glucose elicits a significantly more pronounced insulin response than an intravenous glucose infusion with identical changes of plasma glucose concentrations. The incretin effect is mediated by the gastrointestinal hormones glucose-dependent insulinotropic peptide (GIP) and GLP-1, which are physiologically secreted after a meal, especially after carbohydrate consumption.[179] In healthy individuals the incretin effect is responsible for 50% to 70% of the postprandial insulin secretion.[180] In type 2 diabetes, the incretin effect is diminished, mostly because GIP has lost its insulinotropic activity as a result of chronic hyperglycemia.[181,182] Supraphysiologic concentrations of GLP-1 are able to restore glucose-dependent insulin secretion and to normalize plasma glucose in type 2 diabetes, as long as sufficient beta cell mass is still present. It is interesting to note that GLP-1 also inhibits glucagon secretion in a glucose-dependent manner. This effect also contributes to the glucose normalization observed under supraphysiologic GLP-1 plasma concentrations.[183] During the last decade, additional physiologic effects of GLP-1 were discovered that may help to normalize metabolism in type 2 diabetes.[179] GLP-1 also slows gastric emptying and thereby retards the resorption of carbohydrates, and in rodent models it increases beta cell function and beta cell mass. Like other gastrointestinal hormones, GLP-1 is also found as a neurotransmitter in the brain. GLP-1–containing neurons in the hypothalamus are involved in mediating satiety.[184,185] Novel data also describe cardiovascular effects of GLP-1 that seem to be favorable in type 2 diabetes or in patients with the metabolic syndrome (e.g., improvement of left ventricular function in myocardial infarct models, reduction of BP).[186] The incretin-based therapies for type 2 diabetes with GLP-1 receptor agonists or with dipeptidyl peptidase (DPP-4) inhibitors that elevate endogenous GLP-1 plasma concentrations use these GLP-1 effects.[187]

Beta Cell Mass

Several studies have shown that at the time of type 2 diabetes diagnosis, beta cell mass has already decreased to around 50% of the original beta cell mass and that this amount of beta cell reduction is critical.[188–190] With this reduction in beta cell mass, for many middle-aged or old aged persons, normal glucose metabolism is no longer possible. In persons with marked insulin resistance, moderate loss of beta cell mass may already lead to a manifestation of diabetes. Most patients with type 2 diabetes show a 40% to 50% reduction in beta cell mass compared with a nondiabetic age-matched control group.[191–193] The loss of beta cells in comparison with the loss of other cell types within the pancreatic islet is relatively selective for the beta cells; loss of the glucagon-secreting alpha cells or the somatostatin-producing delta cells is not observed in a comparable quantity in type 2 diabetes.[194] Even though the exact causes for the reduced beta cell mass in type 2 diabetes are not completely elucidated, programmed cell death (apoptosis) seems to play a key pathogenetic role. Secondary factors such as elevated free fatty acid plasma concentrations, oxidative stress, and chronic hyperglycemia (see the later discussion of glucose toxicity) lead to an increased rate of beta cell apoptosis. Other possibilities such as a reduced rate of beta cell proliferation or beta cell neogenesis play most likely only a minor role in the reduction of beta cell mass in type 2 diabetes.[191]

Glucose Toxicity

Chronic hyperglycemia leads to a desensitization of the beta cell toward a glucose stimulus. This effect is also described as glucose toxicity of the beta cell. Glucose toxicity does not seem to be a substantial pathogenetic factor for the development of type 2 diabetes or in early stages of the disease. In later stages of diabetes with overt chronic hyperglycemia it may lead to an additional dysfunction of the beta cell contributing to a further decline of metabolic control.[195] It is interesting to note that the results from the United Kingdom Prospective Diabetes Study (UKPDS) showed comparably progressive beta cell dysfunction in the intensively treated patients as well as in the control group.[190] This finding indicates that plasma glucose concentrations may have less influence on the progressive beta cell dysfunction.

Lipotoxicity

Free fatty acids from alimentary sources or from endogenous pools are also involved in mediating beta cell dysfunction. Elevated free fatty acid concentrations lead to a diminished glucose-dependent insulin secretion.[196] Investigations in vitro in beta cell lines showed an increase of programmed cell death (apoptosis) of the cultured cells under the influence of elevated concentrations of free fatty acids. This effect is observed with saturated fatty acids but not with unsaturated fatty acids. An approximately 20-fold–increased apoptosis rate of beta cells was induced by the fatty acids palmitate and stearate, which are predominantly found in fats from animal sources. Fatty acids from plant sources that are monounsaturated or polyunsaturated such as oleate, palmitoleate, and linoleate did not show the apoptotic effect.

Saturated fatty acids most likely transmit apoptotic signals in beta cells via protein kinase C.[197,198] In epidemiologic studies an association between the nutritional fat composition and beta cell function has been suggested. A correlation between the intake of saturated fatty acids and the incidence of type 2 diabetes has been shown.[199,200]

SUMMARY

This chapter gives insight into the pathophysiology and mechanisms involved in insulin resistance, a paramount characteristic of type 2 diabetes.

On the genetic level, SNPs in genes associated with diabetes risk contribute to altered insulin signaling, insulin secretion, organ function, or organ crosstalk (e.g., among the intestine, the endocrine pancreas, the liver, the brain, and the adipose tissue).

The mechanisms involved in insulin resistance mainly occur after insulin binding to the insulin receptor, with insulin normally mediating metabolic effects via the signaling molecules AKT/PKB, as well as mitogenic effects via the signaling proteins Ras/Raf/MAP kinase. In insulin resistance, reduced cellular insulin action is found with respect to metabolic but not mitogenic effects of insulin. Defects in the insulin signaling cascade are already present in the first steps of the signal transmission in insulin resistance and type 2 diabetes.

The activation of the insulin signal transduction cascade leads to glucose transport into the cell. The insulin effect on the glucose transport system is mediated by a translocation of glucose transporters from the intracellular pools to the plasma membrane and activation of these transporters in the plasma membrane. The glucose transporter GLUT-4 plays a major role. A reduced capacity of insulin-dependent translocation of GLUT-4 to the plasma membrane is observed as a consequence of insulin resistance.

Concerning the crosstalk between various tissues, the adipose tissue and adipocytes contribute to the development of insulin resistance by producing and secreting mediators such as adipokines and cytokines that act on the muscle and other target tissues of insulin action. The visceral adipose tissue is now seen as an endocrine organ with respect to special functions concerning the activation and secretion of numerous hormones and cytokines that mediate insulin resistance and chronic inflammation. Chronic inflammation is associated with an increased risk for macrovascular complications in type 2 diabetes and the metabolic syndrome.

Insulin resistance also leads to lipid accumulation in the muscle and liver, aggravating the metabolic disturbances. In NAFLD and NASH, hepatokines such as fetuin-A contribute to insulin resistance and most likely to the increased cardiovascular risk associated with this condition.

The brain has only recently been recognized as an important organ regulating insulin sensitivity. It contributes to energy expenditure and body weight regulation. Neutralizing insulin effects in the brain in animal experiments leads to hyperphagia and obesity and to a reduced peripheral action of insulin in the liver, indicating an important organ interaction between the brain and the liver.

In addition, defects in insulin secretion and pancreatic islet function contribute to the pathophysiology of type 2 diabetes. Multiple defects involving insulin secretion have been characterized in type 2 diabetes. These include a diminished or absent fast insulin response after a sharp rise in glucose concentration (the so-called "first phase" of insulin secretion), an increase in the secretion of proinsulin, a defect in the insulinotropic action of incretin hormones (i.e., a defect in the crosstalk between the small intestine and the endocrine pancreas), and a defect in the interdependent pulsatile secretions of insulin and glucagon. In addition to genetic backgrounds for these pathophysiologic findings (SNPs in diabetes candidate genes), glucotoxicity, lipotoxicity, and the effects of inflammatory cytokines (predominantly secreted by adipocytes) contribute to the defects in pancreatic beta cell function and also loss of beta cell mass in type 2 diabetes.

References

1. Pierce M, Keen H, Bradley C: Risk of diabetes in offspring of parents with non-insulin-dependent diabetes. *Diabet Med* 12:6, 1995.
2. Newman B, Selby JV, King MC, et al: Concordance for type 2 (non-insulin-dependent) diabetes mellitus in male twins. *Diabetologia* 30:763, 1987.
3. Müssig K, Staiger H, Machicao F, et al: Genetic variants affecting incretin sensitivity and incretin secretion. *Diabetologia* 53:2289, 2010.
4. Staiger H, Machicao F, Fritsche A, et al: Pathomechanisms of type 2 diabetes genes. *Endocr Rev* 30:557, 2009.
5. Lango H, Palmer CN, Morris AD, et al: Assessing the combined impact of 18 common genetic variants of modest effect sizes on type 2 diabetes risk. *Diabetes* 57:3129, 2008.
6. Ng MC, Park KS, Oh B, et al: Implication of genetic variants near TCF7L2, SLC30A8, HHEX, CDKAL1, CDKN2A/B, IGF2BP2, and FTO in type 2 diabetes and obesity in 6,719 Asians. *Diabetes* 57:2226, 2008.
7. Lyssenko V, Jonsson A, Almgren P, et al: Clinical risk factors, DNA variants, and the development of type 2 diabetes. *N Engl J Med* 359:2220, 2008.
8. Meigs JB, Shrader P, Sullivan LM, et al: Genotype score in addition to common risk factors for prediction of type 2 diabetes. *N Engl J Med* 359:2208, 2008.
9. Sparsø T, Grarup N, Andreasen C, et al: Combined analysis of 19 common validated type 2 diabetes susceptibility gene variants shows moderate discriminative value and no evidence of gene-gene interaction. *Diabetologia* 52:1308, 2009.
10. Ling C, Del Guerra S, Lupi R, et al: Epigenetic regulation of PPARGC1A in human type 2 diabetic islets and effect on insulin secretion. *Diabetologia* 51:615–622, 2008.
11. Ling C, Poulsen P, Simonsson S, et al: Genetic and epigenetic factors are associated with expression of respiratory chain component NDUFB6 in human skeletal muscle. *J Clin Invest* 117:3427, 2007.
12. Rönn T, Poulsen P, Hansson O, et al: Age influences DNA methylation and gene expression of COX7A1 in human skeletal muscle. *Diabetologia* 51:1159, 2008.
13. Florez JC, Jablonski KA, McAteer J, et al: Testing of diabetes-associated WFS1 polymorphisms in the diabetes prevention program. *Diabetologia* 51:451, 2008.
14. Frayling TM, Timpson NJ, Weedon MN, et al: A common variant in the FTO gene is associated with body mass index and predisposes to childhood and adult obesity. *Science* 316:889, 2007.
15. Gudmundsson J, Sulem P, Steinthorsdottir V, et al: Two variants on chromosome 17 confer prostate cancer risk, and the one in TCF2 protects against type 2 diabetes. *Nat Genet* 39:977, 2007.
16. Grarup N, Andersen G, Krarup NT, et al: Association testing of novel type 2 diabetes risk alleles in the JAZF1, CDC123/CAMK1D, TSPAN8, THADA, ADAMTS9, and NOTCH2 loci with insulin release, insulin sensitivity, and obesity in a population-based sample of 4,516 glucose-tolerant middle-aged Danes. *Diabetes* 57:2534, 2008.
17. Grarup N, Rose CS, Andersson EA, et al: Studies of association of variants near the HHEX, CDKN2A/B, and IGF2BP2 genes with type 2 diabetes and impaired insulin release in 10,705 Danish subjects: validation and extension of genome-wide association studies. *Diabetes* 56:3105, 2007.
18. Groenewoud MJ, Dekker JM, Fritsche A, et al: Variants of CDKAL1 and IGF2BP2 affect first-phase insulin secretion during hyperglycaemic clamps. *Diabetologia* 51:1659, 2008.
19. Kirchhoff K, Machicao F, Haupt A, et al: Polymorphisms in the TCF7L2, CDKAL1 and SLC30A8 genes are associated with impaired proinsulin conversion. *Diabetologia* 51:597, 2008.
20. Lyssenko V, Nagorny CL, Erdos MR, et al: Common variant in MTNR1B associated with increased risk of type 2 diabetes and impaired early insulin secretion. *Nat Genet* 41:82, 2009.
21. Moore AF, Jablonski KA, McAteer JB, et al: Extension of type 2 diabetes genome-wide association scan results in the diabetes prevention program. *Diabetes* 57:2503, 2008.
22. Munoz J, Lok KH, Gower BA, et al: Polymorphism in the transcription factor 7-like 2 (TCF7L2) gene is associated with reduced insulin secretion in nondiabetic women. *Diabetes* 55:3630, 2006.
23. Nielsen EM, Hansen L, Carstensen B, et al: The E23K variant of Kir6.2 associates with impaired post-OGTT serum insulin response and increased risk of type 2 diabetes. *Diabetes* 52:573, 2003.
24. Palmer ND, Lehtinen AB, Langefeld CD, et al: Association of TCF7L2 gene polymorphisms with reduced acute insulin response in Hispanic Americans. *J Clin Endocrinol Metab* 93:304, 2008.
25. Pascoe L, Frayling TM, Weedon MN, et al: Beta cell glucose sensitivity is decreased by 39% in non-diabetic individuals carrying multiple diabetes-risk alleles compared with those with no risk alleles. *Diabetologia* 51:1989, 2008.
26. Prokopenko I, Langenberg C, Florez JC, et al: Variants in MTNR1B influence fasting glucose levels. *Nat Genet* 41:77, 2009.
27. Rong R, Hanson RL, Ortiz D, et al: Association analysis of variation in/near FTO, CDKAL1, SLC30A8, HHEX, EXT2, IGF2BP2, LOC387761, and CDKN2B with type 2 diabetes and related quantitative traits in Pima Indians. *Diabetes* 58:478, 2009.
28. Sandhu MS, Weedon MN, Fawcett KA, et al: Common variants in WFS1 confer risk of type 2 diabetes. *Nat Genet* 39:951, 2007.
29. Saxena R, Gianniny L, Burtt NP, et al: Common single nucleotide polymorphisms in TCF7L2 are reproducibly associated with type 2 diabetes and reduce the insulin response to glucose in non-diabetic individuals. *Diabetes* 55:2890, 2006.
30. Saxena R, Voight BF, Lyssenko V, et al: Genome-wide association analysis identifies loci for type 2 diabetes and triglyceride levels. *Science* 316:1331, 2007.
31. Scott LJ, Mohlke KL, Bonnycastle LL, et al: A genomewide association study of type 2 diabetes in Finns detects multiple susceptibility variants. *Science* 316:1341, 2007.
32. Sladek R, Rocheleau G, Rung J, et al: A genome-wide association study identifies novel risk loci for type 2 diabetes. *Nature* 445:881, 2007.
33. Sparsø T, Andersen G, Albrechtsen A, et al: Impact of polymorphisms in WFS1 on prediabetic phenotypes in a population-based sample of middle-aged people with normal and abnormal glucose regulation. *Diabetologia* 51:1646, 2008.

34. Staiger H, Machicao F, Kantartzis K, et al: Novel meta-analysis-derived type 2 diabetes risk loci do not determine prediabetic phenotypes. *PLoS One* 3:e3019, 2008.
35. Staiger H, Machicao F, Schäfer SA, et al: Polymorphisms within the novel type 2 diabetes risk locus MTNR1B determine beta-cell function. *PLoS One* 3:e3962, 2008.
36. Staiger H, Machicao F, Stefan N, et al: Polymorphisms within novel risk loci for type 2 diabetes determine beta-cell function. *PLoS One* 2:e832, 2007.
37. Staiger H, Stancáková A, Zilinskaite J, et al: A candidate type 2 diabetes polymorphism near the HHEX locus affects acute glucose-stimulated insulin release in European populations: results from the EUGENE2 study. *Diabetes* 57:514, 2008.
38. Stancáková A, Pihlajamäki J, Kuusisto J, et al: Single nucleotide polymorphism rs7754840 of CDKAL1 is associated with impaired insulin secretion in nondiabetic offspring of type 2 diabetic subjects and in a large sample of men with normal glucose tolerance. *J Clin Endocrinol Metab* 93:1924, 2008.
39. Steinthorsdottir V, Thorleifsson G, Reynisdottir I, et al: A variant in CDKAL1 influences insulin response and risk of type 2 diabetes. *Nat Genet* 39:770, 2007.
40. Unoki H, Takahashi A, Kawaguchi T, et al: SNPs in KCNQ1 are associated with susceptibility to type 2 diabetes in East Asian and European populations. *Nat Genet* 40:1098, 2008.
41. Wegner L, Hussain MS, Pilgaard K, et al: Impact of TCF7L2 rs7903146 on insulin secretion and action in young and elderly Danish twins. *J Clin Endocrinol Metab* 93:4013, 2008.
42. Yasuda K, Miyake K, Horikawa Y, et al: Variants in KCNQ1 are associated with susceptibility to type 2 diabetes mellitus. *Nat Genet* 40:1092, 2008.
43. Zeggini E, Weedon MN, Lindgren CM, et al: Replication of genome-wide association signals in UK samples reveals risk loci for type 2 diabetes. *Science* 316:1336, 2007.
44. Gonzalez-Sanchez JL, Martinez-Larrad MT, et al: K121Q PC-1 gene polymorphism is not associated with insulin resistance in a Spanish population. *Obes Res* 11:603, 2003.
45. Loos RJ, Franks PW, Francis RW, et al: TCF7L2 polymorphisms modulate proinsulin levels and beta-cell function in a British Europid population. *Diabetes* 56:1943, 2007.
46. Stolerman ES, Manning AK, McAteer JB, et al: TCF7L2 variants are associated with increased proinsulin/insulin ratios but not obesity traits in the Framingham Heart Study. *Diabetologia* 52:614, 2009.
47. Kang ES, Park SY, Kim HJ, et al: Effects of Pro12Ala polymorphism of peroxisome proliferator-activated receptor gamma2 gene on rosiglitazone response in type 2 diabetes. *Clin Pharmacol Ther* 78:202, 2005.
48. Wolford JK, Yeatts KA, Dhanjal SK, et al: Sequence variation in PPARG may underlie differential response to troglitazone. *Diabetes* 54:3319, 2005.
49. Blüher M, Lubben G, Paschke R: Analysis of the relationship between the Pro12Ala variant in the PPAR gamma2 gene and the response rate to therapy with pioglitazone in patients with type 2 diabetes. *Diabetes Care* 26:825, 2003.
50. Florez JC, Jablonski KA, Sun MW, et al: Effects of the type 2 diabetes-associated PPARG P12A polymorphism on progression to diabetes and response to troglitazone. *J Clin Endocrinol Metab* 92:1502, 2007.
51. Kimber CH, Doney AS, Pearson ER, et al: TCF7L2 in the Go-DARTS study: evidence for a gene dose effect on both diabetes susceptibility and control of glucose levels. *Diabetologia* 50:1186, 2007.
52. Florez JC, Jablonski KA, Bayley N, et al: TCF7L2 polymorphisms and progression to diabetes in the diabetes prevention program. *N Engl J Med* 355:241, 2006.
53. Pearson ER, Donnelly LA, Kimber C, et al: Variation in TCF7L2 influences therapeutic response to sulfonylureas: a GoDARTs study. *Diabetes* 56:2178, 2007.
54. Matthaei S, Stumvoll M, Kellerer M, et al: Pathophysiology and pharmacological treatment of insulin resistance. *Endocr Rev* 21:585, 2000.
55. Bonora E, Targher G, Alberiche M, et al: Homeostasis model assessment closely mirrors the glucose clamp technique in the assessment of insulin sensitivity: studies in subjects with various degrees of glucose tolerance and insulin sensitivity. *Diabetes Care* 23:57, 2000.
56. Gutt M, Davis CL, Spitzer SB, et al: Validation of the insulin sensitivity index (ISI[0,120]): comparison with other measures. *Diabetes Res Clin Pract* 47:177, 2000.
57. Matsuda M, DeFronzo RA: Insulin sensitivity indices obtained from oral glucose tolerance testing: comparison with the euglycemic insulin clamp. *Diabetes Care* 22:1462, 1999.
58. Stumvoll M, Mitrakou A, Pimenta W, et al: Use of the oral glucose tolerance test to assess insulin release and insulin sensitivity. *Diabetes Care* 23:295, 2000.
59. Fu S, Watkins SM, Hotamisligil GS: The role of endoplasmic reticulum in hepatic lipid homeostasis and stress signaling. *Cell Metab* 15:623, 2012.
60. Nolan CJ, Damm P, Prentki M: Type 2 diabetes across generations: from pathophysiology to prevention and management. *Lancet* 378:169, 2011.
61. Olefsky JM, Glass CK: Macrophages, inflammation, and insulin resistance. *Annu Rev Physiol* 72:219, 2010.
62. Saltiel AR, Kahn CR: Insulin signalling and the regulation of glucose and lipid metabolism. *Nature* 414:799, 2001.
63. Stefan N, Häring HU: The role of hepatokines in metabolism. *Nat Rev Endocrinol* 9:144, 2013.
64. Häring HU: The insulin receptor: signalling mechanism and contribution to the pathogenesis of insulin resistance. *Diabetologia* 34:848, 1991.
65. Kellerer M, Lammers R, Häring HU: Insulin signal transduction: possible mechanisms for insulin resistance. *Exp Clin Endocrinol Diabetes* 107:97, 1999.
66. Lee YH, White MF: Insulin receptor substrate proteins and diabetes. *Arch Pharm Res* 27:361, 2004.
67. Taniguchi CM, Emanuelli B, Kahn CR: Critical nodes in signalling pathways: insights into insulin action. *Nat Rev Mol Cell Biol* 7:85, 2006.
68. Cusi K, Maezono K, Osman A, et al: Insulin resistance differentially affects the PI 3-kinase- and MAP kinase-mediated signaling in human muscle. *J Clin Invest* 105:311, 2000.
69. Pollak M: The insulin and insulin-like growth factor receptor family in neoplasia: an update. *Nat Rev Cancer* 12:159, 2012.
70. Moller DE, Yokota A, Flier JS: Normal insulin-receptor cDNA sequence in Pima Indians with NIDDM. *Diabetes* 38:1496, 1989.
71. O'Rahilly S, Choi WH, Patel P, et al: Detection of mutations in insulin-receptor gene in NIDDM patients by analysis of single-stranded conformation polymorphisms. *Diabetes* 40:777, 1991.
72. Strack V, Bossenmaier B, Stoyanov B, et al: A 973 valine to methionine mutation of the human insulin receptor: interaction with insulin-receptor substrate-1 and Shc in HEK 293 cells. *Diabetologia* 40:1135, 1997.
73. Caro JF, Ittoop O, Pories WJ, et al: Studies on the mechanism of insulin resistance in the liver from humans with noninsulin-dependent diabetes. Insulin action and binding in isolated hepatocytes, insulin receptor structure, and kinase activity. *J Clin Invest* 78:249, 1986.
74. Kellerer M, Sesti G, Seffer E, et al: Altered pattern of insulin receptor isotypes in skeletal muscle membranes of type 2 (non-insulin-dependent) diabetic subjects. *Diabetologia* 36:628, 1993.
75. Klein HH, Vestergaard H, Kotzke G, et al: Elevation of serum insulin concentration during euglycemic hyperinsulinemic clamp studies leads to similar activation of insulin receptor kinase in skeletal muscle of subjects with and without NIDDM. *Diabetes* 344:1310, 1995.
76. Obermaier B, Ermel B, Biemer E, et al: Insulin receptor kinase in human skeletal muscle. *FEBS Lett* 186:85, 1985.
77. Obermaier-Kusser B, White MF, Pongratz DE, et al: A defective intramolecular autoactivation cascade may cause the reduced kinase activity of the skeletal muscle insulin receptor from patients with non-insulin-dependent diabetes mellitus. *J Biol Chem* 264:9497, 1989.
78. Dunaif A: Insulin resistance and the polycystic ovary syndrome: mechanism and implications for pathogenesis. *Endocr Rev* 18:774, 1997.
79. Kellerer M, Coghlan M, Capp E, et al: Mechanism of insulin receptor kinase inhibition in non-insulin-dependent diabetes mellitus patients. Phosphorylation of serine 1327 or threonine 1348 is unaltered. *J Clin Invest* 96:6, 1995.
80. Chibalin AV, Yu M, Ryder JW, et al: Exercise-induced changes in expression and activity of proteins involved in insulin signal transduction in skeletal muscle: differential effects on insulin-receptor substrates 1 and 2. *Proc Natl Acad Sci U S A* 97:38, 2000.
81. Freidenberg GR, Reichart D, Olefsky JM, et al: Reversibility of defective adipocyte insulin receptor kinase activity in non-insulin-dependent diabetes mellitus. Effect of weight loss. *J Clin Invest* 82:1398, 1988.
82. Zierath JR, Krook A, Wallberg-Henriksson H: Insulin action in skeletal muscle from patients with NIDDM. *Mol Cell Biochem* 182:153, 1998.
83. Longo N, Wang Y, Smith SA, et al: Genotype-phenotype correlation in inherited severe insulin resistance. *Hum Mol Genet* 11:1465, 2002.
84. Andreelli F, Laville M, Ducluzeau PH, et al: Defective regulation of phosphatidylinositol-3-kinase gene expression in skeletal muscle and adipose tissue of non-insulin-dependent diabetes mellitus patients. *Diabetologia* 42:358, 1999.
85. Kim YB, Nikoulina SE, Ciaraldi TP, et al: Normal insulin-dependent activation of AKT/protein kinase B, with diminished activation of phosphoinositide 3-kinase, in muscle in type 2 diabetes. *J Clin Invest* 104:733, 1999.
86. Krook A, Björnholm M, Galuska D, et al: Characterization of signal transduction and glucose transport in skeletal muscle from type 2 diabetic patients. *Diabetes* 49:284, 2000.
87. Pratipanawatr W, Pratipanawatr T, Cusi K, et al: Skeletal muscle insulin resistance in normoglycemic subjects with a strong family history of type 2 diabetes is associated with decreased insulin-stimulated insulin receptor substrate-1 tyrosine phosphorylation. *Diabetes* 50:2572, 2001.
88. Marchetti P, Lupi R, Federici M, et al: Insulin secretory function is impaired in isolated human islets carrying the Gly(972)−>Arg IRS-1 polymorphism. *Diabetes* 51:1419, 2002.
89. Pedersen O: Genetics of insulin resistance. *Exp Clin Endocrinol Diabetes* 107:113, 1999.
90. Stumvoll M, Stefan N, Fritsche A, et al: Interaction effect between common polymorphisms in PPAR gamma2 (Pro12Ala) and insulin receptor substrate 1 (Gly972Arg) on insulin sensitivity. *J Mol Med* 80:33, 2002.
91. 'T Hart LM, Nijpels G, Dekker JM, et al: Variations in insulin secretion in carriers of gene variants in IRS-1 and -2. *Diabetes* 51:884, 2002.
92. Joost HG, Bell GI, Best JD, et al: Nomenclature of the GLUT/SLC2A family of sugar/polyol transport facilitators. *Am J Physiol* 282:E974, 2002.
93. Garvey WT, Huecksteadt TP, Matthaei S, et al: Role of glucose transporters in the cellular insulin resistance of type II non-insulin-dependent diabetes mellitus. *J Clin Invest* 81:1528, 1988.
94. Pedersen O, Bak JF, Andersen PH, et al: Evidence against altered expression of GLUT1 or GLUT4 in skeletal muscle of patients with obesity or NIDDM. *Diabetes* 39:865, 1990.
95. Shepherd PR, Kahn BB: Glucose transporters and insulin action–implications for insulin resistance and diabetes mellitus. *N Engl J Med* 341:248, 1999.
96. Sinha MK, Raineri-Maldonado C, Buchanan C, et al: Adipose tissue glucose transporters in NIDDM. Decreased levels of muscle/fat isoform. *Diabetes* 40:472, 1991.
97. Cline GW, Petersen KF, Krssak M, et al: Impaired glucose transport as a cause of decreased insulin-stimulated muscle glycogen synthesis in type 2 diabetes. *N Engl J Med* 341:240, 1999.
98. Williams KV, Price JC, Kelley DE: Interactions of impaired glucose transport and phosphorylation in skeletal muscle insulin resistance. A dose-response assessment using positron emission tomography. *Diabetes* 50:2069, 2001.
99. Kusari J, Verma US, Buse JB, et al: Analysis of the gene sequences of the insulin receptor and the insulin-sensitive glucose transporter (GLUT-4) in patients with common-type non-insulin-dependent diabetes mellitus. *J Clin Invest* 88:1323, 1991.
100. Rosenblatt-Velin N, Lerch R, Papageorgiou I, et al: Insulin resistance in adult cardiomyocytes undergoing dedifferentiation: role of GLUT4 expression and translocation. *FASEB J* 18:872, 2004.
101. Björntorp P: Visceral obesity: a "civilization syndrome". *Obes Res* 1:206, 1993.
102. Després JP, Moorjani S, Lupien PJ, et al: Regional distribution of body fat, plasma lipoproteins, and cardiovascular disease. *Arteriosclerosis* 10:497, 1990.
103. Marniemi J, Kronholm E, Aunola S, et al: Visceral fat and psychosocial stress in identical twins discordant for obesity. *J Intern Med* 251:35, 2002.
104. Baghaei F, Rosmond R, Westberg L, et al: The CYP19 gene and associations with androgens and abdominal obesity in premenopausal women. *Obes Res* 11:578, 2003.
105. Staiger H, Häring HU: Adipocytokines: fat-derived humoral mediators of metabolic homeostasis. *Exp Clin Endocrinol Diabetes* 113:67, 2005.
106. Heni M, Machann J, Staiger H, et al: Pancreatic fat is negatively associated with insulin secretion in individuals with impaired fasting glucose and/or impaired glucose tolerance: a nuclear magnetic resonance study. *Diabetes Metab Res Rev* 26:200, 2010.
107. Machann J, Häring H, Schick F, et al: Intramyocellular lipid and insulin resistance. *Diabetes Obes Metab* 6:239, 2004.
108. Stefan N, Kantartzis K, Häring HU: Causes and metabolic consequences of fatty liver. *Endocr Rev* 29:939, 2008.
109. Tushuizen ME, Bunck MC, Pouwels PJ, et al: Pancreatic fat content and beta-cell function in men with and without type 2 diabetes. *Diabetes Care* 30:2916, 2007.
110. Arner P: Regional adipocity in man. *J Endocrinol* 155:191, 1997.
111. Kadowaki T, Yamauchi T, Kubota N, et al: Adiponectin and adiponectin receptors in insulin resistance, diabetes, and the metabolic syndrome. *J Clin Invest* 116:1784, 2006.
112. Ouchi N, Parker JL, Lugus JJ, et al: Adipokines in inflammation and metabolic disease. *Nat Rev Immunol* 11:85, 2011.
113. Turer AT, Scherer PE: Adiponectin: mechanistic insights and clinical implications. *Diabetologia* 55:2319, 2012.
114. Antoniades C, Antonopoulos AS, Tousoulis D, et al: Adiponectin: from obesity to cardiovascular disease. *Obes Rev* 10:269, 2009.
115. Li S, Shin HJ, Ding EL, et al: Adiponectin levels and risk of type 2 diabetes: a systematic review and meta-analysis. *JAMA* 302:179, 2009.
116. Maury E, Brichard SM: Adipokine dysregulation, adipose tissue inflammation and metabolic syndrome. *Mol Cell Endocrinol* 314:1, 2010.
117. Yamauchi T, Kamon J, Minokoshi Y, et al: Adiponectin stimulates glucose utilization and fatty-acid oxidation by activating AMP-activated protein kinase. *Nat Med* 8:1288, 2002.
118. Mitchell F: Obesity: glypican-4: role in insulin signalling. *Nat Rev Endocrinol* 8:505, 2012.
119. Pedersen BK, Febbraio MA: Muscles, exercise and obesity: skeletal muscle as a secretory organ. *Nat Rev Endocrinol* 8:457, 2012.
120. Utriainen T, Takala T, Luotolahti M, et al: Insulin resistance characterizes glucose uptake in skeletal muscle but not in the heart in NIDDM. *Diabetologia* 41:555, 1998.
121. Jacob S, Machann J, Rett K, et al: Association of increased intramyocellular lipid content with insulin resistance in lean nondiabetic offspring of type 2 diabetic subjects. *Diabetes* 48:1113, 1999.
122. Petersen KF, Shulman GI: Pathogenesis of skeletal muscle insulin resistance in type 2 diabetes mellitus. *Am J Cardiol* 90:11G, 2002.

123. Thamer C, Machann J, Bachmann O, et al: Intramyocellular lipids: anthropometric determinants and relationships with maximal aerobic capacity and insulin sensitivity. *J Clin Endocrinol Metab* 88:1785, 2003.
124. Virkamäki A, Korsheninnikova E, Seppälä-Lindroos A, et al: Intramyocellular lipid is associated with resistance to in vivo insulin actions on glucose uptake, antilipolysis, and early insulin signaling pathways in human skeletal muscle. *Diabetes* 50:2337, 2001.
125. Kelley DE, Goodpaster B, Wing RR, et al: Skeletal muscle fatty acid metabolism in association with insulin resistance, obesity, and weight loss. *Am J Physiol* 277:E1130, 1999.
126. Kelley DE, Goodpaster BH: Skeletal muscle triglyceride. An aspect of regional adiposity and insulin resistance. *Diabetes Care* 24:933, 2001.
127. Lewis GF, Carpentier A, Adeli K, et al: Disordered fat storage and mobilization in the pathogenesis of insulin resistance and type 2 diabetes. *Endocr Rev* 23:201, 2002.
128. Staiger H, Tschritter O, Machann J, et al: Relationship of serum adiponectin and leptin concentrations with body fat distribution in humans. *Obes Res* 11:368, 2003.
129. Hoene M, Weigert C: The stress response of the liver to physical exercise. *Exerc Immunol Rev* 16:163, 2010.
130. Kantartzis K, Thamer C, Peter A, et al: High cardiorespiratory fitness is an independent predictor of the reduction in liver fat during a lifestyle intervention in non-alcoholic fatty liver disease. *Gut* 58:1281, 2009.
131. Goodyear LJ: AMP-activated protein kinase: a critical signaling intermediary for exercise-stimulated glucose transport? *Exerc Sport Sci Rev* 28:113, 2000.
132. Hoene M, Weigert C: The role of interleukin-6 in insulin resistance, body fat distribution and energy balance. *Obes Rev* 9:20, 2008.
133. Pedersen BK: The diseasome of physical inactivity—and the role of myokines in muscle-fat cross talk. *J Physiol* 587(23):5559, 2009.
134. Han SH, Sakuma I, Shin EK, et al: Antiatherosclerotic and anti-insulin resistance effects of adiponectin: basic and clinical studies. *Prog Cardiovasc Dis* 52:126, 2009.
135. Unger RH, Cherrington AD: Glucagonocentric restructuring of diabetes: a pathophysiologic and therapeutic makeover. *J Clin Invest* 122:4, 2012.
136. Groop LC, Bonadonna RC, DelPrato S, et al: Glucose and free fatty acid metabolism in non-insulin-dependent diabetes mellitus. Evidence for multiple sites of insulin resistance. *J Clin Invest* 84:205, 1989.
137. Matsuda M, Defronzo RA, Glass L, et al: Glucagon dose-response curve for hepatic glucose production and glucose disposal in type 2 diabetic patients and normal individuals. *Metabolism* 51:1111, 2002.
138. O'Meara NM, Sturis J, Van Cauter E, et al: Lack of control by glucose of ultradian insulin secretory oscillations in impaired glucose tolerance and in non-insulin-dependent diabetes mellitus. *J Clin Invest* 92:262, 1993.
139. Sanyal AJ, Campbell-Sargent C, Mirshahi F, et al: Nonalcoholic steatohepatitis: association of insulin resistance and mitochondrial abnormalities. *Gastroenterology* 120:1183, 2001.
140. Seppälä-Lindroos A, Vehkavaara S, Häkkinen AM, et al: Fat accumulation in the liver is associated with defects in insulin suppression of glucose production and serum free fatty acids independent of obesity in normal men. *J Clin Endocrinol Metab* 87(3023):87, 2002.
141. Khashab M, Chalasani N: Use of insulin sensitizers in NASH. *Endocrinol Metab Clin North Am* 36:1067, 2007.
142. Chalasani N, Younossi Z, Lavine JE, et al: The diagnosis and management of non-alcoholic fatty liver disease: practice guideline by the American Gastroenterological Association, American Association for the Study of Liver Diseases, and American College of Gastroenterology. *Gastroenterology* 142:1592, 2012.
143. Cohen JC, Horton JD, Hobbs HH: Human fatty liver disease: old questions and new insights. *Science* 332:1519, 2011.
144. Bugianesi E: Non-alcoholic steatohepatitis and cancer. *Clin Liver Dis* 11:191, 2007.
145. Starley BQ, Calcagno CJ, Harrison SA: Nonalcoholic fatty liver disease and hepatocellular carcinoma: a weighty connection. *Hepatology* 51:1820, 2010.
146. Targher G, Day CP, Bonora E: Risk of cardiovascular disease in patients with nonalcoholic fatty liver disease. *N Engl J Med* 363:1341, 2010.
147. Weikert C, Stefan N, Schulze MB, et al: Plasma fetuin-a levels and the risk of myocardial infarction and ischemic stroke. *Circulation* 118:2555, 2008.
148. Havrankova J, Roth J, Brownstein M: Insulin receptors are widely distributed in the central nervous system of the rat. *Nature* 272:827, 1978.
149. Tschritter O, Preissl H, Hennige AM, et al: High cerebral insulin sensitivity is associated with loss of body fat during lifestyle intervention. *Diabetologia* 55:175, 2012.
150. Porte D Jr, Seeley RJ, Woods SC, et al: Obesity, diabetes and the central nervous system. *Diabetologia* 41:863, 1998.
151. Obici S, Feng Z, Karkanias G, et al: Decreasing hypothalamic insulin receptors causes hyperphagia and insulin resistance in rats. *Nat Neurosci* 5:566, 2002.
152. Obici S, Zhang BB, Karkanias G, et al: Hypothalamic insulin signaling is required for inhibition of glucose production. *Nat Med* 8:1376, 2002.
153. Goodner CJ, Walike BC, Koerker DJ, et al: Insulin, glucagon, and glucose exhibit synchronous, sustained oscillations in fasting monkeys. *Science* 195:177, 1977.
154. Pørksen N, Munn S, Steers J, et al: Impact of sampling technique on appraisal of pulsatile insulin secretion by deconvolution and cluster analysis. *Am J Physiol* 269:E478, 1995.
155. Song SH, McIntyre SS, Shah H, et al: Direct measurement of pulsatile insulin secretion from the portal vein in human subjects. *J Clin Endocrinol Metab* 85:4491, 2000.
156. Paolisso G, Scheen AJ, Giugliano D, et al: Pulsatile insulin delivery has greater metabolic effects than continuous hormone administration in man: importance of pulse frequency. *J Clin Endocrinol Metab* 72:607, 1991.
157. O'Rahilly S, Turner RC, Matthews DR: Impaired pulsatile secretion of insulin in relatives of patients with non-insulin-dependent diabetes. *N Engl J Med* 318:1225, 1988.
158. Polonsky KS, Given BD, Hirsch LJ, et al: Abnormal patterns of insulin secretion in non-insulin-dependent diabetes mellitus. *N Engl J Med* 318:1231, 1988.
159. Meier JJ, Pennartz C, Schenker N, et al: Hyperglycaemia is associated with impaired pulsatile insulin secretion: effect of basal insulin therapy. *Diabetes Obes Metab* 15:258, 2013.
160. Menge BA, Grüber L, Jørgensen SM, et al: Loss of inverse relationship between pulsatile insulin and glucagon secretion in patients with type 2 diabetes. *Diabetes* 60:2160, 2011.
161. Bratanova-Tochkova TK, Cheng H, Daniel S, et al: Triggering and augmentation mechanisms, granule pools, and biphasic insulin secretion. *Diabetes* 51:S83, 2002.
162. Daniel S, Noda M, Straub SG, et al: Identification of the docked granule pool responsible for the first phase of glucose-stimulated insulin secretion. *Diabetes* 48:1686, 1999.
163. Porte D Jr, Pupo AA: Insulin responses to glucose: evidence for a two pool system in man. *J Clin Invest* 48:2309, 1969.
164. Rorsman P, Eliasson L, Renström E, et al: The cell physiology of biphasic insulin secretion. *News Physiol Sci* 15:72, 2000.
165. American Diabetes Association: Diagnosis and classification of diabetes mellitus. *Diabetes Care* 36(Suppl 1):S67, 2013.
166. Pfeifer MA, Halter JB, Porte D Jr: Insulin secretion in diabetes mellitus. *Am J Med* 70:579, 1981.
167. Stumvoll M, Fritsche A, Häring HU: Clinical characterization of insulin secretion as the basis for genetic analyses. *Diabetes* 51(Suppl 1):S122, 2002.
168. Stumvoll M, Fritsche A, Stefan N, et al: A 60 minute hyperglycemic clamp is sufficient to assess both phases of insulin secretion. *Horm Metab Res* 32:230, 2000.
169. Luzi L, DeFronzo RA: Effect of loss of first-phase insulin secretion on hepatic glucose production and tissue glucose disposal in humans. *Am J Physiol* 257:E241, 1989.
170. Oheim M, Loerke D, Stühmer W, et al: Multiple stimulation-dependent processes regulate the size of the releasable pool of vesicles. *Eur Biophys J* 28:91, 1999.
171. Vague P, Moulin JP: The defective glucose sensitivity of the B cell in non insulin dependent diabetes. Improvement after twenty hours of normoglycaemia. *Metabolism* 31:139, 1982.
172. Mitrakou A, Kelley D, Veneman T, et al: Contribution of abnormal muscle and liver glucose metabolism to postprandial hyperglycemia in NIDDM. *Diabetes* 39:1381, 1990.
173. Meier JJ, Kjems LL, Veldhuis JD, et al: Postprandial suppression of glucagon secretion depends on intact pulsatile insulin secretion: further evidence for the intraislet insulin hypothesis. *Diabetes* 55:1051, 2006.
174. Temple RC, Carrington CA, Luzio SD, et al: Insulin deficiency in non-insulin-dependent diabetes. *Lancet* 1:293, 1989.
175. Kahn SE, Halban PA: Release of incompletely processed proinsulin is the cause of the disproportionate proinsulinemia of NIDDM. *Diabetes* 46:1725, 1997.
176. Kahn SE, Leonetti DL, Prigeon RL, et al: Proinsulin as a marker for the development of NIDDM in Japanese-American men. *Diabetes* 44:173, 1995.
177. Saad MF, Kahn SE, Nelson RG, et al: Disproportionately elevated proinsulin in Pima Indians with noninsulin-dependent diabetes mellitus. *J Clin Endocrinol Metab* 70:1247, 1990.
178. Rhodes CJ, Alarcón C: What beta-cell defect could lead to hyperproinsulinemia in NIDDM? Some clues from recent advances made in understanding the proinsulin-processing mechanism. *Diabetes* 43:511, 1994.
179. Drucker DJ, Nauck MA: The incretin system: glucagon-like peptide-1 receptor agonists and dipeptidyl peptidase-4 inhibitors in type 2 diabetes. *Lancet* 368:1696, 2006.
180. Nauck MA, Homberger E, Siegel EG, et al: Incretin effects of increasing glucose loads in man calculated from venous insulin and C-peptide responses. *J Clin Endocrinol Metab* 63:492, 1986.
181. Nauck MA, Heimesaat MM, Orskov C, et al: Preserved incretin activity of glucagon-like peptide 1 [7-36 amide] but not of synthetic human gastric inhibitory polypeptide in patients with type-2 diabetes mellitus. *J Clin Invest* 91:301, 1993.
182. Nauck M, Stöckmann F, Ebert R, et al: Reduced incretin effect in type 2 (non-insulin-dependent) diabetes. *Diabetologia* 29:46, 1986.
183. Nauck MA, Kleine N, Orskov C, et al: Normalization of fasting hyperglycaemia by exogenous glucagon-like peptide 1 (7-36 amide) in type 2 (non-insulin-dependent) diabetic patients. *Diabetologia* 36:741, 1993.
184. Gallwitz B: Anorexigenic effects of GLP-1 and its analogues. *Handb Exp Pharmacol* 209:185, 2012.
185. Turton MD, O'Shea D, Gunn I, et al: A role for glucagon-like peptide-1 in the central regulation of feeding. *Nature* 379:69, 1996.
186. Ussher JR, Drucker DJ: Cardiovascular biology of the incretin system. *Endocr Rev* 33:187, 2012.
187. Russell-Jones D, Gough S: Recent advances in incretin-based therapies. *Clin Endocrinol (Oxf)* 77:489, 2012.
188. Kumar AF, Gruessner RW, Seaquist ER: Risk of glucose intolerance and diabetes in hemipancreatectomized donors selected for normal preoperative glucose metabolism. *Diabetes Care* 31:1639, 2008.
189. Menge BA, Tannapfel A, Belyaev O, et al: Partial pancreatectomy in adult humans does not provoke beta-cell regeneration. *Diabetes* 57:142, 2008.
190. UK Prospective Diabetes Study (UKPDS) Group: Intensive blood-glucose control with sulphonylureas or insulin compared with conventional treatment and risk of complications in patients with type 2 diabetes. UK Prospective Diabetes Study (UKPDS) Group. *Lancet* 352:837, 1998.
191. Butler AE, Janson J, Bonner-Weir S, et al: Beta-cell deficit and increased beta-cell apoptosis in humans with type 2 diabetes. *Diabetes* 52:102, 2003.
192. Meier JJ, Menge BA, Breuer TG, et al: Functional assessment of pancreatic beta-cell area in humans. *Diabetes* 58:1595, 2009.
193. Westermark P, Wilander E: The influence of amyloid deposits on the islet volume in maturity onset diabetes mellitus. *Diabetologia* 15:417, 1978.
194. Sakuraba H, Mizukami H, Yagihashi N, et al: Reduced beta-cell mass and expression of oxidative stress-related DNA damage in the islet of Japanese type II diabetic patients. *Diabetologia* 45:85, 2002.
195. Yki-Järvinen H, Esko N, Eero H, et al: Clinical benefits and mechanisms of a sustained response to intermittent insulin therapy in type 2 diabetic patients with secondary drug failure. *Am J Med* 84:185, 1988.
196. Unger RH: Lipotoxic diseases. *Annu Rev Med* 53:319, 2002.
197. Eitel K, Staiger H, Brendel MD, et al: Different role of saturated and unsaturated fatty acids in beta-cell apoptosis. *Biochem Biophys Res Commun* 299:853, 2002.
198. Eitel K, Staiger H, Rieger J, et al: Protein kinase C delta activation and translocation to the nucleus are required for fatty acid-induced apoptosis of insulin-secreting cells. *Diabetes* 52:991, 2003.
199. Meyer KA, Kushi LH, Jacobs DR Jr, et al: Dietary fat and incidence of type 2 diabetes in older Iowa women. *Diabetes Care* 24:1528, 2001.
200. Salmerón J, Hu FB, Manson JE, et al: Dietary fat intake and risk of type 2 diabetes in women. *Am J Clin Nutr* 73:1019, 2001.

3 Type 1 Diabetes
Pathophysiology, Molecular Mechanisms, Genetic Insights

Petter Bjornstad and Marian J. Rewers

Type 1 diabetes mellitus (T1DM) is one of the most prevalent chronic diseases of childhood, affecting more than 1.4 million people in the United States, of whom 150,000 are children.[1,2] Over the past 50 years, the incidence in children has been increasing at a rapid rate of up to 5% per year worldwide—that is, doubling every 20 years.[3] The lifetime risk of developing T1DM now exceeds 1% in North America and Europe. Whereas T1DM accounts for only approximately 5% of diabetes, it is associated with higher per-person morbidity, mortality, and health care costs than type 2 diabetes (T2DM).[4]

T1DM incidence is trimodal, peaking at the ages of 2, 4 to 6, and 10 to 14 years. This pattern may reflect age-specific infections and increased insulin resistance of puberty. Although children are most visibly affected, half of T1DM patients are diagnosed after age 20. There is generally an equal male-to-female distribution of T1DM; however, a slight male predominance has been reported in high-risk populations, and the opposite in low-risk ethnic groups.[5]

The ongoing pandemic of T1DM cannot be attributed to genetics or increasing survival and fecundity of adults with T1DM; a powerful environmental factor or factors must be at play. In this chapter we review the pathophysiology underlying T1DM, and discuss possible mechanisms linking genetic predisposition to environmental triggers in the development of T1DM.

PATHOGENESIS

T1DM is characterized by a long preclinical period of autoimmune attack on the beta cells, carried out by autoreactive T cells and marked by the emergence of autoantibodies against beta cell autoantigens. The process appears to result from loss of tolerance to beta cell autoantigens in genetically susceptible individuals. Several environmental triggers have been implicated, but none have been definitely proven. **Figure 3-1** illustrates the complexity of the pathogenesis underlying T1DM.

The normal pancreas has a large reserve capacity; at least 70% of the functional capacity of the beta cells must be lost before clinical T1DM develops. Studies of human pancreata in patients with established T1DM suggest that a number of beta cells are able to survive the autoimmune insult, but are unable to secrete sufficient amounts of insulin to prevent hyperglycemia. Rodents may generate new beta cell progenitor cells,[6] but there is no evidence for beta cell regeneration in humans with diabetes.

Selective destruction of pancreatic beta cells results in insulinopenia. The impairment in insulin secretion is also partially functional and caused by the inhibition of insulin secretion by cytokines interleukin 1 (IL-1), tumor necrosis factor alpha (TNF-α), TNF-β, and interferon gamma (IFN-γ).[7] Insulin resistance may also play a role in T1DM pathogenesis and cannot be explained simply by obesity or puberty.

After diagnosis, T1DM patients are more insulin resistant than nondiabetic controls despite similar adiposity, body fat composition, and high-density lipoprotein (HDL) cholesterol.[8] Significant insulin resistance has been documented in T1DM patients at or near hemoglobin A1c (HbA1c) targets,[8,9] suggesting that resistance to insulin action on glucose and nonesterified fatty acid suppression are not mediated by prevailing glycemia.[8] In insulin-treated patients, insulin resistance is secondary to prolonged exposure to supraphysiologic levels of exogenous insulin that increase ectopic fat accumulation in liver and skeletal muscles[8] and increase oxidative stress.[10–12] The ectopically accumulated fat and its catabolites are thought to induce insulin resistance via various signaling pathways including mitogen-activated protein kinases (MAPKs), protein kinase C, IκB kinases, S6 kinases, and endoplasmic reticulum stress.[13–15] Chronic insulin resistance increases the risk of diabetic macrovascular and microvascular complications.[8,16–18a]

AUTOIMMUNITY

The nonobese diabetic (NOD) strain of mouse is an essential model of autoimmune T1DM. The advantage of this murine strain is that it develops spontaneous autoimmune diabetes, which shares many similarities with autoimmune type 1 diabetes in human patients. Recent research on this model has provided a wealth of insight into mechanisms likely involved in pathogenesis of T1DM.[19,20]

It is now generally accepted that T1DM arises from a breakdown in self-tolerance to beta cell autoantigens. Chronic T cell–mediated inflammation of the islets results in selective destruction of beta cells and sparing of the alpha, delta, and pancreatic polypeptide cells.[21] Alternative scenarios are possible—for example, an adaptive immune response to persistent infection of the islets where beta cells are particularly sensitive to cytokine IL-1β–mediated killing, and increased expression of class I molecules during local infections may enhance their susceptibility.[22,23]

Autopsy data have shown that destruction is caused by infiltration of the islets by macrophages, dendritic cells, natural

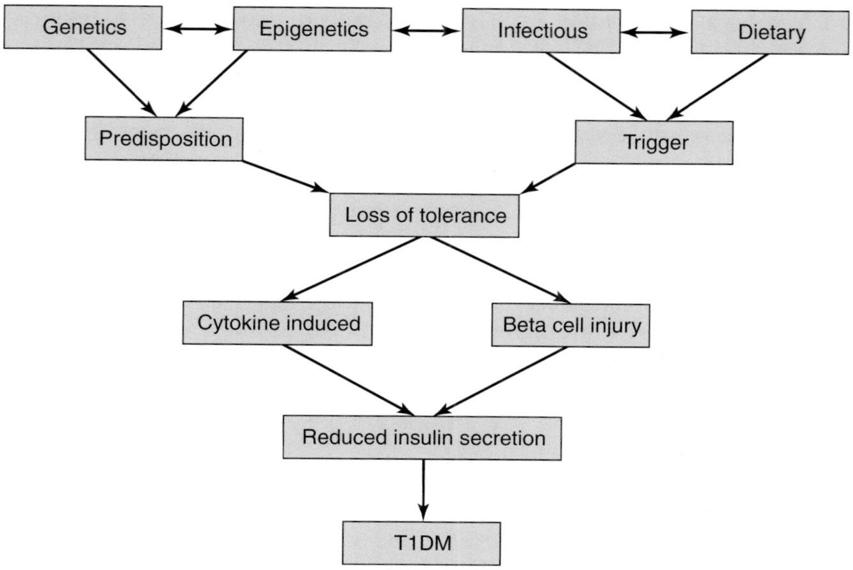

FIGURE 3-1 Diagram showing the complexity of the pathogenesis of type 1 diabetes mellitus (T1DM).

killer cells, and lymphocytes.[24] The T cells are the key players in the autoimmune attack of beta cells, including helper T cells, cytotoxic T cells, and regulatory T cells.[25] Humoral response and autoantibody production do not cause direct beta cell damage, but develop secondary to beta cell damage, and are useful disease markers.

Loss of Tolerance

Immune tolerance is essential to achieve immune homeostasis and self-tolerance. The loss of self-tolerance is the hallmark of T1DM pathogenesis. The establishment of tolerance starts in fetal life and includes both a central and a peripheral arm. Central tolerance is the process whereby immature T and β cells acquire tolerance to self-antigens during maturation within the thymus and bone marrow, respectively. It consists of positive and negative selection. Positive selection is the process of testing T cells for major histocompatibility complex (MHC) restriction. T cells with receptors with weak binding to MHC class I and II are allowed to survive (positively selected). This process is important in that it sets up a system in which all mature T cells will have T cell receptors (TCRs) that recognize antigens presented by MHC. Negative selection is the process whereby T cells that bind with high affinity to MHC class I and II, alone or carrying self-peptides, are eliminated by apoptosis. For central tolerance to be efficient, the negatively selecting stromal elements in the thymus medulla will have to express a large diversity of tissue-restricted antigens (TRAs) that represent as many self-antigens expressed outside of the thymus as necessary to establish and maintain self-tolerance. This is possible by promiscuous gene expression, which is the expression of a highly diverse set of genes in the medullary thymic epithelial cells, otherwise expressed in a strictly tissue-restricted fashion. Except for the involvement of the autoimmune regulator (AIRE), the molecular and cellular regulation of this gene expression pattern is poorly understood. The absence of a single TRA is sufficient to elicit spontaneous autoimmunity.[26]

Under this model, thymus dysfunction could lead to a decrease in the expression of T1DM-related antigens promoting a continuous enrichment of the peripheral T cell repertoire with self-reactive T cells, as well as a decrease in the selection of specific T regulatory cells (Tregs). Thymus transplantation from diabetes-resistant to diabetes-prone rats can prevent insulitis and diabetes; conversely, transplantation of thymus from nonobese diabetic to diabetes-resistant mice induced insulitis.[27,28] All the members of the insulin gene family are expressed in the thymus.[29] In mice, in which two genes code for (pro)insulin (*Ins1* and *Ins2*), *Ins2* is predominantly expressed in the thymus, whereas *Ins1* is dominant in the islet beta cells, which leads to a higher immune tolerance to *Ins2*. *Ins2*$^{-/-}$ cogenic NOD mice have a significantly higher rate of insulitis and diabetes than *Ins1*$^{-/-}$ cogenic NOD mice.[30,31]

Negative thymic selection is not entirely efficient and inadvertently permits the efflux of some autoreactive T cells with low-affinity TCR for self-antigens. To avoid the development of autoimmunity, additional mechanisms are in place. One of these mechanisms is the thymic generation of Tregs, which maintain homeostasis of the immune system and tolerance to self-antigens by controlling self-reactive T cells. The depletion of naturally occurring Tregs elicits multiorgan autoimmune disease, for example, the immunodysregulation polyendocrinopathy enteropathy X-linked (IPEX) syndrome—a rare congenital deficiency of forkhead box P3 (FOXP3) expression in humans.[32] Tregs constitute 10% of CD4$^+$ T cells in the thymus and the periphery and express the IL-2 receptor alpha chain (CD25) and FOXP3 protein.[33] They are initially anergic, but when activated they suppress proliferation and IL-2 production of naïve and memory T cells.[34]

Another mechanism allowing peripheral tolerance to self-antigens involves anergy. When a self-reactive lymphocyte recognizes its cognate antigen on a cell but does not receive the required co-stimulatory signal, it becomes anergized. The cell-surface glycoproteins CD80 (B7-1) and CD86 (B7-2) are essential co-stimulatory molecules, found almost exclusively on professional antigen-presenting cells (APCs). Interaction of these B7 molecules on APCs with CD28 on T cells is required for T cell activation. Moreover, if naïve T cells do become activated, they express an additional receptor called *cytotoxic T lymphocyte–associated 4* (CTLA-4), which has a greater binding affinity for the B7 molecules than CD28.[35] Binding of CTLA-4 to B7 results in a negative signal to the T cells, resulting in inhibition of T cell activity.[36] CTLA-4 is also an important co-stimulatory molecule expressed by T-regulatory cells.[37]

β cell tolerance occurs as a result of clonal deletion through apoptosis of immature β cells reactive to self-antigens. Immature β cells expressing surface IgM that reacts with self-antigens are rendered unresponsive or anergic. Thus, only those β cells that do not react with self-antigens in the bone marrow are allowed to mature and migrate to the periphery where further maturation occurs.

Autoantigens

Several autoantigens have been identified in T1DM and may play an important role in the initiation and progression of the autoimmune injury (**Table 3-1**). Most of the autoantigens are human leukocyte antigen (HLA) A2 restricted, CD8+ T cell epitopes such as proinsulin, glutamic acid decarboxylase (GAD), islet-specific glucose-6-phosphatase catalytic subunit–related protein (IGRP), and islet amyloid polypeptide (IAPP).[38,39] The study of antigens in the development of T1DM is more complicated than initially thought and includes the following concepts: (1) intermolecular spreading of antigenicity; (2) tissue-specific cleavage producing antigenic peptides specific to beta cells; and (3) synergy of multiple islet antigens.

TABLE 3-1 Autoantigens and Autoantibodies

AUTOANTIGEN	DESCRIPTION OF ANTIGEN	ANTIBODY
Insulin	Protein secreted by β cells	IAA
Glutamic acid decarboxylase	Enzyme catalyzing decarboxylation of glutamate to GABA	GADA
Insulinoma-associated protein 2	Neuroendocrine protein	IA-2A
Islet-specific glucose-6-phosphatase catalytic subunit–related protein	Catalytic subunit of glucose-6-phosphatase	IGRPA
Chromogranin A	Protein found in secretory granules in β cells	ChgAA
Zinc transporter 8	β cell–specific cation efflux zinc transporter	ZnT8A

GABA = γ-aminobutyric acid.

With regard to intermolecular spreading of antigenicity, we know that the initial antibody response in T1DM occurs primarily against insulin or GAD, spreading over time to other antigens. Tissue-specific cleavage appears critical to generation of diabetogenic autoantigens. A good example is the cleavage product of chromogranin A (ChgA)—WE-14, which is specifically recognized by the pathogenic BDC2.5 TCR (see later). It may also be necessary for T cells to target multiple beta cell antigens for the development of T1DM to occur (synergy of multiple antigens). For example, the targeting of IGRP by the CD8+ T cells is very diabetogenic, but only in the context of the T cells also targeting insulin peptide B:9-23.[40]

Insulin

Insulin is composed of two peptide chains referred to as the A chain and B chain, which are linked together by two disulfide bonds, and an additional disulfide is formed within the A chain. The A chain consists of 21 amino acids, and the B chain of 30 amino acids. Proinsulin is the prohormone precursor to insulin. C peptide, a 31–amino acid peptide, is cleaved from proinsulin as it is enzymatically converted to insulin. One current leading hypothesis is that insulin itself may be the crucial autoantigen in T1DM. In NOD mice, a single amino acid mutation of insulin peptide 9-23 prevents development of diabetes.[41] Recently, NOD studies have also shown that *only* APCs from islets are able to stimulate anti-B:9-23 T cells.[42] Furthermore, knockouts of the insulin genes in NOD mice greatly influence progression to disease.[31] In addition, the administration of insulin or its B chain can prevent or delay diabetes in susceptible mice during the prediabetic phase. Prospective studies, including the German BABYDIAB and the Finnish Diabetes Prediction and Prevention Study (DIPP), also indicate that autoantibodies against insulin usually emerge before any other antibodies, including anti-GAD65, anti–IA-2, and anti–zinc transporter 8 (ZnT8) (**Table 3-2**).[43-45]

It is astonishing that proinsulin, a protein of only 86 amino acids, contains so many epitopes for a spectrum of HLA class I and class II alleles. T cell reacting epitopes have been demonstrated within insulin A and B chains,[46,47] the C peptide and B-C chain junction, and the C-A chain junction region.[48] Specific CD4+ and CD8+ T cells targeting insulin and precursor epitopes has been reported both in newly diagnosed and in chronic T1DM.[49] CD4+ T cell reactivity has been noted mostly in connection with susceptibility alleles HLA-DR3 and HLA-DR4.[50] CD8+ T cell reactivity, on the other hand, is associated in particular with HLA-A2.[39]

TABLE 3-2 Prospective Cohort Studies of the Natural History of Type 1 Diabetes

	BABYDIAB (GERMANY)	DAISY (COLORADO)	DIPP (FINLAND)	TEDDY (FOUR COUNTRIES)
Year started	1989	1993	1994	2004
First-degree relatives (n)	1650 offspring	1120 offspring siblings	8150	923
General population (n)	–	1422		7754
Persistent islet Ab+ (n)	149	183	537	450*
Diabetes (n)	47	71	320	126†

Note: The BABYDIAB consists of offspring of parents with T1DM. DAISY has two groups: first-degree relatives of T1DM and high-risk individuals from the general population. DIPP screened infants in the general population, including first-degree relatives, for HLA types. Finally, the TEDDY cohort consists of newborns with a first-degree relative with T1DM as well as those from the general population enrolled from six clinical centers in four countries (personal communication from Ziegler, Simell, and Rewers, October 2011).

*As of October 2012, 800 cases expected by 15 years of follow-up.

†As of October 2012, 400 cases expected by 15 years of follow-up.

Ab+ = Autoantibody positive.

Glutamic Acid Decarboxylase

GAD is an enzyme that catalyzes the decarboxylation of glutamate to γ-aminobutyric acid (GABA) and CO_2. GAD isoforms GAD67 and GAD65 are encoded by two different genes, *GAD1* and *GAD2*. *GAD2* is expressed in the pancreas and the brain. The association of GAD65 autoantibodies with T1DM is well known,[51,52] and these autoantibodies were found in 52% of newly diagnosed children in the U.S. SEARCH for Diabetes in Youth study.[53] More recently, GAD has been used as a tolerogenic vaccine to preserve functional beta cells. Unfortunately, GAD65 antigen therapy did not significantly improve clinical outcomes over a 15-month period in a recent randomized controlled trial (RCT).[54]

Insulinoma-Associated Protein 2

Insulinoma-associated protein 2 (IA-2) is a neuroendocrine protein and a member of the tyrosine phosphatase family, with its gene located on chromosome 14.[55] Antibodies against IA-2 appear later than antibodies against insulin or GAD and are associated with progression to diabetes. Ellis and coworkers found anti–IA-2 antibodies in the sera of 58% of newly diagnosed T1DM patients[55]; and, similarly, Dabelea and colleagues identified IA-2A in 60% of newly diagnosed children in the SEARCH cohort.[53]

ZnT8

ZnT8 is a novel autoantigen in T1DM.[56] It is a beta cell–specific cation efflux zinc transporter with its gene located on chromosome 8. The Diabetes Autoimmunity Study in the Young (DAISY) cohort consists of two groups, including first-degree relatives of individuals with T1DM and individuals from the general population who underwent HLA typing of cord blood, and has shown that ZnT8 antibodies are present in 60% to 80% of newly diagnosed T1DM patients (see **Table 3-2**).[57] In addition, 25% of T1DM patients who are negative for autoantibodies to insulin, GAD, IA-2, and islet cells (ICA) tested positive for ZnT8 autoantibodies.[57] Moreover, the DAISY study showed that ZnT8 autoantibodies emerge later than the other insulin autoantibodies.[57] The antibodies have also been shown to decline quickly after diagnosis of T1DM.[58] Howson and colleagues found an association between anti-ZnT8 antibodies and the single-nucleotide polymorphisms (SNPs) rs7522061 and rs9258750A > G in, respectively, the Fc-receptor-like–3 *(FCRL3)* gene and HLA class I locus.[58]

Islet-Specific Glucose-6-Phosphatase Catalytic Subunit–Related Protein

IGRP is an important autoantigen that is selectively expressed in beta cells.[59] IGRP is recognized as an antigen by the CD8+ T cell clone NY8.3.[59] IGRP is not expressed in the thymus in NOD mice, thereby allowing IGRP-reactive T cells to escape into the periphery. For this reason, peripheral tolerance independently confers protection against autoimmunity.[60,61] Krishnamurthy and colleagues successfully showed that peripheral tolerance alone is sufficient to protect NOD8.3 mice from autoimmune diabetes.[62]

Chromogranin A

The chromogranin A (ChgA) gene is located on chromosome 14 and encodes a protein found in secretory granules of many different secretory cell types, including beta cells. It is a precursor pro-protein that is proteolytically processed within the granule to form a variety of peptides, including vasostatin 1 (VS-1; ChgA 1-76, ChgA 29-42), VS-2 (ChgA 1-113), and WE-14 (ChgA 358-371). The functions of these peptides are still not clearly understood. As previously mentioned, ChgA illustrates the importance of tissue-specific cleavage. In fact, a specific cleave of ChgA within the beta cells is essential for T cell binding. The cleavage product WE-14 is tissue-specific, meaning it is specifically produced in the islet cells and recognized by pathogenic BDC2.5 TCR of NOD mice via pockets 5 through 9 of the I-Ag7 MHC class II molecule.[63] Nikoopour and colleagues identified another cleavage product, ChgA 29-42 peptide, as the natural epitope of BDC2.5 CD4+ T cells, and demonstrated induction of diabetes after transfer of ChgA 29-42 activated BDC2.5 splenocytes into NOD/severe combined immunodeficiency (SCID) mice.[64]

In contrast, cells expressing noncleaved ChgA do not effectively produce these autoantigenic peptides and are thus not recognized by T cells. For example, production of WE-4 cleaves four N-terminal amino acids that, if present, would occupy pockets 1 to 4 on the I-Ag7 cMHC class II molecule and thereby block BDC2.5 TCR stimulation.[63]

Adaptive Immune Response
T Cell Response

The development of the destructive pathologic lesion known as *insulitis,* and the steps leading to T1DM in humans, are only partially understood. Immunohistologic examination of pancreatic tissues from patients with T1DM has demonstrated that in contrast to the animal models of spontaneous T1DM, insulitis is rare in humans.[65] When present, anti-islet T-lymphocytes, both CD4+ and CD8+ T cells, beta cells, macrophages, and dendritic cells are found in the inflammatory lesion.[66] CD8+ T lymphocytes represent the largest cell population within the inflammatory infiltrates and are widely recognized as the final effectors in the pathogenesis of T1DM.[25,67] Immunosuppressive drugs specifically directed against T cells delay disease progress,[68] and transfer of anti-islet specific CD4+ and CD8+ T cells can induce diabetes in immune-incompetent recipient NOD mice.[69]

Mechanistic studies involving CD8+ T cell (CTL) killing of human islets have shown that interferons can accelerate human islet killing by inducing expression of MHC class I molecules on beta cells[70] and thereby targeting them for cytotoxic T cell destruction.[71,72] Killing of human islets is shown to be perforin dependent in the absence of cytokines.[73] Further studies have also shown that CTL-mediated killing occurs via caspase-independent pathways in human T1DM.[73] CTLs are also sources of reactive oxygen species (ROSs) and proinflammatory cytokines. Because beta cells have a low capacity for disposing of ROSs generated from mitochondrial metabolism compared with other tissues,[74,75] ROSs could act as soluble mediators of beta cell death in T1DM.[76] CD4+ T cells, on the other hand, recognize peptides presented by MHC class II molecules and participate in the destruction of beta cells directly by the production of cytokines, and indirectly by the activation of local innate cells, such as macrophages and dendritic cells.[77] T cell–derived cytotoxicity in mouse models occurs via nitric oxide (NO)–dependent necrosis with very little contribution from apoptosis.[78] Conversely, in humans, preventing inducible NO synthase function does not consistently prevent beta cell destruction.[79] There is also evidence that apoptosis is an important pathway of cytolysis.[80]

Mitochondria in beta cells are essential for several cellular processes, including glucose-stimulated insulin secretion. These organelles are also important regulators of cell death. TNF-α– and IFN-γ–induced cell death depends on functional mitochondria, evident by the mitochondrial DNA (mtDNA)–deficient cells being resistant to cytokine killing.[81,82] Apoptosis is also a very energy-demanding process, and it is hypothesized that inhibition of adenosine triphosphate (ATP) production by endogenous inhibitors of oxidative phosphorylation may cause the switch from apoptosis to necrosis in metabolically suppressed cells (i.e., beta cells pre-T1DM) that have already been signaled for apoptotic cell death. In addition, mitochondria are an important source of cellular ROSs that can lead to caspase-dependent apoptosis in beta cells.[83]

Endoplasmic reticulum is also an organelle that is essential in the normal beta cell physiology. Beta cells are very prone to endoplasmic reticulum stress, as evidenced by the many mutations that affect insulin protein folding. The additional viral protein synthesis in a virally infected beta cell may cause endoplasmic reticulum stress that would not only saturate the cell's ability to replenish stored insulin pools, but also make it vulnerable to apoptosis and direct T cell lysis.[84]

Cytokines

Cytokines play an essential role in the pathogenesis of T1DM, and IFN-γ, TNF-α, and IL-1β have been particularly well studied. Immunohistologic samples from patients with T1DM demonstrate IFN-γ–secreting lymphocytes in the islets.[85] TNF-α– and IL-β–producing macrophages and dendritic cells have been identified in pancreatic islets in patients with recent-onset T1DM.[86] Human islets have been shown to be particularly sensitive to combinations of IL-1β, TNF-α, and IFN-γ. For example, addition of TNF-α to human islets inhibits beta cell function and, when combined with IFN-γ, causes reduced beta cell viability.[87] Cytokines have also been implicated in determining whether the immune response of CD4[+] T cells to an antigen is predominantly cellular (Th1) or humoral (Th2). T1DM is believed to be a Th-1 associated disease. Cytokines not only are able to control the type of immune response mounted, but also alter the expression of many proteins in the beta cells, including insulin. IFN-γ stimulates the expression of MHC class I molecules in islet beta cells, which is illustrated well by the prevention of insulitis in NOD mice after treatment with antibodies to IFN-γ.[88] IL-1 stimulates the expression of protective proteins including ganglioside and superoxide dismutase, both thought to be involved in the recovery of beta cell injury.[89] It has also recently become apparent that insulinopenia in T1DM is not solely a result of beta cell destruction, but also is secondary to a reversible beta cell dysfunction caused by inflammatory cytokines.

Antibody Response

Autoantibodies could theoretically injure beta cells by antibody-dependent complement cytotoxicity or by targeting NK cells to beta cell antigens, but induction of T1DM in animal models has been shown to be dependent on T cells.[90] Consequently the pathogenic significance of T1DM-related antibodies is very low, and the real effectors of beta cell autoimmune destruction are self-reactive CD4[+] and CD8[+] T cells.[68]

Extending these observations to the clinical context, even though antibodies are not required for the development T1DM, they are valuable prognostic markers for disease risk. The fact that autoantibodies also appear several years before the clinical onset of T1DM when insulin secretion is normal also makes them very useful in predicting the window of opportunity to potentially prevent the disease in the future.[91] As they are also the most reliable diagnostic test, testing for autoantibodies is now an essential part of the T1DM workup. In the Childhood Diabetes in Finland (DiMe) study, a prospectively family study in Finland in which serum samples were obtained at the diagnosis of T1DM from probands and siblings, 91% of 758 children and adolescents younger than 15 years with newly diagnosed T1DM tested positive for at least two antibodies, and 71% for three or more.[92]

More recently, in the multicenter SEARCH for Diabetes in Youth study, 74% of 2291 newly diagnosed cases of diabetes in patients younger than 20 years showed autoantibody positivity (positive for either glutamic acid decarboxylase antibodies [GADA] or insulinoma associated-2 autoantibodies [IA-2A]).[53] Wenzlau and colleagues showed that by testing for circulating antibodies to ZnT8A in combination with the three other antibodies (GADA, IA-2A, and IAA), one is able to detect up to 98% of individuals at disease onset.[57]

Human studies have demonstrated an important role of B lymphocytes as APCs in T1DM.[93] In addition, β cell deficiency by gene targeting and β cell depletion by specific antibodies have been shown to prevent the development of T1DM in NOD mice.[94]

Innate Immune System Response

There is growing evidence that the innate immune system also plays an important role in the pathogenesis of T1DM, conferring protection in the early stages, and is later involved in precipitating the disease (**Table 3-3**).

Macrophages, in particular, have shown to be important contributors in the pathogenesis of T1DM. Preventing the influx of macrophages into the pancreas of NOD mice has been shown to abort the induction of T1DM.[95,96] Macrophages in NOD mice function differently than in non-obese resistant (NOR) mice, with regard to both cytokine production and phagocytosis, producing higher levels of proinflammatory IL-12, IL-1β, and TNF-α cytokines[86,97] and demonstrating impaired phagocytosis of apoptotic beta cells.[98]

TABLE 3-3 Innate Immune Cells

TYPE OF CELL	ROLE IN T1DM PATHOGENESIS	REFERENCE
Macrophages	Producing proinflammatory cytokines and impaired phagocytosis of apoptotic β cells	86, 95–98
Dendritic cells	Peripheral immune tolerance by inducing expansion of Treg cells	99, 100
Plasmacytoid dendritic cells	Conversion of naïve CD4[+] T cells to Treg cells	103
Natural killer cells	Inverse relation with Treg cells and associated with coxsackievirus B infection	105, 107, 108
Invariant natural killer cells	Recognize glycolipid antigens, and induction of these cells has shown to protect against T1DM development in NOD mice	109, 110, 111

Dendritic cells are implicated as important contributors to peripheral immune tolerance[99] by being able to induce expansion of Tregs.[100] Studies in NOD mice have shown that induction of dendritic cells with granulocyte colony-stimulating factor (G-CSF) expands Treg cells and thereby suppresses beta cell autoimmunity.[101] The plasmacytoid subpopulation of dendritic cells has a protective role in the pathogenesis of T1DM.[102] Plasmacytoid dendritic cells have specifically been implicated in the conversion of naïve CD4+ T cells to Treg cells, which are key contributors to ensuring peripheral immune tolerance and preventing T1DM.[103]

Natural killer cells are also implicated in the pathogenesis of T1DM and have been detected in the pancreases of NOD mice and in the pancreases of patients with T1DM.[104] Again, their role in T1DM pathogenesis is complex; studies have shown both a protective and a deleterious role of these innate cells. Impaired natural killer cell function has been documented in lymphoid tissues of NOD mice.[105] Conversely, the depletion of Treg cells in NOD mice is associated with an exacerbation of natural killer cell activation in the pancreas and is concomitant with disease onset.[106] The presence of natural killer cells in the pancreas of T1DM patients has also been associated with coxsackievirus B infection.[107,108] Furthermore, natural killer cells are thought to be key cellular players in the pathogenesis of T1DM induced by coxsackievirus infection in mouse models.[107,108]

An unusual subpopulation of natural killer cells that has also been implicated in the pathogenesis of T1DM is the invariant natural killer T cells. This is a group of T cells that recognizes glycolipid antigens presented by the HLA class I–related CD1d molecule. These T cells play a regulatory role in the immune system, and many studies have demonstrated their protective role against T1DM.[109,110] Induction of invariant natural killer T cells by glycolipids (e.g., α-galactosylceramide) may prevent T1DM development in NOD mice.[111]

ETIOLOGY

The cause of immune susceptibility in the pathogenesis of T1DM is still unknown, but it is very likely that both genetic and environmental factors are essential contributors to the autoimmune destruction of pancreatic beta cells.

Genetics

T1DM is a polygenic disease that does not fit any mendelian pattern of inheritance. This is exemplified well by the fact that siblings of patients with T1DM have a 15-fold greater risk of developing T1DM compared with the general population, and the concordance rate for T1DM in monozygotic twins is greater than 50%, compared with 6% to 10% concordance in dizygotic twins.[112] Susceptibility and protective genes have been identified at more than 40 loci. Carrying a susceptibility gene increases the risk for T1DM, but does not automatically imply that the person will develop the disease. By far the most important T1DM risk genes are found in the HLA region located on chromosome 6p21. This locus accounts for up to 30% to 65% of genetic T1DM susceptibility.[113] Non-HLA T1DM loci have a smaller but important effect on T1DM susceptibility; most appear to primarily affect the immune system and particularly T cells.[114]

TABLE 3-4 HLA Genes

HLA GENE	SUBTYPES	ROLE IN T1DM PATHOGENESIS	REFERENCE
HLA I	HLA-A, HLA-B, HLA-C	Expressed on all nucleated cells, permitting CD8+ T cell recognition	118
HLA II	HLA-DR, HLA-DQ, HLA-DP	Expressed exclusively on professional antigen-presenting cells capable of activating CD4+ T lymphocytes	113, 116, 117
HLA III		Not directly involved in antigen presentation, but important components of the immune system	120

HLA Genes

The major histocompatibility (HLA) genes make up cell-surface proteins involved in antigen presentation (**Table 3-4**). They are also among the most polymorphic in the human genome, which confers a heterozygous advantage allowing the presentation of a larger variety of antigens to the immune system and thus providing greater protection from new pathogens. HLA class II molecules (HLA-DR, HLA-DQ, and HLA-DP) are expressed exclusively on B lymphocytes, dendritic cells, and macrophages—professional APCs capable of activating CD4+ T lymphocytes. In contrast, HLA class I molecules (HLA-A, HLA-B, and HLA-C) are expressed on all nucleated cells, permitting CD8+ (cytolytic) T cell recognition. HLA class III proteins are not directly involved in antigen presentation, but still make up important components of the immune system.

Diabetes susceptibility is related to peptide-binding characteristics of the various HLA gene products, but exactly how HLA molecules confer susceptibility to selective autoimmune-mediated beta cell destruction is unknown. One possible explanation is that susceptibility-conferring HLA molecules initiate autoimmunity by binding diabetogenic self-antigens and presenting them efficiently to T lymphocytes. In contrast, protective HLA molecules would bind these peptides and present them to the immune system less efficiently. Another, more plausible alternative is that poor binding and presentation of self-antigens (e.g., pre-proinsulin, GAD, IA-2A, and ZnT8) in the thymus results in an ineffective central tolerance of diabetogenic self-antigens and thus breakdown of self-tolerance.[114]

T1DM is most strongly associated with the polymorphisms of six of the genes of the HLA class II locus IDDM1: HLA-DRB1, HLA-DRA1, HLA-DQB1, HLA-DQA1, HLA-DPB1, and HLA-DPA1. Specific combinations of these alleles are associated with a spectrum from highly susceptible to highly protective genotypes. The highest risk genotype, HLA-DR3, DQB1*0201/DR4,DQB1*0302, is present in 2.4% of the general population and 25% to 40% of T1DM patients, and is associated with an earlier onset of T1DM. The risk of developing T1DM with this genotype is approximately 1 in 15, compared with a risk of 1 in 300 in the general population.[115] The next highest-risk genotypes are those homozygous for polymorphisms in DR4 or DR3. At least one of the two highest-risk haplotypes—DR3-DQA1*0501-DQB1*0201 and DR4-DQA1*0301-DQB1*0302—is present in more than 90% of patients with T1DM.[113,116] On the other hand, the HLA-DQA1*0102 and DQB1*0602 alleles confer protection from T1DM.[117]

DIABETES MELLITUS

HLA class I genes also include both susceptibility and protective alleles. The HLA-B*39 allele is associated with progression to T1DM in children positive for either one or two autoantibodies.[118] HLA-A*24 is associated with more aggressive islet destruction, and conversely HLA-A*03 and HLA-A*11 appear to confer protection against T1DM development.[118] Overexpression of HLA class I molecules by the beta cells is thought to be an important event preceding insulitis.[119]

The HLA class III region comprises gene products involved in the activation cascades of the complement system, hormonal synthesis, inflammation, cell stress, extracellular matrix organization, and immunoglobulin superfamily members.[120] Polymorphisms in the *AIF-1* gene have been shown to be significantly associated with T1DM susceptibility after conditioning on HLA-DRB1, HLA-DQB1, HLA-A, and HLA-B alleles.[121]

Non-HLA Genes

Despite being the most significant genetic locus in T1DM, HLA alleles cannot account for the entire genetic predisposition of this disease. The fact that T1DM has increased by approximately 3% per year worldwide over the past three decades,[122] despite a decrease in patients with the high-risk HLA-DR3/4 genotype, suggests the importance of non-HLA-related alleles and other environmental factors in T1DM pathogenesis.[123] Numerous non-HLA genes have been identified to be associated with T1DM risk; the most extensively investigated include insulin gene *(INS)*, cytotoxic T lymphocyte–associated 4 gene *(CTLA-4)*, protein tyrosine phosphatase nonreceptor type 22 gene *(PTPN22)*, and IL-2 receptor alpha gene *(IL2RA)* (**Table 3-5**).

Insulin Gene

Insulin-dependent diabetes mellitus 2 (IDDM2) represents a genetic susceptibility locus for T1DM within *INS*, which is located on chromosome 11p15.5, and accounts for 10% of familial clustering.[124] The genetic risk conferred by mutations within the insulin gene is a result of its role as a primary initiating autoantigen in T1DM.[125,126]

The *INS* gene is transcribed and translated in the thymus, which is essential for central immunologic tolerance. The IDDM2 locus gives rise to a variable number of tandem repeats (VNTR) at the promoter end of *INS*. The number of repeats ranges from 25 to approximately 200, and the alleles of the proinsulin gene are classified by total size. Type I insulin VNTR consists of 26 to 63 repeats, type II of 64 to 140, and type III of 141 to 209.[127,128] The number of VNTRs appears to correlate with the risk for developing T1DM. For that reason, type I confers susceptibility; patients homozygous for type I have lower levels of insulin expression in the thymus[125,126] and higher titers of insulin autoantibodies.[129] Conversely, VNTR

type III protects carriers from T1DM.[125,126] The mechanistic explanation is that VNTRs regulate the expression of insulin in the thymus by affecting the AIRE, a transcription factor, binding to its promoter region.[130] Type I VNTRs will induce lower transcription of insulin in the thymus, where central tolerance to autoantigens operates, resulting in reduced tolerance—that is, less efficient elimination by negative selection of insulin-reactive T cells, and increased risk of T1DM development.

Cytotoxic T Lymphocyte–Associated Protein 4 Gene

The *CTLA-4* gene is located on chromosome 2q33, and its polymorphisms have been shown to contribute to T1DM susceptibility.[131] The CTLA-4–encoded molecule is a co-stimulatory receptor involved in the IL-2 receptor signaling pathway and plays an important role in the regulation of peripheral tolerance.[132] It is expressed by Tregs and functions as a negative regulator of T cell activation; binding of CTLA-4 to B7 results in inhibition of T cell activity.[133] In particular, variations in the concentrations of soluble CTLA-4 protein and the +49 G/G polymorphism have been associated with T1DM risk.[134]

Protein Tyrosine Phosphatase Nonreceptor Type 22 Gene

The protein tyrosine phosphatase nonreceptor type 22 *(PTPN22)* gene is located on chromosome 1p13[135] and is strongly associated with T1DM as well as other autoimmune diseases.[135] The *PTPN22* gene encodes the lymphoid-specific protein tyrosine phosphatase (LYP), which inhibits T cell activation by dephosphorylating essential kinases in T cell signaling, including lymphocyte-specific protein tyrosine kinase (LCK) and zeta-chain-associated protein kinase 70 (ZAP70).[114] There is a strong association between polymorphisms of the *PTPN22* gene and T1DM risk.[136] The 1858 T variant is also independently associated with the development of persistent islet autoimmunity among individuals with the high-risk HLA genotype for T1DM.[137] The 1858 T variant results in a missense mutation, R620W, which causes gain of function.[138] This variant of PTPN22 is unable to bind the signaling molecule Csk, allowing the accumulation of large numbers of self-reactive T cells and contributing to autoimmunity.

Interferon Induced with Helicase C Domain 1 Gene

The interferon induced with helicase C domain 1 *(IFIH1)* gene is located on chromosome 2q and has been associated with T1DM in genome-wide association studies.[139] A possible mechanism explaining T1DM susceptibility is that the cytoplasmic helicase senses and initiates antiviral activity against picornaviruses by increasing interferon production and class I HLA expression.[140] This increased expression enables the cytotoxic CD8+ T cells to recognize both

TABLE 3-5 Non-HLA Genes

HLA GENE	LOCATION	ROLE IN T1DM PATHOGENESIS	REFERENCE
Insulin gene *(INS)*	Chromosome 11p15.5	Primary initiating autoantigen in T1DM	124, 125, 126
Cytotoxic T lymphocyte–associated protein 4 gene *(CTLA4)*	Chromosome 2q33	Polymorphisms shown to contribute to T1DM susceptibility because of its role in regulation of peripheral tolerance	131, 132
Protein tyrosine phosphatase nonreceptor type 22 gene *(PTPN22)*	Chromosome 1p13	Strongly associated with T1DM and other autoimmune diseases	135
Interferon induced with helicase C domain 1 gene *(IFIH1)*	Chromosome 2q	Associated with T1DM in genome-wide association studies	139
Interleukin 2 receptor alpha subunit gene *(IL2RA)*	Chromosome 10p15.1	Implicated in several autoimmune diseases, including T1DM	142

viral and beta cell antigens, which may result in beta cell apoptosis.[141]

Interleukin 2 Receptor Alpha Subunit Gene

The *IL2RA* gene is located on chromosome 10p15.1.[142] This gene encodes the expression of CD25 on regulatory and memory T cells and is implicated in a number of autoimmune disorders, including T1DM.[142] The expression of CD25 is important for suppressing T cell proliferation, and unregulated expression may cause uninhibited T cell proliferation and predispose to autoimmunity.[143] Both a susceptible (SS) and a protective (P1P1) haplotype for *IL2RA* have been identified, and recent studies have shown that the SS haplotype is associated with decreased IL-2 responsiveness and FOXP3 expression by Tregs, both important in modulating self-tolerance.[144]

Epigenetics

Epigenetics refers to modifications to the genome that do not involve a change in the actual nucleotide sequence. The most common mechanisms include DNA methylation and chromatin remodeling. Uniparental disomy (imprinting) is an example of epigenetics in which there is silencing of either the maternal or the paternal allele at one or more genetic loci. Offspring of affected fathers have a 6% to 7% risk of developing T1DM, more than double that of affected mothers,[145] suggesting an imprinting effect. Epigenetics is increasingly recognized as a possible molecular mechanism for gene-environment interactions. Miao and colleagues found that CTLA-4 had a different H3K9me2 methylation pattern in T1DM lymphocytes versus normal.[146] They also noted significant variations in histone H3K9Ac levels at the promoter regions of *HLA-DRB1* and *HLA-DQB1* genes in monocytes between T1DM patients and healthy controls.[147] Fradin and colleagues found consistent methylation differences between T1DM patients and nondiabetic controls at CpG sites at the proximal part of the *INS* gene promoter.[148] The fact that epigenetics is implicated in immune tolerance was recently illustrated by Bettini and colleagues. Their study showed that epigenetic modifications of *FOXP3* resulted in abnormal Treg function, Treg cell insufficiency, and rapid acceleration of diabetes in a murine model.[149]

Environmental Factors

It is well accepted that environmental factors play an important role in the pathogenesis of T1DM. The potential mechanisms include direct beta cell toxicity, the triggering of beta cell autoimmunity, molecular mimicry, and induction of insulin resistance. The Environmental Determinants of Diabetes in the Young (TEDDY) study, a large multicenter study, is currently under way to identify environmental factors predisposing to or protective against islet autoimmunity and T1DM and will, it is hoped, add insight into both dietary and infectious triggers.[150]

Dietary Factors

Islet autoantibodies start emerging during the first year of life, suggesting that early life exposure(s) may be pivotal.[45] Consequently, infant and childhood dietary factors have been implicated as a vehicle of environmental triggers in the pathogenesis of the disease (**Table 3-6**).

Exposure to cow's milk (CM) in early neonatal life has received considerable attention. In the DiMe study, high

TABLE 3-6 Dietary Factors

DIETARY FACTOR	ROLE IN T1DM PATHOGENESIS	REFERENCES
Cow's milk	The DiMe study showed a strong association between consumption of cow's milk and T1DM.	151
Breast feeding	Early studies suggest that breast feeding for prolonged periods confers protection from developing T1DM.	156
Gluten	Gluten has been incriminated as an important diabetogenic agent, but the BABYDIET study showed no effect of gluten elimination on development of islet autoimmunity.	159, 164
Vitamin D	Finnish birth-cohort study showed that high-dose vitamin D supplements in infancy are associated with a decrease in risk of T1DM development.	165, 166
Omega-3 fatty acids	Higher intake was associated with lower risk of T1DM development.	169, 170

consumption of CM protein was strongly associated with the emergence of beta cell autoantibodies and progression to clinical T1DM in initially unaffected siblings of children with T1DM.[151] In the Finnish Dietary Intervention Trial for the Prevention of Type 1 Diabetes (FINDIA), infants were randomized to receive either CM formula, a whey-based hydrolyzed formula, or a whey-based formula free of bovine insulin, and those infants who received formula free of bovine insulin were significantly less likely to have autoantibodies at age 3 years than the infants who were fed CM.[152] More recently, the association between CM intake and beta cell autoimmunity has also been shown to be more marginal.[153]

Several mechanisms have been proposed to explain the link between CM proteins and beta cell autoimmunity. Bovine serum albumin is structurally very similar to islet protein p69, and a misdirected immune response against this protein may explain the immune-mediated beta cell injury.[154] In addition, infants fed CM-based formulas have significantly higher titers of antibodies to bovine insulin, and for that reason it has been theorized that early exposure to CM results in immunization to bovine insulin, a molecule that differs structurally from human insulin in only three amino acid positions.[155]

Early reports have suggested that children who were exclusively breast fed for prolonged periods as infants are at lower risk of developing T1DM.[156] The proposed mechanism of protection is decreased gut permeability and enterovirus infection protection.[157] This has not been confirmed in more recent studies that found no association of breast feeding or duration of breast feeding and emergence of beta cell autoantibodies.[158] For that reason the causal relationship still remains unclear. The ongoing Trial to Reduce IDDM in the Genetically at Risk (TRIGR) has randomized infants at increased risk of T1DM, at weaning, to receive either an extensively hydrolyzed formula or a conventional CM-based formula. Follow-up analysis is expected in 2014.

Gluten has also been incriminated as an important diabetogenic agent.[159] Two prospective studies have shown an association between introduction of cereals in infancy and early beta cell autoimmunity.[160,161] These studies found beta cell autoimmune susceptibility with introduction of gluten in the first 3 months of life compared with introduction in the first 4 to 6 months.[160,161] The temporal association may be explained by immaturity of the gut and immune system in at-risk individuals.[162] Two small-scale studies showed that a gluten-free diet had no effect on beta cell autoimmunity but was associated with increased endogenous insulin secretion in family members at risk of T1DM.[159,163] More recently, a randomized clinical trial as part of the BABYDIET study, a primary prevention trial involving children with a first-degree relative with T1DM, showed no effect of gluten elimination on development of islet autoimmunity in genetically at-risk children.[164]

Vitamin D deficiency has also been implicated as a risk factor for T1DM.[165] Results reported by a Finnish study found that regular high-dose vitamin D supplements in infancy were associated with a decrease risk compared with no supplementation.[165] On the other hand, Finland, which is one of the areas in the world with the highest incidence of T1DM, reports an uptake of 80% for vitamin D supplements in children up to the age of 1 year.[166] There is also a striking difference in the annual incidence rate of T1DM in the neighboring populations of Finland and Russian Karelia (42/100,000 compared with 7.8/100,000), with no difference reported in the circulating vitamin D concentrations in pregnant women and schoolchildren.[167] Furthermore, Simpson and colleagues showed that neither vitamin D nor 25-hydroxyvitamin D (25[OH]D) levels were associated with risk of islet autoimmunity or T1DM in the DAISY population.[168]

Omega-3 fatty acids have also been reported to play a protective role in the development of T1DM. Studies have showed that higher omega-3 fatty acid intake is associated with lower risk of beta cell autoimmunity. In a case-cohort study based on the DAISY population, omega-3 fatty acid intake between the ages of 1 and 6 years was associated with lower risk of islet-autoimmunity.[169] A similar study from Norway supported these findings by showing that children with T1DM were less likely to have been given cod liver oil during infancy.[170]

Infectious Factors

Viruses, including herpesviruses,[171] mumps virus,[172] rubella virus,[173,174] retroviruses,[175] and in particular enteroviruses, have been implicated in the development of T1DM (**Table 3-7**). In animal models, viral infections can both promote and diminish autoimmunity. Viruses can initiate autoimmunity by at least four mechanisms (**Fig. 3-2**):

1. Molecular mimicry between viral proteins and autoantigens (e.g., PC2 protein of coxsackievirus mimics GAD65; rubella virus capsid protein mimics 52-kd islet protein; rotavirus mimics GAD and IA-2; cytomegalovirus mimics 38-kd islet protein; VP0 capsid protein in enterovirus mimics IAR/IA-2 tyrosine phosphatase)
2. Release of autoantigens following beta cell cytokine-induced injury, which are subsequently taken up by APCs and presented to T cells
3. Cytokine-induced upregulation of MHC and co-stimulatory molecules on APCs, enabling them to present self-peptides in immunogenic form to T cells
4. Interference with central and peripheral self-tolerance

Enteroviruses belong to the picornavirus family of RNA viruses. The proposed mechanism of how enterovirus contributes to the self-reactive process includes activation of interferon production, overexpression of class I HLA molecules, and chemokine-induced inflammation. Multiple studies have reported increased frequency of enteroviral RNA in patients with newly diagnosed T1DM.[176,177] Perinatal exposure to enterovirus may play a role in the pathogenesis of T1DM. Elfving and colleagues showed an increased prevalence of antienterovirus IgM in pregnant mothers whose children later developed T1DM during childhood; however, the known confounding effect of HLA-DR3/4 was not accounted for in their studies.[178–180]

The Australian BABYDIAB study followed approximately 500 babies with a first-degree relative with T1DM from birth, and found that rotavirus seroconversion was linked with the appearance of an increase in islet antibodies compared with HLA and age-matched controls.[181] These findings were not confirmed in prospective studies in Finland and Colorado.

Viral infections during childhood may also play a role in the development of immunoregulatory mechanisms that protect against diabetes.[182] The hygiene hypothesis proposes that improved hygiene in the Western World has led to a decline in immunity to common infections and increased incidence of autoimmunity. In other words, with early infectious exposures, young children build appropriate immune responses to pathogens. This idea is also supported by the findings that daycare attendance in early infancy confers protection against development of childhood diabetes.[183] The relationship between viral infection and autoimmunity appears to be temporal; studies have shown that enteroviral infections before weaning are beneficial and infections after are associated with susceptibility for T1DM development.[184–186] Vaccinations have not been associated with development of T1DM.[187,188]

In the last few years research has shed light on possible mechanistic pathways linking genetic predisposition to viral infections in the pathogenesis of T1DM. A good example is the *OAS1* gene, which encodes an antiviral enzyme that may induce beta cell damage through RNase L–mediated degradation of cellular RNA. Polymorphisms of *OAS1* produce an enzyme that is thought to result in a reduced apoptosis-mediated antiviral response, causing more extensive beta cell damage and initiation of autoimmune attack.[189] Another example is the *IFIH1* gene, which also encodes an RNA-activated apoptosis protein, and is associated with increased production of type 1 interferons that may contribute to the autoimmune attack of beta cells.[190,191] Polymorphisms of *IFIH1* confer both susceptibility and

TABLE 3-7 Viruses

VIRUSES	DESCRIPTION	REFERENCES
Enteroviruses	Multiple studies have reported increased frequency of enteroviral RNA in patients with newly diagnosed T1DM. In particular, coxsackievirus B4 is strongly associated with islet autoimmunity.	175, 176, 177
Rubella	Perinatal exposure may play a role in the pathogenesis of T1DM.	173, 174
Herpesviruses	These viruses are associated with autoimmune disease, occasionally with diabetes.	171
Mumps	Earlier reports indicate association with T1DM, but this remains controversial.	172
Rotavirus	Australian BABYDIAB study reports autoimmunity following rotavirus infection.	181

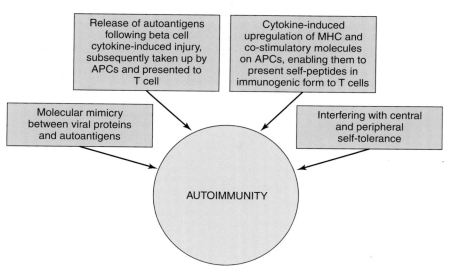

FIGURE 3-2 **Viral-induced β cell autoimmunity.** APC = Antigen presenting cells; MHC = major histocompatibility complex.

protection. IFIH1 alleles associated with higher IFIH1 levels are associated with an increased risk of developing T1DM, whereas protective IFIH1 alleles are linked with a decreased expression of *IFIH1*, and consequently a lower risk of T1DM.

Although the conclusion is controversial, studies have shown that susceptibility to the diabetogenic coxsackievirus B4 may be genetically predisposed, being restricted by HLA-DR and HLA-DQ alleles.[192] The HLA-DR3 allele has also been associated with enteroviral persistence in T1DM.[193] Whether HLA alleles provide a link between genetic susceptibility and viral triggers is still unclear and warrants further investigation.

Other Environmental Factors

Many other environmental factors have been proposed to be involved in the pathogenesis of T1DM. Increased weight gain in infancy has been reported to be an important risk factor,[174] but this has not been confirmed in larger studies. Children who develop T1DM have been shown to be both heavier and taller in infancy than their nondiabetic peers.[194]

Psychological stress may also constitute a trigger in the development of T1DM. Children with T1DM are, according to some studies, more exposed to stressful situations than controls.[195,196] The stress is especially frequent 2 years preceding diagnosis, and it may be the associated changes in hormonal and neuronal signals that contribute to the development of T1DM in genetically susceptible individuals.[197]

A potential protective factor is the microbiome, defined as the constellation of microorganisms that reside on the surface of skin, in the saliva and oral mucosa, in the conjunctiva, and in the gastrointestinal tracts, as shown in a study in NOD mice in which probiotic administration prevented T1DM.[198] In another study BB-DP rats were given *Lactobacillus* strains isolated from BB-DR rats and showed a reduced rate of diabetes development.[199]

SUMMARY

Significant advances have been recently made in our understanding of the etiopathogenesis of T1DM. We are also finally beginning to explore some possible mechanistic pathways linking genetic predisposition and exogenous triggers.

Interruption of the disease process remains the long-term goal of T1DM research. Environmental modification likely offers the most powerful strategy for effective prevention. Most of our knowledge is derived from NOD mouse models. Although no animal model is able to fully describe the complexity of human T1DM, these models have allowed invaluable insight into the pathogenesis. Still, care is required in applying these findings to humans because many of them are unconfirmed, and for that reason there is a need for large prospective studies of high-risk children to gain further insight into environmental triggers in human T1DM and better understanding of infectious and genetic predispositions.

References

1. Liese AD, Hirsch T, von Mutius E, Weiland SK: Burden of overweight in Germany: prevalence differences between former East and West German children, *Eur J Public Health* 16 (5):526–531, 2006.
2. Rewers M, Norris J, Dabelea D: Epidemiology of type 1 diabetes mellitus, *Adv Exp Med Biol* 552:219–246, 2004.
3. Forlenza GP, Rewers M: The epidemic of type 1 diabetes: what is it telling us? *Curr Opin Endocrinol Diabetes Obes* 18(4):248–251, 2011.
4. Rewers M: Challenges in diagnosing type 1 diabetes in different populations, *Diabetes Metab J* 36 (2):90–97, 2012.
5. Gale EA, Gillespie KM: Diabetes and gender, *Diabetologia* 44(1):3–15, 2001.
6. Xu X, D'Hoker J, Stangé G, et al: Beta cells can be generated from endogenous progenitors in injured adult mouse pancreas, *Cell* 132(2):197–207, 2008.
7. Rabinovitch A: An update on cytokines in the pathogenesis of insulin-dependent diabetes mellitus, *Diabetes Metab Rev* 14(2):129–151, 1998.
8. Schauer IE, Snell-Bergeon JK, Bergman BC, et al: Insulin resistance, defective insulin-mediated fatty acid suppression, and coronary artery calcification in subjects with and without type 1 diabetes: the CACTI study, *Diabetes* 60(1):306–314, 2011.
9. Nadeau KJ, Regensteiner JG, Bauer TA, et al: Insulin resistance in adolescents with type 1 diabetes and its relationship to cardiovascular function, *J Clin Endocrinol Metab* 95 (2):513–521, 2010.
10. Liu HY, Cao SY, Hong T, et al: Insulin is a stronger inducer of insulin resistance than hyperglycemia in mice with type 1 diabetes mellitus (T1DM), *J Biol Chem* 284(40):27090–27100, 2009.
11. Perseghin G, Lattuada G, Danna M, et al: Insulin resistance, intramyocellular lipid content, and plasma adiponectin in patients with type 1 diabetes, *Am J Physiol Endocrinol Metab* 285(6): E1174–E1181, 2003.
12. Pospisilik JA, Knauf C, Joza N, et al: Targeted deletion of AIF decreases mitochondrial oxidative phosphorylation and protects from obesity and diabetes, *Cell* 131(3):476–491, 2007.
13. Ye J: Role of insulin in the pathogenesis of free fatty acid-induced insulin resistance in skeletal muscle, *Endocr Metab Immune Disord Drug Targets* 7(1):65–74, 2007.
14. Wullaert A, van Loo G, Heyninck K, Beyaert R: Hepatic tumor necrosis factor signaling and nuclear factor-kappaB: effects on liver homeostasis and beyond, *Endocr Rev* 28(4):365–386, 2007.
15. Kaneto H, Matsuoka TA, Katakami N, et al: Oxidative stress and the JNK pathway are involved in the development of type 1 and type 2 diabetes, *Curr Mol Med* 7(7):674–686, 2007.
16. Rodrigues TC, Veyna AM, Haarhues MD, et al: Obesity and coronary artery calcium in diabetes: the coronary artery calcification in type 1 diabetes (CACTI) study, *Diabetes Technol Ther* 13 (10):991–996, 2011.
17. Orchard TJ, Olson JC, Erbey JR, et al: Insulin resistance-related factors, but not glycemia, predict coronary artery disease in type 1 diabetes: 10-year follow-up data from the Pittsburgh Epidemiology of Diabetes Complications Study, *Diabetes Care* 26(5):1374–1379, 2003.
18. Nadeau KJ, Zeitler PS, Bauer TA, et al: Insulin resistance in adolescents with type 2 diabetes is associated with impaired exercise capacity, *J Clin Endocrinol Metab* 94(10):3687–3695, 2009.
18a. Bjornstad P, Snell-Bergeon JK, Rewers M, et al: Early diabetic nephropathy: a complication of reduced insulin sensitivity in type 1 diabetes, *Diabetes Care* 36(11):3678–3683, 2013. http://dx.doi.org/10.2337/dc13-0631.

19. Atkinson MA, Leiter EH: The NOD mouse model of type 1 diabetes: as good as it gets? *Nat Med* 5 (6):601–604, 1999.

20. Anderson MS, Bluestone JA: The NOD mouse: a model of immune dysregulation, *Annu Rev Immunol* 23:447–485, 2005.

21. Hanafusa T, Miyazaki A, Miyagawa J, et al: Examination of islets in the pancreas biopsy specimens from newly diagnosed type 1 (insulin-dependent) diabetic patients, *Diabetologia* 33 (2):105–111, 1990.

22. Buteau J, Shlien A, Foisy S, Accili D: Metabolic diapause in pancreatic beta-cells expressing a gain-of-function mutant of the forkhead protein Foxo1, *J Biol Chem* 282(1):287–293, 2007.

23. Greenbaum CJ, Prigeon RL, D'Alessio DA: Impaired beta-cell function, incretin effect, and glucagon suppression in patients with type 1 diabetes who have normal fasting glucose, *Diabetes* 51(4):951–957, 2002.

24. Foulis AK, Liddle CN, Farquharson MA, et al: The histopathology of the pancreas in type 1 (insulin-dependent) diabetes mellitus: a 25-year review of deaths in patients under 20 years of age in the United Kingdom, *Diabetologia* 29(5):267–274, 1986.

25. Bluestone JA, Herold K, Eisenbarth G: Genetics, pathogenesis and clinical interventions in type 1 diabetes, *Nature* 464(7293):1293–1300, 2010.

26. DeVoss J, Hou Y, Johannes K, et al: Spontaneous autoimmunity prevented by thymic expression of a single self-antigen, *J Exp Med* 203(12):2727–2735, 2006.

27. Georgiou HM, Bellgrau D: Thymus transplantation and disease prevention in the diabetes-prone Bio-Breeding rat, *J Immunol* 142(10):3400–3405, 1989.

28. Georgiou HM, Mandel TE: Induction of insulitis in athymic (nude) mice. The effect of NOD thymus and pancreas transplantation, *Diabetes* 44(1):49–59, 1995.

29. Ashton-Rickardt PG, Bandeira A, Delaney JR, et al: Evidence for a differential avidity model of T cell selection in the thymus, *Cell* 76(4):651–663, 1994.

30. Thébault-Baumont K, Dubois-Laforgue D, Krief P, et al: Acceleration of type 1 diabetes mellitus in proinsulin 2-deficient NOD mice, *J Clin Invest* 111(6):851–857, 2003.

31. Moriyama H, Abiru N, Paronen J, et al: Evidence for a primary islet autoantigen (preproinsulin 1) for insulitis and diabetes in the nonobese diabetic mouse, *Proc Natl Acad Sci U S A* 100 (18):10376–10381, 2003.

32. Wildin RS, Ramsdell F, Peake J, et al: X-linked neonatal diabetes mellitus, enteropathy and endocrinopathy syndrome is the human equivalent of mouse scurfy, *Nat Genet* 27(1):18–20, 2001.

33. d'Hennezel E, Bin Dhuban K, Torgerson T, Piccirillo CA: The immunogenetics of immune dysregulation, polyendocrinopathy, enteropathy, X linked (IPEX) syndrome, *J Med Genet* 49 (5):291–302, 2012.

34. Itoh M, Takahashi T, Sakaguchi N, et al: Thymus and autoimmunity: production of CD25+CD4+ naturally anergic and suppressive T cells as a key function of the thymus in maintaining immunologic self-tolerance, *J Immunol* 162(9):5317–5326, 1999.

35. Collins AV, Brodie DW, Gilbert RJ, et al: The interaction properties of costimulatory molecules revisited, *Immunity* 17(2):201–210, 2002.

36. Linsley PS, Brady W, Urnes M, et al: CTLA-4 is a second receptor for the B cell activation antigen B7, *J Exp Med* 174(3):561–569, 1991.

37. Read S, Malmstrom V, Powrie F: Cytotoxic T lymphocyte-associated antigen 4 plays an essential role in the function of CD25(+)CD4(+) regulatory cells that control intestinal inflammation, *J Exp Med* 192(2):295–302, 2000.

38. Panagiotopoulos C, Qin H, Tan R, et al: Identification of a beta-cell-specific HLA class I restricted epitope in type 1 diabetes, *Diabetes* 52(11):2647–2651, 2003.

39. Marron MP, Graser RT, Chapman HD, Serreze DV: Functional evidence for the mediation of diabetogenic T cell responses by HLA-A2.1 MHC class I molecules through transgenic expression in NOD mice, *Proc Natl Acad Sci U S A* 99(21):13753–13758, 2002.

40. Atkinson MA, Bluestone JA, Eisenbarth GS, et al: How does type 1 diabetes develop? The notion of homicide or beta-cell suicide revisited, *Diabetes* 60(5):1370–1379, 2011.

41. Nakayama M, Beilke JN, Jasinski JM, et al: Priming and effector dependence on insulin B:9-23 peptide in NOD islet autoimmunity, *J Clin Invest* 117(7):1835–1843, 2007.

42. Mohan JF, Levisetti MG, Calderon B, et al: Unique autoreactive T cells recognize insulin peptides generated within the islets of Langerhans in autoimmune diabetes, *Nat Immunol* 11(4):350–354, 2010.

43. Ziegler AG, Hummel M, Schenker M, Bonifacio E: Autoantibody appearance and risk for development of childhood diabetes in offspring of parents with type 1 diabetes: the 2-year analysis of the German BABYDIAB study, *Diabetes* 48(3):460–468, 1999.

44. Kukko M, Kimpimäki T, Korhonen S, et al: Dynamics of diabetes-associated autoantibodies in young children with human leukocyte antigen-conferred risk of type 1 diabetes recruited from the general population, *J Clin Endocrinol Metab* 90(5):2712–2717, 2005.

45. Kimpimäki T, Kupila A, Hämäläinen AM, et al: The first signs of beta-cell autoimmunity appear in infancy in genetically susceptible children from the general population: the Finnish Type 1 Diabetes Prediction and Prevention Study, *J Clin Endocrinol Metab* 86 (10):4782–4788, 2001.

46. Durinovic-Belló I, Boehm BO, Ziegler AG: Predominantly recognized proInsulin T helper cell epitopes in individuals with and without islet cell autoimmunity, *J Autoimmun* 18(1):55–66, 2002.

47. Durinovic-Belló I, Schlosser M, Riedl M, et al: Pro- and anti-inflammatory cytokine production by autoimmune T cells against preproinsulin in HLA-DRB1*04, DQ8 type 1 diabetes, *Diabetologia* 47(3):439–450, 2004.

48. Semana G, Gausling R, Jackson RA, Hafler DA: T cell autoreactivity to proinsulin epitopes in diabetic patients and healthy subjects, *J Autoimmun* 12(4):259–267, 1999.

49. Alleva DG, Crowe PD, Jin L, et al: A disease-associated cellular immune response in type 1 diabetics to an immunodominant epitope of insulin, *J Clin Invest* 107(2):173–180, 2001.

50. Ouyang Q, Standifer NE, Qin H, et al: Recognition of HLA class I-restricted beta-cell epitopes in type 1 diabetes, *Diabetes* 55(11):3068–3074, 2006.

51. Atkinson MA, Eisenbarth GS: Type 1 diabetes: new perspectives on disease pathogenesis and treatment, *Lancet* 358(9277):221–229, 2001.

52. Baekkeskov S, Aanstoot HJ, Christgau S, et al: Identification of the 64 K autoantigen in insulin-dependent diabetes as the GABA-synthesizing enzyme glutamic acid decarboxylase, *Nature* 347(6289):151–156, 1990.

53. Dabelea D, Pihoker C, Talton JW, et al: Etiological approach to characterization of diabetes type, *Diabetes Care* 34(7):1628–1633, 2011.

54. Ludvigsson J, Krisky D, Casas R, et al: GAD65 antigen therapy in recently diagnosed type 1 diabetes mellitus, *N Engl J Med* 366(5):433–442, 2012.

55. Ellis TM, Schatz DA, Ottendorfer EW, et al: The relationship between humoral and cellular immunity to IA-2 in IDDM, *Diabetes* 47(4):566–569, 1998.

56. Énée É, Kratzer R, Arnoux JB, et al: ZnT8 is a major CD8+ T cell–recognized autoantigen in pediatric type 1 diabetes, *Diabetes* 61(7):1779–1784, 2012.

57. Wenzlau JM, Juhl K, Yu L, et al: The cation efflux transporter ZnT8 (Slc30A8) is a major autoantigen in human type 1 diabetes, *Proc Natl Acad Sci U S A* 104(43):17040–17045, 2007.

58. Howson JM, Krause S, Stevens H, et al: Genetic association of zinc transporter 8 (ZnT8) autoantibodies in type 1 diabetes cases, *Diabetologia*: 1–7, 2012.

59. Lieberman SM, Evans AM, Han B, et al: Identification of the β cell antigen targeted by a prevalent population of pathogenic CD8+ T cells in autoimmune diabetes, *Proc Natl Acad Sci U S A* 100 (14):8384–8388, 2003.

60. Gardner JM, Devoss JJ, Friedman RS, et al: Deletional tolerance mediated by extrathymic aire-expressing cells, *Science* 321(5890):843–847, 2008.

61. Han B, Serra P, Yamanouchi J, et al: Developmental control of CD8+ T cell-avidity maturation in autoimmune diabetes, *J Clin Invest* 115(7):1879, 2005.

62. Krishnamurthy B, Chee J, Jhala G, et al: Complete diabetes protection despite delayed thymic tolerance in NOD8.3 TCR transgenic mice due to antigen-induced extrathymic deletion of T cells, *Diabetes* 61(2):425–435, 2012.

63. Stadinski BD, Delong T, Reisdorph N, et al: Chromogranin A is an autoantigen in type 1 diabetes, *Nat Immunol* 11(3):225–231, 2010.

64. Nikoopour E, Sandrock C, Huszarik K, et al: Cutting edge: vasostatin-1–derived peptide ChgA29–42 is an antigenic epitope of diabetogenic BDC2.5 T cells in nonobese diabetic mice, *J Immunol* 186(7):3831–3835, 2011.

65. In't Veld P: Insulitis in human type 1 diabetes: the quest for an elusive lesion, *Islets* 3(4):131–138, 2011.

66. Hanafusa T, Imagawa A: Insulitis in human type 1 diabetes, *Ann N Y Acad Sci* 1150:297–299, 2008.

67. Kolb H, Kolb-Bachofen V, Roep BO: Autoimmune versus inflammatory type I diabetes: a controversy? *Immunol Today* 16(4):170–172, 1995.

68. Roep BO: The role of T-cells in the pathogenesis of type 1 diabetes: from cause to cure, *Diabetologia* 46(3):305–321, 2003.

69. Lehuen A, Diana J, Zaccone P, Cooke A: Immune cell crosstalk in type 1 diabetes, *Nat Rev Immunol* 10(7):501–513, 2010.

70. Seewaldt S, Thomas HE, Ejrnaes M, et al: Virus-induced autoimmune diabetes: most beta-cells die through inflammatory cytokines and not perforin from autoreactive (anti-viral) cytotoxic T-lymphocytes, *Diabetes* 49(11):1801–1809, 2000.

71. Foulis AK, Farquharson MA, Hardman R: Aberrant expression of class II major histocompatibility complex molecules by B cells and hyperexpression of class I major histocompatibility complex molecules by insulin containing islets in type 1 (insulin-dependent) diabetes mellitus, *Diabetologia* 30(5):333–343, 1987.

72. Itoh N, Hanafusa T, Miyazaki A, et al: Mononuclear cell infiltration and its relation to the expression of major histocompatibility complex antigens and adhesion molecules in pancreas biopsy specimens from newly diagnosed insulin-dependent diabetes mellitus patients, *J Clin Invest* 92 (5):2313–2322, 1993.

73. Campbell PD, Estella E, Dudek NL, et al: Cytotoxic T-lymphocyte-mediated killing of human pancreatic islet cells in vitro, *Hum Immunol* 69(9):543–551, 2008.

74. Tiedge M, Lortz S, Drinkgern J, Lenzen S: Relation between antioxidant enzyme gene expression and antioxidative defense status of insulin-producing cells, *Diabetes* 46 (11):1733–1742, 1997.

75. Lenzen S, Drinkgern J, Tiedge M: Low antioxidant enzyme gene expression in pancreatic islets compared with various other mouse tissues, *Free Radic Biol Med* 20(3):463–466, 1996.

76. Pi J, Zhang Q, Fu J, et al: ROS signaling, oxidative stress and Nrf2 in pancreatic beta-cell function, *Toxicol Appl Pharmacol* 244(1):77–83, 2010.

77. Mathis D, Vence L, Benoist C: Beta-cell death during progression to diabetes, *Nature* 414 (6865):792–798, 2001.

78. Liu D, Pavlovic D, Chen MC, et al: Cytokines induce apoptosis in beta-cells isolated from mice lacking the inducible isoform of nitric oxide synthase (iNOS–/–), *Diabetes* 49(7):1116–1122, 2000.

79. Rabinovitch A, Suarez-Pinzon WL, Strynadka K, et al: Human pancreatic islet beta-cell destruction by cytokines is independent of nitric oxide production, *J Clin Endocrinol Metab* 79(4):1058–1062, 1994.

80. Grunnet LG, Aikin R, Tonnesen MF, et al: Proinflammatory cytokines activate the intrinsic apoptotic pathway in beta-cells, *Diabetes* 58(8):1807–1815, 2009.

81. Lightfoot YL, Chen J, Mathews CE: Role of the mitochondria in immune-mediated apoptotic death of the human pancreatic beta cell line betaLox5, *PLoS One* 6(6):e20617, 2011.

82. Rabinovitch A, Suarez-Pinzon W, Strynadka K, et al: Transfection of human pancreatic islets with an anti-apoptotic gene (bcl-2) protects beta-cells from cytokine-induced destruction, *Diabetes* 48(6):1223–1229, 1999.

83. Mehmeti I, Gurgul-Convey E, Lenzen S, Lortz S: Induction of the intrinsic apoptosis pathway in insulin-secreting cells is dependent on oxidative damage of mitochondria but independent of caspase-12 activation, *Biochim Biophys Acta* 1813(10):1827–1835, 2011.

84. Lightfoot YL, Chen J, Mathews CE: Immune-mediated beta-cell death in type 1 diabetes: lessons from human beta-cell lines, *Eur J Clin Invest* 42(11):1244–1251, 2012.

85. Rabinovitch A, Suarez-Pinzon WL: Cytokines and their roles in pancreatic islet beta-cell destruction and insulin-dependent diabetes mellitus, *Biochem Pharmacol* 55(8):1139–1149, 1998.

86. Uno S, Imagawa A, Okita K, et al: Macrophages and dendritic cells infiltrating islets with or without beta cells produce tumour necrosis factor-alpha in patients with recent-onset type 1 diabetes, *Diabetologia* 50(3):596–601, 2007.

87. Soldevila G, Buscema M, Doshi M, et al: Cytotoxic effect of IFN-gamma plus TNF-alpha on human islet cells, *J Autoimmun* 4(2):291–306, 1991.

88. Kay TW, Campbell IL, Oxbrow L, Harrison LC: Overexpression of class I major histocompatibility complex accompanies insulitis in the non-obese diabetic mouse and is prevented by anti-interferon-gamma antibody, *Diabetologia* 34(11):779–785, 1991.

89. Eizirik DL, Sandler S, Palmer JP: Repair of pancreatic beta-cells. A relevant phenomenon in early IDDM? *Diabetes* 42(10):1383–1391, 1993.

90. Martin S, Wolf-Eichbaum D, Duinkerken G, et al: Development of type 1 diabetes despite severe hereditary B-lymphocyte deficiency, *N Engl J Med* 345(14):1036–1040, 2001.

91. Schatz D, Cuthbertson D, Atkinson M, et al: Preservation of C-peptide secretion in subjects at high risk of developing type 1 diabetes mellitus—a new surrogate measure of non-progression? *Pediatr Diabetes* 5(2):72–79, 2004.

92. Savola K, Bonifacio E, Sabbah E, et al: IA-2 antibodies—a sensitive marker of IDDM with clinical onset in childhood and adolescence. Childhood Diabetes in Finland Study Group, *Diabetologia* 41(4):424–429, 1998.

93. Pescovitz MD, Greenbaum CJ, Krause-Steinrauf H, et al: Rituximab, B-lymphocyte depletion, and preservation of beta-cell function, *N Engl J Med* 361(22):2143–2152, 2009.

94. Hu CY, Rodriguez-Pinto D, Du W, et al: Treatment with CD20-specific antibody prevents and reverses autoimmune diabetes in mice, *J Clin Invest* 117(12):3857–3867, 2007.

95. Hutchings PR, Cooke A: The transfer of autoimmune diabetes in NOD mice can be inhibited or accelerated by distinct cell populations present in normal splenocytes taken from young males, *J Autoimmun* 3(2):175–185, 1990.

96. Jun HS, Yoon CS, Zbytnuik L, et al: The role of macrophages in T cell-mediated autoimmune diabetes in nonobese diabetic mice, *J Exp Med* 189(2):347–358, 1999.

97. Alleva DG, Pavlovich RP, Grant C, et al: Aberrant macrophage cytokine production is a conserved feature among autoimmune-prone mouse strains: elevated interleukin (IL)-12 and an imbalance in tumor necrosis factor-alpha and IL-10 define a unique cytokine profile in macrophages from young nonobese diabetic mice, *Diabetes* 49(7):1106–1115, 2000.

98. O'Brien BA, Huang Y, Geng X, et al: Phagocytosis of apoptotic cells by macrophages from NOD mice is reduced, *Diabetes* 51(8):2481–2488, 2002.

99. Ueno H, Klechevsky E, Morita R, et al: Dendritic cell subsets in health and disease, *Immunol Rev* 219:118–142, 2007.

100. Tang Q, Bluestone JA: The Foxp3+ regulatory T cell: a jack of all trades, master of regulation, *Nat Immunol* 9(3):239–244, 2008.

101. Kared H, Masson A, Adle-Biassette H, et al: Treatment with granulocyte colony-stimulating factor prevents diabetes in NOD mice by recruiting plasmacytoid dendritic cells and functional CD4(+) CD25(+) regulatory T-cells, *Diabetes* 54(1):78–84, 2005.
102. Diana J, Griseri T, Lagaye S, et al: NKT cell-plasmacytoid dendritic cell cooperation via OX40 controls viral infection in a tissue-specific manner, *Immunity* 30(2):289–299, 2009.
103. Diana J, Gahzarian L, Simoni Y, Lehuen A: Innate immunity in type 1 diabetes, *Discov Med* 11 (61):513–520, 2011.
104. Brauner H, Elemans M, Lemos S, et al: Distinct phenotype and function of NK cells in the pancreas of nonobese diabetic mice, *J Immunol* 184(5):2272–2280, 2010.
105. Carnaud C, Gombert J, Donnars O, et al: Protection against diabetes and improved NK/NKT cell performance in NOD.NK1.1 mice congenic at the NK complex, *J Immunol* 166(4):2404–2411, 2001.
106. Feuerer M, Shen Y, Littman DR, et al: How punctual ablation of regulatory T cells unleashes an autoimmune lesion within the pancreatic islets, *Immunity* 31(4):654–664, 2009.
107. Alba A, Planas R, Clemente X, et al: Natural killer cells are required for accelerated type 1 diabetes driven by interferon-beta, *Clin Exp Immunol* 151(3):467–475, 2008.
108. Flodström M, Maday A, Balakrishna D, et al: Target cell defense prevents the development of diabetes after viral infection, *Nat Immunol* 3(4):373–382, 2002.
109. Novak J, Griseri T, Beaudoin L, Lehuen A: Regulation of type 1 diabetes by NKT cells, *Int Rev Immunol* 26(1–2):49–72, 2007.
110. Novak J, Lehuen A: Mechanism of regulation of autoimmunity by iNKT cells, *Cytokine* 53 (3):263–270, 2011.
111. Forestier C, Takaki T, Molano A, et al: Improved outcomes in NOD mice treated with a novel Th2 cytokine-biasing NKT cell activator, *J Immunol* 178(3):1415–1425, 2007.
112. Redondo MJ, Jeffrey J, Fain PR, et al: Concordance for islet autoimmunity among monozygotic twins, *N Engl J Med* 359(26):2849–2850, 2008.
113. Noble JA, Valdes AM, Cook M, et al: The role of HLA class II genes in insulin-dependent diabetes mellitus: molecular analysis of 180 Caucasian, multiplex families, *Am J Hum Genet* 59 (5):1134–1148, 1996.
114. Pociot F, Akolkar B, Concannon P, et al: Genetics of type 1 diabetes: what's next? *Diabetes* 59 (7):1561–1571, 2010.
115. Rewers M, Bugawan TL, Norris JM, et al: Newborn screening for HLA markers associated with IDDM: diabetes autoimmunity study in the young (DAISY), *Diabetologia* 39(7):807–812, 1996.
116. Aly TA, Ide A, Jahromi MM, et al: Extreme genetic risk for type 1A diabetes, *Proc Natl Acad Sci U S A* 103(38):14074–14079, 2006.
117. Pugliese A, Gianani R, Moromisato R, et al: HLA-DQB1*0602 is associated with dominant protection from diabetes even among islet cell antibody-positive first-degree relatives of patients with IDDM, *Diabetes* 44(6):608–613, 1995.
118. Lipponen K, Gombos Z, Kiviniemi M, et al: Effect of HLA class I and class II alleles on progression from autoantibody positivity to overt type 1 diabetes in children with risk-associated class II genotypes, *Diabetes* 59(12):3253–3256, 2010.
119. Zehn D, Bevan MJ: T cells with low avidity for a tissue-restricted antigen routinely evade central and peripheral tolerance and cause autoimmunity, *Immunity* 25(2):261–270, 2006.
120. Complete sequence and gene map of a human major histocompatibility complex. The MHC sequencing consortium, *Nature* 401(6756):921–923, 1999.
121. Eike MC, Olsson M, Undlien DE, et al: Genetic variants of the HLA-A, HLA-B and AIF1 loci show independent associations with type 1 diabetes in Norwegian families, *Genes Immun* 10 (2):141–150, 2009.
122. Onkamo P, Väänänen S, Karvonen M, Tuomilehto J: Worldwide increase in incidence of Type I diabetes—the analysis of the data on published incidence trends, *Diabetologia* 42 (12):1395–1403, 1999.
123. Steck AK, Rewers MJ: Genetics of type 1 diabetes, *Clin Chem* 57(2):176–185, 2011.
124. Bell GI, Horita S, Karam JH: A polymorphic locus near the human insulin gene is associated with insulin-dependent diabetes mellitus, *Diabetes* 33(2):176–183, 1984.
125. Pugliese A, Zeller M, Fernandez A Jr, , et al: The insulin gene is transcribed in the human thymus and transcription levels correlated with allelic variation at the INS VNTR-IDDM2 susceptibility locus for type 1 diabetes, *Nat Genet* 15(3):293–297, 1997.
126. Vafiadis P, Bennett ST, Todd JA, et al: Insulin expression in human thymus is modulated by INS VNTR alleles at the IDDM2 locus, *Nat Genet* 15(3):289–292, 1997.
127. Bennett ST, Lucassen AM, Gough SC, et al: Susceptibility to human type 1 diabetes at IDDM2 is determined by tandem repeat variation at the insulin gene minisatellite locus, *Nat Genet* 9 (3):284–292, 1995.
128. Lucassen AM, Julier C, Beressi JP, et al: Susceptibility to insulin dependent diabetes mellitus maps to a 4.1 kb segment of DNA spanning the insulin gene and associated VNTR, *Nat Genet* 4(3):305–310, 1993.
129. Durinovic-Belló I, Wu RP, Gersuk VH, et al: Insulin gene VNTR genotype associates with frequency and phenotype of the autoimmune response to proinsulin, *Genes Immun* 11 (2):188–193, 2010.
130. Anderson MS, Venanzi ES, Klein L, et al: Projection of an immunological self shadow within the thymus by the aire protein, *Science* 298(5597):1395–1401, 2002.
131. Zhernakova A, Eerligh P, Barrera P, et al: CTLA4 is differentially associated with autoimmune diseases in the Dutch population, *Hum Genet* 118(1):58–66, 2005.
132. Wing K, Onishi Y, Prieto-Martin P, et al: CTLA-4 control over Foxp3+ regulatory T cell function, *Science* 322(5899):271–275, 2008.
133. Kolar P, Knieke K, Hegel JK, et al: CTLA-4 (CD152) controls homeostasis and suppressive capacity of regulatory T cells in mice, *Arthritis Rheum* 60(1):123–132, 2009.
134. Rydén A, Bolmeson C, Jonson CO, et al: Low expression and secretion of circulating soluble CTLA-4 in peripheral blood mononuclear cells and sera from type 1 diabetic children, *Diabetes Metab Res Rev* 28(1):84–96, 2012.
135. Bottini N, Musumeci L, Alonso A, et al: A functional variant of lymphoid tyrosine phosphatase is associated with type I diabetes, *Nat Genet* 36(4):337–338, 2004.
136. Lempainen J, Hermann R, Veijola R, et al: Effect of the PTPN22 and INS risk genotypes on the progression to clinical type 1 diabetes after the initiation of β-cell autoimmunity, *Diabetes* 61 (4):963–966, 2012.
137. Steck AK, Zhang W, Bugawan TL, et al: Do non-HLA genes influence development of persistent islet autoimmunity and type 1 diabetes in children with high-risk HLA-DR, DQ genotypes? *Diabetes* 58(4):1028–1033, 2009.
138. Vang T, Congia M, Macis MD, et al: Autoimmune-associated lymphoid tyrosine phosphatase is a gain-of-function variant, *Nat Genet* 37(12):1317–1319, 2005.
139. Liu S, Wang H, Jin Y, et al: IFIH1 polymorphisms are significantly associated with type 1 diabetes and IFIH1 gene expression in peripheral blood mononuclear cells, *Hum Mol Genet* 18 (2):358–365, 2009.
140. Kato H, Takeuchi O, Sato S, et al: Differential roles of MDA5 and RIG-I helicases in the recognition of RNA viruses, *Nature* 441(7089):101–105, 2006.
141. von Herrath M: Diabetes: a virus-gene collaboration, *Nature* 459(7246):518–519, 2009.
142. Vella A, Cooper JD, Lowe CE, et al: Localization of a type 1 diabetes locus in the IL2RA/CD25 region by use of tag single-nucleotide polymorphisms, *Am J Hum Genet* 76(5):773–779, 2005.
143. Salomon B, Lenschow DJ, Rhee L, et al: B7/CD28 costimulation is essential for the homeostasis of the CD4+CD25+ immunoregulatory T cells that control autoimmune diabetes, *Immunity* 12 (4):431–440, 2000.
144. Garg G, Tyler JR, Yang JH, et al: Type 1 diabetes-associated IL2RA variation lowers IL-2 signaling and contributes to diminished CD4+CD25+ regulatory T cell function, *J Immunol* 188 (9):4644–4653, 2012 May 1.
145. Warram JH, Krolewski AS, Gottlieb MS, Kahn CR: Differences in risk of insulin-dependent diabetes in offspring of diabetic mothers and diabetic fathers, *N Engl J Med* 311(3):149–152, 1984.
146. Miao F, Smith DD, Zhang L, et al: Lymphocytes from patients with type 1 diabetes display a distinct profile of chromatin histone H3 lysine 9 dimethylation: an epigenetic study in diabetes, *Diabetes* 57(12):3189–3198, 2008.
147. Miao F, Chen Z, Zhang L, et al: Profiles of epigenetic histone post-translational modifications at type 1 diabetes susceptible genes, *J Biol Chem* 287(20):16335–16345, 2012.
148. Fradin D, Le Fur S, Mille C, et al: Association of the CpG methylation pattern of the proximal insulin gene promoter with type 1 diabetes, *PLoS One* 7(5):e36278, 2012.
149. Bettini ML, Pan F, Bettini M, et al: Loss of epigenetic modification driven by the Foxp3 transcription factor leads to regulatory T cell insufficiency, *Immunity* 36(5):717–730, 2012.
150. Rewers M, Barriga K, Baxter J, et al: The environmental determinants of diabetes in the young (TEDDY) study, *Ann N Y Acad Sci* 1150:1–13, 2008.
151. Virtanen SM, Hyppönen E, Läärä E, et al: Cow's milk consumption, disease-associated autoantibodies and type 1 diabetes mellitus: a follow-up study in siblings of diabetic children. Childhood Diabetes in Finland Study Group, *Diabet Med* 15(9):730–738, 1998.
152. Vaarala O, Ilonen J, Ruohtula T, et al: Removal of bovine insulin from cow's milk formula and early initiation of beta-cell autoimmunity in the FINDIA pilot study, *Arch Pediatr Adolesc Med,* 2012, p. archpediatrics, 608–614, 2011.
153. Virtanen SM, Nevalainen J, Kronberg-Kippilä C, et al: Food consumption and advanced beta cell autoimmunity in young children with HLA-conferred susceptibility to type 1 diabetes: a nested case-control design, *Am J Clin Nutr* 95(2):471–478, 2012.
154. Karjalainen J, Martin JM, Knip M, et al: A bovine albumin peptide as a possible trigger of insulin-dependent diabetes mellitus, *N Engl J Med* 327(5):302–307, 1992.
155. Vaarala O, Knip M, Paronen J, et al: Cow's milk formula feeding induces primary immunization to insulin in infants at genetic risk for type 1 diabetes, *Diabetes* 48(7):1389–1394, 1999.
156. Kimpimäki T, Erkkola M, Korhonen S, et al: Short-term exclusive breastfeeding predisposes young children with increased genetic risk of Type I diabetes to progressive beta-cell autoimmunity, *Diabetologia* 44(1):63–69, 2001.
157. Sadeharju K, Knip M, Virtanen SM, et al: Maternal antibodies in breast milk protect the child from enterovirus infections, *Pediatrics* 119(5):941–946, 2007.
158. Couper JJ, Steele C, Beresford S, et al: Lack of association between duration of breast-feeding or introduction of cow's milk and development of islet autoimmunity, *Diabetes* 48(11):2145–2149, 1999.
159. Hummel M, Bonifacio E, Naserke HE, Ziegler AG: Elimination of dietary gluten does not reduce titers of type 1 diabetes-associated autoantibodies in high-risk subjects, *Diabetes Care* 25 (7):1111–1116, 2002.
160. Norris JM, Barriga K, Klingensmith G, et al: Timing of initial cereal exposure in infancy and risk of islet autoimmunity, *JAMA* 290(13):1713–1720, 2003.
161. Ziegler AG, Schmid S, Huber D, et al: Early infant feeding and risk of developing type 1 diabetes-associated autoantibodies, *JAMA* 290(13):1721–1728, 2003.
162. Norris JM: Infant and childhood diet and type 1 diabetes risk: recent advances and prospects, *Curr Diab Rep* 10(5):345–349, 2010.
163. Pastore MR, Bazzigaluppi E, Belloni C, et al: Six months of gluten-free diet do not influence autoantibody titers, but improve insulin secretion in subjects at high risk for type 1 diabetes, *J Clin Endocrinol Metab* 88(1):162–165, 2003.
164. Hummel S, Pflüger M, Hummel M, et al: Primary dietary intervention study to reduce the risk of islet autoimmunity in children at increased risk for type 1 diabetes, *Diabetes Care* 34 (6):1301–1305, 2011.
165. Hyppönen E, Läärä E, Reunanen A, et al: Intake of vitamin D and risk of type 1 diabetes: a birth-cohort study, *Lancet* 358(9292):1500–1503, 2001.
166. Räsänen M, Kronberg-Kippilä C, Ahonen S, et al: Intake of vitamin D by Finnish children aged 3 months to 3 years in relation to sociodemographic factors, *Eur J Clin Nutr* 60(11):1317–1322, 2006.
167. Viskari H, Kondrashova A, Koskela P, et al: Circulating vitamin D concentrations in two neighboring populations with markedly different incidence of type 1 diabetes, *Diabetes Care* 29(6):1458–1459, 2006.
168. Simpson M, Brady H, Yin X, et al: No association of vitamin D intake or 25-hydroxyvitamin D levels in childhood with risk of islet autoimmunity and type 1 diabetes: the Diabetes Autoimmunity Study in the Young (DAISY), *Diabetologia* 54(11):2779–2788, 2011.
169. Norris JM, Yin X, Lamb MM, et al: Omega-3 polyunsaturated fatty acid intake and islet autoimmunity in children at increased risk for type 1 diabetes, *JAMA* 298(12):1420–1428, 2007.
170. Stene LC, Joner G: Use of cod liver oil during the first year of life is associated with lower risk of childhood-onset type 1 diabetes: a large, population-based, case-control study, *Am J Clin Nutr* 78 (6):1128–1134, 2003.
171. Sairenji T, Daibata M, Sorli CH, et al: Relating homology between the Epstein-Barr virus BOLF1 molecule and HLA-DQw8 beta chain to recent onset type 1 (insulin-dependent) diabetes mellitus, *Diabetologia* 34(1):33–39, 1991.
172. Hyöty H, Hiltunen M, Reunanen A, et al: Decline of mumps antibodies in type 1 (insulin-dependent) diabetic children and a plateau in the rising incidence of type 1 diabetes after introduction of the mumps-measles-rubella vaccine in Finland. Childhood Diabetes in Finland Study Group, *Diabetologia* 36(12):1303–1308, 1993.
173. Ginsberg-Fellner F, Witt ME, Yagihashi S, et al: Congenital rubella syndrome as a model for type 1 (insulin-dependent) diabetes mellitus: increased prevalence of islet cell surface antibodies, *Diabetologia* 27(Suppl):87–89, 1984.
174. Akerblom HK, Knip M: Putative environmental factors in Type 1 diabetes, *Diabetes Metab Rev* 14 (1):31–67, 1998.
175. Conrad B, Weidmann E, Trucco G, et al: Evidence for superantigen involvement in insulin-dependent diabetes mellitus aetiology, *Nature* 371(6495):351–355, 1994.
176. Clements GB, Galbraith DN, Taylor KW: Coxsackie B virus infection and onset of childhood diabetes, *Lancet* 346(8969):221–223, 1995.
177. Nairn C, Galbraith DN, Taylor KW, Clements GB: Enterovirus variants in the serum of children at the onset of type 1 diabetes mellitus, *Diabet Med* 16(6):509–513, 1999.
178. Elfving M, Svensson J, Oikarinen S, et al: Maternal enterovirus infection during pregnancy as a risk factor in offspring diagnosed with type 1 diabetes between 15 and 30 years of age, *Exp Diabetes Res* 2008:271958, 2008.
179. Dahlquist GG, Boman JE, Juto P: Enteroviral RNA and IgM antibodies in early pregnancy and risk for childhood-onset IDDM in offspring, *Diabetes Care* 22(2):364–365, 1999.
180. Dahlquist GG, Ivarsson S, Lindberg B, Forsgren M: Maternal enteroviral infection during pregnancy as a risk factor for childhood IDDM. A population-based case-control study, *Diabetes* 44(4):408–413, 1995.
181. Couper JJ: Environmental triggers of type 1 diabetes, *J Paediatr Child Health* 37(3):218–220, 2001.
182. Bach JF: Infections and autoimmune diseases, *J Autoimmun* 25(Suppl):74–80, 2005.
183. McKinney PA, Okasha M, Parslow RC, et al: Early social mixing and childhood Type 1 diabetes mellitus: a case-control study in Yorkshire, UK, *Diabet Med* 17(3):236–242, 2000.
184. Tracy S, Drescher KM: Coxsackievirus infections and NOD mice: relevant models of protection from, and induction of, type 1 diabetes, *Ann N Y Acad Sci* 1103:143–151, 2007.

185. Lönnrot M, Korpela K, Knip M, et al: Enterovirus infection as a risk factor for beta-cell autoimmunity in a prospectively observed birth cohort: the Finnish Diabetes Prediction and Prevention Study, *Diabetes* 49(8):1314–1318, 2000.

186. Hyöty H, Hiltunen M, Knip M, et al: A prospective study of the role of coxsackie B and other enterovirus infections in the pathogenesis of IDDM. Childhood Diabetes in Finland (DiMe) Study Group, *Diabetes* 44(6):652–657, 1995.

187. Blom L, Nystrom L, Dahlquist G: The Swedish childhood diabetes study. Vaccinations and infections as risk determinants for diabetes in childhood, *Diabetologia* 34(3):176–181, 1991.

188. Infections and vaccinations as risk factors for childhood type 1 (insulin-dependent) diabetes mellitus: a multicentre case-control investigation. EURODIAB Substudy 2 Study Group, *Diabetologia* 43(1):47–53, 2000.

189. Field LL, Bonnevie-Nielsen V, Pociot F, et al: OAS1 splice site polymorphism controlling antiviral enzyme activity influences susceptibility to type 1 diabetes, *Diabetes* 54(5):1588–1591, 2005.

190. Yoneyama M, Kikuchi M, Matsumoto K, et al: Shared and unique functions of the DExD/H-box helicases RIG-I, MDA5, and LGP2 in antiviral innate immunity, *J Immunol* 175(5):2851–2858, 2005.

191. Meylan E, Tschopp J, Karin M: Intracellular pattern recognition receptors in the host response, *Nature* 442(7098):39–44, 2006.

192. D'Alessio DJ: A case-control study of group B coxsackievirus immunoglobulin M antibody prevalence and HLA-DR antigens in newly diagnosed cases of insulin-dependent diabetes mellitus, *Am J Epidemiol* 135(12):1331–1338, 1992.

193. Oikarinen S, Martiskainen M, Tauriainen S, et al: Enterovirus RNA in blood is linked to the development of type 1 diabetes, *Diabetes* 60(1):276–279, 2011.

194. Hyppönen E, Kenward MG, Virtanen SM, et al: Infant feeding, early weight gain, and risk of type 1 diabetes. Childhood Diabetes in Finland (DiMe) Study Group, *Diabetes Care* 22(12):1961–1965, 1999.

195. Sepa A, Wahlberg J, Vaarala O, et al: Psychological stress may induce diabetes-related autoimmunity in infancy, *Diabetes Care* 28(2):290–295, 2005.

196. Robinson N, Lloyd CE, Fuller JH, Yateman NA: Psychosocial factors and the onset of type 1 diabetes, *Diabet Med* 6(1):53–58, 1989.

197. Karavanaki K, Tsoka E, Liacopoulou M, et al: Psychological stress as a factor potentially contributing to the pathogenesis of type 1 diabetes mellitus, *J Endocrinol Invest* 31(5):406–415, 2008.

198. Calcinaro F, Dionisi S, Marinaro M, et al: Oral probiotic administration induces interleukin-10 production and prevents spontaneous autoimmune diabetes in the non-obese diabetic mouse, *Diabetologia* 48(8):1565–1575, 2005.

199. Valladares R, Sankar D, Li N, et al: *Lactobacillus johnsonii* N6.2 mitigates the development of type 1 diabetes in BB-DP rats, *PLoS One* 5(5):e10507, 2010.

4 The Metabolic Syndrome
Prevalence and Controversies in Clinical Context

Frank Pistrosch, Frank Schaper, and Markolf Hanefeld

The metabolic syndrome (MetS) is defined as clustering of metabolic components that occur together more often than by chance alone and predispose to atherosclerotic vascular disease and diabetes. First descriptions of associated metabolic diseases occurred at the beginning of the last century when Kylin reported a connection between hyperglycemia, hypertension, and gout.[1] Thus, the intention with the introduction of MetS was primarily to get a clinical tool or common term for an interrelated cluster of metabolic diseases. Later, Vague realized the central role of android obesity in this cluster of diseases and connected MetS with atherosclerotic vascular disease.[2] This then was extended to "plurimetabolic syndrome," associated with increased risk of cardiovascular disease (CVD), by Crepaldi and colleagues.[3] In 1981 the first definition of MetS was published, connecting classical interrelated metabolic diseases with hypertension and atherosclerotic vascular diseases:

"The metabolic syndrome represents the common prevalence of obesity, hyper- and dys-lipoproteinaemia, maturity onset diabetes (type 2), gout and hypertension associated with increased incidence of atherosclerotic vascular disease, fatty liver and gallstones that develop on the basis of genetic susceptibility combined with over-nutrition and physical inactivity. If this working hypothesis can be confirmed it provides the basis for integrated diagnostics and prevention of this cluster of diseases, which is of central importance for health care."[4]

Despite these clear descriptions of the main components of MetS that might identify individuals at higher risk of atherosclerotic vascular disease that extend beyond classic risk factors—for example, age, sex, low-density lipoprotein (LDL) cholesterol, and smoking—the clinical and scientific usefulness of the concept of MetS is still an issue of debate. The main reason for this controversy might be the lack of a generally accepted definition of the syndrome: simple clinical measures are used to identify complex disorders, and cutoff limits were defined without sufficient epidemiologic data.

With the introduction of arbitrary cutoff limits for accepted components, there are now different definitions put forth by international and national institutions, including the World Health Organization (WHO),[5] the American Heart Association (AHA) and U.S. National Institutes of Health

National Heart, Lung, and Blood Institute (NHLBI),[6] and the International Diabetes Federation (IDF) (**Table 4-1**).[7]

The consequence of these different definitions based on arbitrary cutoff limits was a different estimation of the prevalence of patients with MetS.[8,9] Moreover, MetS according to IDF criteria had only a weak relationship to cardiovascular risk, because it was focused on insulin resistance, obesity, and dysglycemia as risk factors for diabetes. Thus it was not surprising that the usefulness of the concept was questioned in a joint statement of the ADA and the European Association for the Study of Diabetes (EASD).[10]

To overcome confusion and the waste of resources resulting from competing parallel investigations, a unifying concept and definitions were recently adopted (see **Table 4-1**).[11]

Here we analyze the association of MetS with CVD according to the primary idea behind a syndrome that is a tool to search for other components interrelated with the lead trait or disease.

ASSOCIATION BETWEEN METABOLIC SYNDROME AND CARDIOVASCULAR DISEASE IN THE POPULATION

The global prevalence of MetS in the adult population varies from 15% to 50%. The estimated prevalence is affected by multiple factors such as age, sex, nutrition habits, lifestyle factors, socioeconomic conditions, and ethnicity as major determinants in addition to variability in the proposed definitions.[12,13]

MetS is not an absolute risk indicator because it does not involve many of the factors that determine absolute cardiovascular risk—for example, smoking, age, sex, and LDL cholesterol level.[11] Therefore it is not surprising that the usefulness of MetS as an independent cardiovascular risk indicator is a matter of controversy.

Most studies have revealed an increased risk for the development of CVD associated with MetS.[14–19] A meta-analysis of 36 longitudinal studies found a hazard ratio of 1.78 (95% confidence interval [CI] 1.58-2.00) for incident CVD events and death in individuals with MetS.[17] An analysis of the Framingham database also demonstrated an increased age-adjusted CVD risk of 2.88 (95% CI 1.99-4.16) for men and 2.25 (95% CI 1.31-3.88) for women with MetS.[18]

TABLE 4-1 Definitions of Metabolic Syndrome According to WHO, AHA/NHLBI, and IDF at the Beginning of the 21st Century and Consensus Statement 2009

WHO (1999)[5]	AHA/NHLBI (2005)[6]	IDF (2005)[7]	CONSENSUS STATEMENT CRITERIA (2009)[11]
NGT: Two criteria plus insulin resistance (highest quartiles of HOMA-IR) IFG or IGT: Two criteria	Three or more criteria	Central obesity as precondition Waist: Male ≥94 cm Female ≥80 cm Plus two or more criteria	
Dyslipidemia: TG ≥1.7 mmol/L (150 mg/dL) and/or HDL-C ↓: Male <0.9 (35 mg/dL) Female <1.0 mmol/L (40 mg/dL) Hypertension: ≥140/90 mm Hg Obesity: BMI >30 kg/m² WHR: Male >0.9 Female >0.85 Microalbuminuria: ≥20 µg/min	Hypertriglyceridemia: TG ≥1.7 mmol/L (150 mg/dL) or Rx HDL-C ↓: Male <1.04 (40 mg/dL) Female <1.29 mmol/L (50 mg/dL) Hypertension: ≥130/85* mm Hg or Rx Central obesity: Male ≥102 cm Female ≥88 cm WC Fasting PG: ≥6.1 mmol/L (110 mg/dL) or Rx	Hypertriglyceridemia: TG ≥1.7 mmol/L (150 mg/dL) or Rx HDL-C ↓: Male <1.04 (40 mg/dL) Female <1.29 mmol/L (50 mg/dL) or Rx Elevated blood pressure: ≥130/85* mm Hg or Rx Fasting PG: ≥5.6 mmol/L (100 mg/dL) (OGTT recommended)	Hypertriglyceridemia: TG ≥1.7 mmol/L (150 mg/dL) HDL-C ↓: Male <1.03 (40 mg/dL) Female: <1.29 mmol/L (50 mg/dL) Blood pressure: ≥130/85 mmHg Obesity/waist: depends on country-specific definitions Fasting PG: ≥5.6 mmol/L (100 mg/dL) or Rx

AHA=American Heart Association; BMI=body mass index; HDL-C=high-density lipoprotein cholesterol; HOMA-IR=homeostatic model assessment, insulin resistance; IDF=International Diabetes Federation; IFG=impaired fasting glucose; IGT=impaired glucose tolerance; NGT=normal glucose tolerance; NHLBI=National Heart, Lung, and Blood Institute; OGTT=oral glucose tolerance test; PG=plasma glucose; TG=triglycerides; WC=waist circumference; WHO=World Health Organization; WHR=waist-to-hip ratio.
*Systolic and/or diastolic.

Obviously there is an association between the increase of CVD risk and the number of features of MetS.[19] Recently published data from a large population-based meta-analysis that included more than 900,000 patients showed a twofold increase in cardiovascular events and a 1.5-fold increase in all-cause mortality rates in patients with MetS. The cardiovascular risk was still high in patients with MetS but without diabetes.[20] MetS according to National Cholesterol Education Program—Adult Treatment Panel III (NCEP-ATP III) criteria could also be confirmed to be associated with CVD in Asian populations.[21,22]

There are few contradictory studies. In two large prospective studies, Sattar and colleagues[23] found that MetS had only a weak or no association with cardiovascular risk in an elderly population representative of the United Kingdom. In these prospective studies, however, MetS was a major risk factor for type 2 diabetes. Therefore the authors concluded that there is no common soil for diabetes and CVD based on MetS classification. Overall, there is sufficient evidence that patients with MetS are at twice the risk of developing CVD over the next 5 to 10 years,[11] and in all related studies there was an approximately twofold higher prevalence of MetS in comparable cohorts with major CVDs (coronary heart disease, cerebrovascular disease, stroke).[24,25]

It is interesting to see that in the United States, obesity, diabetes, and coronary heart disease develop in parallel, with some lag time for development of coronary heart disease (**Table 4-2**).[16]

The same phenomenon can be observed in the process of globalization and westernization in numerous other countries.[26]

The next question that arises is whether the outcome of CVD might be associated with MetS. In the Acute Coronary Syndrome (ACS) Israeli Survey, the outcomes of 1060 patients with ACS have been evaluated. Multivariable analysis identified MetS as a strong independent predictor of 30-day and 1-year mortality after ACS events, with hazard ratios of 2.54 (95% CI 1.22-5.31) and 1.96 (95% CI 1.18-3.24), respectively.[27]

In a study of 633 consecutive patients hospitalized with acute myocardial infarction, patients with (n=290) and without (n=343) MetS were compared. Acute myocardial infarction characteristics and left ventricular ejection fraction at admission were not statistically different between the groups. In-hospital case fatality was higher in patients with MetS compared with those without, as was the incidence of severe heart failure (Killip class II or greater). In multivariable analysis, MetS was a strong and independent predictor of severe heart failure, but not in-hospital death. Analysis of the predictive value of each of the five MetS components for severe heart failure showed that hyperglycemia was the major predictor (odds ratio [OR] 3.31; 95% CI 1.86-5.87).[28] These data demonstrate a worse outcome of CVD in patients with MetS.

There are fewer data available concerning MetS and cerebrovascular disease. A 14-year longitudinal cohort study comprising 1131 men (114 [10%] with and 1017 without MetS) has shown that MetS was associated with all types of stroke (OR 2.05 (95% CI, 1.03 to 4.11)); 65 strokes occurred during the monitoring, 47 of which were ischemic.[29]

After a 14-year follow-up in 2097 individuals with initial high prevalence of MetS (men 30.3%, women 24.7%), 75 men and 55 women sustained the first stroke. The age-adjusted relative risk of stroke in individuals with diabetes and MetS was high (OR 3.28; 95% CI 1.82-5.92), higher than that of any other MetS phenotype. In this study, with a high prevalence of MetS, MetS was also an independent risk factor for stroke in individuals without diabetes.[30]

ASSOCIATIONS BETWEEN METABOLIC SYNDROME AND INTERMEDIATE MARKERS OF CARDIOVASCULAR DISEASE

In a meta-analysis of data from patients with quantitative coronary angiography who underwent intravascular ultrasound, MetS was crudely associated with increased

TABLE 4-2 Prevalence of the Metabolic Syndrome According to Criteria of the National Cholesterol Education Program—Adult Treatment Panel III (NCEP-ATP-III); 1998 and 1999 World Health Organization Criteria, Diabetes (DM) and Coronary Heart Disease (CHD) by Age Group among U.S. Population ≥20 years

AGE	1998 WHO (N = 35.8 M)	1999 WHO (N = 41.3 M)	NCEP-ATP-III (N = 48.4 M)	DM (N = 14.0 M)	CHD (N = 12.2 M)
20-29 years (36 M)	4.9%	4.9%	6.0%	0.5%	1.9%
30-39 years (42 M)	11.0%	11.1%	14.2%	2.0%	3.4%
40-49 years (42 M)	19.3%	21.2%	24.6%	5.0%	4.5%
50-59 years (30 M)	28.5%	32.4%	36.5%	12.9%	7.5%
60-69 years (20 M)	35.3%	42.0%	48.1%	17.7%	11.9%
70-79 years (16 M)	35.0%	44.3%	48.4%	18.4%	16.1%
80+ years (9 M)	22.4%	27.7%	43.3%	15.5%	17.9%

Data from Alexander CM, Landsman PB, Teutsch SM, et al: NCEP-defined metabolic syndrome, diabetes, and prevalence of coronary heart disease among NHANES III participants age 50 years and older, *Diabetes* 52:1210; 2003.

progression of plaque atheroma volume.[31] The main independent predictive factors for progression were hypertriglyceridemia (OR 1.26; 95% CI 1.06-1.49) and a body mass index exceeding 30 kg/m² (OR 1.18; 95% CI 1.00-1.40). However, after adjusting for these two components, MetS itself disappeared as an independent predictor for plaque atheroma progression. This is in line with studies from Sundström and colleagues,[32] who reported that MetS did not predict cardiovascular mortality independently of its individual components. This illustrates that the components of MetS have partially overlapping pathophysiologic mechanisms. Therefore their total combined effect could be less than the sum of individual effects.

In the Nijmegen Biomedical Study several noninvasive measurements of atherosclerosis were performed in 1517 participants aged 50 to 70 years with and without MetS.[33] Participants with MetS by NCEP-ATP III criteria were characterized by increased subclinical atherosclerosis compared with participants without any trait of MetS, as reflected by increased pulse wave velocity, increased carotid intimamedia thickness (IMT), and thicker carotid plaques. The number of MetS traits was strongly associated with the severity of subclinical atherosclerosis. It is interesting to note that noninvasive measurements of atherosclerosis were already notably worse when one or two traits of MetS were present, with increasing prevalence and severity when four or five traits were present.

Carotid IMT and plaque volume were examined by ultrasound in a total of 166 individuals (73 with MetS versus 93 without MetS).[34] Increased IMT was observed in patients with versus without MetS (0.818 mm versus 0.746 mm; P < 0.05), as well as increased total plaque volume (125 ± 26 versus 77.3 ± 17.0 mm³, respectively; P = 0.039). The higher the number of risk factors that characterize MetS, the greater the increase in the IMT.

In a cross-sectional study, MetS (n = 95) was associated with an increased common carotid IMT thickness of more than 16% (P = 0.002) and increased arterial stiffness of more than 32% (P = 0.012) compared with patients without MetS (n = 376).[35]

CARDIOVASCULAR DISEASES AND METABOLIC SYNDROME IN PATIENTS WITH ABNORMAL GLUCOSE TOLERANCE

It is a consistent finding that type 2 diabetes is present in more than 70% of patients with MetS.[36,37] In the Diabetes in Germany (DIG) study, a population-based observational study with more than 4000 patients, more than 75% had MetS by NCEP-ATP III criteria; most of them had three or four MetS component criteria (**Table 4-3**).[38] Among individual permuted phenotypes, the triplet of hypertension plus obesity and hypertriglyceridemia was the most commonly observed criterion identifying participants with MetS.

Already patients with impaired glucose tolerance (IGT) exhibit an increase in prevalence of MetS compared with subjects with normal glucose tolerance in the same age range. Approximately every second subject with IGT is diagnosed with MetS.[39,40]

Dysglycemia as a cardiovascular risk factor develops along a continuum up to the upper normal range for fasting and postprandial plasma glucose levels.[41,42] There exists overwhelming evidence that cardiovascular events and progression of vascular lesions in diabetes strongly depend on the presence of comorbidities such as hypertension and dyslipidemia—two major traits of MetS. As shown in **Table 4-3**, hypertension and hypertriglyceridemia are the most frequent single traits in type 2 diabetes patients in Germany.

With the dominance of hypertension and lipids as single risk factors, it is not surprising that different phenotypes or combinations of MetS bear different cardiovascular risks. In the DIG study the highest risk for all combinations that are displayed in **Table 4-4** was for those patients with three or more component criteria that included hypertension with any combination of two or more other traits. In all combinations with hypertension, women had a higher cardiovascular risk than men. However, quartets and quintets of component MetS criteria had no higher risk than triplets. This may be biased by small numbers of quartets and quintets. Overall, MetS was associated with an adjusted odds ratio of 1.38 (CI 1.04-1.82) for men and 1.67 (CI 1.08-2.59) for women.

TABLE 4-3 Prevalence of Metabolic Syndrome (NCEP-ATP III) and Its Traits in Type 2 Diabetes Patients: the Diabetes in Germany Study (DIG)

TRAITS	PREVALENCE (%)		
	Total	**Male**	**Female**
Obesity*	49.8	44.4	55.9
Hypertension	91.3	91.3	91.4
Hypertriglyceridemia	55.4	56.5	54.1
Low HDL-C	9.3	10.0	8.4
Only diabetes	2.4	2.6	2.2
Plus 1 trait	20.5	21.5	19.3
Plus 2 traits	35.3	36.4	34.1
Plus 3 traits	27.2	25.1	29.5
Plus 4 traits	4.0	4.2	3.8
Overall MetS	74.4	73.2	75.8

HDL-C = high-density lipoprotein cholesterol; HTG = hypertriglyceridemia; NCEP-ATP III = National Cholesterol Education Program—Adult Treatment Panel III.
*Difference by gender $P \leq 0.001$; χ^2 test. Obesity: body mass index exceeding 30 kg/m². Data from Hanefeld M, Koehler C, Gallo S, et al: Impact of the individual components of the metabolic syndrome and their different combinations on the prevalence of atherosclerotic vascular disease in type 2 diabetes: the Diabetes in Germany (DIG) study, *Cardiovasc Diabetol* 6:13, 2007.

As demonstrated in **Figure 4-1**, hypertension in the DIG study is the most important single risk factor for cardiovascular disease in type 2 diabetes, with an odds ratio twice of that of MetS per se. This, however, is not an argument against the clinical usefulness of MetS as a construct in the setting of type 2 diabetes. In the DIG study, stepwise regression analysis to determine significance of MetS together with major established risk factors confirms overall MetS, age, male sex, LDL cholesterol levels, and smoking as independent risk factors.[38] The lesson from this and other studies is that a careful consideration of all traits of MetS in patients with type 2 diabetes is highly clinically relevant and can be used as guide for patient-centered treatment.

COMMON SOIL FOR METABOLIC SYNDROME AND CARDIOVASCULAR DISEASE?

MetS has risen to increased clinical consideration and scrutiny together with the worldwide epidemic of obesity and diabetes. However, the pathophysiologic mechanisms leading to a cluster of metabolic diseases are not completely understood.[43] Although insulin resistance is the core abnormality of individuals with MetS,[44] there is insufficient evidence for a causal link between the two.[45]

A common hypothesis describes metabolic susceptibility as a central factor for the development of MetS (**Fig. 4-2**). This metabolic susceptibility is determined by polygenic variability of individuals[46] but also genetic defects of insulin signaling or dysfunctional adipose tissue and gene-environment interactions.[47,48] Once a sedentary lifestyle with decreased physical activity and high-calorie diet leads to the acquisition of body fat and development of overweight and obesity, a susceptible individual is at high risk to develop MetS.

Although several factors influence the development of MetS (see **Fig. 4-2**), abdominal obesity seems to be a prerequisite for its development,[49,50] and central obesity might causally link MetS with CVD.[47] Dysfunctional visceral adipose tissue is associated with increased secretion of inflammatory cytokines such as interleukin 6 (IL-6), tumor necrosis factor alpha (TNF-α), and resistin and a decrease in the anti-inflammatory adipokine adiponectin.[51,52] Whether the inflammatory response of the visceral adipose tissue is primarily induced by intracellular fat accumulation or by infiltration of activated macrophages is still a matter of debate.[53]

Inflammatory cytokines are involved in the induction of endothelial dysfunction and insulin resistance.[47] Furthermore, the insulin-resistant state of obesity is characterized by increased plasma levels of free fatty acids that have cardiotoxic effects and impair the production of endothelial vasodilators.[54,55]

TABLE 4-4 Odds Ratios (95% Confidence Intervals) for Cardiovascular Disease of Different Phenotypes of Metabolic Syndrome in the Diabetes in German Study Population by Sex (NCEP-ATP III Criteria)

PHENOTYPE	TOTAL POPULATION	MALES	FEMALES
Triads			
DM + HBP + LHDL	5.67 (2.84-11.31)	4.25 (1.92-9.41)	10.90 (2.51-47.46)
DM + HBP + HTG	5.64 (2.29-13.87)	4.96 (1.80-13.71)	8.78 (1.21-63.91)
DM + HBP + Obes	6.17 (2.51-15.16)	6.11 (2.22-16.85)	9.19 (1.26-66.82)
DM + LHDL + HTG	1.14 (0.82-1.58)	0.85 (0.55-1.31)	1.78 (1.07-2.96)
DM + LHDL + Obes	0.90 (0.59-1.37)	0.54 (0.29-1.01)	1.76 (0.97-3.19)
DM + HTG + Obes	0.96 (0.79-1.17)	0.91 (0.71-1.17)	1.20 (0.86-1.68)
Quartets			
DM + HBP + LHDL + HTG	1.21 (0.87-1.69)	0.90 (0.58-1.39)	1.90 (1.13-3.20)
DM + HBP + LHDL + Obes	0.95 (0.62-1.46)	0.56 (0.30-1.04)	1.92 (1.05-3.50)
DM + HBP + HTG + Obes	1.01 (0.82-1.23)	0.93 (0.72-1.21)	1.29 (0.92-1.79)
DM + LHDL + HTG + Obes	0.86 (0.54-1.38)	0.47 (0.23-0.95)	1.85 (0.97-3.52)
Quintet			
DM + HBP + LHDL + HTG + Obes	0.92 (0.57-1.47)	0.49 (0.24-1.00)	2.03 (1.06-3.87)
Overall MetS	1.41 (1.12-1.78)	1.38 (1.04-1.82)	1.67 (1.08-2.59)

DM = diabetes mellitus; HBP = high blood pressure; HTG = hypertriglyceridemia; LHDL = low high-density lipoprotein cholesterol; NCEP-ATP III, National Cholesterol Education Program—Adult Treatment Panel III; Obes = obesity.
Data from Hanefeld M, Koehler C, Gallo S, et al: Impact of the individual components of the metabolic syndrome and their different combinations on the prevalence of atherosclerotic vascular disease in type 2 diabetes: the Diabetes in Germany (DIG) study, *Cardiovasc Diabetol* 6:13, 2007.

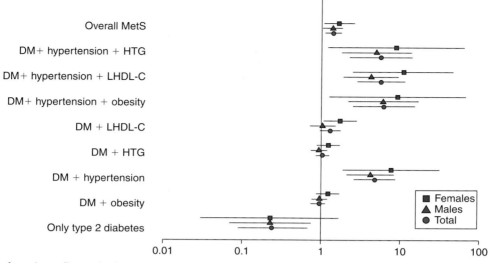

FIGURE 4-1 Odds ratios for major cardiovascular diseases by traits and phenotypes of the metabolic syndrome in patients with type 2 diabetes. *(Modified from from Hanefeld M, Koehler C, Gallo S, et al: Impact of the individual components of the metabolic syndrome and their different combinations on the prevalence of atherosclerotic vascular disease in type 2 diabetes: the Diabetes in Germany [DIG] study,* Cardiovasc Diabetol *6:13, 2007.)*

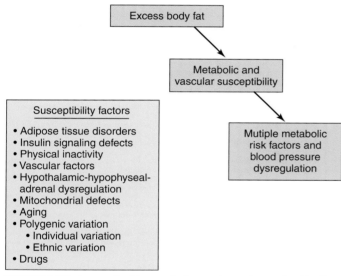

FIGURE 4-2 Pathogenesis of the metabolic-vascular syndrome. *(Modified from Cornier MA, Dabelea D, Hernandez TL, et al: The metabolic syndrome,* Endocr Rev *29:777, 2008.)*

Despite this complex pathophysiology as soil for MetS and associated diseases, we also have to keep in mind the strong impact of lifestyle and environment on the development of both MetS and cardiovascular disease. Therefore, if we consider a possible common soil for MetS and cardiovascular disease, we have to focus not on a one-dimensional genetic or pathophysiologic axis but on lifestyle changes accompanied by rapid behavioral and cultural transitions and mitigation of socioeconomic stress in the process of globalization and westernization.[26,56] As a prominent example, a close correlation between job stress and MetS was shown in the prospective Whitehall II population-based cohort study that was established in 1985 among 10,308 London-based civil servants who were 35 to 55 years of age at baseline.[57] Socioeconomic support and social status were assessed by questionnaires several times during 14 years of follow-up. The age-adjusted odds ratio for MetS

after adjustment for grade of stress exposure in the highest grade was more than 2, versus low and moderate exposure.

A high social gradient for MetS that could not be explained by behavioral factors was reported from a subgroup analysis of the Copenhagen City Heart Study, a population-based cohort study that included 3462 women and 2576 men.[58,59] In general, lower-class people have higher risk for development of MetS and cardiovascular disease, as demonstrated during the transition period in Eastern bloc countries.[60]

Thus we find the common soil for MetS and cardiovascular diseases in times of globalization in a metabolic susceptibility as well as in an unhealthy lifestyle, in changes of socio-economic conditions, and in environmental factors.

METABOLIC SYNDROME AS GUIDE FOR PATIENT-CENTERED TREATMENT

As previously discussed, *metabolic syndrome* is a simple term for a heterogenic cluster of interrelated diseases with complex interaction with cardiovascular disease. However, there are core elements of a common soil, such as nutrition, physical activity, social behavior, and stress, as a basis for therapeutic lifestyle intervention. (See also Chapter 12.)

Beyond lifestyle, consideration for individualized drug treatment or interventional measures such as bariatric surgery targeting modification of each of the traits of MetS may be clinically prudent (see Chapter 6), and the presence or absence of prevalent cardiovascular conditions and their complications can be used as guide for a patient-centered yet integrated approach.

Lifestyle modification should always be the primary intervention to prevent the development of the components of MetS or to reduce the risk of CVD if MetS is already present. (See Chapter 12.)

A post hoc analysis of the prospective Diabetes Prevention Program (DPP) that included overweight people with both IGT and increased fasting glucose demonstrated a significant 41% reduction in the incidence of MetS after lifestyle modification compared with no intervention. Among those participants without MetS at baseline, 53% of the placebo group but only 38% of the lifestyle group developed MetS during the follow-up period of 2.8 years.[61] A recent multicenter trial from Spain assessed the effects of a Mediterranean diet on the incidence of CVD in 7447 persons with cardiovascular risk factors; 61.4% met the criteria for MetS at baseline. After a median follow-up of 4.8 years, the hazard ratio (HR) for CVD events was 0.7 (95% CI 0.54-0.92) for the group assigned to a Mediterranean diet with extra-virgin olive oil compared with the control group. The greatest risk reduction was observed in people with components of MetS (e.g., hypertension, abdominal adiposity, dyslipidemia).[62]

Pharmacotherapy with glucose-lowering drugs can prevent the development of type 2 diabetes in people with IGT or increased fasting glucose (see Chapter 6). This has been demonstrated for metformin, acarbose, and thiazolidinediones.[63] In the DPP trial, metformin therapy reduced the incidence of type 2 diabetes by 31% and the incidence of MetS by 17%.[61,64] Comparable results regarding the prevention of type 2 diabetes was demonstrated with acarbose in the Study to Prevent Non–Insulin-Dependent Diabetes Mellitus (STOP-NIDDM). People with IGT were assigned to treatment with either acarbose or placebo. After a mean follow-up of 3.3 years, the number needed to treat to prevent one case of newly diagnosed diabetes in patients with MetS was 5.8 versus 16.5 in those without MetS.[65] In addition, acarbose reduced the incidence of hypertension compared with placebo (HR 0.59 [95% CI 0.39-0.9]).[66] Thiazolidinediones have also been considered for use in people with MetS because they target a number of its components by improvement of glycemic control and insulin sensitivity; however, in contrast to metformin or acarbose, thiazolidinediones have been associated with adverse outcomes, especially congestive heart failure and weight gain, which have limited their use in clinical practice.

In a subgroup analysis of the Antihypertensive and Lipid-Lowering Treatment to Prevent Heart Attack Trial (ALLHAT), which evaluated metabolic, cardiovascular, and renal outcomes in nondiabetic individuals with or without MetS who were assigned to initial hypertension treatment with a thiazide-like diuretic (chlorthalidone), a calcium channel blocker (amlodipine), or an angiotensin-converting enzyme (ACE) inhibitor (lisinopril), treatment with chlorthalidone was associated with significantly higher risk for development of type 2 diabetes in the presence of MetS compared with the treatment with lisinopril.[67]

Thus consideration for use of specific glucose-lowering and blood pressure medications might be guided by the presence or absence of traits of MetS, because pleiotropic effects of such therapies may be used for an integrated approach to this cluster of interrelated conditions. However, no rigorous outcome data are available to place into clinical context such drug-induced progression to diabetes versus drug efficacy with regard to important clinical outcomes.

In addition to the metabolic abnormalities that determine the diagnostic criteria of MetS, there are clinical diseases and biochemical risk factors frequently associated with MetS (e.g., nonalcoholic fatty liver disease, sleep apnea, erectile dysfunction, albuminuria, hyperuricemia, increased biomarkers of low-grade inflammation; **Box 4-1**).[68-72] Some of these comorbidities might further increase the cardiovascular risk related to traits of MetS. Therefore, looking for comorbidities and their treatment should be an essential part of good clinical practice.

 BOX 4-1 Diseases and Emerging Risk Factors Related to the Metabolic Syndrome

Nonalcoholic fatty liver

Sleep apnea

Albuminuria

Minor sexual, neural, and psychological abnormalities

Social depression

Increased subclinical inflammation

Endothelial dysfunction

Increased intima-media thickness

Thrombophilia

In conclusion, currently available data support the evolving concept of MetS as the center of a complex network of cardiovascular risk factors that goes beyond the traditional CVD risk factors. The concept provides an integrated approach for screening, diagnostic testing, prevention, and treatment of diseases associated with MetS in the context of a patient-centered treatment strategy to prevent cardiovascular disease.

References

1. Kylin ES: Hypertonie-Hyperglykämie-Hyperurikämiesyndrom, *Zentralblatt für Innere Medizin* 44:1923.
2. Vague J: The degree of masculine differentiation of obesities: a factor determining predisposition to diabetes, atherosclerosis, gout, and uric calculous disease, *Am J Clin Nutr* 4:20–34, 1956.
3. Avagaro P, et al: Association of hyperlipidemia, diabetes mellitus and mild obesity, *Acta diabetol Let* 4:572–590, 1967.
4. Hanefeld M, Leonhardt W: Das metabolische syndrome, *Dt Gesundh Wesen* 36:545–551, 1981.
5. Alberti KG, Zimmet PZ: Definition, diagnosis and classification of diabetes mellitus and its complications. Part 1: diagnosis and classification of diabetes mellitus provisional report of a WHO consultation, *Diabet Med* 15(7):539–553, 1998.
6. Grundy SM, Cleeman JI, Daniels SR, et al: American Heart Association, National Heart, Lung, and Blood Institute: Diagnosis and management of the metabolic syndrome: an American Heart Association/National Heart, Lung, and Blood Institute scientific statement, *Circulation* 112 (17):2735–2752, 2005.
7. Alberti KG, Zimmet P, Shaw J: IDF Epidemiology Task Force Consensus Group. The metabolic syndrome: a new worldwide definition, *Lancet* 366:1059–1062, 2005.
8. Moebus S, Hanisch JU, Aidelsburger P, et al: Impact of 4 different definitions used for the assessment of the prevalence of the Metabolic Syndrome in primary healthcare: the German Metabolic and Cardiovascular Risk Project (GEMCAS), *Cardiovasc Diabetol* 6:22, 2007, 6.
9. Qiao Q, Laatikainen T, Zethelius B, et al: Comparison of definitions of metabolic syndrome in relation to the risk of developing stroke and coronary heart disease in Finnish and Swedish cohorts, *Stroke* 40(2):337–343, 2009.
10. Kahn R, Buse J, Ferrannini E, Stern M: American Diabetes Association, European Association for the Study of Diabetes: The metabolic syndrome: time for a critical appraisal: joint statement from the American Diabetes Association and the European Association for the Study of Diabetes, *Diabetes Care* 28(9):2289–2304, 2005.
11. Alberti KG, Eckel RH, Grundy SM, et al: Harmonizing the metabolic syndrome: a joint interim statement of the International Diabetes Federation Task Force on Epidemiology and Prevention; National Heart, Lung, and Blood Institute; American Heart Association; World Heart Federation; International Atherosclerosis Society; and International Association for the Study of Obesity, *Circulation* 120(16):1640–1645, 2009.
12. Cameron AJ, Shaw JE, Zimmet PZ: The metabolic syndrome: prevalence in worldwide populations, *Endocrinol Metab Clin North Am* 33:351–375, 2004.
13. Wilson PW, Meigs JB: Cardiometabolic risk: a Framingham perspective, *Int J Obes (Lond)* 32 (Suppl 2):17–20, 2008.
14. Jeppesen J, Hansen TW, Rasmussen S, et al: Insulin resistance, the metabolic syndrome and risk of incident cardiovascular disease: a population based study, *J Am Coll Cardiol* 49:2112–2119, 2007.
15. Isomaa B, Almgren P, Tuomi T, et al: Cardiovascular morbidity and mortality associated with the metabolic syndrome, *Diabetes Care* 24:683–689, 2001.
16. Alexander CM, Landsman PB, Teutsch SM, et al: NCEP-defined metabolic syndrome, diabetes, and prevalence of coronary heart disease among NHANES III participants age 50 years and older, *Diabetes* 52(5):1210–1214, 2003.
17. Gami AS, Witt BJ, Howard DE, et al: Metabolic syndrome and risk of incident cardiovascular events and death: a systematic review and meta-analysis, *J Am Coll Cardiol* 49:403–414, 2007.
18. Wilson PW, D'Agostino RB, Parise H, et al: Metabolic syndrome as a precursor of cardiovascular disease and type 2 diabetes mellitus, *Circulation* 112(20):3066–3072, 2005.
19. Hong Y, Jin X, Mo J, et al: Metabolic syndrome, its preeminent clusters, incidence coronary heart disease and all cause mortality—results of prospective analysis for the Atherosclerosis Risk in Communities study, *J Intern Med* 262:113–122, 2007.
20. Mottillo S, Filion KB, Genest J, et al: The metabolic syndrome and cardiovascular risk a systematic review and meta-analysis, *J Am Coll Cardiol* 56(14):1113–1132, 2010.
21. Jia WP, Xiang KS, Chen L, et al: A comparison of the application of two working definitions of metabolic syndrome in Chinese population, *Zhonghua Yi Xue Za Zhi* 84(7):534–538, 2004.
22. Cameron AJ, Zimmet PZ, Soderberg S, et al: The metabolic syndrome as a predictor of incident diabetes mellitus in Mauritius, *Diabet Med* 24(12):1460–1469, 2007.
23. Sattar N, McConnachie A, Shaper AG, et al: Can metabolic syndrome usefully predict cardiovascular disease and diabetes? Outcome data from two prospective studies, *Lancet* 371 (9628):1927–1935, 2008.
24. Grundy SM: Metabolic syndrome pandemic, *Arterioscler Thromb Vasc Biol* (4):629–636, 2008.

testing can also be used. A recent statement by the International Expert Committee of the World Health Organization (WHO) has advocated that an HbA1c of 6.5% (48 mmol/mol) or higher can now be used to define T2DM.[44] However, there is no clear consensus on how or whether HbA1c should be used to classify diabetes risk below this level.[45] The American Diabetes Association (ADA) tentatively suggested that an HbA1c value of 5.7% to 6.4% indicates a high risk of T2DM, whereas an international expert committee suggested a range of 6.0% to 6.4%.[34,46] The latter range was also recently endorsed by the National Institute for Health and Care Excellence (NICE) in the United Kingdom, which now recommends that HbA1c be used to identify those with a high risk of T2DM and that patients with a value of 6.0% to 6.4% be referred to a T2DM prevention program.[33] Prospective data from the United Kingdom support the use of 6.0% to 6.4% to define an at-risk category, because individuals in this group were found to have a risk of future T2DM that was twice that in individuals with a value of 5.5% to 5.9%.[18] However, other data from Germany suggest that an HbA1c threshold of 5.7% is likely to have the best sensitivity and specificity for detection of future T2DM risk[45] but demonstrate that the combination of HbA1c and the 1-hour plasma glucose concentration after a 75-g oral glucose load in predicting future T2DM risk was significantly better in a multivariable model than either one of them alone. The 1-hour plasma glucose concentration has previously been shown to be a strong predictor of T2DM risk[47] and also other chronic disease[48] but has major logistical issues. Furthermore, the optimal HbA1c cut point for identifying individuals at increased diabetes risk is 5.7%[45] and not 6.0% as originally suggested by the ADA Expert Committee.[46] If HbA1c exceeding 6.0% had been used to identify individuals at increased risk for future T2DM, only about one third of patients who developed T2DM would have been identified. Thus, use of an HbA1c cut point of 5.7% together with the 1-hour plasma glucose concentration[45] would identify many additional high-risk individuals who could benefit from an intervention program.[45]

The most cost-efficient way to balance resources against risk has yet to be determined. In the meantime, the balance that is struck may depend to a large extent on pragmatic considerations, particularly financial constraints.[38] It is acknowledged that, along with strategies for identification and intervention for those with a high risk of a widely prevalent condition such as T2DM, it is also fundamentally important to use initiatives that are aimed at shifting the distribution of known risk factors, such as BMI in adults or BMI percentiles in childhood and waist circumference within the population as a whole.[49] Strategies for primary prevention on a public health level and high-risk strategies need to work in parallel.[39]

Physical Activity

Epidemiologic, experimental, and randomized controlled clinical study trial-level evidence has consistently demonstrated that levels of physical activity are centrally involved in the regulation of glucose homeostasis, independent of other factors including adiposity.[50,51] A modest increase in walking activity, toward levels that are consistent with the minimum recommendations, significantly improved 2-hour postload glucose levels by 23 mg/dL over 12 months in high-risk overweight and obese individuals despite the

absence of any significant change in body weight or waist circumference.[52] This may correspond to a greater than 60% reduction in risk of developing T2DM within 24 months.[53] These findings were consistent with findings from other studies,[26] but replication of the results is needed and attempts are under way. Although the promotion of physical activity is a cornerstone of effective T2DM prevention programs, the role of physical inactivity in helping identify T2DM risk is less clear and more problematic for several reasons. First, physical inactivity is highly prevalent among the general population; it has consistently been shown that 50% to 80% of the population in both developed and developing countries fails to meet the minimum recommendations for health.[54] Indeed, when physical activity levels are objectively measured, rather than by subjective self-report, around 95% of the population fail to meet the minimum requirements for health, making inactivity a near universal condition.[54] Therefore commonly used definitions of physical inactivity do not provide a clear mechanism for stratifying diabetes risk. Second, methods that rely on self-reporting by individuals of their activity levels are highly inaccurate and unreliable. For example, an internationally used and validated self-reported measure of physical activity described as little as 10% of the variation in objectively measured levels through accelerometry[55]; in contrast, simple measures of adiposity, such as BMI and waist circumference, are reasonably accurate on a population level. For these reasons, self-recording levels of physical (in)activity has not been shown to add to the predictive power of diabetes risk scores or to be useful when incorporated into other methods of quantifying diabetes risk. However, it is important that physical inactivity, as with other lifestyle variables, be considered for the individual assessments of T2DM risk.[18]

To be successful, lifestyle intervention programs should focus on types of physical activity that are acceptable to most of the population. Walking has consistently been shown to be the most popular choice of physical activity, including in those with a high risk of T2DM.[26] Indeed, walking for 150 min/wk during leisure time is associated with a 60% reduction in the relative risk of T2DM compared with those that did little or no walking in their leisure time.[26] Of importance, walking is associated with fewer barriers than other forms of physical activity in black and minority ethnic populations dwelling in developed countries, such as South Asians.[56]

Wearing a pedometer and keeping a daily step log have been widely advocated as effective self-regulatory strategies in the promotion of increased ambulatory activity, and their use has consistently been shown to successfully promote increased physical activity.[57] The success of pedometer interventions is centered on the pedometer's ability to raise awareness of current activity levels, provide objective feedback to the individual, and facilitate clear and simple goal setting. To be effective, it is essential that realistic and personalized step-per-day goals be used; goals that are too ambitious can often be demotivating and lead to failure. Sedentary individuals (fewer than 5000 steps/day) should initially aim for an average increase in ambulatory activity of around 2000 steps/day conducted at a moderate to vigorous intensity, which is roughly equivalent to an additional 150 minutes of walking activity per week.[58] Alternatively, the categories of ambulatory activity shown in **Table 5-1** can be used to guide lifestyle interventions. For example, those in the sedentary or inactive categories could initially

TABLE 5-1 Physical Activity Categories Based on Steps per Day

CATEGORY	STEPS PER DAY
Sedentary	<5,000
Low (typical of daily activity excluding volitional activity)	5,000-7,499
Moderate (likely to incorporate the equivalent of around 30 minutes of moderate-intensity physical activity per day)	7,500-9,999
High (likely to incorporate the equivalent of around 45 minutes of moderate-intensity physical activity)	10,000-12,499
Very high (likely to incorporate the equivalent of over 45 minutes of moderate-intensity physical activity)	>12,500

Data from Tudor-Locke and Bassett, 2004.[58]

aim to increase their ambulatory activity by at least 2000 steps/day. Those in the moderate category could be encouraged to try and enter the high category, and those achieving the high or very high categories should be helped to at least maintain their activity levels. For people who have significant barriers to walking, such as joint problems, alternative forms of physical activity, such as cycling, water aerobics, or swimming, should be encouraged.

Nutritional Aspects

Obesity is one of the most important risk factors for T2DM, and population trends in obesity and T2DM run in parallel.[59] The pathophysiology of adiposity with regard to the development of T2DM is not fully understood; however, several mechanisms that may interact have been identified. Adipose tissue, especially the tissue surrounding internal organs (visceral fat), is today regarded as an active endocrine organ that secretes a variety of proinflammatory adipokines that act at both the local and the systemic levels.[60] Cornier and colleagues have reported that increasing adipose tissue mass leads to changes in the secretion of these adipokines as well as increased turnover of free fatty acids, which bring on insulin resistance, the harbinger of metabolic disturbances leading to T2DM.[61]

Even though the basic cause of excess body fat accumulation is an imbalance between energy intake (i.e., dietary intake) and expenditure, the factors predisposing to the development of overweight and obesity are multifactorial and poorly understood. Nevertheless, regular physical activity, high dietary intake of fiber, and reduced intake of energy-dense micronutrient-poor foods were identified by WHO as lifestyle targets for reducing obesity.[62] In the DPS, the dietary energy density was found to be associated with achieved weight reduction,[14] which supports the intuitive recommendation to increase foods with low energy density such as vegetables and fruits to increase satiety while reducing total energy intake. An increased understanding of these mechanisms will be helpful in providing prioritization of behavioral targets for future prevention programs.

Nutritional Recommendations

For most people, weight reduction is difficult to sustain. Fortunately, T2DM prevention studies have shown that changing one's lifestyle is effective without significant weight reduction.[10,12,52] An important contributor is physical activity; however, the composition of diet seems to be important as well. Epidemiologic studies have suggested that several dietary factors may either increase diabetes risk (e.g., intake

of refined grains, red and processed meat, and sugar-sweetened beverages; heavy alcohol consumption) or decrease it (e.g., intake of whole-grain cereal, vegetables, legumes, nuts, dairy, and coffee; moderate alcohol consumption), independently of body weight change.[18] The suggested mechanisms behind these observations include improvement of insulin secretion and/or insulin resistance as a result of reduced glycemia and lipidemia, reduced ectopic fat, reduced low-grade inflammation, changes in cell membrane phospholipids, and improvement of intestinal peptide secretion.[18]

In addition to weight reduction and increased physical activity, the Finnish DPS aimed at reduced total and saturated fat intake and increased fiber density of the diet.[63] The post hoc analyses showed that T2DM risk reduction was clearly associated with the achievement of these lifestyle goals. In the U.S. DPP study, dietary goals were reduced energy intake (to achieve weight reduction) and reduced total fat.[28] The T2DM prevention studies from China, India, and Japan aimed at reduced fat, energy, alcohol, and refined carbohydrates and increased fiber.[10,12,13] A recent study from Spain showed that adoption of a Mediterranean diet, characterized by a high intake of vegetables, fruits, legumes, extra virgin olive oil, nuts, fish, whole grains, and red wine, also decreases T2DM incidence remarkably,[64] without body weight reduction.

A pragmatic way to prevent T2DM therefore would be to focus on diet composition and physical activity. A strict diet emphasizing dietary restriction and avoidance of certain food groups (e.g., sources of fat or carbohydrates) and aiming solely at weight reduction may be more efficient for achieving weight loss in the short term, but may not be sustainable in the long run.[65] Diet may well vary according to food culture, food availability, and personal preferences and yet follow the same general principles:

- High intake of vegetables and fruits should be encouraged.
- Grain products should mainly be unrefined, with high natural fiber content.
- Vegetable sources of fat with low saturated fat content (such as olive oil) should be preferred.
- As a source of protein, nuts, legumes, dairy products, and fish should be favored and red meat limited.
- The intake of highly processed foods (e.g., processed meat, sweetened beverages, confectionery) should be limited.

The Right Intervention for the Person at Risk

Supporting Behavior Change

As described earlier, there seem to be several possible routes to nonpharmacologic diabetes prevention, but a common factor is the need to support sustained changes in lifestyle behaviors. However, achieving the required changes reliably is challenging. Both clinical intervention programs[66] and "real-world" diabetes prevention programs demonstrate wide variation in their ability to deliver weight loss or changes in physical activity.[18] It is therefore of importance to be able to characterize the components of lifestyle interventions that are reliably associated with increased effectiveness (**Fig. 5-2**). Only by understanding what makes interventions effective can we design diabetes prevention programs that will deliver the expected benefits and optimize cost-effectiveness in scalable, real world prevention programs.

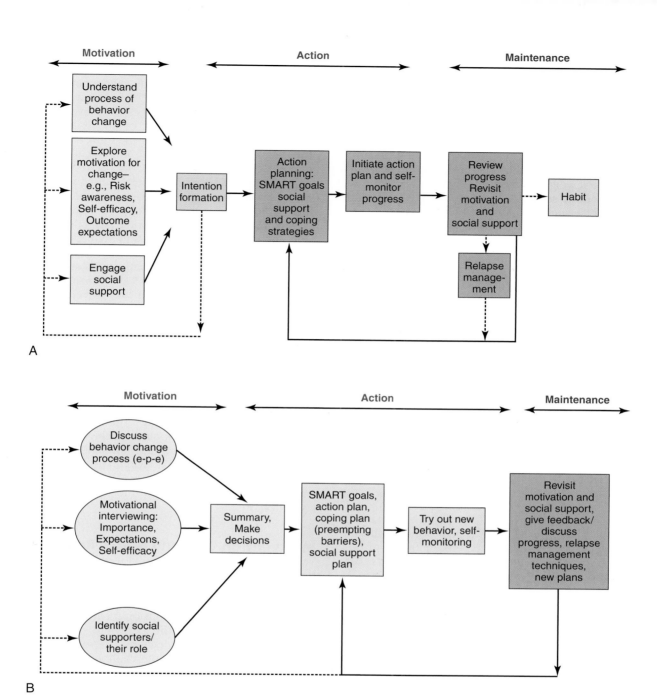

FIGURE 5-2 Behavior change model and behavior change techniques based on SMART goals: *Specific, Measurable, Achievable, Relevant, Time* related.[66] e-p-e = elicit-provide-elicit (a technique for patient-centered information exchange).

A recent analysis of reviews systematically examined a wide range of evidence from existing high-quality reviews of RCTs of interventions to support changes in diet and/or physical activity in people at high risk of developing T2DM.[67] Based on the grading of 129 analyses that related intervention characteristics to effectiveness, evidence-based recommendations were developed. These recommendations are broadly consistent with other recent international guidelines for supporting lifestyle change in people with high cardiovascular risk with T2DM[68] and obesity.[69]

Applying these recommendations may help to guide the selection of intervention components in a way that maximizes the likely effectiveness of diabetes prevention programs. However, it is worth noting that the evidence base

on the best strategies for supporting behavior change is far from complete. Individuals with high T2DM risk from different backgrounds and cultures may be responsive to a number of different strategies that modify the cognitive, social, and emotional processes that underpin their lifestyle behaviors. There are also a number of possible modes of intervention beyond persuasive face-to-face interaction, including modification of the physical environment and changes in food pricing or regulation and taxation. Hence, there may be considerable opportunities to further increase the efficiency and cost-effectiveness of programs to support lifestyle behavior change (see also **Chapter 12**).

Considerable attention is also needed to address the issue of maintenance of lifestyle changes. Long-term follow-up of

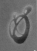

weight loss interventions shows a clear pattern of weight regain over 5 to 10 years, even in the successful diabetes prevention research studies.[29,65] It is likely that when weight loss is achieved through changes in diet or physical activity that are challenging for people to adhere to or that they do not enjoy, these changes will not be sustainable in the long term. Recent data from a meta-analysis of multiple long-term cohort studies indicate that a habitual energy imbalance of an excess of only 50 to 100 kcal/day seems sufficient to cause the gradual weight gain observed in most adults. Consequently, "modest, sustained changes in lifestyle could mitigate or reverse such an energy imbalance." Hence, promoting a series of small changes that people can easily live with, rather than dramatic changes in diet or activity, may be a strategy worth further investigation.

RECOMMENDATIONS FOR TYPE 2 DIABETES PREVENTION PRACTICE

The European Union supported the IMAGE project (Development and Implementation of a European Guideline and Training Standards for Diabetes Prevention), a multiprofessional initiative to develop practice recommendations for diabetes prevention practice.[18] More than 100 experts in this field worked for 2.5 years to prepare an evidence-based guideline for T2DM prevention,[37] a toolkit for diabetes prevention practice,[38] a guideline for evaluation and quality management in T2DM prevention,[70] and a European training curriculum for prevention managers.[71]

The major output of the IMAGE project—relevant for prevention practice—is the practical diabetes prevention guideline called "Toolkit for the Prevention of Type 2 Diabetes." This toolkit is developed for all professionals involved in diabetes prevention: those working in primary health care services, physicians, physical activity experts, dietitians, nurses, and teachers, but also stakeholders and politicians. The Toolkit condenses the essence of what is necessary to build up the management of a diabetes prevention program, with financial, intervention-related, and quality assurance aspects, and refers to the latest evidence in diabetes prevention. The core of the Toolkit describes elements of an effective lifestyle intervention program and gives the core goals of lifestyles (behavior, physical activity, and diet) and finishes with an overview of how to evaluate intervention programs and how to establish quality assurance. It provides several recommendations that may help in planning and implementing T2DM prevention programs worldwide.[4,20,72]

The Toolkit provides a good balance between clear, accurate information and practical guidance; it is not, however, intended to be a comprehensive source of information. Specifically, detailed instructions about how to achieve and maintain weight reduction, which is one of the main issues in T2DM prevention, are not given because local and national guidelines as well as other sources of information are available elsewhere. Furthermore, intervention delivery staff members are assumed to have basic knowledge about, for example, diet and physical activity and their health effects and about supporting behavior change. Finally, the Toolkit is not designed to be used to provide intervention materials to be delivered directly to those participating in prevention interventions, although it does contain some examples of information sheets and materials that might be used with participants.

Contents of the Type 2 Diabetes Prevention Toolkit

The Toolkit starts with an executive summary including the rationale for T2DM prevention.[38] It is followed by a chapter representing the background (T2DM prevalence, risk factors, consequences, evidence of successful prevention) and giving instructions about the planning and development of prevention programs and the identification and recruitment of participants at high risk for T2DM. One of the core items of the Toolkit is the description of what to do and how to do it. Behavior change is a process that requires individual attention and effective communication to achieve motivation, self-monitoring, sustained support, and other intervention to prevent and manage relapses (see **Fig. 5-2**). This section includes a model of intervention including empowerment and patient-centered messages. It is followed by key messages on behaviors (physical activity and diet) that are important in prevention of T2DM (**Tables 5-2** and **5-3** and **Box 5-1**), and practical advice for patient-centered counseling. The focus is on long-term, sustainable lifestyle changes.

A brief guide for evaluation and quality assurance in reference to the quality and outcome indicators is included. This section is followed by a consideration of possible risks and adverse effects. The IMAGE Toolkit main text ends with a positive mission statement, emphasizing what can be achieved if we work together. The appendices give the reader a set of easy-to-use tools including a checklist for prevention program development, templates for goal setting and for food and physical activity diaries, an example of a risk-screening questionnaire (the FINDRISC questionnaire), and a template for evaluation and quality assurance data collection.[38]

Intervention Cost and Scarce Resources

There is clearly tension between the evidence-based recommendation for maximizing intervention intensity (number or frequency of contacts) and the practical availability of resources (suitably trained staff and funding) for diabetes prevention. However, this tension might be reduced in several ways. These include the following:

· *Using group-based interventions.* There are several good examples of group-based interventions that produce levels of weight loss similar to those in the large diabetes prevention studies, at least in the short term.[73,74] Group-based intervention also costs less than individual intervention.
· *Reducing staff costs.* Lifestyle interventions can be delivered successfully by a range of staff, including physicians, nurses, dietitians and nutritionists, exercise specialists, and nonprofessionals.[67] More research is needed to define the range of personal skills and type of training required to maintain program effectiveness.[71]
· *Applying self-delivered and Internet-based approaches.* This type of intervention could potentially provide a low-cost solution for a considerable subgroup of the population and may be a useful supplement for face-to-face programs. Given the success of such approaches to support smoking cessation[75] and recovery from depression,[76] it should in theory be possible to use them to support changes in diet and physical activity. Although a number of programs are under evaluation, more robust evidence on effectiveness is still needed before this approach can be endorsed.

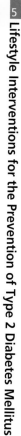

TABLE 5-2 The FITT Recommendations: General Guidelines for Individuals of Moderate Fitness[38]

FITT PRINCIPLE		AEROBIC ENDURANCE TRAINING	RESISTANCE TRAINING
Frequency	How often	3 ×/wk (minimum) Max 2-day gap between training sessions	2-3 ×/wk
Intensity	How hard	(a) Light to moderate (40%-60% Vo$_2$ max/50%-70% HRmax) (e.g., brisk walking—5-6 km/hr) Slightly increased breathing rate (b) Vigorous (e.g., jogging—8-10 km/hr) Increased breathing rate and sweating	Light to moderate (slight muscular fatigue)
Time	How long	(a) Light to moderate 45-60 min (total >150 min/wk) (b) Vigorous 30-40 min (total >90 min/wk)	One to three sets of 8-15 repetitions for each exercise
Type	What kind	Walking, jogging, cycling, swimming, hiking, skiing	Approximately eight different strength exercises using the major muscles of the body (e.g., with fitness machines, resistance bands, or just with your own body weight)

HRmax = Maximum heart rate as assessed by a cardiac stress test (or similar); Vo$_2$max = maximum rate of oxygen consumption as measured during incremental exercise testing.

TABLE 5-3 The EAT CLEVER Principle—Brief Practical Advice for Counselors to Be Applied Within the Framework of National Dietary Recommendations[38]

	EAT CLEVER
Estimation of the dietary pattern compared with the recommendations	Use the food diary or interview to help your patient become aware of his or her dietary pattern and food consumption. Compare dietary intake with the recommendations. Consider special needs, resources, and readiness to change food habits.
Aims in the long and short term	Discuss both short- and long-term goals: What is your patient willing and able to do at the moment? Help to set practical, achievable targets and proceed with small steps. Make a plan with your patient.
Tools, guidance, and support	What types of tools, guidance, support, or skills are needed and available? Involving the family and friends and participating in group counseling are worth considering.
Composition of the diet	A diet high in sugar and other refined carbohydrates and low in fiber content or high in saturated and *trans* fats may increase the risk for diabetes and other related disorders. Whole grains and moderate amounts of coffee and alcohol may decrease the risk. Encourage the use of herbs and spices to reduce salt. Refer to national nutrition recommendations, but consider the special requirements of people with high diabetes risk, such as the improvement of the components of the metabolic syndrome. Take into account any additional disease the patient may have.
Lifestyle for the whole life	Diet is influenced by culture; religion; ethical, physiologic, psychological, social, and economic aspects; availability of food items; and individual likes and dislikes. Help the patient to find his or her own healthy way of life. Lifestyle change is a process and relapses are part of it. Help your patient to learn from these experiences to develop successful strategies over time.
Energy	Excessive energy intake causes weight gain. If the patient is overweight, make a plan with her or him to support gradual weight loss (step by step). Focus on substituting foods with high saturated fat and/or refined carbohydrate content with lower-energy items. How many meals and snacks, beverages and alcohol included, does he or she have during a day and night? Some regularity in the daily meal plan helps to control over-eating.
Variety	Emphasize variety instead of restriction. A health-promoting diet provides satiety and pleasure as well as protective nutrients. Encourage patients to try new foods. Give advice on how to read food labels. This can help your patient to feel more confident and expand his or her healthy food choices.
Evaluation	Evaluation and self-monitoring help in achieving and maintaining new food habits. Body weight and/or waist circumference should be measured regularly. Encourage your patient to use a food diary or some other methods to monitor eating habits: the number of meals and snacks, the amounts of certain food stuffs, such as vegetables, whole grains, sugar, alcoholic beverages, vegetable oil and/or fat, and so on.
Risks management	Dietary guidance must be based on evidence from nutrition and behavioral sciences. Focus on the big picture: Changing one aspect in the diet affects many others. Strict restrictions and "crash dieting" may lead to an unhealthy diet, and can cause damage in the long term as well as psychological and social harm. A multidisciplinary team, including a registered dietitan and a psychologist, can give essential support to avoid these risks.

- *Developing standardized recommendation for diabetes prevention practice.*[37,38] Applying the recommendations on supporting behavior change should enhance the efficiency of lifestyle intervention programs.
- *Disclosing the economic benefits of diabetes prevention.*[77] Economic modeling indicates that group-based diabetes prevention interventions in the United States would provide a return on investment within a 3-year time frame. This has resulted in the release of significant resources in the United States from government and health maintenance organizations.
- *Taking advantage of expertise.* To deliver prevention programs on a large scale, we need to identify a sufficient number of people with the expertise and experience to

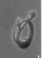
BOX 5-1 Nutrition and Dietary Guidance for Sustained Diabetes Prevention[38]

GOALS FOR FOOD INTAKE	GOALS FOR LONG-TERM NUTRIENT INTAKE
• Consuming fruit, vegetables, and legumes in abundance (≥500 g or five portions per day)	• Energy intake balanced with physical activity levels to achieve or maintain healthy body weight
• Choosing whole grains in all cereal products	• Total fat 25 to 35 E%* (60 to 80 g/day with 2000 kcal daily intake level), of which saturated or trans fat is 10 E% or less
• Limiting sugar to ≤50 g/day, including sugar in food and beverages	• Dietary fiber 25 to 35 g/day
• Consuming vegetable oil and/or soft margarines and/or nuts as the primary source of fat	• Salt (NaCl) ≤6 g/day
• Limiting butter, other saturated fat, and partially hydrogenated fats	• Alcohol ≤5 E%*
• Choosing low-fat milk and meat products	
• Consuming fish regularly (≥2 times per week)	
• Consuming alcoholic beverages in moderation (≤2 drinks/day for men and ≤1 drink/day for women) if at all	
• Other goals according to individual needs (e.g., body weight, diseases, medications, age)	

*E% = Proportion of total energy.

design and deliver them. Investing in high-quality training would seem to be essential for the implementation of successful programs.[71]

· *Maximizing the uptake of both screening and intervention.* Further research is needed in this area, but this may require multimedia approaches, involvement of multiple sectors (public health, voluntary sector, commercial and workplace programs, health care, and social care), and the use of social marketing techniques to target messages to appropriate population subgroups.

· *Ensuring sustainability of funding and support within both health care and political arenas.* This will require a sustained focus and willingness to invest in preventive health care. The United Nations summit on noncommunicable diseases has helped to present an opportunity to more firmly and sustainably establish diabetes prevention on the global health agenda.[78]

· *Developing quality management systems.* Quality management systems are needed to provide continuous benchmarking and monitoring of the effectiveness of prevention programs.[70]

· *Further improving the technology to support behavior change.* This could be achieved by establishing "networks of practice" so that we can learn how to improve the efficiency of interventions from practice or real-world experience as well as from developments in theory and research. The global network Active in Diabetes Prevention (www.activeindiabetesprevention.com) provides a forum for exchanging knowledge and intervention materials as well as educational standards and recommendations for prevention practice.

Improving Effectiveness in Type 2 Diabetes Diabetes Prevention Practice

One of the challenges in developing intervention programs for diabetes prevention is to find the right intervention that has the highest probability to be successful in the individual with high T2DM risk. This strongly varies among different individuals. In today's practice, we should aim to be using standardized and structured intervention programs that we apply to all the people at risk that we have identified in a prevention plan. By this approach, we accept that sometimes only 20% of the people achieve the highest effect and that in 80% of the people the program may be less efficient.[79] It is possible to increase the probability of success by developing intervention programs that follow a behavior change model. Such a model was developed as part of the IMAGE project, wherein patients are seen as being in three stages[37,66]:

· The stage of motivation
· The stage of action
· The stage of maintenance

The development of intervention programs following this behavior change model may generate a higher efficacy because of an increase in flexibility in program execution (see also **Chapter 12**). The key point in the IMAGE project was that the behavior change model was accompanied by a collection of behavioral techniques for supporting the lifestyle changes (see **Fig. 5-2**). Specific tools and techniques for each stage of the behavior change model were elicited from more than 300 studies[66] and shown to be effective. The prevention manager can choose the techniques needed for the intervention in several stages. The use of the techniques allows a much more widespread implementation of an intervention plan and may be one step away from focusing only on structured and standardized intervention concepts by allowing a higher degree of flexibility of the intervention manager and focusing more on individual needs and preferences.

This behavior change model then was further developed by a working group derived from the IMAGE project.[18,66] Daily practice in performing intervention shows that even the intervention planning, by focusing on the behavior change model, misses an effect in a large number of people receiving the intervention. One of the difficulties is associated with the use of standardized programs that follow a standardized curriculum. Furthermore, difficulties also arise from the fact that most of the intervention programs do not include different preferences and interests of the people receiving the intervention. This is followed by different stages of morbidity[81] that also define different preferences and interests that can be a barrier to an effect of a program if someone with very low risk is sitting together in an intervention group with someone having a very high risk and different preferences and interests. Based on this background, the further development of intervention programs must take this information into account to develop an assessment to identify the most suitable intervention characteristics for a person at risk.

Prevention Managers

As part of the IMAGE project, a curriculum for the training of prevention managers was also developed.[71] The purpose was to develop common European learning goals, teaching methods, and contents as well as teaching material for the training of health care professionals who want to carry out lifestyle interventions for T2DM prevention (Prevention

Managers T2DM). With this curriculum, for the first time, standardized state-of-the art training for health care professionals interested in offering preventive intervention can be performed Europe-wide in a comparable and consistent way. This is particularly useful because a standardized method to train the trainers for T2DM prevention can also pilot the same strategies for the prevention of other chronic diseases. All materials needed to train a prevention manager are freely available at www.virtualpreventioncenter.com. National institutions, such as universities or associations interested in the training of eligible health care professionals, are encouraged to download the specific teaching materials and follow the curriculum for the training of prevention managers.

The idea behind the curriculum for the training of diabetes prevention managers was to develop a standardized training curriculum for people coming from different professional disciplines who together want to deliver coordinated interventions for the prevention of T2DM. Currently 11 European countries and more than 20 extra-European countries have started to train prevention managers following the IMAGE curriculum.

MOVING DIABETES PREVENTION INTO PRACTICE

A challenging step is to translate the research findings into nationwide or regional diabetes prevention programs that translate the research findings to real-life health care settings. Finland has led the way with FIN-D2D, a large-scale implementation covering a quarter of the Finnish population.[82] Another landmark was the profusion of published implementation trials including Good Ageing in Lahti Region (GOAL) and the Saxon Diabetes Prevention Program in Europe,[83] the Greater Green Triangle Diabetes Prevention Project in Australia, the Walking away from Type 2 Diabetes program in the United Kingdom,[81,84] and programs in Indianapolis, Pittsburgh, and Montana in the United States.[4,85] A great challenge will be the scaling up from these implementation trials to sizeable regional and national programs.

Political support is needed, and this requires the development of a national or international action plan for diabetes prevention, which needs involvement of a number of stakeholders at governmental and nongovernmental levels. Furthermore, the presentation of the evidence in the field of diabetes prevention on the scientific and practical level as well as the training of people to deliver preventive intervention are required.

Steps in Development of a Prevention Program

Basic Science in Diabetes Prevention

Exploration of the molecular physiology of the prevention of T2DM is key to both understanding the pathobiologic mechanisms of diabetes prevention and also developing targeted intervention programs with improved outcomes. Growing evidence suggests that insulin resistance in a normoglycemic person is the key processor of the development of T2DM risk (see also **Chapter 2**).[30] The role of visceral fat mass and visceral obesity seems to be a key trigger for the development of insulin resistance (see also **Chapter 6**).[87] The visceral fat secreted adipokine profile directly influences inflammatory processes and insulin resistance development, which then altogether directly influence diabetes risk.[88] Furthermore,

increasing levels of circulating insulin and proinsulin seem to be a major factor in triggering T2DM development and subsequent cardiovascular disease and cardiovascular morbidity. Understanding these pathophysiologic mechanisms will make it necessary to explore the genetic basis of the regulation of insulin resistance and to understand visceral obesity and the combined pathophysiology behind it. Current evidence from genome-wide association studies explains a small proportion of T2DM pathophysiology (see also **Chapter 2**).[89,90] However, current investigations suggest that there is a link between genetic susceptibility and the outcome in preventive interventions.[91,92] Furthermore, results from basic prevention studies show that there is a substantial proportion of people at risk for T2DM who do not respond to an intervention or do not benefit from an intervention, even without T2DM development. A significant challenge in the future is development of pathophysiology-targeted prevention programs, as well as identification of nonresponders to preventive interventions.

Efficacy in Diabetes Prevention

To test intervention concepts and to generate evidence about intervention structures, T2DM prevention programs have to be tested in ideal RCT settings. In recent years considerable evidence has shown that sustained lifestyle change enables a significant ability to prevent or delay T2DM.[15,93] A number of large randomized clinical trials have shown that interventions focusing on improved physical activity and nutritional intake along with strategies and supports for behavior change enabled up to 58% prevention of T2DM. Furthermore, use of traditionally known diabetes drugs enables prevention of T2DM (see also **Chapter 6**).[15,27] Lifestyle interventions and drug treatment do not show an additive effect; unfortunately, there is conflicting evidence about the combination. Lifestyle intervention was more effective in older adults and less effective in obese people than the drug metformin. Metformin was more effective in younger, heavier people and women with a history of gestational diabetes mellitus (GDM) in the DPP.[15] By summarizing the efficacy of interventions for diabetes prevention, we have learned that the prevention of diabetes is effective and feasible, but we have also identified barriers and the challenging task of how to implement this knowledge.[94]

The efficacy of diabetes prevention programs may be strongly influenced by pathophysiologic differences. There is a huge variation in the conversion from IGT to T2DM, and the trigger mechanisms are not completely understood. The higher the conversion rate is, and the higher the prevalence of impaired glucose metabolism in the population, the greater the efficacy of prevention programs. Because the prevalence of IGT is increasing in almost all populations, the efficacy of T2DM prevention programs may increase in the future.[18]

Effectiveness in Diabetes Prevention

After evidence has been obtained from RCTs, it is necessary to translate this knowledge into real-world settings. This generates a number of new challenges and makes it necessary to start a critical discussion about necessity and practicability of what was done in the RCTs and what is applicable to real-world settings. A number of translation studies have tried to do this and have found ways to reduce costs and achieve the same or similar weight loss as in the RCTs. There are challenges in moving from RCTs to real-world implementation in diabetes prevention. One issue is screening to identify individuals at high risk. It is unrealistic to believe that performing two oral glucose tolerance tests for screening, which is done in some countries, can be appropriate for prevention programs in real-world settings, except in very high-risk individuals in the medical environment. A number of translational trials have been performed in several parts of the world, with different experiences. The implementation design often depends on limited financial resources and is driven by the circumstances in the environment to enable screening and intervention. Therefore the translational trials are often driven by the practical need for diabetes prevention and the dimensions of the clinical and public health problem in the environment. They adjust screening procedures and interventions to fit the existing environments, driven by the hypothesis to test the feasibility and applicability of an intervention program to the real-world setting.[40] The subsequent translation studies of the U.S. DPP have shown that by delivering the program in a group setting (instead of one-on-one) and using lower-cost trained health educators and community organization staff, the program can be delivered effectively and cost-effectively.[95]

Efficiency of Diabetes Prevention

After having learned from the implementation trials and having put together practical evidence from effectiveness studies, the next challenge is to modify the programs or their implementation to achieve the biggest impact for the most people who need the intervention. The efficacy research studies are often applicable only to a limited part of the population, and studies often include a relatively small number of people. The effectiveness trials are more likely to use a more broadly defined high-risk population, but the interventions that have been proven to be effective in real-world settings still may not address factors that will scale the intervention to reach the most people. At this stage, for the first time, policy perspectives and plans for cost-effective expansion of the intervention are taken into account. RCTs or effectiveness trials cannot tell us how to achieve the best effect for most of the people; this requires networking with a number of specialists and stakeholders from neighboring fields in medicine and public health and with expertise in fields such as management, economics, and policy development.

For programs to be efficient in the prevention of T2DM on a population level, political support on local and national levels to build national diabetes prevention plans is needed. These plans help relevant players and stakeholders to network to agree on a concerted plan of action involving different societal and personal resources to enable an efficient and wide-reaching T2DM prevention program.

Availability of Diabetes Prevention

After the efficiency of T2DM prevention has been addressed through a practical framework of stakeholders, and with political support and the necessary resources to enable a population-based impact, it is necessary to address program availability, accessibility, and capacity. Availability includes an adequate number of programs with easy access in the community, the existence of adequate personnel resources to train the prevention managers, and an adequate number of prevention managers. The development of the European curriculum for the training of prevention mangers is a relevant achievement to standardize intervention procedures

and to develop "train the trainer" strategies. As part of the National Diabetes Prevention Program, the United States has developed the Diabetes Training and Technical Assistance Center at Emory University to help train master trainers and lifestyle coaches and coordinate training efforts.[95] Policies that support adequate resources and coordination are important at this stage and support from scientists and medical experts in the field to drive the right political decisions and program availability is vital.

The industrialization of T2DM prevention programs becomes a relevant challenge. The Danish example of the tax on saturated fatty acids is an effective model for T2DM prevention on a national scale, but the intervention failed because of political reasons and the missing pan-European policy. The industrialization can also be achieved by adequate and intensified training of medical professional and health care workers to conduct T2DM prevention programs and to build a framework to implement business solutions for T2DM prevention. The extensive growth of new media and mobile health solutions may help to make healthy lifestyle information more available throughout the population, but also to enable mobile health intervention concepts. We have to accept that no one solution will address the needs of a large population. We will need a number of solutions providing adequate care and attention for T2DM prevention, based on target populations, individual prevalence, readiness to change lifestyle, environmental and regional aspects, and many more factors.[18]

Distribution of Diabetes Prevention

Even the best program will fail if it cannot reach people at increased risk.[83] Any preventive action will have to be performed in the environment in which the people at increased risk live and work.[3,96] Structures and policies to identify high-risk individuals and manage intervention follow-up and evaluation have to be established. Scientific evaluation standards based on the RCTs need to be translated into the public health care setting with careful management of considerably more limited resources. This has been achieved in Europe by the international IMAGE consortium with a quality management structure.[70] In the United States, the National Diabetes Prevention Program includes a recognition program that sets standards that help ensure program quality and consistency. The U.S. Centers for Disease Control and Prevention (CDC) is responsible for conducting this program and reporting on the distribution and quality of the diabetes prevention program across the United States.[95]

National Initiatives

Along with European level support, national governments and health care organizations are increasingly developing tailored national policies and guidance aimed at the prevention of chronic disease. For example, Finland has adopted a regional systematic whole-system approach across all sectors of the health care community, including primary care, pharmacy, and community settings, to the prevention of T2DM.[82] In the United Kingdom, the National Health Service Health Check program has been rolled out nationally and aims to screen all individuals aged 45 to 70 years for the risk of chronic disease and to treat high-risk individuals accordingly (www. healthcheck.nhs.uk).[86] In addition, new NICE guidance has been published that provides a blueprint for the prevention of T2DM in the community and primary care.[33] A similar program is under way in Germany. A health check for

Adipose tissue

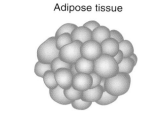

Oxidative stress modulation
Adipocytokine release
Inhibition of adipocyte differentiation
 in vitro
↑ Adiponectin and leptin levels
↑ PPAR - α receptor
Weight gain

Pancreas

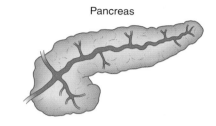

Impaired insulin secretion
Impaired pancreatic blood flow
Islet cell fibrosis and death
Impaired first-phase insulin release
Alpha$_1$-adrenergic receptor blockade

Muscle

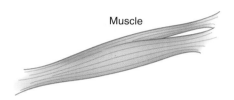

Impaired peripheral glucose uptake
Enhanced insulin resistance
↓ Glucose transporter 4
↑ Post-receptor activity of insulin
↑ PPAR-α receptor
Alpha$_1$-adrenergic receptor blockade
Vasodilatation

Liver

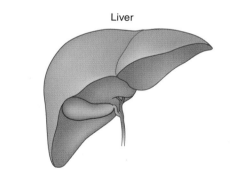

↓ Cytokine release
↑ Hepatic fat content
Inhibition of isoprenoid biosynthesis
↓ Glucose transporter 4
Oxidative stress medulation

Vessel

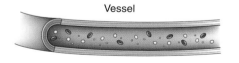

Oxidative stress modulation
↑ Potassium levels
Anti-inflammatory activity
Enhanced nitric oxide synthesis
↓ LDL-C oxidation

FIGURE 6-1 Potential mechanisms by which pharmacologic therapies may affect glycemic control. LDL-C = Low-density lipoprotein cholesterol; PPAR-α = peroxisome proliferator-activated receptor alpha.

Despite these clinical benefits, many physicians are reluctant to prescribe beta blockers because of perceived negative metabolic effects (**Box 6-3**). However, beta blockers should not be considered a homogenous class of agents. Beta blockers consist of nonvasodilating and vasodilating agents, which differ in terms of their mechanisms of action and effects on glucose and lipid metabolism. Treatment with nonvasodilating beta blockers is associated with an increased propensity of patients with hypertension to develop diabetes. A substudy of the Atherosclerosis Risk in Communities (ARIC) observational cohort study, which included 3804 patients with hypertension, demonstrated that patients treated with nonvasodilating beta blockers had a 28% higher risk of developing diabetes than patients on no pharmacologic treatment for hypertension.[35] Patients receiving thiazide diuretics, ACE inhibitors, or calcium

DIABETES MELLITUS

BOX 6-3 Potential Deleterious Metabolic Effects of Beta Blockers

- Reduced glycemic control
- Masking of hypoglycemia
- Deterioration in insulin resistance
  - Decreased blood flow to muscles, reducing peripheral insulin-stimulated glucose uptake
  - Interference with insulin secretion from pancreatic beta cells
  - Decrement in the first phase of insulin secretion
- Weight gain
- Dyslipidemia

channel antagonists were not at significantly higher or lower risk for subsequent diabetes than untreated patients.[35] Similarly, the Losartan Intervention for Endpoint Reduction in Hypertension (LIFE) randomized trial demonstrated in 9193 patients that the risk of developing diabetes was 25% lower among patients with hypertension and left ventricular hypertrophy who received losartan-based therapy than among patients who received atenolol-based therapy.[36]

Nonvasodilating beta blockers (atenolol, metoprolol, pindolol, and propranolol) reduce blood pressure in association with a cardiac output reduction and may increase or have no appreciable influence on peripheral vascular resistance.[37] Nonvasodilating beta blockers include first- and second-generation agents. First-generation beta blockers (propranolol) block both beta$_1$- and beta$_2$-adrenergic receptors (nonselective beta blockade), whereas second-generation beta blockers (atenolol and metoprolol) specifically target beta$_1$-adrenergic receptors (cardioselective beta blockade).[38] Nonvasodilating beta blockers significantly decrease insulin sensitivity by approximately 14% to 33% among patients with hypertension.[39,40] Studies have shown increases in glucose concentrations with the use of atenolol alone,[41,42] metoprolol,[43] or propranolol,[44,45] although other studies have shown no changes in glucose levels with atenolol[46–48] or propranolol.[49,50] However, glucose levels at a particular timepoint may not reflect long-term changes in glucose metabolism as reflected by hemoglobin A1c (HbA1c). As an example, after 6 months of treatment, once-daily metoprolol did not affect fasting plasma glucose but significantly increased HbA1c levels by a relative increase of 5% from baseline in patients with hypertension.[51]

In contrast, vasodilating beta blockers (carvedilol, labetalol, and nebivolol) reduce peripheral vascular resistance but have little or no effect on cardiac output. Numerous studies have shown that vasodilating beta blockers are associated with more favorable effects on glucose and lipid profiles than nonvasodilating beta blockers.[52] Bisoprolol, a beta$_1$-selective adrenergic blocker, was reported to have a neutral effect on glucose and insulin levels during a glucose tolerance test after 24 weeks of treatment at 5 to 10 mg/day in 13 patients with hypertension.[53]

Although the specific mechanisms have not been identified, several have been postulated to explain the negative effects of nonvasodilating beta blockers on glucose and lipid metabolism, most of which relate to their hemodynamic effects. Treatment with nonvasodilating beta blockers, which block either the beta$_1$-adrenergic receptor or the beta$_1$- and beta$_2$-adrenergic receptors, results in unopposed alpha$_1$-adrenergic receptor activity (which can induce vasoconstriction), decreased blood flow to the muscles, and reduced insulin-stimulated glucose uptake in the periphery.[54,55] Nonvasodilating beta blockers may also interfere

with insulin secretion from pancreatic beta cells. Moreover, beta blockers may decrease the first phase of insulin secretion (potentially an important predictor of diabetes) via impairment of beta$_2$-mediated insulin release.[54,56] Weight gain also has been noted in patients who received nonvasodilating beta blockers[57,58] and is closely linked to an increased risk for developing diabetes.[59] Increased peripheral blood flow from the action of vasodilating beta blockers may result in efficient glucose dispersal to the skeletal muscles, thereby facilitating insulin sensitivity.[37] The mechanisms responsible for the beneficial effects of vasodilating beta blockers on glucose and lipid metabolism are not entirely understood but may include alpha$_1$-adrenergic receptor blockade, vasodilation, reduced oxidative stress, anti-inflammatory activity, and lack of weight gain.[52,60,61]

In the Glycemic Effects in Diabetes Mellitus: Carvedilol-Metoprolol Comparison in Hypertensives (GEMINI) trial, the metabolic effects of carvedilol and metoprolol were compared in 1235 patients with type 2 diabetes and hypertension. The use of carvedilol in the presence of RAAS blockade was not deleterious to glycemic control and improved some components of the metabolic syndrome relative to metoprolol.[62] On the other hand, metoprolol significantly increased HbA1c levels from baseline (absolute increase of 0.15%), in contrast to carvedilol (0.02%) with an absolute difference between the groups of 0.13% ($P = 0.004$ for carvedilol versus metoprolol).[62] Statistically significant improvement was observed in insulin sensitivity with carvedilol (−9.1%) but not statistically significant with metoprolol (−2.0%). In this trial, metoprolol-treated patients experienced a significant weight gain (1.2 ± 0.16 kg) compared with carvedilol-treated patients (0.17 ± 0.19 kg).[63] In another study, a group of patients treated with metoprolol had an increase in body weight of 1.8 kg after 2 months of treatment. In contrast, no significant weight gain was found in the group of patients treated with carvedilol.[64] This is in accordance with the weight gain seen after treatment with beta blockers in large clinical trials.[65] In the presence of heart failure, carvedilol was shown to be associated with improved survival (the Carvedilol or Metoprolol European Trial [COMET]) and with fewer cases of new-onset diabetes compared with metoprolol.[66,67]

Carvedilol and nebivolol enhance nitric oxide synthesis and thus mediate endothelial-dependent vasodilation.[68–71] Carvedilol is associated with antioxidant activity, possibly because of stimulation of endothelial nitric oxide production or reduced nitric oxide inactivation.[72,73] Carvedilol also inhibits low-density lipoprotein cholesterol (LDL-C) oxidation, potentially reducing the accumulation of oxidized LDL-C in vessel walls and subsequent vascular damage.[74] Furthermore, carvedilol has been shown to protect against reactive oxygen species via scavenging of free radicals, suppression of free radical generation, and prevention of ferric ion-induced oxidation.[72,73] Carvedilol treatment reduced proinflammatory markers, including plasma C-reactive protein and monocyte chemotactic protein 1, in patients with hypertension and diabetes.[73]

Nebivolol is considered to have a neutral effect on metabolic parameters in patients with hypertension,[7] but among 80 patients with hypertension, nebivolol significantly reduced baseline insulin levels and insulin resistance versus metoprolol after 6 months of treatment.[75] In a larger, open-label study involving 328 patients with hypertension, compared with baseline, nebivolol significantly reduced fasting glucose, total cholesterol, and triglyceride levels.[76] Another large, open-label study involving 2838 patients with hypertension and diabetes showed that after 3 months of nebivolol treatment, significant reductions were observed from baseline in fasting glucose, HbA1c, total cholesterol, LDL-C, and triglyceride levels, with an increase in high-density lipoprotein cholesterol (HDL-C).[77] Several small studies have demonstrated that labetalol treatment compared with other antihypertensive therapies is associated with neutral effects on glucose and lipid metabolism in patients with essential hypertension.[78,79]

Thiazide Diuretics

Thiazide diuretics can result in various undesired biochemical changes, and in general increase glucose and insulin resistance. Thiazides have been shown to increase fasting glucose levels and impair glucose tolerance curves in many long-term studies.[80–82] The effect on glucose tolerance is usually reversible if the thiazide is stopped,[83] and the effect on blood glucose levels is dose related.[83]

The mechanistic underpinning of these effects is not well understood. Thiazide-induced hypokalemia, as well as effects on other pathophysiologic pathways, may explain these metabolic disturbances, such as increased visceral adiposity, hyperuricemia, decreased glucose metabolism, and pancreatic beta cell hyperpolarization.[84] Whereas many large randomized, prospective clinical trials show an association between thiazide use and increased blood glucose, findings are mixed regarding the association with new-onset diabetes. Many issues must be considered in evaluating these associations in these trials, including the following:

- Most are post hoc findings and were not adequately powered to assess this association.
- New-onset diabetes was defined differently in many studies.
- Many studies had follow-up durations of only a few years, which may not be long enough to fully assess prolonged hyperglycemia.
- Comparing drug classes is difficult because of differing study designs.[85]

A meta-analysis of clinical trials revealed that of all antihypertensives assessed, beta blockers and thiazide diuretics are associated with the highest risk of diabetes. This analysis found that thiazides are associated with higher risk of diabetes than placebo and, along with beta blockers, had the highest risk of all major classes of antihypertensives.[86] The pathophysiologic process accounting for these effects may be mediated through influence on potassium balance and circulating potassium levels. It has been reported that potassium infusions causing more than a 1- to 1.5-mEq/L elevation in plasma potassium enhance insulin release twofold to threefold compared with basal levels.[87] The relationship between potassium and glucose homeostasis is central because many believe that thiazide-induced potassium depletion drives hyperglycemia.[88] Actually, a meta-analysis of 59 clinical studies showed a significant correlation between thiazide-induced potassium depletion and increased blood glucose levels, as well as a correlation between potassium supplementation (or concomitant use of potassium-sparing agents) and attenuation of hyperglycemia.[89] In addition, a secondary analysis of the Systolic Hypertension in the Elderly Program (SHEP) investigated the relationship between serum potassium and thiazide-induced diabetes.[90] The risk for developing diabetes was increased in the first year of thiazide treatment.[90] In addition, independent of drug treatment, each 0.5-mEq/L decrease in serum potassium was associated with a 45% increased risk for development of diabetes throughout the course of the study.[90] A retrospective analysis of an extended follow-up of the SHEP trial was recently reported.[91] After a mean follow-up period of 14.3 years, patients treated with thiazide were more likely to develop new-onset diabetes. However, new-onset diabetes that developed in patients treated with thiazide diuretics was not associated with significantly increased cardiovascular or total mortality.

Alteration in fat distribution is another possible mechanism for thiazide-induced dysglycemia. Patients treated with 25 to 50 mg of thiazide daily had significant reductions in insulin sensitivity, compared with those treated with candesartan or placebo.[92] Serum potassium levels were significantly lower in patients taking thiazide, but levels in all groups remained within normal limits.[92] While taking thiazide, patients also developed a significantly higher hepatic fat content, and a significant correlation was found between hepatic fat content and decreased insulin sensitivity.[92] Whether decreased insulin sensitivity was a result of this visceral fat accumulation or vice versa is not clear. Low-grade inflammation assessed with C-reactive protein was also significantly increased with thiazide treatment,[92] suggesting a possible role for inflammation in the development of insulin resistance. Of clinical interest is that patients with abdominal obesity are more likely to experience new-onset diabetes with thiazide treatment than those without abdominal obesity.[93,94] In older studies of thiazide diuretics, the dosage (or equivalent in vitro concentration) used was 50 mg of thiazide or more. Today, clinicians do not often prescribe doses greater than 25 mg of thiazide or its equivalent. Of note, findings from the Antihypertensive and Lipid-Lowering Treatment to Prevent Heart Attack Trial (ALLHAT) diabetes extension study suggest that thiazide-related incident diabetes has less adverse long-term CVD impact than incident diabetes that develops while patients are taking amlopidine or lisinopril.[95]

Calcium Channel Blockers

In 16,176 hypertensive patients with CAD enrolled in the International Verapamil SR Trandolapril Study (INVEST), a verapamil-based treatment regimen was associated with a decrease in the incidence of type 2 diabetes from 8.2% to 7.0% compared with an atenolol-based regimen.[96] Diabetes incidence was not a predefined endpoint in this study, and no adjustment was made for concomitant therapies, which could potentially affect diabetes incidence. In ALLHAT, the risk of incident diabetes at 4 years of follow-up was 9.3% with the calcium channel blocker amlodipine and 7.8% with the ACE inhibitor lisinopril.[97]

High-dose calcium channel blocker therapy can inhibit insulin release, but this effect is generally not seen with usual therapeutic doses.[98,99] Impaired insulin release appears to be counterbalanced by increased peripheral glucose uptake, such that the predominant effect of these agents is metabolically neutral or favorable.[98,100] Evidence from animal models suggests that vasodilation and improved peripheral blood flow may explain the potential improvement in insulin sensitivity seen with calcium channel blockade.[101] Thus, calcium channel blockers appear to have a neutral or slightly favorable effect on glucose metabolism.

Niacin

Niacin is known to increase insulin resistance and have adverse effects on blood glucose levels, but to have favorable effects on plasma lipids and lipoproteins. Niacin reduces plasma triglycerides, increases HDL-C, and reduces LDL-C modestly. Concerns have been raised about use of niacin in diabetic patients because of its adverse effects on insulin resistance and blood glucose levels.[102,103]

Reports from the Assessment of Diabetes Control and Evaluation of the Efficacy Niaspan Trial (ADVENT),[104] the Arterial Disease Multiple Intervention Trial (ADMIT),[105] and the HDL-Atherosclerosis Treatment Study (HATS)[106] have shown that the modest increase in glucose level caused by niacin treatment could be easily counteracted by adjusting the diet, amount of exercise, and dose of glucose-lowering medication. During the follow-up period in the Atherothrombosis Intervention in Metabolic Syndrome with Low HDL/High Triglycerides: Impact on Global Health Outcomes (AIM-HIGH) trial, the dose of the study drug was reduced in 6.3% of the patients in the niacin group and 3.4% of the patients in the placebo group ($P < 0.001$). Increased glucose level was the primary reason for dose reduction in 5 (0.3%) and 10 (0.6%) patients (placebo versus niacin, respectively). The study drug was discontinued in 25.4% of the patients in the niacin group and in 20.1% of the patients in the placebo group ($P < 0.001$). The primary reason for discontinuation because of increased glucose level was reported in 14 (0.8%) and 29 (1.7%) patients (placebo versus niacin, respectively).[107] During HATS, there was a 20% rise in insulin levels in the groups taking niacin. This finding was accompanied by a 2% to 3% increase in fasting glucose levels. In patients with diabetes,[106] glucose levels increased by approximately 15% by 3 months in those receiving niacin, but returned to baseline by 8 months. Changes in glucose-lowering medications were permitted, but no data were provided. Glycemic control among patients with diabetes returned to pretreatment values after 8 months, probably because of better diabetes management.[106] The changes in blood glucose with extended-release (ER) niacin are typically modest and transient and more prevalent in patients with diabetes.[104,105] On average, the rise in HbA1c levels is small and can be managed by titrating hypoglycemic therapy, but blood glucose levels should be closely monitored in patients with difficult-to-treat diabetes.

The Heart Protection Study 2—Treatment of HDL to Reduce the Incidence of Vascular Events (HPS2-THRIVE) study, a large randomized trial that comprising 25,673 patients tested the use of extended-release niacin and the antiflushing agent laropiprant for the reduction of major vascular events, did not find a significantly reduced risk of major vascular events in patients with well-controlled LDL-C levels. The failure of niacin in the HPS2-THRIVE study was first announced in late December 2012. In light of these findings, the role of extended-release niacin for the prevention of CVD should be reconsidered, given the side effects of niacin including a 25% increased risk of new-onset diabetes and the difficulties in controlling glucose level when patients are taking niacin.[108]

Statins

Statin therapy, particularly high-dose therapy, is associated with increased diabetes risk.[109,110] These study observations are supported by results from two meta-analyses including over 100,000 participants demonstrating that long-term statin intake was associated with increased risk of new-onset diabetes.[111,112] Several meta-analyses have been conducted to elucidate the effect of statins on glucose metabolism.[111,113,114] Treatment with statins has been associated with a 9% increase in the risk of developing diabetes without any clear differential effect among individual statins.[111,113] However, the overall data available strongly suggest that the reduction in CVD events outweighs the minor effect on glucose homeostasis.[115,116] In contrast, it has been suggested that various statins may affect glucose metabolism differentially.[114,117]

Pravastatin appeared to improve insulin sensitivity, whereas simvastatin was associated with an adverse effect on glucose metabolism.[114] Also, atorvastatin and rosuvastatin nonsignificantly worsened insulin sensitivity.[114] Rosuvastatin administration in hypercholesterolemic patients with impaired fasting glucose was associated with a dose-dependent increase in insulin resistance.[118,119]

The mechanisms by which statins may impair glucose metabolism are not fully understood. Several mechanisms may be responsible for these diabetogenic effects (**Box 6-4**).[120] One possibility is a statin-mediated decrease in various metabolic products of the mevalonate pathway, such as the isoprenoids farnesyl pyrophosphate or geranylgeranyl pyrophosphate. These isoprenoid molecules have been linked with the upregulation of the membrane transport protein glucose transporter 4 (GLUT-4) in 3 T3-L1 adipocytes, thus augmenting glucose uptake.[121] In type 2 diabetic mice and human patients treated for 3 months, atorvastatin impaired glucose tolerance and GLUT-4 expression by inhibiting isoprenoid biosynthesis.[122] In addition, a possible role for the small guanosine triphosphate (GTP) binding proteins as regulators of glucose-mediated insulin secretion by beta cells has been suggested.[123] Statins, by inhibiting 3-hydroxy-3-methylglutaryl-coenzyme A (HMG-CoA) reductase, decrease the production of these substances. High doses of lipophilic statins decreased insulin secretion from beta cell lines, mediated either by the inhibition of HMG-CoA reductase or direct cytotoxicity.[124] Therefore the lipophilicity of individual statins may influence their effects on glucose metabolism. Statins, particularly the lipophilic compounds, have been shown to inhibit glucose-induced cytosolic Ca^{2+} elevations and insulin secretion as a result of blockade of L-type Ca^{2+} channels in rat islet beta cells.[125] Simvastatin attenuates increases in cardiorespiratory fitness and skeletal muscle mitochondrial content when combined with exercise training in overweight or obese patients at risk of the metabolic syndrome.[126] However, this opposes the observed effects of rosuvastatin, which is known to be a hydrophilic molecule. A protective effect of pravastatin,

---

BOX 6-4 Potential Mechanisms by Which Statins May Impair Glucose Metabolism

Decrement in various metabolic products of the mevalonate pathway
- ↓ Isoprenoid farnesyl pyrophosphate
- ↓ Geranylgeranyl pyrophosphate

↓ Glucose transporter 4 expression

↓ Protein isoprenylation and affect on the distribution of several small G proteins
- ↓ Potentiation of nutrient-induced insulin secretion by bombesin and vasopressin

↓ Insulin secretion from beta cell lines
- Blockade of L-type Ca^{2+} channels in animal models

($13,243) are more than five times that of a patient without diabetes ($2560).[234] The largest components of costs are hospital inpatient care (50%), medication and supplies (12%), retail prescriptions to treat complications (11%), and physician office visits (9%).[234] Advantages of bariatric surgery with regard to diabetes translate into considerable economic benefits. Surgery costs for laparoscopic surgery may fully be recovered after 26 months. These data suggest that surgical therapy is clinically more effective and ultimately less expensive than standard therapy for diabetes patients with BMI of 35 kg/m^2 or higher.[235] This has also been reported in Canada, where health care system coverage differs from the United States. The initial costs of surgery can be amortized over 3.5 years.[236]

Observed metabolic effects following some procedures implicate weight-independent antidiabetes mechanisms.[226,227] These benefits result in part from mechanisms beyond reduced food intake and body weight because glycemic improvements precede substantial weight loss. Mingrone and colleagues[230] found that all the surgical patients achieved glycemic control without diabetes medications within only 15 days after surgery. Schauer and colleagues[229] reported that diabetes medication use decreased postoperatively, long before maximum weight loss occurred. Recent studies corroborate a growing body of evidence showing that weight-independent mechanisms contribute to diabetes remission after some bariatric procedures.[227,237] This notion is based primarily on (1) the early postoperative effects of RYGB surgery on glycemic control, (2) the long-term efficacy of different surgical procedures on resolution of type 2 diabetes, (3) the effect of duodenojejunal bypass (DJB) surgery, which bypasses the upper gastrointestinal tract but causes minimal weight loss, (4) the hormonal response to glucose or mixed-meal ingestion, and (5) upper gastrointestinal tract bypass in rodent models. Operations that reroute chyme in such a way that the duodenum and proximal jejunum are bypassed, resulting in chyme delivery directly to the jejunum, may be a promising pathophysiologic avenue in diabetes management.

Nonsurgical Duodenal Exclusion

An alternative approach would be to duplicate the effects of the gastric bypass or BPD procedure by diverting chyme from the proximal small intestine. The duodenojejunal bypass liner (DJBL) is an endoscopically placed and removable intestinal liner developed to achieve duodenal exclusion and promoting significant weight loss beyond a minimal sham. The DJBL is a 60-cm impermeable fluoropolymer device, which, after endoscopic deployment in the proximal duodenum, functions to prevent partially digested food from contacting the proximal intestine, similar to RYGB but without gastric restriction. Bile and pancreatic secretions pass along the outer wall of the liner and mix with the chyme exiting distal to the liner into the jejunum. Mean weight loss averages approximately 10 kg after 12 weeks with diabetes remission in several patients.[238–240] There seems to be a procedural learning curve of five to seven procedures.[240] Most DJBL-related adverse events are mild or moderate in the implantation patients. Many of the adverse events occurring within the first 2 weeks likely reflect adaptation to the DJBL. Mild bleeding is an expected adverse event associated with the anchoring of the device in the gastric pylorus.

SUMMARY

Regarding cardiovascular medications, although not definitive, the available evidence from bench research and clinical studies suggests a potentially beneficial effect on diabetes incidence for inhibitors of the RAAS system, a neutral effect for calcium channel blockers, and a detrimental effect for thiazide diuretics, nonvasodilating beta blockers, niacin, and statins. Vasodilating beta blockers have a number of favorable glycometabolic effects, although their effect in incident diabetes has not been fully explored.

Potentially diabetogenic agents should not be denied to patients with compelling indications for these drugs because of concerns that blood glucose levels will increase. Indeed, beta blockers have been well proven to lower cardiovascular morbidity and mortality in post–myocardial infarction and in chronic systolic heart failure patients. They should be considered among first-line agents in such patient populations. In patients with diabetes and nephropathy, ACE inhibitors or ARBs are considered to be first-line therapy. In patients without nephropathy, ACE inhibitors were associated with a reduction in cardiovascular morbidity and mortality in patients with diabetes. Because hypertensive patients with impaired fasting glucose or impaired glucose tolerance are commonly obese with several comorbidities, many will require multidrug antihypertensive therapy. Therefore, the choice of initial agent is not as important as ensuring that blood pressure treatment goals are achieved. The diabetogenic potential of thiazide diuretics and nonvasodilating beta blockers can be minimized by using the lowest effective dose possible. In addition, minimizing hypokalemia with thiazides and using alpha$_1$-adrenergic receptor–selective agents or agents with concomitant beta$_2$-blocking activity will also limit the detrimental effects of thiazides and beta blockers on blood glucose levels. The European Society of Hypertension and European Society of Cardiology guidelines note that, compared with nonvasodilating beta blockers, vasodilating beta blockers have fewer or no dysmetabolic effects and are less likely to cause new-onset diabetes.[241] In addition, the American Association of Clinical Endocrinologists guidelines state that third-generation beta blockers (carvedilol and nebivolol) induce vasodilation and increase insulin sensitivity and, as a result, are particularly appropriate for the treatment of patients with diabetes.[242] Management of dyslipidemia is also very important in patient with diabetes. Statins should not be withheld on the basis of a potential, small risk of new-onset diabetes emerging during long-term therapy.

Several other large global trials have clearly shown that noncardiovascular drug therapies, including metformin, acarbose, and glitazones, can also reduce the incidence of diabetes. Some of these trials also reported a significant increase in the probability of regression of dysglycemia to normoglycemia. All of the completed diabetes prevention trials studied individuals during a period of 3 to 4 years, after which formal application of the intervention was stopped. However, because diabetes is a lifelong disease, whether the effect of a relatively short exposure to a diabetes prevention intervention is sustained is clearly clinically important.

Bariatric surgery with its substantial weight loss reduces the incidence of diabetes in overweight insulin-resistant patients and is associated with remission of diabetes in a large percentage of patients. Although bariatric surgery appears to be an effective means for preventing and/or reversing type 2 diabetes, it cannot be considered a practical response to the worldwide epidemic of diabetes. In addition, bariatric surgery is associated with the potential for both immediate and long-term adverse metabolic consequences. In considering the usefulness of bariatric surgery, it is also important to recognize that long-term follow-up is required before a beneficial therapeutic effect can be assigned in patients with diabetes because of the potential for weight regain that has been observed after some surgical procedures.

Overall, the most important goal in the management of patients with type 2 diabetes should be the attainment of treatment targets according to guidelines and the institution of therapies that have been proven to reduce cardiovascular morbidity and mortality. One must keep in mind that most patients with diabetes are overweight or obese and will require more than one drug to achieve blood pressure targets and high doses of statins to achieve lipid targets. In these individuals, the choice of initial therapy is less important than ensuring that risk factors are treated in a timely and aggressive fashion. Management of obesity is also pivotal in patients with diabetes.

References

1. Chobanian AV, Bakris GL, Black HR, et al: Seventh report of the Joint National Committee on Prevention, Detection, Evaluation, and Treatment of High Blood Pressure, *Hypertension* 42 (6):1206–1252, 2003.
2. Johnson ML, Pietz K, Battleman DS, et al: Prevalence of comorbid hypertension and dyslipidemia and associated cardiovascular disease, *Am J Manag Care* 10(12):926–932, 2004.
3. Garcia-Puig J, Ruilope LM, Luque M, et al: Glucose metabolism in patients with essential hypertension, *Am J Med* 119(4):318–326, 2006.
4. Mitrakou A, Kelley D, Veneman T, et al: Contribution of abnormal muscle and liver glucose metabolism to postprandial hyperglycemia in NIDDM, *Diabetes* 39(11):1381–1390, 1990.
5. Ferrannini E, Simonson DC, Katz LD, et al: The disposal of an oral glucose load in patients with non-insulin-dependent diabetes, *Metabolism* 37(1):79–85, 1988.
6. U.K. prospective diabetes study 16. Overview of 6 years' therapy of type II diabetes: a progressive disease. U.K. Prospective Diabetes Study Group, *Diabetes* 44(11):1249–1258, 1995.
7. Fonseca VA: Effects of beta-blockers on glucose and lipid metabolism, *Curr Med Res Opin* 26 (3):615–629, 2010.
8. Cowie CC, Harris MI, Silverman RE, et al: Effect of multiple risk factors on differences between blacks and whites in the prevalence of non-insulin-dependent diabetes mellitus in the United States, *Am J Epidemiol* 137(7):719–732, 1993.
9. Egede LE, Dagogo-Jack S: Epidemiology of type 2 diabetes: focus on ethnic minorities, *Med Clin North Am* 89(5):949–975, 2005, viii.
10. McNeely MJ, Boyko EJ: Type 2 diabetes prevalence in Asian Americans: results of a national health survey, *Diabetes Care* 27(1):66–69, 2004.
11. Brancati FL, Kao WH, Folsom AR, et al: Incident type 2 diabetes mellitus in African American and white adults: the Atherosclerosis Risk in Communities Study, *JAMA* 283(17):2253–2259, 2000.
12. Shai I, Jiang R, Manson JE, et al: Ethnicity, obesity, and risk of type 2 diabetes in women: a 20-year follow-up study, *Diabetes Care* 29(7):1585–1590, 2006.
13. Haffner SM, Hazuda HP, Mitchell BD, et al: Increased incidence of type II diabetes mellitus in Mexican Americans, *Diabetes Care* 14(2):102–108, 1991.
14. Cowie CC, Rust KF, Byrd-Holt DD, et al: Prevalence of diabetes and impaired fasting glucose in adults in the U.S. population: National Health and Nutrition Examination Survey 1999–2002, *Diabetes Care* 29(6):1263–1268, 2006.
15. Cowie CC, Rust KF, Ford ES, et al: Full accounting of diabetes and pre-diabetes in the U.S. population in 1988–1994 and 2005–2006, *Diabetes Care* 32(2):287–294, 2009.
16. Cowie CC, Rust KF, Byrd-Holt DD, et al: Prevalence of diabetes and high risk for diabetes using A1C criteria in the U.S. population in 1988–2006, *Diabetes Care* 33(3):562–568, 2010.
17. Harris MI, Flegal KM, Cowie CC, et al: Prevalence of diabetes, impaired fasting glucose, and impaired glucose tolerance in U.S. adults. The Third National Health and Nutrition Examination Survey, 1988–1994, *Diabetes Care* 21(4):518–524, 1998.
18. Nichols GA, Arondekar B, Herman WH: Medical care costs one year after identification of hyperglycemia below the threshold for diabetes, *Med Care* 46(3):287–292, 2008.
19. Nichols GA, Brown JB: Higher medical care costs accompany impaired fasting glucose, *Diabetes Care* 28(9):2223–2229, 2005.
20. Dall TM, Zhang Y, Chen YJ, et al: The economic burden of diabetes, *Health Aff (Millwood)* 29 (2):297–303, 2010.
21. Zhang Y, Dall TM, Mann SE, et al: The economic costs of undiagnosed diabetes, *Popul Health Manag* 12(2):95–101, 2009.
22. Colditz GA, Willett WC, Rotnitzky A, et al: Weight gain as a risk factor for clinical diabetes mellitus in women, *Ann Intern Med* 122(7):481–486, 1995.
23. Chan JM, Rimm EB, Colditz GA, et al: Obesity, fat distribution, and weight gain as risk factors for clinical diabetes in men, *Diabetes Care* 17(9):961–969, 1994.
24. Yusuf S, Gerstein H, Hoogwerf B, et al: Ramipril and the development of diabetes, *JAMA* 286 (15):1882–1885, 2001.
25. Vermes E, Ducharme A, Bourassa MG, et al: Enalapril reduces the incidence of diabetes in patients with chronic heart failure: insight from the Studies Of Left Ventricular Dysfunction (SOLVD), *Circulation* 107(9):1291–1296, 2003.
26. Braunwald E, Domanski MJ, Fowler SE, et al: Angiotensin-converting-enzyme inhibition in stable coronary artery disease, *N Engl J Med* 351(20):2058–2068, 2004.
27. Pfeffer MA, Swedberg K, Granger CB, et al: Effects of candesartan on mortality and morbidity in patients with chronic heart failure: the CHARM-Overall programme, *Lancet* 362(9386):759–766, 2003.
28. Lithell H, Hansson L, Skoog I, et al: The Study on Cognition and Prognosis in the Elderly (SCOPE): principal results of a randomized double-blind intervention trial, *J Hypertens* 21 (5):875–886, 2003.
29. Julius S, Kjeldsen SE, Weber M, et al: Outcomes in hypertensive patients at high cardiovascular risk treated with regimens based on valsartan or amlodipine: the VALUE randomised trial, *Lancet* 363(9426):2022–2031, 2004.
30. Padwal R, Laupacis A: Antihypertensive therapy and incidence of type 2 diabetes: a systematic review, *Diabetes Care* 27(1):247–255, 2004.
31. Jandeleit-Dahm KA, Tikellis C, Reid CM, et al: Why blockade of the renin-angiotensin system reduces the incidence of new-onset diabetes, *J Hypertens* 23(3):463–473, 2005.
32. Sharma AM, Janke J, Gorzelniak K, et al: Angiotensin blockade prevents type 2 diabetes by formation of fat cells, *Hypertension* 40(5):609–611, 2002.
33. Kon V, Jabs K: Angiotensin in atherosclerosis, *Curr Opin Nephrol Hypertens* 13(3):291–297, 2004.
34. Benson SC, Pershadsingh HA, Ho CI, et al: Identification of telmisartan as a unique angiotensin II receptor antagonist with selective PPARgamma-modulating activity, *Hypertension* 43 (5):993–1002, 2004.
35. Gress TW, Nieto FJ, Shahar E, et al: Hypertension and antihypertensive therapy as risk factors for type 2 diabetes mellitus. Atherosclerosis Risk in Communities Study, *N Engl J Med* 342 (13):905–912, 2000.
36. Dahlof B, Devereux RB, Kjeldsen SE, et al: Cardiovascular morbidity and mortality in the Losartan Intervention For Endpoint reduction in hypertension study (LIFE): a randomised trial against atenolol, *Lancet* 359(9311):995–1003, 2002.
37. Messerli FH, Grossman E: beta-Blockers in hypertension: is carvedilol different? *Am J Cardiol* 93 (9A):7B–12B, 2004.
38. Frishman WH: A historical perspective of the development of B-Adrenergic blockers, *J Clin Hypertens* 9(Suppl. s4):19–27, 2007.
39. Jacob S, Rett K, Wicklmayr M, et al: Differential effect of chronic treatment with two beta-blocking agents on insulin sensitivity: the carvedilol-metoprolol study, *J Hypertens* 14(4): 489–494, 1996.
40. Lithell HO: Effect of antihypertensive drugs on insulin, glucose, and lipid metabolism, *Diabetes Care* 14(3):203–209, 1991.
41. Aberg H, Morlin C, Lithell H: Different long-term metabolic effects of enalapril and atenolol in patients with mild hypertension. EGTA Group, *J Hum Hypertens* 9(2):149–153, 1995.
42. Helgeland A, Strommen R, Hagelund CH, et al: Enalapril, atenolol, and hydrochlorothiazide in mild to moderate hypertension. A comparative multicentre study in general practice in Norway, *Lancet* 1(8486):872–875, 1986.
43. Jacob S, Klimm HJ, Rett K, et al: Effects of moxonidine vs. metoprolol on blood pressure and metabolic control in hypertensive subjects with type 2 diabetes, *Exp Clin Endocrinol Diabetes* 112(6):315–322, 2004.
44. Berglund G, Andersson O, Widgren B: Low-dose antihypertensive treatment with a thiazide diuretic is not diabetogenic. A 10-year controlled trial with bendroflumethiazide, *Acta Med Scand* 220(5):419–424, 1986.
45. Propranolol or hydrochlorothiazide alone for the initial treatment of hypertension. IV. Effect on plasma glucose and glucose tolerance. Veterans Administration Cooperative Study Group on Antihypertensive Agents, *Hypertension* 7(6 Pt 1):1008–1016, 1985.
46. Sourgens H, Schmidt J, Derendorf H: Comparison of talinolol and atenolol effects on blood pressure in relation to lipid and glucose metabolic parameters. Results from the TALIP study, *Int J Clin Pharmacol Ther* 41(1):22–29, 2003.
47. Chrysant SG, Chappel C, Farnham DJ, et al: Antihypertensive and metabolic effects of single and combined atenolol regimens, *J Clin Pharmacol* 32(1):61–65, 1992.
48. Ruilope LM: Comparison of a new vasodilating beta-blocker, carvedilol, with atenolol in the treatment of mild to moderate essential hypertension, *Am J Hypertens* 7(2):129–136, 1994.
49. Bagatin J, Sardelic S, Pivac N, et al: Comparison of chlorthalidone, propranolol and bopindolol in six-month treatment of arterial hypertension, *Int J Clin Pharmacol Res* 18(2):73–78, 1998.
50. Perez-Stable EJ, Coates TJ, Baron RB, et al: Comparison of a lifestyle modification program with propranolol use in the management of diastolic hypertension, *J Gen Intern Med* 10(8):419–428, 1995.
51. Haenni A, Lithell H: Treatment with a beta-blocker with beta 2-agonism improves glucose and lipid metabolism in essential hypertension, *Metabolism* 43(4):455–461, 1994.
52. Pedersen ME, Cockcroft JR: The vasodilatory beta-blockers, *Curr Hypertens Rep* 9(4):269–277, 2007.
53. Owada A, Suda S, Hata T, et al: The effects of bisoprolol, a selective beta1-blocker, on glucose metabolism by long-term administration in essential hypertension, *Clin Exp Hypertens* 23 (4):305–316, 2001.
54. Sarafidis PA, Bakris GL: Antihypertensive treatment with beta-blockers and the spectrum of glycaemic control, *QJM* 99(7):431–436, 2006.
55. Tang WH: A critical review of anti-adrenergic therapy in patients with heart failure and diabetes mellitus, *Vasc Health Risk Manag* 3(5):639–645, 2007.
56. DeFronzo RA, Mandarino L, Ferrannini E: Metabolic and molecular pathogenesis of type 2 diabetes mellitus. In DeFronzo RA, Ferrannini E, Keen H, Zimmet P, editors: *International textbook of diabetes mellitus*, ed 3., Chichester, UK, 2004, John Wiley & Sons Ltd, pp 359–373.
57. Efficacy of atenolol and captopril in reducing risk of macrovascular and microvascular complications in type 2 diabetes: UKPDS 39. UK Prospective Diabetes Study Group, *BMJ* 317 (7160):713–720, 1998.
58. Rossner S, Taylor CL, Byington RP, et al: Long term propranolol treatment and changes in body weight after myocardial infarction, *BMJ* 300(6729):902–903, 1990.
59. Ko DT, Hebert PR, Coffey CS, et al: Beta-blocker therapy and symptoms of depression, fatigue, and sexual dysfunction, *JAMA* 288(3):351–357, 2002.
60. Egan BM, Basile J, Chilton RJ, et al: Cardioprotection: the role of beta-blocker therapy, *J Clin Hypertens (Greenwich)* 7(7):409–416, 2005.
61. Bell DS: Optimizing treatment of diabetes and cardiovascular disease with combined alpha, beta-blockade, *Curr Med Res Opin* 21(8):1191–1200, 2005.
62. Bakris GL, Fonseca V, Katholi RE, et al: Metabolic effects of carvedilol vs metoprolol in patients with type 2 diabetes mellitus and hypertension: a randomized controlled trial, *JAMA* 292 (18):2227–2236, 2004.
63. Messerli FH, Bell DS, Fonseca V, et al: Body weight changes with beta-blocker use: results from GEMINI, *Am J Med* 120(7):610–615, 2007.
64. Kveiborg B, Hermann TS, Major-Pedersen A, et al: Metoprolol compared to carvedilol deteriorates insulin-stimulated endothelial function in patients with type 2 diabetes - a randomized study, *Cardiovasc Diabetol* 9:21, 2010.
65. Pischon T, Sharma AM: Use of beta-blockers in obesity hypertension: potential role of weight gain, *Obes Rev* 2(4):275–280, 2001.
66. Poole-Wilson PA, Swedberg K, Cleland JG, et al: Comparison of carvedilol and metoprolol on clinical outcomes in patients with chronic heart failure in the Carvedilol Or Metoprolol European Trial (COMET): randomised controlled trial, *Lancet* 362(9377):7–13, 2003.
67. Torp-Pedersen C, Metra M, Charlesworth A, et al: Effects of metoprolol and carvedilol on pre-existing and new onset diabetes in patients with chronic heart failure: data from the Carvedilol Or Metoprolol European Trial (COMET), *Heart* 93(8):968–973, 2007.
68. Agabiti RE, Rizzoni D: Metabolic profile of nebivolol, a beta-adrenoceptor antagonist with unique characteristics, *Drugs* 67(8):1097–1107, 2007.
69. Kozlovski VI, Lomnicka M, Chlopicki S: Nebivolol and carvedilol induce NO-dependent coronary vasodilatation that is unlikely to be mediated by extracellular ATP in the isolated guinea pig heart, *Pharmacol Rep* 58(Suppl):103–110, 2006.

70. Giugliano D, Marfella R, Acampora R, et al: Effects of perindopril and carvedilol on endothelium-dependent vascular functions in patients with diabetes and hypertension, *Diabetes Care* 21 (4):631–636, 1998.
71. González M I: Adrenoreceptors, endothelial function, and lipid profile: effects of atenolol, doxazosin, and carvedilol, *Coron Artery Dis* 5(11):909–918, 1994.
72. Toda N: Vasodilating beta-adrenoceptor blockers as cardiovascular therapeutics, *Pharmacol Ther* 100(3):215–234, 2003.
73. Dandona P, Ghanim H, Brooks DP: Antioxidant activity of carvedilol in cardiovascular disease, *J Hypertens* 25(4):731–741, 2007.
74. Maggi E, Marchesi E, Covini D, et al: Protective effects of carvedilol, a vasodilating beta-adrenoceptor blocker, against in vivo low density lipoprotein oxidation in essential hypertension, *J Cardiovasc Pharmacol* 27(4):532–538, 1996.
75. Celik T, Iyisoy A, Kursaklioglu H, et al: Comparative effects of nebivolol and metoprolol on oxidative stress, insulin resistance, plasma adiponectin and soluble P-selectin levels in hypertensive patients, *J Hypertens* 24(3):591–596, 2006.
76. Kusljugic Z, Divkovic K, Barakovic F, et al: Effects of nebivolol on artery hypertension—multicentre study Bosnia and Herzegovina, *Bosn J Basic Med Sci* 5(1):42–51, 2005.
77. Schmidt AC, Graf C, Brixius K, et al: Blood pressure-lowering effect of nebivolol in hypertensive patients with type 2 diabetes mellitus: the YESTONO study, *Clin Drug Investig* 27(12):841–849, 2007.
78. Ohman KP, Weiner L, von Schenck H, et al: Antihypertensive and metabolic effects of nifedipine and labetalol alone and in combination in primary hypertension, *Eur J Clin Pharmacol* 29 (2):149–154, 1985.
79. Siwach SB, Dahiya SS, Seth S, et al: Effect of atenolol and labetalol on serum lipids, *J Assoc Physicians India* 41(5):293–294, 1993.
80. Adverse reactions to bendrofluazide and propranolol for the treatment of mild hypertension. Report of Medical Research Council Working Party on Mild to Moderate Hypertension, *Lancet* 2(8246):539–543, 1981.
81. Medical Research Council trial of treatment of hypertension in older adults: principal results. MRC Working Party, *BMJ* 304(6824):405–412, 1992.
82. Amery A, Birkenhager W, Brixko P, et al: Glucose intolerance during diuretic therapy in elderly hypertensive patients. A second report from the European Working Party on high blood pressure in the elderly (EWPHE), *Postgrad Med J* 62(732):919–924, 1986.
83. Ramsay LE, Yeo WW, Jackson PR: Diabetes, impaired glucose tolerance and insulin resistance with diuretics, *Eur Heart J* 13(Suppl G):68–71, 1992.
84. Duarte JD, Cooper-DeHoff RM: Mechanisms for blood pressure lowering and metabolic effects of thiazide and thiazide-like diuretics, *Expert Rev Cardiovasc Ther* 8(6):793–802, 2010.
85. Sica DA: Diuretic-related side effects: development and treatment, *J Clin Hypertens (Greenwich)* 6(9):532–540, 2004.
86. Elliott WJ, Meyer PM: Incident diabetes in clinical trials of antihypertensive drugs: a network meta-analysis, *Lancet* 369(9557):201–207, 2007.
87. Bia MJ, DeFronzo RA: Extrarenal potassium homeostasis, *Am J Physiol* 240(4):F257–F268, 1981.
88. Carter BL, Einhorn PT, Brands M, et al: Thiazide-induced dysglycemia: call for research from a working group from the national heart, lung, and blood institute, *Hypertension* 52(1):30–36, 2008.
89. Zillich AJ, Garg J, Basu S, et al: Thiazide diuretics, potassium, and the development of diabetes: a quantitative review, *Hypertension* 48(2):219–224, 2006.
90. Shafi T, Appel LJ, Miller ER III, , et al: Changes in serum potassium mediate thiazide-induced diabetes, *Hypertension* 52(6):1022–1029, 2008.
91. Kostis JB, Wilson AC, Freudenberger RS, et al: Long-term effect of diuretic-based therapy on fatal outcomes in subjects with isolated systolic hypertension with and without diabetes, *Am J Cardiol* 95(1):29–35, 2005.
92. Eriksson JW, Jansson PA, Carlberg B, et al: Hydrochlorothiazide, but not Candesartan, aggravates insulin resistance and causes visceral and hepatic fat accumulation: the mechanisms for the diabetes preventing effect of Candesartan (MEDICA) Study, *Hypertension* 52(6): 1030–1037, 2008.
93. Cooper-DeHoff RM, Wen S, Beitelshees AL, et al: Impact of abdominal obesity on incidence of adverse metabolic effects associated with antihypertensive medications, *Hypertension* 55 (1):61–68, 2010.
94. Neeland IJ, Turer AT, Ayers CR, et al: Dysfunctional adiposity and the risk of prediabetes and type 2 diabetes in obese adults, *JAMA* 308(11):1150–1159, 2012.
95. Barzilay JI, Davis BR, Pressel SL, et al: Long-term effects of incident diabetes mellitus on cardiovascular outcomes in people treated for hypertension: the ALLHAT Diabetes Extension Study, *Circ Cardiovasc Qual Outcomes* 5(2):153–162, 2012.
96. Pepine CJ, Handberg EM, Cooper-DeHoff RM, et al: A calcium antagonist vs a non-calcium antagonist hypertension treatment strategy for patients with coronary artery disease. The International Verapamil-Trandolapril Study (INVEST): a randomized controlled trial, *JAMA* 290(21): 2805–2816, 2003.
97. Major outcomes in high-risk hypertensive patients randomized to angiotensin-converting enzyme inhibitor or calcium channel blocker vs diuretic: The Antihypertensive and Lipid-Lowering Treatment to Prevent Heart Attack Trial (ALLHAT), *JAMA* 288(23):2981–2997, 2002.
98. Houston MC: The effects of antihypertensive drugs on glucose intolerance in hypertensive nondiabetics and diabetics, *Am Heart J* 115(3):640–656, 1988.
99. Lender D, Arauz-Pacheco C, Breen L, et al: A double blind comparison of the effects of amlodipine and enalapril on insulin sensitivity in hypertensive patients, *Am J Hypertens* 12(3):298–303, 1999.
100. Trost BN, Weidmann P: Effects of calcium antagonists on glucose homeostasis and serum lipids in non-diabetic and diabetic subjects: a review, *J Hypertens Suppl* 5(4):S81–S104, 1987.
101. Pitre M, Gaudreault N, Santure M, et al: Isradipine and insulin sensitivity in hypertensive rats, *Am J Physiol* 276(6 Pt 1):E1038–E1048, 1999.
102. Alvarsson M, Grill V: Impact of nicotinic acid treatment on insulin secretion and insulin sensitivity in low and high insulin responders, *Scand J Clin Lab Invest* 56(6):563–570, 1996.
103. Poynten AM, Gan SK, Kriketos AD, et al: Nicotinic acid-induced insulin resistance is related to increased circulating fatty acids and fat oxidation but not muscle lipid content, *Metabolism* 52 (6):699–704, 2003.
104. Grundy SM, Vega GL, McGovern ME, et al: Efficacy, safety, and tolerability of once-daily niacin for the treatment of dyslipidemia associated with type 2 diabetes: results of the assessment of diabetes control and evaluation of the efficacy of niaspan trial, *Arch Intern Med* 162(14): 1568–1576, 2002.
105. Elam MB, Hunninghake DB, Davis KB, et al: Effect of niacin on lipid and lipoprotein levels and glycemic control in patients with diabetes and peripheral arterial disease: the ADMIT study: A randomized trial. Arterial Disease Multiple Intervention Trial, *JAMA* 284(10): 1263–1270, 2000.
106. Zhao XQ, Morse JS, Dowdy AA, et al: Safety and tolerability of simvastatin plus niacin in patients with coronary artery disease and low high-density lipoprotein cholesterol (The HDL Atherosclerosis Treatment Study), *Am J Cardiol* 93(3):307–312, 2004.
107. Boden WE, Probstfield JL, Anderson T, et al: Niacin in patients with low HDL cholesterol levels receiving intensive statin therapy, *N Engl J Med* 365(24):2255–2267, 2011.
108. High patient compliance with nicacin/laropiprant in large clinical trial: interim safety and tolerability results from HPS-2 THRIVE study released at 2012 ESC congress: drug trends in cardiology, *Cardiovasc J Afr* 23(8):471, 2012.
109. Preiss D, Sattar N: Statins and the risk of new-onset diabetes: a review of recent evidence, *Curr Opin Lipidol* 22(6):460–466, 2011.
110. Culver AL, Ockene IS, Balasubramanian R, et al: Statin use and risk of diabetes mellitus in postmenopausal women in the Women's Health Initiative, *Arch Intern Med* 172(2):144–152, 2012.
111. Sattar N, Preiss D, Murray HM, et al: Statins and risk of incident diabetes: a collaborative meta-analysis of randomised statin trials, *Lancet* 375(9716):735–742, 2010.
112. Rajpathak SN, Kumbhani DJ, Crandall J, et al: Statin therapy and risk of developing type 2 diabetes: a meta-analysis, *Diabetes Care* 32(10):1924–1929, 2009.
113. Mills EJ, Wu P, Chong G, et al: Efficacy and safety of statin treatment for cardiovascular disease: a network meta-analysis of 170,255 patients from 76 randomized trials, *QJM* 104(2):109–124, 2011.
114. Baker WL, Talati R, White CM, et al: Differing effect of statins on insulin sensitivity in non-diabetics: a systematic review and meta-analysis, *Diabetes Res Clin Pract* 87(1):98–107, 2010.
115. Ridker PM, Pradhan A, MacFadyen JG, et al: Cardiovascular benefits and diabetes risks of statin therapy in primary prevention: an analysis from the JUPITER trial, *Lancet* 380(9841):565–571, 2012.
116. Anderson TJ, Gregoire J, Hegele RA, et al: 2012 update of the Canadian Cardiovascular Society guidelines for the diagnosis and treatment of dyslipidemia for the prevention of cardiovascular disease in the adult, *Can J Cardiol* 29(2):151–167, 2013.
117. Freeman DJ, Norrie J, Sattar N, et al: Pravastatin and the development of diabetes mellitus: evidence for a protective treatment effect in the West of Scotland Coronary Prevention Study, *Circulation* 103(3):357–362, 2001.
118. Kostapanos MS, Milionis HJ, Agouridis AD, et al: Rosuvastatin treatment is associated with an increase in insulin resistance in hyperlipidaemic patients with impaired fasting glucose, *Int J Clin Pract* 63(9):1308–1313, 2009.
119. Rizos CV, Milionis HJ, Kostapanos MS, et al: Effects of rosuvastatin combined with olmesartan, irbesartan, or telmisartan on indices of glucose metabolism in Greek adults with impaired fasting glucose, hypertension, and mixed hyperlipidemia: a 24-week, randomized, open-label, prospective study, *Clin Ther* 32(3):492–505, 2010.
120. Koh KK, Sakuma I, Quon MJ: Differential metabolic effects of distinct statins, *Atherosclerosis* 215 (1):1–8, 2011.
121. Chamberlain LH: Inhibition of isoprenoid biosynthesis causes insulin resistance in 3 T3-L1 adipocytes, *FEBS Lett* 507(3):357–361, 2001.
122. Nakata M, Nagasaka S, Kusaka I, et al: Effects of statins on the adipocyte maturation and expression of glucose transporter 4 (SLC2A4): implications in glycaemic control, *Diabetologia* 49 (8):1881–1892, 2006.
123. Li G, Regazzi R, Roche E, et al: Blockade of mevalonate production by lovastatin attenuates bombesin and vasopressin potentiation of nutrient-induced insulin secretion in HIT-T15 cells. Probable involvement of small GTP-binding proteins, *Biochem J* 289(Pt 2):379–385, 1993.
124. Ishikawa M, Okajima F, Inoue N, et al: Distinct effects of pravastatin, atorvastatin, and simvastatin on insulin secretion from a beta-cell line, MIN6 cells, *J Atheroscler Thromb* 13(6):329–335, 2006.
125. Yada T, Nakata M, Shiraishi T, et al: Inhibition by simvastatin, but not pravastatin, of glucose-induced cytosolic Ca2+ signalling and insulin secretion due to blockade of L-type Ca2+ channels in rat islet beta-cells, *Br J Pharmacol* 126(5):1205–1213, 1999.
126. Mikus CR, Boyle LJ, Borengasser SJ, et al: Simvastatin impairs exercise training adaptations, *J Am Coll Cardiol* 62(8):709–714, 2013.
127. Deushi M, Nomura M, Kawakami A, et al: Ezetimibe improves liver steatosis and insulin resistance in obese rat model of metabolic syndrome, *FEBS Lett* 581(29):5664–5670, 2007.
128. Hiramitsu S, Ishiguro Y, Matsuyama H, et al: The effects of ezetimibe on surrogate markers of cholesterol absorption and synthesis in Japanese patients with dyslipidemia, *J Atheroscler Thromb* 17(1):106–114, 2010.
129. Yagi S, Akaike M, Aihara K, et al: Ezetimibe ameliorates metabolic disorders and microalbuminuria in patients with hypercholesterolemia, *J Atheroscler Thromb* 17(2):173–180, 2010.
130. Garg A, Grundy SM: Cholestyramine therapy for dyslipidemia in non-insulin-dependent diabetes mellitus. A short-term, double-blind, crossover trial, *Ann Intern Med* 121(6):416–422, 1994.
131. Zieve FJ, Kalin MF, Schwartz SL, et al: Results of the glucose-lowering effect of WelChol study (GLOWS): a randomized, double-blind, placebo-controlled pilot study evaluating the effect of colesevelam hydrochloride on glycemic control in subjects with type 2 diabetes, *Clin Ther* 29(1):74–83, 2007.
132. Yamakawa T, Takano T, Utsunomiya H, et al: Effect of colestimide therapy for glycemic control in type 2 diabetes mellitus with hypercholesterolemia, *Endocr J* 54(1):53–58, 2007.
133. Goldberg RB, Fonseca VA, Truitt KE, et al: Efficacy and safety of colesevelam in patients with type 2 diabetes mellitus and inadequate glycemic control receiving insulin-based therapy, *Arch Intern Med* 168(14):1531–1540, 2008.
134. Fonseca VA, Rosenstock J, Wang AC, et al: Colesevelam HCl improves glycemic control and reduces LDL cholesterol in patients with inadequately controlled type 2 diabetes on sulfonylurea-based therapy, *Diabetes Care* 31(8):1479–1484, 2008.
135. Bays HE, Goldberg RB, Truitt KE, et al: Colesevelam hydrochloride therapy in patients with type 2 diabetes mellitus treated with metformin: glucose and lipid effects, *Arch Intern Med* 168 (18):1975–1983, 2008.
136. Tziomalos K, Athyros VG, Mikhailidis DP: Colesevelam improves glycemic control and lipid management in inadequately controlled type 2 diabetes mellitus, *Nat Clin Pract Endocrinol Metab* 5(1):16–17, 2009.
137. Rosenstock J, Fonseca VA, Garvey WT, et al: Initial combination therapy with metformin and colesevelam for achievement of glycemic and lipid goals in early type 2 diabetes, *Endocr Pract* 16(4):629–640, 2010.
138. Jialal I, Abby SL, Misir S, et al: Concomitant reduction in low-density lipoprotein cholesterol and glycated hemoglobin with colesevelam hydrochloride in patients with type 2 diabetes: a pooled analysis, *Metab Syndr Relat Disord* 7(3):255–258, 2009.
139. Handelsman Y, Abby SL, Jin X, et al: Colesevelam HCl improves fasting plasma glucose and lipid levels in patients with prediabetes, *Postgrad Med* 121(6):62–69, 2009.
140. Handelsman Y, Goldberg RB, Garvey WT, et al: Colesevelam hydrochloride to treat hypercholesterolemia and improve glycemia in prediabetes: a randomized, prospective study, *Endocr Pract* 16(4):617–628, 2010.
141. Levy P, Jellinger PS: The potential role of colesevelam in the management of prediabetes and type 2 diabetes mellitus, *Postgrad Med* 122(3 Suppl):1–8, 2010.
142. Vega GL, Dunn FL, Grundy SM: Effect of colesevelam hydrochloride on glycemia and insulin sensitivity in men with the metabolic syndrome, *Am J Cardiol* 108(8):1129–1135, 2011.
143. Younk LM, Davis SN: Evaluation of colesevelam hydrochloride for the treatment of type 2 diabetes, *Expert Opin Drug Metab Toxicol* 8(4):515–525, 2012.
144. Tenenbaum A, Motro M, Fisman EZ, et al: Peroxisome proliferator-activated receptor ligand bezafibrate for prevention of type 2 diabetes mellitus in patients with coronary artery disease, *Circulation* 109(18):2197–2202, 2004.
145. Anderlova K, Dolezalova R, Housova J, et al: Influence of PPAR-alpha agonist fenofibrate on insulin sensitivity and selected adipose tissue-derived hormones in obese women with type 2 diabetes, *Physiol Res* 56(5):579–586, 2007.
146. Fabbrini E, Mohammed BS, Korenblat KM, et al: Effect of fenofibrate and niacin on intrahepatic triglyceride content, very low-density lipoprotein kinetics, and insulin action in obese subjects with nonalcoholic fatty liver disease, *J Clin Endocrinol Metab* 95(6):2727–2735, 2010.
147. Tenenbaum A, Motro M, Fisman EZ: Dual and pan-peroxisome proliferator-activated receptors (PPAR) co-agonism: the bezafibrate lessons, *Cardiovasc Diabetol* 4:14, 2005.

148. Peters JM, Aoyama T, Burns AM, et al: Bezafibrate is a dual ligand for PPARalpha and PPARbeta: studies using null mice, *Biochim Biophys Acta* 1632(1–3):80–89, 2003.
149. Drew BG, Duffy SJ, Formosa MF, et al: High-density lipoprotein modulates glucose metabolism in patients with type 2 diabetes mellitus, *Circulation* 119(15):2103–2111, 2009.
150. Fryirs MA, Barter PJ, Appavoo M, et al: Effects of high-density lipoproteins on pancreatic beta-cell insulin secretion, *Arterioscler Thromb Vasc Biol* 30(8):1642–1648, 2010.
151. Barter PJ, Rye KA, Tardif JC, et al: Effect of torcetrapib on glucose, insulin, and hemoglobin A1c in subjects in the Investigation of Lipid Level Management to Understand its Impact in Atherosclerotic Events (ILLUMINATE) trial, *Circulation* 124(5):555–562, 2011.
152. Barter PJ, Caulfield M, Eriksson M, et al: Effects of torcetrapib in patients at high risk for coronary events, *N Engl J Med* 357(21):2109–2122, 2007.
153. Garg R, Hurwitz S, Williams GH, et al: Aldosterone production and insulin resistance in healthy adults, *J Clin Endocrinol Metab* 95(4):1986–1990, 2010.
154. Raheja P, Price A, Wang Z, et al: Spironolactone prevents chlorthalidone-induced sympathetic activation and insulin resistance in hypertensive patients, *Hypertension* 60(2):319–325, 2012.
155. Corry DB, Tuck ML: The effect of aldosterone on glucose metabolism, *Curr Hypertens Rep* 5(2): 106–109, 2003.
156. Ogilvie RI: Antilipolytic effect of digoxin in the forearm of man, *J Clin Endocrinol Metab* 36 (3):568–575, 1973.
157. Ogilvie RI, Klassen GA: Metabolic effect and uptake of (3 H)digoxin in the forearm of man, *Clin Sci* 42(5):567–577, 1972.
158. Gerstein HC, Yusuf S, Bosch J, et al: Effect of rosiglitazone on the frequency of diabetes in patients with impaired glucose tolerance or impaired fasting glucose: a randomised controlled trial, *Lancet* 368(9541):1096–1105, 2006.
159. Hanley AJ, Zinman B, Sheridan P, et al: Effect of Rosiglitazone and Ramipril on {beta} -cell function in people with impaired glucose tolerance or impaired fasting glucose: the DREAM trial, *Diabetes Care* 33(3):608–613, 2010.
160. Gerstein HC, Mohan V, Avezum A, et al: Long-term effect of rosiglitazone and/or ramipril on the incidence of diabetes, *Diabetologia* 54(3):487–495, 2011.
161. Boyko EJ, Gerstein HC, Mohan V, et al: Effects of ethnicity on diabetes incidence and prevention: results of the Diabetes REduction Assessment with ramipril and rosiglitazone Medication (DREAM) trial, *Diabet Med* 27(11):1226–1232, 2010.
162. DeFronzo RA, Tripathy D, Schwenke DC, et al: Pioglitazone for diabetes prevention in impaired glucose tolerance, *N Engl J Med* 364(12):1104–1115, 2011.
163. Ratner RE: An update on the Diabetes Prevention Program, *Endocr Pract* 12(Suppl 1):20–24, 2006.
164. Knowler WC, Fowler SE, Hamman RF, et al: 10-year follow-up of diabetes incidence and weight loss in the Diabetes Prevention Program Outcomes Study, *Lancet* 374(9702):1677–1686, 2009.
165. West DS, Elaine PT, Bursac Z, et al: Weight loss of black, white, and Hispanic men and women in the Diabetes Prevention Program, *Obesity (Silver Spring)* 16(6):1413–1420, 2008.
166. Within-trial cost-effectiveness of lifestyle intervention or metformin for the primary prevention of type 2 diabetes, *Diabetes Care* 26(9):2518–2523, 2003.
167. Palmer AJ, Roze S, Valentine WJ, et al: Intensive lifestyle changes or metformin in patients with impaired glucose tolerance: modeling the long-term health economic implications of the diabetes prevention program in Australia, France, Germany, Switzerland, and the United Kingdom, *Clin Ther* 26(2):304–321, 2004.
168. Padwal R, Majumdar SR, Johnson JA, et al: A systematic review of drug therapy to delay or prevent type 2 diabetes, *Diabetes Care* 28(3):736–744, 2005.
169. Khattab S, Mohsen IA, Aboul FI, et al: Can metformin reduce the incidence of gestational diabetes mellitus in pregnant women with polycystic ovary syndrome? Prospective cohort study, *Gynecol Endocrinol* 27(10):789–793, 2011.
170. Glueck CJ, Wang P, Goldenberg N, et al: Pregnancy outcomes among women with polycystic ovary syndrome treated with metformin, *Hum Reprod* 17(11):2858–2864, 2002.
171. Glueck CJ, Goldenberg N, Wang P, et al: Metformin during pregnancy reduces insulin, insulin resistance, insulin secretion, weight, testosterone and development of gestational diabetes: prospective longitudinal assessment of women with polycystic ovary syndrome from preconception throughout pregnancy, *Hum Reprod* 19(3):510–521, 2004.
172. Gilbert C, Valois M, Koren G: Pregnancy outcome after first-trimester exposure to metformin: a meta-analysis, *Fertil Steril* 86(3):658–663, 2006.
173. Khattab S, Mohsen IA, Foutouh IA, et al: Metformin reduces abortion in pregnant women with polycystic ovary syndrome, *Gynecol Endocrinol* 22(12):680–684, 2006.
174. Glueck CJ, Phillips H, Cameron D, et al: Continuing metformin throughout pregnancy in women with polycystic ovary syndrome appears to safely reduce first-trimester spontaneous abortion: a pilot study, *Fertil Steril* 75(1):46–52, 2001.
175. Glueck CJ, Sieve L, Zhu B, et al: Plasminogen activator inhibitor activity, 4G5G polymorphism of the plasminogen activator inhibitor 1 gene, and first-trimester miscarriage in women with polycystic ovary syndrome, *Metabolism* 55(3):345–352, 2006.
176. Jakubowicz DJ, Iuorno MJ, Jakubowicz S, et al: Effects of metformin on early pregnancy loss in the polycystic ovary syndrome, *J Clin Endocrinol Metab* 87(2):524–529, 2002.
177. Vanky E, Salvesen KA, Heimstad R, et al: Metformin reduces pregnancy complications without affecting androgen levels in pregnant polycystic ovary syndrome women: results of a randomized study, *Hum Reprod* 19(8):1734–1740, 2004.
178. Yang W, Lin L, Qi J: The preventive effect of acarbose and metformin on the IGT population from becoming diabetes mellitus: a 3-year multicentral prospective study, *Chinese Journal of Endocrinology & Metabolism* 3:131–134, 2001.
179. Chiasson JL, Josse RG, Gomis R, et al: Acarbose for prevention of type 2 diabetes mellitus: the STOP-NIDDM randomised trial, *Lancet* 359(9323):2072–2077, 2002.
180. Chiasson JL, Josse RG, Gomis R, et al: Acarbose treatment and the risk of cardiovascular disease and hypertension in patients with impaired glucose tolerance: the STOP-NIDDM trial, *JAMA* 290 (4):486–494, 2003.
181. Torgerson JS, Hauptman J, Boldrin MN, et al: XENical in the prevention of diabetes in obese subjects (XENDOS) study: a randomized study of orlistat as an adjunct to lifestyle changes for the prevention of type 2 diabetes in obese patients, *Diabetes Care* 27(1):155–161, 2004.
182. Heymsfield SB, Segal KR, Hauptman J, et al: Effects of weight loss with orlistat on glucose tolerance and progression to type 2 diabetes in obese adults, *Arch Intern Med* 160(9): 1321–1326, 2000.
183. Sharma AM, Pischon T, Hardt S, et al: Hypothesis: Beta-adrenergic receptor blockers and weight gain: A systematic analysis, *Hypertension* 37(2):250–254, 2001.
184. Scholze J, Grimm E, Herrmann D, et al: Optimal treatment of obesity-related hypertension: the Hypertension-Obesity-Sibutramine (HOS) study, *Circulation* 115(15):1991–1998, 2007.
185. Opie LH, Schall R: Old antihypertensives and new diabetes, *J Hypertens* 22(8):1453–1458, 2004.
186. Mason JM, Dickinson HO, Nicolson DJ, et al: The diabetogenic potential of thiazide-type diuretic and beta-blocker combinations in patients with hypertension, *J Hypertens* 23(10):1777–1781, 2005.
187. Leucht S, Burkard T, Henderson J, et al: Physical illness and schizophrenia: a review of the literature, *Acta Psychiatr Scand* 116(5):317–333, 2007.
188. Bresee LC, Majumdar SR, Patten SB, et al: Prevalence of cardiovascular risk factors and disease in people with schizophrenia: a population-based study, *Schizophr Res* 117(1):75–82, 2010.
189. Saha S, Chant D, McGrath J: A systematic review of mortality in schizophrenia: is the differential mortality gap worsening over time? *Arch Gen Psychiatry* 64(10):1123–1131, 2007.
190. Laursen TM: Life expectancy among persons with schizophrenia or bipolar affective disorder, *Schizophr Res* 131(1–3):101–104, 2011.
191. Weinmann S, Read J, Aderhold V: Influence of antipsychotics on mortality in schizophrenia: systematic review, *Schizophr Res* 113(1):1–11, 2009.
192. Rosack J: FDA to require diabetes warning on antipsychotics, *Psychiatr News* 38(20):1–27, 2012.
193. Mitchell AJ, Delaffon V, Vancampfort D, et al: Guideline concordant monitoring of metabolic risk in people treated with antipsychotic medication: systematic review and meta-analysis of screening practices, *Psychol Med* 42(1):125–147, 2012.
194. Mitchell AJ, Malone D, Doebbeling CC: Quality of medical care for people with and without comorbid mental illness and substance misuse: systematic review of comparative studies, *Br J Psychiatry* 194(6):491–499, 2009.
195. Desai MM, Rosenheck RA, Druss BG, et al: Mental disorders and quality of diabetes care in the veterans health administration, *Am J Psychiatry* 159(9):1584–1590, 2002.
196. Dixon LB, Kreyenbuhl JA, Dickerson FB, et al: A comparison of type 2 diabetes outcomes among persons with and without severe mental illnesses, *Psychiatr Serv* 55(8):892–900, 2004.
197. Jones LE, Clarke W, Carney CP: Receipt of diabetes services by insured adults with and without claims for mental disorders, *Med Care* 42(12):1167–1175, 2004.
198. Goldberg RW, Kreyenbuhl JA, Medoff DR, et al: Quality of diabetes care among adults with serious mental illness, *Psychiatr Serv* 58(4):536–543, 2007.
199. Alberti KG, Eckel RH, Grundy SM, et al: Harmonizing the metabolic syndrome: a joint interim statement of the International Diabetes Federation Task Force on Epidemiology and Prevention; National Heart, Lung, and Blood Institute; American Heart Association; World Heart Federation; International Atherosclerosis Society; and International Association for the Study of Obesity, *Circulation* 120(16):1640–1645, 2009.
200. Meyer JM, Nasrallah HA, McEvoy JP, et al: The Clinical Antipsychotic Trials Of Intervention Effectiveness (CATIE) Schizophrenia Trial: clinical comparison of subgroups with and without the metabolic syndrome, *Schizophr Res* 80(1):9–18, 2005.
201. Nasrallah HA, Meyer JM, Goff DC, et al: Low rates of treatment for hypertension, dyslipidemia and diabetes in schizophrenia: data from the CATIE schizophrenia trial sample at baseline, *Schizophr Res* 86(1–3):15–22, 2006.
202. Itoh Z: Motilin and clinical application, *Peptides* 18(4):593–608, 1997.
203. Mochiki E, Inui A, Satoh M, et al: Motilin is a biosignal controlling cyclic release of pancreatic polypeptide via the vagus in fasted dogs, *Am J Physiol* 272(2Pt 1):G224–G232, 1997.
204. Shiba Y, Mizumoto A, Satoh M, et al: Effect of nonpeptide motilin agonist EM523 on release of gut and pancreatic hormones in conscious dogs, *Gastroenterology* 110(1):241–250, 1996.
205. Ueno N, Inui A, Asakawa A, et al: Erythromycin improves glycaemic control in patients with Type II diabetes mellitus, *Diabetologia* 43(4):411–415, 2000.
206. Peeters TL: Erythromycin and other macrolides as prokinetic agents, *Gastroenterology* 105(6): 1886–1899, 1993.
207. Friis-Moller N, Sabin CA, Weber R, et al: Combination antiretroviral therapy and the risk of myocardial infarction, *N Engl J Med* 349(21):1993–2003, 2003.
208. Worm SW, De WS, Weber R, et al: Diabetes mellitus, preexisting coronary heart disease, and the risk of subsequent coronary heart disease events in patients infected with human immunodeficiency virus: the Data Collection on Adverse Events of Anti-HIV Drugs (D:A:D Study), *Circulation* 119(6):805–811, 2009.
209. Tebas P: Insulin resistance and diabetes mellitus associated with antiretroviral use in HIV-infected patients: pathogenesis, prevention, and treatment options, *J Acquir Immune Defic Syndr* 49(Suppl 2):S86–S92, 2008.
210. Deshpande AD, Harris-Hayes M, Schootman M: Epidemiology of diabetes and diabetes-related complications, *Phys Ther* 88(11):1254–1264, 2008.
211. Brown TT, Tassiopoulos K, Bosch RJ, et al: Association between systemic inflammation and incident diabetes in HIV-infected patients after initiation of antiretroviral therapy, *Diabetes Care* 33 (10):2244–2249, 2010.
212. Grinspoon S: Diabetes mellitus, cardiovascular risk, and HIV disease, *Circulation* 119(6): 770–772, 2009.
213. Wand H, Calmy A, Carey DL, et al: Metabolic syndrome, cardiovascular disease and type 2 diabetes mellitus after initiation of antiretroviral therapy in HIV infection, *AIDS* 21(18):2445–2453, 2007.
214. Carr A, Samaras K, Thorisdottir A, et al: Diagnosis, prediction, and natural course of HIV-1 protease-inhibitor-associated lipodystrophy, hyperlipidaemia, and diabetes mellitus: a cohort study, *Lancet* 353(9170):2093–2099, 1999.
215. Brown TT, Li X, Cole SR, et al: Cumulative exposure to nucleoside analogue reverse transcriptase inhibitors is associated with insulin resistance markers in the Multicenter AIDS Cohort Study, *AIDS* 19(13):1375–1383, 2005.
216. Kanaya AM, Herrington D, Vittinghoff E, et al: Glycemic effects of postmenopausal hormone therapy: the Heart and Estrogen/progestin Replacement Study. A randomized, double-blind, placebo-controlled trial, *Ann Intern Med* 138(1):1–9, 2003.
217. Manson JE, Rimm EB, Colditz GA, et al: A prospective study of postmenopausal estrogen therapy and subsequent incidence of non-insulin-dependent diabetes mellitus, *Ann Epidemiol* 2 (5):665–673, 1992.
218. Rossi R, Origliani G, Modena MG: Transdermal 17-beta-estradiol and risk of developing type 2 diabetes in a population of healthy, nonobese postmenopausal women, *Diabetes Care* 27 (3):645–649, 2004.
219. Zhang Y, Howard BV, Cowan LD, et al: The effect of estrogen use on levels of glucose and insulin and the risk of type 2 diabetes in American Indian postmenopausal women: the strong heart study, *Diabetes Care* 25(3):500–504, 2002.
220. Hammond CB, Jelovsek FR, Lee KL, et al: Effects of long-term estrogen replacement therapy. I. Metabolic effects, *Am J Obstet Gynecol* 133(5):525–536, 1979.
221. Gabal LL, Goodman-Gruen D, Barrett-Connor E: The effect of postmenopausal estrogen therapy on the risk of non-insulin-dependent diabetes mellitus, *Am J Public Health* 87(3): 443–445, 1997.
222. Amed S, Dean HJ, Panagiotopoulos C, et al: Type 2 diabetes, medication-induced diabetes, and monogenic diabetes in Canadian children: a prospective national surveillance study, *Diabetes Care* 33(4):786–791, 2010.
223. Dabelea D, Bell RA, D'Agostino RB Jr. et al: Incidence of diabetes in youth in the United States, *JAMA* 297(24):2716–2724, 2007.
224. Haines L, Wan KC, Lynn R, et al: Rising incidence of type 2 diabetes in children in the U.K, *Diabetes Care* 30(5):1097–1101, 2007.
225. Poirier P, Cornier MA, Mazzone T, et al: Bariatric surgery and cardiovascular risk factors: a scientific statement from the American Heart Association, *Circulation* 123(15): 1683–1701, 2011.
226. Thaler JP, Cummings DE: Minireview: hormonal and metabolic mechanisms of diabetes remission after gastrointestinal surgery, *Endocrinology* 150(6):2518–2525, 2009.
227. Rubino F, Schauer PR, Kaplan LM, et al: Metabolic surgery to treat type 2 diabetes: clinical outcomes and mechanisms of action, *Annu Rev Med* 61:393–411, 2010.
228. Dixon JB, O'Brien PE, Playfair J, et al: Adjustable gastric banding and conventional therapy for type 2 diabetes: a randomized controlled trial, *JAMA* 299(3):316–323, 2008.
229. Schauer PR, Kashyap SR, Wolski K, et al: Bariatric surgery versus intensive medical therapy in obese patients with diabetes, *N Engl J Med* 366(17):1567–1576, 2012.
230. Mingrone G, Panunzi S, De GA, et al: Bariatric surgery versus conventional medical therapy for type 2 diabetes, *N Engl J Med* 366(17):1577–1585, 2012.

6

231. Buchwald H, Avidor Y, Braunwald E, et al: Bariatric surgery: a systematic review and meta-analysis, *JAMA* 292(14):1724–1737, 2004.

232. Sjostrom L, Lindroos AK, Peltonen M, et al: Lifestyle, diabetes, and cardiovascular risk factors 10 years after bariatric surgery, *N Engl J Med* 351(26):2683–2693, 2004.

233. Buchwald H, Estok R, Fahrbach K, et al: Weight and type 2 diabetes after bariatric surgery: systematic review and meta-analysis, *Am J Med* 122(3):248–256, 2009.

234. Campbell RK, Martin TM: The chronic burden of diabetes, *Am J Manag Care* 15(9 Suppl):S248–S254, 2009.

235. Klein S, Ghosh A, Cremieux PY, et al: Economic impact of the clinical benefits of bariatric surgery in diabetes patients with BMI >/=35 kg/m(2), *Obesity (Silver Spring)* 19(3):581–587, 2011.

236. Sampalis JS, Liberman M, Auger S, et al: The impact of weight reduction surgery on health-care costs in morbidly obese patients, *Obes Surg* 14(7):939–947, 2004.

237. Sandoval D: Bariatric surgeries: beyond restriction and malabsorption, *Int J Obes (Lond)* 35 (Suppl 3):S45–S49, 2011.

238. Rodriguez-Grunert L, Galvao Neto MP, Alamo M, et al: First human experience with endoscopically delivered and retrieved duodenal-jejunal bypass sleeve, *Surg Obes Relat Dis* 4(1):55–59, 2008.

239. Tarnoff M, Rodriguez L, Escalona A, et al: Open label, prospective, randomized controlled trial of an endoscopic duodenal-jejunal bypass sleeve versus low calorie diet for pre-operative weight loss in bariatric surgery, *Surg Endosc* 23(3):650–656, 2009.

240. Gersin KS, Rothstein RI, Rosenthal RJ, et al: Open-label, sham-controlled trial of an endoscopic duodenojejunal bypass liner for preoperative weight loss in bariatric surgery candidates, *Gastrointest Endosc* 71(6):976–982, 2010.

241. Mancia G, De BG, Dominiczak A, et al: 2007 Guidelines for the management of arterial hypertension: the Task Force for the management of arterial hypertension of the European Society of Hypertension (ESH) and of the European Society of Cardiology (ESC), *Eur Heart J* 28(12):1462–1536, 2007.

242. Torre JJ, Bloomgarden ZT, Dickey RA, et al: American Association of Clinical Endocrinologists Medical Guidelines for Clinical Practice for the diagnosis and treatment of hypertension, *Endocr Pract* 12(2):193–222, 2006.

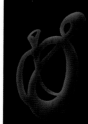

PART II

DIABETES AND ATHEROSCLEROSIS

7

Epidemiology of Coronary and Peripheral Atherosclerosis in Diabetes

Wolfgang Koenig

PREVALENCE OF IMPAIRED GLUCOSE METABOLISM IN PATIENTS WITH MANIFEST ATHEROSCLEROSIS

In patients with manifest coronary heart disease (CHD), based on the Ludwigshafen Risk and Cardiovascular Health (LURIC) study, approximately 20% of men and 25% of women had previously diagnosed diabetes. Newly detected diabetes was present in another 15% of men and approximately 10% of women.[1] More detailed data on the prevalence of abnormal glucose regulation in patients with manifest CHD across Europe were collected in the Euro Heart Survey on Diabetes and the Heart.[2] This survey involved 110 centers in 25 countries, recruiting more than 4000 patients referred to a cardiologist because of suspected coronary artery disease (CAD), including acute coronary syndrome (ACS) patients and those with stable symptoms. Of these patients, 31% had manifest diabetes. In 1920 patients without known diabetes, an oral glucose tolerance test (OGTT) was performed. The prevalence of impaired glucose tolerance (IGT) in those with ACS was 36%, with an additional 22% having newly detected diabetes. The corresponding figures in those with stable CAD were 37% and 14%, respectively. In another study[3] from Spain, in 662 consecutive patients admitted to the hospital without a previous diagnosis of diabetes who were referred for coronary intervention in 2005 and 2006, the prevalence of diabetes was 45%. Analyses of more than 120,000 patients from randomized clinical trials in the late 1990s, at least 30% of them coming from the United States, revealed a prevalence of diabetes of 23% in women and 15% in men.[4] Yet this certainly represents an underestimation as a result of selection bias and, most commonly, absence of systematic screening for incident diabetes.

Impaired glucose homeostasis (IGH) is also prevalent in this population. IGH comprises impaired fasting glucose (IFG) and IGT. IFG has been defined as a fasting glucose range of 110 to 126 mg/dL, and fasting glucose tolerance is pathologic if it exceeds 140 mg/dL according to 2-hour glucose levels after oral intake of 75 g of glucose (OGTT). Prevalence of these two entities may vary in different populations and may also not be consistently present in the same individual.

In the previously mentioned study[3] from Spain in 662 consecutive patients without a previous diagnosis of diabetes who were referred for coronary intervention in 2005 and 2006, IGT was present in 24.5%, yet IFG was seen in only 1%. Thus again, more than two thirds of this population with manifest atherosclerotic disease had an abnormal glucose metabolism. In the LURIC study in patients with manifest CHD, approximately 20% of men and 15% of women showed an abnormal OGTT result. Putting these figures into perspective, approximately two thirds of patients with manifest cardiovascular disease (CVD) had impaired glucose metabolism, as results from the LURIC study have shown.[1]

Thus, impaired glucose metabolism including manifest type 2 diabetes, pathologic oral glucose tolerance, and

IFG are prevalent in patients with manifest atherosclerosis. In particular, manifest type 2 diabetes is at least twice as frequent in CHD patients compared with those free of CHD.

DIABETES MELLITUS AND SUBCLINICAL ATHEROSCLEROSIS

Subclinical atherosclerosis represents the early manifestation of vascular disease without clinical symptoms. It can be assessed in all three major vascular beds by noninvasive but also by invasive imaging techniques. For carotid atherosclerosis, measurement of the intima-media thickness (IMT) or the presence of plaque on high-resolution transcutaneous ultrasound represents the method of choice. In the coronary vascular bed, computed tomography (CT) seems promising, but more precise data can be gathered by several invasive techniques such as intravascular ultrasound (IVUS) or optical coherence tomography (OCT).[5] For the peripheral vascular bed, transcutaneous ultrasound and the ankle-brachial index (ABI) can be used (**Fig. 7-1**).[6] It has been well documented that the presence of subclinical atherosclerosis is associated with a higher incidence of clinical manifestations, yet in a number of studies the incremental value for risk prediction of these clinical manifestations (e.g., for IMT) above and beyond various risk scores such as the Framingham risk model did not yield clinically relevant results.[7] At present, evidence is accumulating that coronary calcium scoring by CT may be superior to various blood biomarkers and also may produce significant incremental value over and above risk scoring.[8] Epidemiologic data on the prevalence of subclinical coronary atherosclerosis and its association with incident CVD, as well as with all-cause mortality, have been published from several studies. One of the largest is the Cardiovascular Health Study (CHS), in which 1343 patients with diabetes, 1432 patients with IGT, and 2421 normoglycemic patients were identified by World Health Organization (WHO) criteria at the baseline examination in 1989-1990 and were followed on average for 6.4 years. Diabetic patients showed a higher prevalence of clinical and subclinical CVD at baseline, and the presence of subclinical disease was strongly related to CHD, stroke, and heart failure. This was particularly pronounced in diabetic patients, in whom the incidence of CHD and stroke was increased almost twofold in those presenting with subclinical disease versus those without (**Fig. 7-2**). A similar relative increase in all three endpoints, but on a lower level, was seen in patients with IGT.[9] Brohall and colleagues[10] published a systematic review of the relevance of carotid IMT in patients with type 2 diabetes mellitus and IGT and focused on the differences between IMT in diabetic patients with IGT versus controls. They included 23 studies with 20,111 patients. Among those were 4019 with diabetes and 1110 with IGT. In 20 of the 23 studies, diabetic patients showed an increased IMT compared with individuals in the reference group, whereas in patients with IGT, the increase in IMT was approximately one third of that observed in patients with diabetes. These findings suggest an older vascular age in diabetic patients of approximately 10 years, and further conclusions drawn from this review estimated an increased relative risk for myocardial infarction (MI) and stroke in the presence of diabetes of almost 40%.

Several studies have looked into carotid atherosclerosis in the setting of the metabolic syndrome. Prospective data from the Bruneck study[11] examined 888 patients aged 40 to 79 years, among whom 303 fulfilled the WHO criteria and 152 fulfilled the National Cholesterol Education Program—Adult Treatment Panel III (NCEP-ATP III) criteria for metabolic syndrome. Five-year changes in carotid status and its relation to incident fatal and nonfatal CHD were assessed. Patients with metabolic syndrome showed increased 5-year incidence and progression of carotid atherosclerosis, and also the incidence of clinical events was increased twofold compared with controls. This has recently been confirmed in the Multi-Ethnic Study of Atherosclerosis (MESA), in which individuals with metabolic syndrome or diabetes had a higher incidence and absolute progression of coronary artery calcification (CAC) compared with patients without diabetes. In addition, progression predicted future CHD events.[12]

Several studies also assessed the prevalence of CAC in various populations. Data from the Dallas Heart Study, a large population-based study in which the individual and joint associations among metabolic syndrome, diabetes, and atherosclerosis as defined by CAC were assessed, suggested that both metabolic syndrome and diabetes mellitus are independently associated with an increased prevalence of atherosclerosis, with the highest prevalence seen in those fulfilling both criteria.[13] In another study, by Wong and colleagues,[14] 1823 patients aged 23 to 79 years were screened for CAC. Of these patients, 279 had metabolic syndrome and 150 had diabetes mellitus. Prevalence of CAC clearly increased from the reference group to those with metabolic syndrome or diabetes, with 53.5%, 58.8%, and 75.3%, respectively, among men and 37.6%, 50.8%, and 52.6%, respectively, among women. CAC also increased with the number of components of the metabolic syndrome (0 to 5) from 34% to 58%. Risk assessment by the Framingham score estimated 41% of patients with metabolic syndrome as having a more than 20% per 10 years increased risk for CHD or a CAC greater than 75% for age and gender. Diabetic patients had a higher incidence and progression of CAC, and progression of CAC predicted clinical CHD events (**Fig. 7-3**). More recently, Elkeles and colleagues[15] prospectively evaluated CAC score as a predictor for cardiovascular events in type 2 diabetes based on 589 patients from the PREDICT study. Follow-up was 4 years, and first CHD and stroke events were identified as primary endpoints. The CAC score was found to be a highly significant independent predictor, with a doubling of calcium being associated with a 32% increase in risk of events—which only slightly decreased in multivariable analysis considering traditional risk factors, and even after adjustment for homocysteine, c-reactive protein (CRP), and the homeostasis model assessment (HOMA) index. The only variable that predicted primary endpoints independently of CAC scoring was the HOMA index. CAC scoring contributed significantly to improved discrimination over and above the Framingham CHD risk score as well as the United Kingdom Prospective Diabetes Study (UKPDS) CHD and CVD risk scores, with an increase in the area under the curve on average of 0.1 (0.63 to 0.73).

Thus, among various measures of subclinical disease, CAC scoring may represent the most promising tool to improve risk prediction in asymptomatic patients with type 2 diabetes mellitus.

SCREENING FOR SUBCLINICAL ATHEROSCLEROSIS

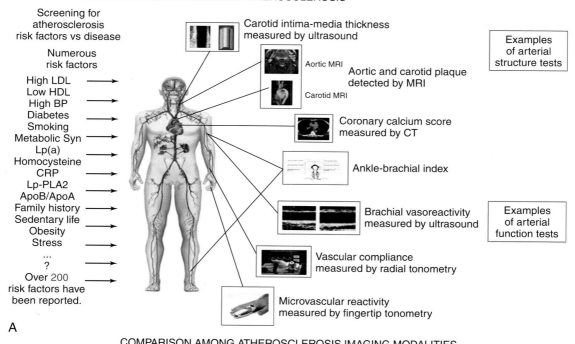

A

COMPARISON AMONG ATHEROSCLEROSIS IMAGING MODALITIES

	Imaging targets	Resolution	Radiation	Invasiveness	Advantages and disadvantages
Coronary angiography	Coronary lumen	0.4 mm	Yes	Yes	Two-dimensional silhouette of lumen only, associated with cardiovascular events, accepted surrogate for expanded indication
IVUS	Coronary arterial wall	0.08–0.10 mm	No	Yes, catheter	Tomographic, volumetric assessment of changes in plaque burden and vascular remodeling with excellent resolution
Carotid ultrasound	cIMT and plaque	0.15 mm	No	No	Wide availability, wide clinical trial experience, low cost, technically demanding; further validation of 3D plaque assessment required
Coronary CT	Coronary lumen and wall	0.4 mm	Yes	No	Rapid acquisition, limited image resolution for plaque burden, radiation exposure
MRI	Carotid lumen and wall	0.5–1.0 mm	No	No	Plaque characterization possible, no validation with clinical events
PET	Metabolic activity in carotids and aorta	4 mm	Yes	No	Limited image resolution, limited ability to visualize coronary arteries, no validation with clinical events
OCT	Coronary arterial lumen and wall	Excellent, 0.01 mm	No	Yes, catheter	Best image resolution, limited depth of view Requires flushing of lumen
NIRS	Tissue spectral contrast (chemical assessment)	1 mm	No	Yes, catheter	Link to plaque status not clear, images difficult to interpret, limited spatial registration
NIR fluorescence	Exogenous molecular contrast	1 mm	No	Yes, catheter and injection of molecular compound	Limited depth of view due to blood absorption, may require flushing; high potential for molecular imaging; depends on targeted compound approval for humans

B

FIGURE 7-1 A, Screening for patients at risk for cardiovascular complications. **B,** Comparison of atherosclerosis imaging modalities. (*A from Koenig W: Circulation 116:3-5, 2007, reprinted from Naghavi M, Falk E, Hecht HS, et al: Vulnerable plaque to vulnerable patiet—Part III: Executive summary of the Screening for Heart Attach Prevention and Education (SHAPE) Task Force report.* Am J Cardiol *98(Suppl):2H-15H, 2006, with permission from Elsevier. Copyright 2006. B modified from Tardif JC, Lesage F, Harel F, et al: Imaging biomarkers in atherosclerosis trials,* Circ Cardiovasc Imaging *4:319-333, 2011.)*

II

DIABETES AND ATHEROSCLEROSIS

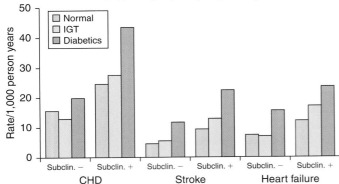

INCIDENT CV EVENTS BY DM STATUS AND
SUBCLINICAL/CLINICAL CVD AT STUDY ENTRY
CHS, N = 5,201, >65 years, FU 6.4 years

FIGURE 7-2 Diabetes status and presence of subclinical and clinical CVD at baseline and incidence of specific events among men and women in the CHS. DM = Diabetes mellitus. *(Modified from Kuller LH, Velentgas P, Barzilay J, et al: Diabetes mellitus: subclinical cardiovascular disease and risk of incident cardiovascular disease and all-cause mortality,* Arterioscler Thromb Vasc Biol *20:823-829, 2000.)*

CLINICAL MANIFESTATIONS OF ATHEROSCLEROSIS IN PREDIABETES, METABOLIC SYNDROME, AND TYPE 2 DIABETES

Coronary Heart Disease Risk of Patients with Prediabetes

Probably the earliest sound epidemiologic evidence of an association between prediabetes and CHD incidence as well as cardiovascular mortality comes from the Busselton study in Australia.[16] In this study, blood glucose and serum levels of insulin were measured 1 hour after an oral glucose load in addition to conventional cardiovascular risk factors. Six-year incidence of CHD and 12-year mortality from CHD and CVD were calculated in relation to baseline parameters. In men aged 60 to 69 years, having borderline or high levels of serum insulin after the 1-hour challenge showed a positive association with 6-year incidence of CHD, 12-year mortality from CHD, and 12-year mortality from CVD with risk ratios of 2.0, 2.3, and 2.4, respectively. Elevated serum insulin was

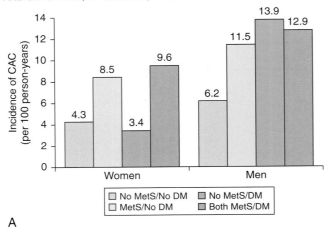

INCIDENCE OF CAC (PER 100 PERSON YR) ACCORDING TO MetS
AND DM STATUS, BY GENDER, AMONG PERSONS w/o BASELINE CAC

A

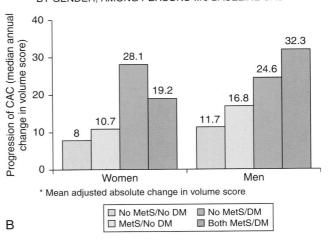

PROGRESSION OF CAC* ACCORDING TO MetS AND DM STATUS,
BY GENDER, AMONG PERSONS w/o BASELINE CAC

* Mean adjusted absolute change in volume score

B

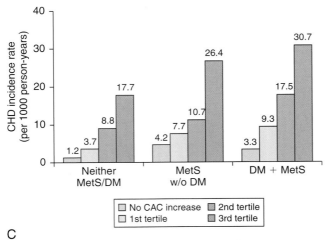

CHD EVENT RATES (PER 1000 PERSON-YEARS) ACCORDING TO
TERTILE OF CAC PROGRESSION BY PRESENCE OF MetS AND DM

C

FIGURE 7-3 A, Incidence of CAC (per 100 person-years) according to metabolic syndrome (MetS) and diabetes (DM) status by gender among persons without baseline CAC. **B,** Progression of CAC (mean unadjusted absolute change in volume score) according to MetS and DM status by gender in persons without baseline CAC. **C,** CHD event rates (per 1000 person-years) according to tertile of CAC progression by presence of MetS and DM. Data are not shown for persons with DM without MetS because of an insufficient number of CHD events. *(Modified from Wong ND, Nelson JC, Granston T, et al: Metabolic syndrome, diabetes, and incidence and progression of coronary calcium: the Multiethnic Study of Atherosclerosis study,* JACC Cardiovasc Imaging *5:358-366, 2012.)*

independently associated with cardiovascular mortality in all men, whereas in women no association could be found. Further evidence of an association between prediabetes and CVD came from two studies from Finland.[17] These authors studied 3267 men aged 40 to 59 years from the Social Insurance Institution's Coronary Heart Disease Study and 1059 men aged 30 to 59 years from the Helsinki Policemen Study. An OGTT was carried out in both studies, and in addition in the Helsinki Policemen Study plasma insulin was measured. In the first study, 4-year mortality from CHD and 4-year incidence of nonfatal MI did not show an association with 1-hour postload plasma glucose. However, in the Helsinki Policemen Study, 1-hour postload blood glucose, but not fasting or 2-hour postload blood glucose, predicted 5-year incidence of CHD endpoints in multivariable analysis. However, 1-hour and 2-hour postload plasma insulin levels both predicted CHD risk even after glucose measurements from the OGTTs were controlled for. The study of men born in 1913 and 1923 also assessed insulin resistance, as estimated with the HOMA equation, and other risk factors for CHD in elderly men and followed them for 8 years.[18] Compared with patients with known diabetes, who had a 2.5-fold increased risk for CHD, there was a 2.2-fold and a 2.4-fold risk among those in the highest compared with the lowest quintile of insulin resistance and fasting insulin, respectively. Further data from the Framingham Heart Study found that IFG was associated with CHD risk in women but not in men.[19] In a first systematic review by Ford and colleagues[20] based on 18 publications, IFG and IGT both were associated with only modest increases in risk for CVD. This was confirmed by two recent, more extensive meta-analyses from the Emerging Risk Factors Collaboration (ERFC) (**Fig. 7-4**),[21,22] which reported data on fasting blood glucose concentration, risk of vascular disease, but also cause-specific death in almost 700,000 and 820,000 people from 102 and 97 prospective studies, respectively. In patients without diabetes, fasting blood glucose concentrations above 100 mg/dL were associated with major causes of death, but not concentrations between 70 and 100 mg/dL. The same held true for incident CHD and stroke.

In aggregate, these data indicate that fasting blood glucose is only modestly associated with risk of vascular disease and that a level exceeding 100 mg/dL but not between 70 and 100 mg/dL is associated with death. Insulin levels may be superior in the prediction of vascular outcome in prediabetic patients.

Coronary Heart Disease Risk of Patients with Metabolic Syndrome

During the past 10 years, a large number of studies have reported on the association between the metabolic syndrome and total mortality as well as CVD morbidity and mortality. Data have come from diverse populations and have included varying definitions; however, in most studies, WHO, International Diabetes Federation (IDF), and ATP III definitions have been used. At present, there is still ongoing controversy regarding whether or not the metabolic syndrome as a whole presents incremental information above and beyond the accumulation of individual risk factors. (See also Chapter 4.)

Probably the most frequently cited report is by Lakka and colleagues[23] from the Kuopio Ischaemic Heart Disease Risk Factor (KIHD) study (**Fig. 7-5**), a population-based prospective cohort of 1209 Finnish men aged 42 to 60 years who were initially free of CVD, cancer, and diabetes. In contrast to other studies, this early study used four different definitions of the metabolic syndrome and found a prevalence ranging from 8.8% to 14.3%. During an 11.4-year follow-up, men with metabolic syndrome as defined by NCEP criteria were 2.5

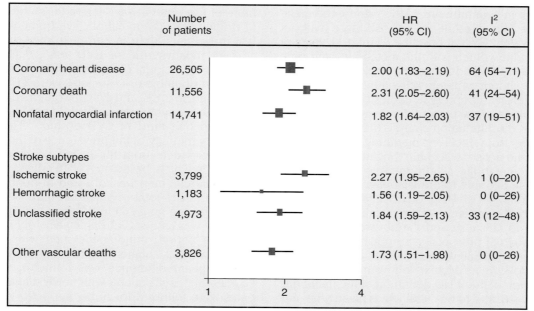

HAZARD RATIOS (HRs) FOR VASCULAR OUTCOMES IN PEOPLE WITH versus THOSE WITHOUT DIABETES AT BASELINE

	Number of patients		HR (95% CI)	I² (95% CI)
Coronary heart disease	26,505		2.00 (1.83–2.19)	64 (54–71)
Coronary death	11,556		2.31 (2.05–2.60)	41 (24–54)
Nonfatal myocardial infarction	14,741		1.82 (1.64–2.03)	37 (19–51)
Stroke subtypes				
Ischemic stroke	3,799		2.27 (1.95–2.65)	1 (0–20)
Hemorrhagic stroke	1,183		1.56 (1.19–2.05)	0 (0–26)
Unclassified stroke	4,973		1.84 (1.59–2.13)	33 (12–48)
Other vascular deaths	3,826		1.73 (1.51–1.98)	0 (0–26)

FIGURE 7-4 Hazard ratios (HRs) for vascular outcomes in people with versus those without diabetes at baseline. CI = Confidence interval; I² = statistic for heterogeneity. *(Modified from Emerging Risk Factors Collaboration; Sarwar N, Gao P, Seshasai SR, et al: Diabetes mellitus, fasting blood glucose concentration, and risk of vascular disease: a collaborative meta-analysis of 102 prospective studies, Lancet 375:2215-2222, 2010.)*

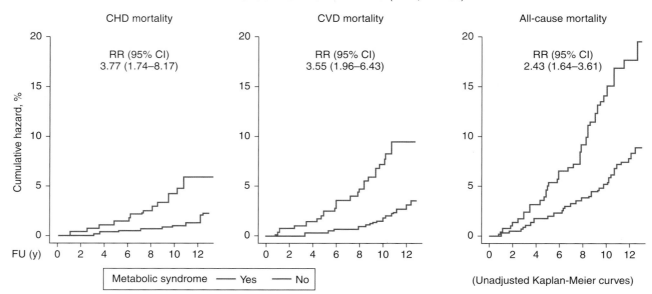

FIGURE 7-5 The metabolic syndrome and total and cardiovascular disease mortality in middle-aged men; unadjusted Kaplan-Meier hazard curves. CI = Confidence interval; RR = relative risk. *(Data from Lakka HM, Laaksonen DE, Lakka TA, et al: The metabolic syndrome and total and cardiovascular disease mortality in middle-aged men, JAMA 288:2709-2716, 2002.)*

times more likely to die of CHD in multivariable analysis than those defined by WHO criteria. The metabolic syndrome as defined by WHO was associated with a 2.6-fold increase in CVD mortality and a 1.9 times higher all-cause mortality. In the Botnia Study from Finland and Sweden, 4400 patients aged 35 to 70 years were studied. Risk for CHD and stroke was increased threefold in patients with metabolic syndrome, and cardiovascular mortality was markedly increased when the WHO definition was used. Microalbuminuria as an individual component was the strongest risk factor for cardiovascular death.[24] Among 12,089 black and white middle-aged individuals in the Atherosclerosis Risk in Communities (ARIC) study, the metabolic syndrome was present in 23% of those without diabetes or prevalent CVD at baseline. During 11 years of follow-up, men and women with the metabolic syndrome were approximately 1.5 and 2 times more likely to develop CHD than those without symptoms after adjustment for age, smoking, low-density lipoprotein cholesterol, and race. Similar associations were present for incident ischemic stroke. However, discrimination analysis based on the area under the curve from receiver operating characteristic (ROC) analysis did not show a clinical significant improvement once the metabolic syndrome was added to the Framingham Risk Score.[25] In the Diabetes Epidemiology: Collaborative Analysis of Diagnostic Criteria in Europe (DECODE) study,[26] prevalence of the metabolic syndrome and its relation to all-cause and cardiovascular mortality were investigated in 11 prospective European cohorts comprising 6156 men and 5356 women without diabetes in the age range of 30 to 89 years. Median follow-up was 8.8 years. A modified version of the WHO definition of the metabolic syndrome was used, and to be classified as having the metabolic syndrome, patients had to have hyperinsulinemia and two or more of the following: obesity, hypertension, dyslipidemia, or impaired glucose regulation. The age-standardized prevalence of the metabolic syndrome was 15.7% in men and 14.2% in women, and hazard ratios for all-cause and cardiovascular mortality in patients with metabolic syndrome were 1.44 and 2.26 in men and 1.38 and 2.78 in women, respectively, after adjustments for age, blood cholesterol, and smoking. Data from the Framingham Heart Study provided a slightly different picture. In 3323 middle-aged patients, the prevalence of the metabolic syndrome was determined as the presence or absence of abdominal obesity, low high-density lipoprotein cholesterol (HDL-C), high triglycerides, hypertension, and IFG, and follow-up was 8 years. The presence of three or more of five criteria was seen in 26.8% of men and 16.6% of women; thus the metabolic syndrome was more prevalent in U.S. men than in European men. In men, the age-adjusted relative risk for CVD was 2.9 (for CHD it was 2.5), and for incident diabetes mellitus it was 6.9. The population attributable risk estimates were 34%, 29%, and 62% in men and 16%, 8%, and 47% in women, respectively. Thus the metabolic syndrome in this U.S. population accounted for up to one third of CVD events.[27] The considerable regional variability of the prevalence of the metabolic syndrome is evident from the Italian Longitudinal Study on Aging,[28] in which, based on ATP III criteria, the prevalence in nondiabetic men was 26% and in nondiabetic women was 15.5%. The total population comprised 5632 individuals in the age range 65 to 84 years at baseline, and CVD mortality was assessed during 4 years of follow-up. During this time period, nondiabetic men with metabolic syndrome had a 12% higher CVD mortality than those without; no significant difference was found in women. In the UKPDS 78,[29] 5102 patients with newly diagnosed type 2 diabetes were followed for a median of 10 years. Metabolic syndrome was based on ATP III, WHO, IDF, and the European Group for the Study of Insulin Resistance criteria, and was found in 61%, 38%, 54%, and 24%, respectively.

RR AND 95% CI FOR MS AND INCIDENT CV EVENTS AND DEATH IN STUDIES USING MV MODELS

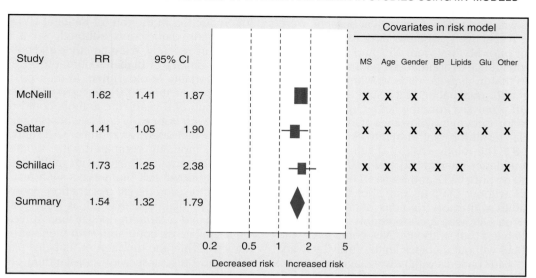

FIGURE 7-6 Relative risk (RR) and 95% confidence interval (CI) for metabolic syndrome and incident cardiovascular events and death in studies that simultaneously included metabolic syndrome and some of its components into multivariable (MV) models. BP = Blood pressure; MS = metabolic syndrome. *(Modified from Gami AS, Witt BJ, Howard DE, et al: Metabolic syndrome and risk of incident cardiovascular events and death: a systematic review and meta-analysis of longitudinal studies,* J Am Coll Cardiol 49:403-414, 2007.)

Patients with metabolic syndrome had an increased risk for CVD compared with those without (the risk in those without metabolic syndrome was between 23% and 33%, depending on the definition used). However, the positive predictive value of the metabolic syndrome for CVD was only 13% to 39%. Based on such poor discrimination with respect to CVD, the authors concluded that the metabolic syndrome may be of limited clinical value for CVD risk stratification in patients with type 2 diabetes. Finally, in the Rancho Bernardo Study,[30] 977 men and 1141 women aged 40 to 94 years were recruited from 1984 to 1987 and followed for mortality for a maximum of 20 years. Various cardiometabolic biomarkers such as adiponectin, leptin, ghrelin, interleukin 6 (IL-6), and CRP were measured, and the ATP III definition of the metabolic syndrome was used. There was a crude 65% increased risk for CHD in those with metabolic syndrome. This association did not significantly decrease after adjustment for adiponectin, leptin, and ghrelin but was attenuated by 25% after adjustment for IL-6 and CRP. Thus the authors concluded that these adiposity-signaling hormones and markers of inflammation explain little of the association between the metabolic syndrome and CHD mortality. Finally, in a systematic review and meta-analysis of longitudinal studies, Gami and colleagues[31] found 37 eligible studies with 43 cohorts. The association between metabolic syndrome and cardiovascular events was stronger in women, in studies enrolling lower-risk individuals, and in studies using the WHO definition. Most important, the association remained statistically significant after adjustment for traditional cardiovascular risk factors, with a relative risk of 1.54 (**Fig. 7-6**).

Thus, despite an ongoing controversy, the aggregate data suggest a modest independent association between the metabolic syndrome and incidence of various cardiovascular outcomes. In addition to its potential role as a risk marker, the metabolic syndrome may serve as an important educational tool.

Coronary Heart Disease Risk of Patients with Type 2 Diabetes (Diabetes as a Coronary Heart Disease Equivalent)

The pronounced increased risk of diabetic patients for CVD was first reported in 1979 based on 20 years of surveillance of the Framingham cohort, which revealed a twofold to threefold increased risk of atherosclerotic complications in various vascular beds, the strongest impact being seen on intermittent claudication.[32] The study with the greatest impact on our awareness of an increased risk for cardiovascular complications in patients with diabetes, which consecutively led to the notion of diabetes as a CHD equivalent, came from a population-based case-control study published by Haffner and colleagues (**Fig. 7-7**).[33] Based on a 7-year

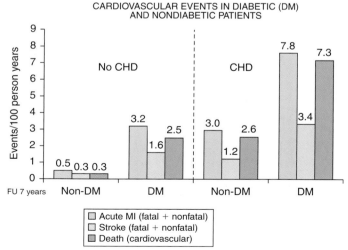

FIGURE 7-7 Incidence of cardiovascular events during a 7-year follow-up in relation to history of MI in patients with type 2 diabetes and in nondiabetic patients. *(Data from Haffner SM, Lehto S, Rönnemaa T, et al. Mortality from coronary heart disease in patients with type 2 diabetes and in nondiabetic patients with and without prior myocardial infarction,* N Engl J Med 339:229-234, 1998.)

follow-up of 1373 nondiabetic patients and 1059 diabetic patients, the incidence rates for nonfatal and fatal MI in nondiabetic patients with and without prior MI at baseline were 18.8% and 3.5%, respectively, whereas in diabetic patients with and without prior MI they were 45% and 22%, respectively. Thus, the incidence in nondiabetic patients with prior MI was similar to that in diabetic patients without prior MI. This was also seen for nonfatal and fatal stroke and for cardiovascular death. Analyses from the large Organization to Assess Strategies for Ischemic Syndromes (OASIS) registry provided a similar result for total mortality as an outcome variable (**Fig. 7-8**). The relative risk of death over 2 years was 1.99 (95% confidence interval [CI] 1.52-2.60) for patients with diabetes and no prior CVD, and it was 1.71 (95% CI 1.44-2.04) for patients without diabetes but prior CVD.[34] However, further studies with more rigorous definitions of MI patients and diabetes showed a considerably lower risk in patients with diabetes but without CVD compared with patients after MI but without diabetes. In the study by Evans and colleagues,[35] 3402 patients with newly diagnosed type 2 diabetes and 5350 patients in the post–acute MI period were recruited and followed for more than 10 years. Compared with patients with diabetes, the post-MI group had an almost threefold increased risk of death and an approximately threefold increased risk of hospitalization with a recurrent MI. This result was supported by data from the population-based ARIC study,[36] in which 13,719 African American and white men and women in the age range 45 to 74 years were studied from 1987 to 1989. In multivariable models, patients with a history of MI but without diabetes at baseline had a 1.9-times risk of fatal and nonfatal MI and a 1.8-times increased risk of CHD mortality compared with patients with diabetes without a prior history of MI. Yet stroke risk was similar between diabetic patients without MI and nondiabetic patients with MI. These data suggest that patients with diabetes are at increased risk for cardiovascular complications, but this risk is lower and not identical to the one of patients who have already experienced a CHD event. Looking at trends of cardiovascular complications in diabetic patients,[37] despite the increased risk compared with patients without diabetes, those with diabetes had an approximately 50% reduction in the rate of incident CVD, as was seen in nondiabetic participants although on a higher absolute level. More recently, Wannamethee and colleagues[38] looked into the impact of diabetes duration on CVD risk and all-cause mortality in older men. In their prospective analysis based on more than 4000 men aged 60 to 79 years of age with a follow-up of 9 years, the authors could demonstrate that patients with both early and late onset of diabetes had a significantly increased risk of major CHD and CVD events and all-cause mortality compared with nondiabetic men who had no history of MI, even with multivariable adjustments including novel risk biomarkers such as CRP, von Willebrand factor, and renal dysfunction. However, men with early-onset diabetes, defined as onset before the age of 60 years and a duration longer than 10 years, had a somewhat similar risk compared with men with prior MI without diabetes. Thus the duration of diabetes plays an important role, and only those with longstanding disease, based on these data, may be considered to have a CHD equivalent (**Fig. 7-9**).

These epidemiologic data are supported by mechanistic studies coming from a prospective registry of diabetic patients undergoing diagnostic coronary angiography and IVUS in whom, in addition to the presence and extension of plaque as assessed by grayscale information, an IVUS-derived modality, virtual histology (VH), was used. Patients with diabetes duration of 10 years or longer showed a greater plaque burden in most diseased segments; also, the proportion of IVUS-defined thin-cap fibroatheroma (TCFA) in those with longstanding diabetes was greater than in those with diabetes duration of less than 10 years. This association was present even with multivariable adjustments taking into account clinical characteristics and treatment modalities.[39]

An earlier meta-analysis[40] based on 37 prospective cohorts comprising almost 450,000 patients showed that the rate of fatal CHD was higher in patients with diabetes than in those without (5.4% versus 1.6%). In addition, this meta-analysis confirmed data from the Framingham study that women with diabetes have a 50% higher risk for a fatal CHD than men, which may be explained to some extent by a more extensive adverse risk profile and in addition by differences in treatment. Two more recent meta-analyses by the ERFC (**Fig. 7-10**)[21,22] clearly demonstrated that diabetes was associated with a twofold excess risk for a wide range of vascular diseases independently from conventional risk factors. This study was based on almost 700,000 patients from whom individual data were available and in whom more than 50,000 fatal and nonfatal vascular outcomes had occurred. Of note, in addition to adjustment for conventional risk factors, in this meta-analysis, data on inflammatory and renal markers were also available that did not significantly attenuate the association. This large database also clearly showed that the impact of diabetes is not restricted to vascular complications such as CHD, stroke, peripheral artery disease (PAD), and vascular death, but diabetes also affects a variety of other causes of death including cancers, infectious diseases, renal and liver disease, and finally mental disorders.

In addition to the solid evidence from numerous long-term prospective epidemiologic studies showing that the presence of diabetes mellitus is associated with adverse vascular and nonvascular outcomes, there are also detailed

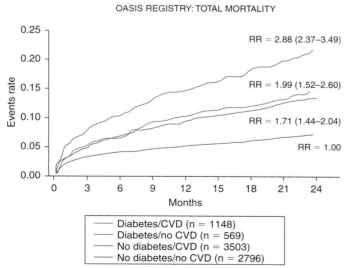

FIGURE 7-8 Total mortality: cumulative event curves for patients with and without diabetes in relation to previously known CVD. (*Modified from Malmberg K, Yusuf S, Gerstein HC, et al: Impact of diabetes on long-term prognosis in patients with unstable angina and non–Q-wave myocardial infarction: results of the OASIS (Organization to Assess Strategies for Ischemic Syndromes) Registry, Circulation 102:1014-1019, 2000.*)

DURATION OF DIABETES IN MEN w/o PREV. MI AND ADJ. HRs OF MAJOR CVD EVENTS AND ALL-CAUSE MORTALITY

	Duration of Diabetes Mellitus in Years		
	0–1	2–7	≥ 8
No. of participants	202	103	109
CVD events			
Rate per 1000 person-years (No. of events)	20.3(32)	19.7(16)	36.6(29)
Age-adjusted HR (95% CI)	1 [Reference]	1.14(0.78–1.67)	1.39(0.98–1.96)
Adjusted HR (95% CI)*	1 [Reference]	1.19(0.79–1.80)	1.49(1.03–2.16)
All-cause mortality			
Rate per 1000 person-years (No. of events)	38.0(60)	44.4(36)	66.9(53)
Age-adjusted HR (95% CI)	1 [Reference]	1.10(0.85–1.43)	1.35(1.06–1.70)
Adjusted HR (95% CI)*	1 [Reference]	1.10(0.83–1.47)	1.39(1.07–1.79)

Abbreviations: CI, confidence interval; CVD, cardiovascular disease; HR, hazards ratio; MI, myocardial infarction. CVD events include nonfatal MI or CVD deaths.
*Adjusted for age, smoking, alcohol consumption, social class, body mass index, physical activity, stroke, systolic blood pressure, high-density lipoprotein and total cholesterol levels, low forced expiratory volume in 1 second, estimated glomerular filtration rate, C-reactive protein level, and von Willebrand factor level.

Rates per 1000 person-years, men aged 60–79 yrs

FIGURE 7-9 Duration of diabetes in 414 diabetic men without previous MI aged 60 to 79 years and rates per 1000 person-years and adjusted HRs of major CVD events and all-cause mortality. *(Modified from Wannamethee SG, Shaper AG, Whincup PH, et al: Impact of diabetes on cardiovascular disease risk and all-cause mortality in older men: influence of age at onset, diabetes duration, and established and novel risk factors,* Arch Intern Med *171:404-410, 2011.)*

HAZARD RATIOS FOR CHD AND ISCHEMIC STROKE BY
BASELINE FASTING BLOOD GLUCOSE CONCENTRATION

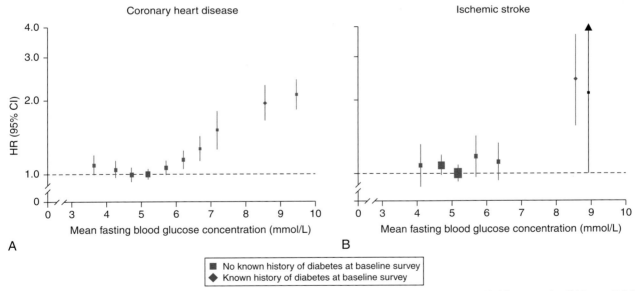

No known history of diabetes at baseline survey
Known history of diabetes at baseline survey

FIGURE 7-10 Hazard ratios for coronary heart disease and ischemic stroke by baseline fasting blood glucose concentration. *(Modified from Emerging Risk Factors Collaboration; Sarwar N, Gao P, Seshasai SR, et al: Diabetes mellitus, fasting blood glucose concentration, and risk of vascular disease: a collaborative meta-analysis of 102 prospective studies,* Lancet *375:2215-2222, 2010.)*

data regarding long-term metabolic control, as assessed by hemoglobin A1c (HbA1c), in patients with type 2 diabetes and its association with macrovascular complications such as MI, stroke, amputation, and total mortality. Such data were reported first from UKPDS 35.[41] In this large prospective study the incidence of clinical complications was significantly associated with glycemia, demonstrating that each

1% reduction in mean HbA1c was associated with reductions in risk of 21% for any endpoint related to diabetes, 21% for deaths, and 40% for MI. Thus the degree of hyperglycemia seems to be strongly related to vascular outcome and all-cause mortality. These data were confirmed in another population-based cohort study from Norfolk, United Kingdom: the European Prospective Investigation into Cancer

DIABETES AND ATHEROSCLEROSIS

II

and Nutrition (EPIC).[42] The database comprised 4662 men aged 45 to 79 years who had HbA1c measured at baseline in 1995 to 1997 and were followed until 1999. The primary outcome of interest was a composite of mortality from all causes, CVD, and ischemic heart disease. Men with manifest diabetes had a 3.5-fold increased risk of death from all causes, a more than 8-fold increased risk for cardiovascular mortality, and a 10-fold increased risk for CHD compared with patients with an HbA1c of less than 5%. However, within several categories of HbA1c from below 5% to above 7%, there was a gradual increase for all of the above-mentioned endpoints, suggesting that even in the normal upper range of HbA1c an increased risk of death or nonfatal coronary complications is present. Data from the large ARIC study based on more than 11,000 African American or white adults also demonstrated that HbA1c values at baseline were associated with newly diagnosed diabetes and cardiovascular outcomes (**Fig. 7-11**). Similar to EPIC Norfolk, this study also showed an

increased risk for diabetes and cardiovascular outcome even in the normal range for HbA1c, but the increase in risk was particularly pronounced in those with an HbA1c of 6.5% or greater. Similar results were found for CHD and for stroke.[43] However, in one study with a high prevalence of diabetes, the Strong Heart Study,[44] in which HbA1c and fasting plasma glucose were measured in more than 4500 Native American adults, neither HbA1c nor fasting blood glucose added to conventional cardiovascular risk factors in the prediction of CHD or total CVD.

To summarize, there is clear evidence from a large number of well-controlled prospective epidemiologic studies, that the presence of type 2 diabetes is associated with an approximately twofold increased risk for various cardiovascular complications. In those with diabetes, the long-term control of glucose metabolism seems to play an important role because a strong relationship has been seen in several studies between HbA1c levels and cardiovascular outcome as well as total mortality.

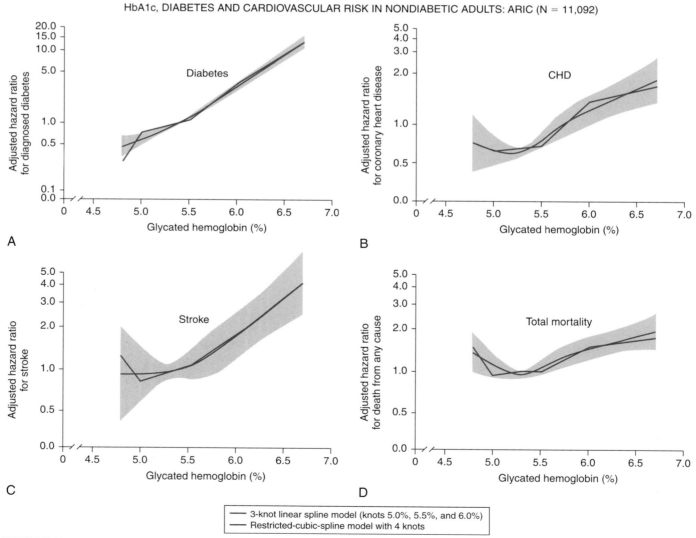

HbA1c, DIABETES AND CARDIOVASCULAR RISK IN NONDIABETIC ADULTS: ARIC (N = 11,092)

— 3-knot linear spline model (knots 5.0%, 5.5%, and 6.0%)
— Restricted-cubic-spline model with 4 knots

FIGURE 7-11 Adjusted HRs for self-reported diagnosed diabetes and CHD, ischemic stroke, and death from any cause, according to the baseline glycated hemoglobin value. (*Data from Selvin E, Steffes MW, Zhu H, et al: Glycated hemoglobin, diabetes, and cardiovascular risk in nondiabetic adults,* N Engl J Med *362:800-811, 2010.*)

SHORT-TERM AND LONG-TERM PROGNOSIS AFTER ACUTE MYOCARDIAL INFARCTION IN PATIENTS WITH PATHOLOGIC GLUCOSE METABOLISM AND AFTER CORONARY INTERVENTIONS OR WITH HEART FAILURE

An ACS, in particular MI (non–ST-segment MI [NSTEMI] or ST-segment MI [STEMI]) is associated with a profound stimulation of the sympathetic nerve system (SNS). Because the SNS adversely affects glucose metabolism, a number of studies have looked into admission blood glucose in patients without manifest diabetes and its relation to in-hospital complications and long-term outcome. Stranders and colleagues[45] studied 846 patients for a median of 15 months. An increase of 18 mg/dL in admission blood glucose was associated with a 4% increase in mortality in nondiabetic and 5% in diabetic patients. Thus, admission blood glucose was similarly associated with long-term risk in nondiabetic as well as diabetic patients. This result is not surprising, given the fact that abnormal glucose tolerance and the metabolic syndrome are common risk factors in patients with acute MI. In one study, two thirds of patients after an MI had abnormal glucose tolerance at discharge compared with only 35% in controls.[46] In another study, almost 50% showed metabolic syndrome on admission to the hospital with an ACS, which was a strong and independent predictor of in-hospital case fatality but also severe heart failure.[47] In a nationwide sample of elderly patients (n = 142,000) hospitalized for acute MI in the United States from 1994 to 1996, higher glucose levels were clearly associated with a greater risk for 30-day mortality in patients without known diabetes compared with those with diabetes. In contrast, among diabetic patients, higher mortality was observed only in those with very high glucose levels (>240 mg/dL) (**Table 7-1**).[48] In a population-based MI registry, MONICA/KORA Augsburg, the authors studied admission blood glucose levels in 1631 nondiabetic and 659 diabetic patients and related admission levels to 30-day as well as 1- and 3-year case fatality. Blood glucose levels on admission were divided into quartiles, and patients without known diabetes in the top quartile (≥150 mg/dL) showed an almost threefold risk of death during in-hospital stay in multivariable analysis. In patients with type 2 diabetes mellitus, a similar relationship

was seen in age- and gender-adjusted analysis, but once treatment was taken into account, as well as in-hospital complications, there was only a trend for an increased in-hospital case fatality that was no longer statistically significant. With regard to 1- and 3-year outcomes after exclusion of those who died within 28 days, only a nonsignificant trend was seen in patients without diabetes, whereas no effect was found in diabetic patients. After 3 years, no association with increased risk of death was seen for patients without or with diabetes.[49] Data from the same population-based registry[50] have demonstrated in more than 2200 patients admitted with MI from 1985 to 1992 an increased 28-day as well as 5-year mortality in diabetic patients versus nondiabetic patients (12.6% versus 7.3% at 28 days). Five-year mortality was increased by 64% in diabetic patients compared with non–diabetic patients. McGuire and colleagues[51] demonstrated in 12,142 patients from the Global Use of Strategies to Open Occluded Arteries in Acute Coronary Syndromes (GUSTO-IIb) study presenting with the whole spectrum of ACS that diabetic patients had an increased overall risk of death or reinfarction, whether they presented with STEMI or NSTEMI, at 30 days and at 6 months. Furthermore, a large number of observational studies and reports from large randomized trials consistently have shown an increased risk for adverse cardiovascular outcomes in patients with the admission diagnosis of diabetes during in-hospital stay or long term.[34,52–54]

In addition, diabetes was a strong predictor of adverse outcome in patients admitted with an ACS who underwent coronary revascularization either by percutaneous coronary intervention (PCI) or coronary artery bypass grafting (CABG).[55] Similar data have been reported from the Prevention of Restenosis with Tranilast and Its Outcomes (PRESTO) trial for PCI in stable patients[56] and from a large dataset of stable patients who underwent CABG.[57] Finally, in 1241 patients with congestive heart failure,[58] a statistically significant impact of diabetes on cardiac survival was seen. Specifically, diabetes was an independent predictor of cardiovascular mortality in ischemic patients but not in nonischemic patients.

In summary, patients with known IGT, metabolic syndrome, manifest type 2 diabetes, or even stress-induced hyperglycemia during an acute coronary event are at

TABLE 7-1 Effect of Admission Glucose on Mortality After Multivariable Adjustment

	HR* (95% CI)			
	Glucose >110-140 mg/dL	Glucose >110-170 mg/dL	Glucose >170-240 mg/dL	Glucose >240 mg/dL
All Patients†				
30-day mortality	1.13 (1.08-1.19)	1.31 (1.24-1.38)	1.52 (1.44-1.60)	1.77 (1.68-1.87)
1-year mortality	1.07 (1.03-1.10)	1.17 (1.13-1.21)	1.31 (1.27-1.36)	1.46 (1.41-1.52)
In Patients Without Known Diabetes‡				
30-day mortality	1.17 (1.11-1.24)	1.37 (1.29-1.44)	1.63 (1.54-1.73)	1.87 (1.75-2.00)
1-year mortality	1.09 (1.05-1.13)	1.20 (1.16-1.25)	1.37 (1.31-1.43)	1.56 (1.48-1.63)
In Patients With Diabetes§				
30-day mortality	0.90 (0.78-1.04)	0.99 (0.86-1.13)	1.09 (0.97-1.24)	1.32 (1.17-1.49)
1-year mortality	0.96 (0.87-1.06)	0.95 (0.86-1.04)	1.04 (0.96-1.14)	1.16 (1.07-1.26)

*Risk-adjusted hazard ratio (HR) with its respective 95% CI.
†All patients with admission glucose ≤110 mg/dL (referent group).
‡Patients without recognized diabetes and admission glucose ≤110 mg/dL (referent group).
§Patients with diabetes and admission glucose ≤110 mg/dL (referent group).
Data from Kosiborod M, Rathore SS, Inzucchi SE, et al: Admission glucose and mortality in elderly patients hospitalized with acute myocardial infarction: implications for patients with and without recognized diabetes, *Circulation* 111:3078-3086, 2005.

increased risk for short-term and long-term complications including vascular death. Diabetes mellitus also remains a strong risk factor for adverse outcome in coronary interventions such as PCI and CABG whether during an emergency situation or in stable patients. Finally, in patients with complications from MI, such as congestive heart failure, diabetes represents a strong risk factor for future outcome, in particular in ischemic cardiomyopathy.

PERIPHERAL ARTERIAL DISEASE AND DIABETES

Early data from the Framingham study have previously suggested that diabetes may be particularly strongly related to peripheral arterial disease (PAD).[32] The risk for PAD is usually twofold to fourfold increased in diabetic compared with nondiabetic patients.[59] Similar to associations observed between diabetes and CAD, the duration and severity of diabetes determine the incidence and extent of PAD.[60] Of note, as also seen in the coronary arterial tree, PAD associated with diabetes is usually characterized by more diffuse and more distal lesions than in patients without diabetes. Data from the large National Health and Nutrition Examination Survey (NHANES) study (1999 to 2204) in a total of 7058 patients 40 years and older showed the highest prevalence of PAD among older adults, non-Hispanics, blacks, and women. In multivariable analysis, in particular diabetes but also hypertension, chronic kidney disease, and smoking were strong risk factors after age, gender, and racial and ethnic differences were taken into account.[61] On a national U.S. level, approximately 2.4 million to 3.6 million diabetic patients have PAD.[62] Based on noninvasive assessment using the ABI, approximately 20% to 30% of patients with diabetes have prevalent PAD (defined as an ABI below 0.9). Similar to associations in the coronary arterial tree, in UKPDS the duration of diabetes and the degree of glycemic control were independent risk factors for PAD.[63] In addition, African Americans and patients of Hispanic descent with diabetes were at increased risk of PAD.[64] Approximately one fourth of diabetic patients with PAD demonstrate progression of symptoms over a 5-year period and an amputation rate of approximately 4%. Whereas in general, PAD symptoms are stable, there is a striking increase in CHD events over the same time period with a 20% nonfatal MI and stroke rate and a 30% death rate.[65] Clearly, the prevalence of PAD differs in relation to the comorbidity present in the individual patient. Thus, increased prevalence of PAD has been reported in patients with diabetes mellitus and arterial hypertension and in particular with chronic kidney disease or even more pronounced end-stage renal disease. Furthermore, in these subgroups the degree of blood glucose control as assessed by HbA1c was strongly increased, with risk of development of PAD and finally the necessity for limb amputation.[66]

In summary, diabetes is associated with an increased risk of PAD, and the degree of blood glucose control is associated with the severity of outcome. However, most diabetic patients have asymptomatic PAD and only approximately 20% are symptomatic. In terms of vessel distribution, PAD is more diffuse and distally located. A clustering of additional risk factors in diabetic patients may strongly contribute to more extensive and severe PAD.

DIABETES AND CORONARY HEART DISEASE IN WOMEN

Since the first publications from Framingham, the risk of coronary or in general cardiovascular complications has been reported to be higher in women compared with men by approximately 50%. In addition, during the acute phase of an ischemic event, the risk of death is higher in women than in men despite taking into account age and potential differences in treatment strategies. There are several well-controlled prospective epidemiologic studies that have looked into gender differences in diabetic patients with regard to fatal or nonfatal cardiovascular outcome. In the Rancho Bernardo Study,[67] during a 14-year follow-up in men and women aged 40 to 79 years, the relative risk for ischemic heart disease in diabetic versus nondiabetic patients was 1.8 in men and 3.3 in women after adjustment for age, and 1.9 in men and 3.3 in women after adjustment for age, systolic blood pressure, cholesterol, body mass index (BMI), and cigarette smoking. This gender difference may largely be explained by a persistently more favorable survival rate of women than men without diabetes. Yet, no convincing pathophysiologic explanation had been suggested. In the British Regional Heart Study and the British Women's Heart Health Study, Wannamethee and colleagues[68] looked into a large panel of traditional and more novel risk markers such as insulin resistance, inflammation, activated coagulation, and endothelial dysfunction in 7529 men and women aged 60 to 79 years with no previous MI. Nondiabetic women clearly tended to have a more favorable risk factor profile—which, however, was attenuated in the diabetic state. Waist circumference, BMI, level of von Willebrand factor, white blood cell count, insulin resistance, diastolic blood pressure, HDL-C, tissue plasminogen activator (t-PA), and factor VIII level differed more between diabetic and nondiabetic women than between diabetic and nondiabetic men. Thus the more extensive risk factor profile in women may account for the increased risk of CVD. It is interesting to note that in the Heart and Estrogen/Progestin Replacement Study (HERS)[69] in women with CHD, hormonal replacement reduced the incidence of diabetes by 35%. The intake of estrogen and progestin in postmenopausal women improved their metabolic profile, but based on other adverse effects, in particular an increase in breast cancer incidence,[70] hormonal replacement cannot be recommended for this purpose. Further data suggest a particularly increased risk in women with diabetes who developed complications after MI such as congestive heart failure. In a study of more than 900 patients, of whom 41% were female, the increased risk of death in diabetic patients appeared to be particularly prominent in women.[71]

In summary, data from several epidemiologic studies and registries indicate that women with diabetes have a higher risk for cardiovascular complications during the acute event but also long term. This may at least in part be a result of the well-known age difference in the occurrence of a first MI between genders, but may also be a result of late diagnosis of acute ischemic events in women and also of differences in treatment strategies—which, at present, are diminishing. In addition, in particular in elderly women the risk factor profile seems to be more extensive than in diabetic men, which may provide an additional explanation for differences in relevant outcomes. However, other gender-specific differences may still play a role, but this area needs further investigation.

DIABETES AND ATHEROSCLEROTIC COMPLICATIONS: GEOGRAPHIC AND ETHNIC DIFFERENCES

Because of the obesity epidemic and the rapid acquisition of the Western lifestyle in many Asian countries and Latin-America, the prevalence and incidence of diabetes are increasing dramatically worldwide, with a much more profound increase in former developing countries compared with established industrialized societies. An increase of 42% has been estimated for the time period between 1995 and 2025 in developed countries, and an approximately 170% increase in developing countries during the same time period. Thus in 2025 there will be more than 300 million people with diabetes in the adult population worldwide, with approximately 230 million in developing countries and approximately 70 million in developed countries.[72] In 2025 the highest prevalence will be seen in former socialist economies of Europe, in countries in the Middle East, in Latin-America and the Caribbean, in India, and finally in Western societies with prevalence rates of 6% to 9%. In terms of absolute numbers, the Middle East and India will be leading, followed by Western countries, China, and Latin America. More recent global estimates based on larger studies from 91 countries suggest that in the population aged 20 to 79 years there will be an increase in the prevalence of diabetes from 6.4% in 2010 (285 million adults) to 7.7% (439 million adults) in 2030. Developing countries will face a 70% increase compared with a 20% increase in industrialized societies.[73] As a consequence, subclinical atherosclerosis and clinical complications from atherosclerosis will increase dramatically.

Thus there are pronounced geographic and ethnic differences in type 2 diabetes incidence, which may be explained by different socioeconomic situations and cultural conditions but also by the well-known susceptibility for insulin resistance in Southeast Asians.

References

1. Winkelmann BR, Marz W, Boehm BO, et al: Rationale and design of the LURIC study—a resource for functional genomics, pharmacogenomics and long-term prognosis of cardiovascular disease, *Pharmacogenomics* 2:S1, 2001.
2. Bartnik M, Ryden L, Ferrari R, et al: The prevalence of abnormal glucose regulation in patients with coronary artery disease across Europe. The Euro Heart Survey on diabetes and the heart, *Eur Heart J* 25:1880, 2004.
3. de la Hera JM, Delgado E, Hernandez E, et al: Prevalence and outcome of newly detected diabetes in patients who undergo percutaneous coronary intervention, *Eur Heart J* 30:2614, 2009.
4. Khot UN, Khot MB, Bajzer CT, et al: Prevalence of conventional risk factors in patients with coronary heart disease, *JAMA* 290:898, 2003.
5. Tardif JC, Lesage F, Harel F, et al: Imaging biomarkers in atherosclerosis trials, *Circ Cardiovasc Imaging* 4:319, 2011.
6. Fowkes FG, Murray GD, Butcher I, et al: Ankle brachial index combined with Framingham Risk Score to predict cardiovascular events and mortality: a meta-analysis, *JAMA* 300:197, 2008.
7. Den Ruijter HM, Peters SA, Anderson TJ, et al: Common carotid intima-media thickness measurements in cardiovascular risk prediction: a meta-analysis, *JAMA* 308:796, 2012.
8. Yeboah J, McClelland RL, Polonsky TS, et al: Comparison of novel risk markers for improvement in cardiovascular risk assessment in intermediate-risk individuals, *JAMA* 308:788, 2012.
9. Kuller LH, Velentgas P, Barzilay J, et al: Diabetes mellitus: subclinical cardiovascular disease and risk of incident cardiovascular disease and all-cause mortality, *Arterioscler Thromb Vasc Biol* 20:823, 2000.
10. Brohall G, Oden A, Fagerberg B: Carotid artery intima-media thickness in patients with type 2 diabetes mellitus and impaired glucose tolerance: a systematic review, *Diabet Med* 23:609, 2006.
11. Bonora E, Kiechl S, Willeit J, et al: Carotid atherosclerosis and coronary heart disease in the metabolic syndrome: prospective data from the Bruneck study, *Diabetes Care* 26:1251, 2003.
12. Wong ND, Nelson JC, Granston T, et al: Metabolic syndrome, diabetes, and incidence and progression of coronary calcium: the Multiethnic Study of Atherosclerosis study, *JACC Cardiovasc Imaging* 5:358, 2012.
13. Chen K, Lindsey JB, Khera A, et al: Independent associations between metabolic syndrome, diabetes mellitus and atherosclerosis: observations from the Dallas Heart study, *Diab Vasc Dis Res* 5:96, 2008.
14. Wong ND, Sciammarella MG, Polk D, et al: The metabolic syndrome, diabetes, and subclinical atherosclerosis assessed by coronary calcium, *J Am Coll Cardiol* 41:1547, 2003.
15. Elkeles RS, Godsland IF, Feher MD, et al: Coronary calcium measurement improves prediction of cardiovascular events in asymptomatic patients with type 2 diabetes: the PREDICT study, *Eur Heart J* 29:2244, 2008.
16. Welborn TA, Wearne K: Coronary heart disease incidence and cardiovascular mortality in Busselton with reference to glucose and insulin concentrations, *Diabetes Care* 2:154, 1979.
17. Pyorala K: Relationship of glucose tolerance and plasma insulin to the incidence of coronary heart disease: results from two population studies in Finland, *Diabetes Care* 2:131, 1979.
18. Welin L, Bresater LE, Eriksson H, et al: Insulin resistance and other risk factors for coronary heart disease in elderly men. The study of men born in 1913 and 1923, *Eur J Cardiovasc Prev Rehabil* 10:283, 2003.
19. Levitzky YS, Pencina MJ, d'Agostino RB, et al: Impact of impaired fasting glucose on cardiovascular disease: the Framingham Heart study, *J Am Coll Cardiol* 51:264, 2008.
20. Ford ES, Zhao G, Li C: Pre-diabetes and the risk for cardiovascular disease: a systematic review of the evidence, *J Am Coll Cardiol* 55:1310, 2010.
21. Emerging Risk Factors Collaboration, Sarwar N, Gao P, et al: Diabetes mellitus, fasting blood glucose concentration, and risk of vascular disease: a collaborative meta-analysis of 102 prospective studies, *Lancet* 375:2215, 2010.
22. Emerging Risk Factors Collaboration, Seshasai SR, Kaptoge S, et al: Diabetes mellitus, fasting glucose, and risk of cause-specific death, *N Engl J Med* 364:829, 2011.
23. Lakka HM, Laaksonen DE, Lakka TA, et al: The metabolic syndrome and total and cardiovascular disease mortality in middle-aged men, *JAMA* 288:2709, 2002.
24. Isomaa B, Almgren P, Tuomi T, et al: Cardiovascular morbidity and mortality associated with the metabolic syndrome, *Diabetes Care* 24:683, 2001.
25. McNeill AM, Rosamond WD, Girman CJ, et al: The metabolic syndrome and 11-year risk of incident cardiovascular disease in the atherosclerosis risk in communities study, *Diabetes Care* 28:385, 2005.
26. Hu G, Qiao Q, Tuomilehto J, et al: Prevalence of the metabolic syndrome and its relation to all-cause and cardiovascular mortality in nondiabetic European men and women, *Arch Intern Med* 164:1066, 2004.
27. Wilson PW, d'Agostino RB, Parise H, et al: Metabolic syndrome as a precursor of cardiovascular disease and type 2 diabetes mellitus, *Circulation* 112:3066, 2005.
28. Maggi S, Noale M, Gallina P, et al: Metabolic syndrome, diabetes, and cardiovascular disease in an elderly Caucasian cohort: the Italian longitudinal study on aging, *J Gerontol A Biol Sci Med Sci* 61:505, 2006.
29. Cull CA, Jensen CC, Retnakaran R, et al: Impact of the metabolic syndrome on macrovascular and microvascular outcomes in type 2 diabetes mellitus: United Kingdom Prospective Diabetes Study 78, *Circulation* 116:2119, 2007.
30. Langenberg C, Bergstrom J, Scheidt-Nave C, et al: Cardiovascular death and the metabolic syndrome: role of adiposity-signaling hormones and inflammatory markers, *Diabetes Care* 29:1363, 2006.
31. Gami AS, Witt BJ, Howard DE, et al: Metabolic syndrome and risk of incident cardiovascular events and death: a systematic review and meta-analysis of longitudinal studies, *J Am Coll Cardiol* 49:403, 2007.
32. Kannel WB, McGee DL: Diabetes and cardiovascular disease. The Framingham study, *JAMA* 241:2035, 1979.
33. Haffner SM, Lehto S, Ronnemaa T, et al: Mortality from coronary heart disease in subjects with type 2 diabetes and in nondiabetic subjects with and without prior myocardial infarction, *N Engl J Med* 339:229, 1998.
34. Malmberg K, Yusuf S, Gerstein HC, et al: Impact of diabetes on long-term prognosis in patients with unstable angina and non-Q-wave myocardial infarction: results of the OASIS (Organization to Assess Strategies for Ischemic Syndromes) registry, *Circulation* 102:1014, 2000.
35. Evans JM, Wang J, Morris AD: Comparison of cardiovascular risk between patients with type 2 diabetes and those who had had a myocardial infarction: cross sectional and cohort studies, *BMJ* 324:939, 2002.
36. Lee CD, Folsom AR, Pankow JS, et al: Cardiovascular events in diabetic and nondiabetic adults with or without history of myocardial infarction, *Circulation* 109:855, 2004.
37. Fox CS, Coady S, Sorlie PD, et al: Trends in cardiovascular complications of diabetes, *JAMA* 292:2495, 2004.
38. Wannamethee SG, Shaper AG, Whincup PH, et al: Impact of diabetes on cardiovascular disease risk and all-cause mortality in older men: influence of age at onset, diabetes duration, and established and novel risk factors, *Arch Intern Med* 171:404, 2011.
39. Lindsey JB, House JA, Kennedy KF, et al: Diabetes duration is associated with increased thin-cap fibroatheroma detected by intravascular ultrasound with virtual histology, *Circ Cardiovasc Interv* 2:543, 2009.
40. Huxley R, Barzi F, Woodward M: Excess risk of fatal coronary heart disease associated with diabetes in men and women: meta-analysis of 37 prospective cohort studies, *BMJ* 332:73, 2006.
41. Stratton IM, Adler AI, Neil HA, et al: Association of glycaemia with macrovascular and microvascular complications of type 2 diabetes (UKPDS 35): prospective observational study, *BMJ* 321:405, 2000.
42. Khaw KT, Wareham N, Luben R, et al: Glycated haemoglobin, diabetes, and mortality in men in Norfolk cohort of European prospective investigation of cancer and nutrition (EPIC-Norfolk), *BMJ* 322:1, 2001.
43. Selvin E, Steffes MW, Zhu H, et al: Glycated hemoglobin, diabetes, and cardiovascular risk in nondiabetic adults, *N Engl J Med* 362:800, 2010.
44. Wang H, Shara NM, Lee ET, et al: Hemoglobin A1c, fasting glucose, and cardiovascular risk in a population with high prevalence of diabetes: the strong heart study, *Diabetes Care* 34:1952, 2011.
45. Stranders I, Diamant M, van Gelder RE, et al: Admission blood glucose level as risk indicator of death after myocardial infarction in patients with and without diabetes mellitus, *Arch Intern Med* 164:982, 2004.
46. Bartnik M, Malmberg K, Hamsten A, et al: Abnormal glucose tolerance—a common risk factor in patients with acute myocardial infarction in comparison with population-based controls, *J Intern Med* 256:288, 2004.
47. Zeller M, Steg PG, Ravisy J, et al: Prevalence and impact of metabolic syndrome on hospital outcomes in acute myocardial infarction, *Arch Intern Med* 165:1192, 2005.
48. Kosiborod M, Rathore SS, Inzucchi SE, et al: Admission glucose and mortality in elderly patients hospitalized with acute myocardial infarction: implications for patients with and without recognized diabetes, *Circulation* 111:3078, 2005.
49. Beck JA, Meisinger C, Heier M, et al: Effect of blood glucose concentrations on admission in nondiabetic versus diabetic patients with first acute myocardial infarction on short- and long-term mortality (from the MONICA/KORA Augsburg Myocardial Infarction Registry), *Am J Cardiol* 104:1607, 2009.
50. Lowel H, Koenig W, Engel S, et al: The impact of diabetes mellitus on survival after myocardial infarction: can it be modified by drug treatment? Results of a population-based myocardial infarction register follow-up study, *Diabetologia* 43:218, 2000.
51. McGuire DK, Emanuelsson H, Granger CB, et al: Influence of diabetes mellitus on clinical outcomes across the spectrum of acute coronary syndromes. Findings from the GUSTO-IIb study. GUSTO IIb Investigators, *Eur Heart J* 21:1750, 2000.
52. Aguilar D, Solomon SD, Kober L, et al: Newly diagnosed and previously known diabetes mellitus and 1-year outcomes of acute myocardial infarction: the VALsartan In Acute myocardial iNfarcTion (VALIANT) trial, *Circulation* 110:1572, 2004.
53. Bartnik M, Malmberg K, Norhammar A, et al: Newly detected abnormal glucose tolerance: an important predictor of long-term outcome after myocardial infarction, *Eur Heart J* 25:1990, 2004.
54. Timmer JR, Ottervanger JP, Thomas K, et al: Long-term, cause-specific mortality after myocardial infarction in diabetes, *Eur Heart J* 25:926, 2004.

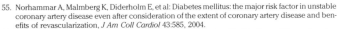

55. Norhammar A, Malmberg K, Diderholm E, et al: Diabetes mellitus: the major risk factor in unstable coronary artery disease even after consideration of the extent of coronary artery disease and benefits of revascularization, *J Am Coll Cardiol* 43:585, 2004.

56. Mathew V, Gersh BJ, Williams BA, et al: Outcomes in patients with diabetes mellitus undergoing percutaneous coronary intervention in the current era: a report from the Prevention of REStenosis with Tranilast and its Outcomes (PRESTO) trial, *Circulation* 109:476, 2004.

57. Lauruschkat AH, Arnrich B, Albert AA, et al: Prevalence and risks of undiagnosed diabetes mellitus in patients undergoing coronary artery bypass grafting, *Circulation* 112:2397, 2005.

58. De GP, Lamblin N, Mouquet F, et al: Impact of diabetes mellitus on long-term survival in patients with congestive heart failure, *Eur Heart J* 25:656, 2004.

59. Newman AB, Siscovick DS, Manolio TA, et al: Ankle-arm index as a marker of atherosclerosis in the Cardiovascular Health Study. Cardiovascular Heart Study (CHS) Collaborative Research Group, *Circulation* 88(837)1993.

60. Jude EB, Oyibo SO, Chalmers N, et al: Peripheral arterial disease in diabetic and nondiabetic patients: a comparison of severity and outcome, *Diabetes Care* 24:1433, 2001.

61. Eraso LH, Fukaya E, Mohler ER III, et al: Peripheral arterial disease, prevalence and cumulative risk factor profile analysis, *Eur J Prev Cardiol* 2012.

62. Marso SP, Hiatt WR: Peripheral arterial disease in patients with diabetes, *J Am Coll Cardiol* 47:921, 2006.

63. Adler AI, Stevens RJ, Neil A, et al: UKPDS 59: hyperglycemia and other potentially modifiable risk factors for peripheral vascular disease in type 2 diabetes, *Diabetes Care* 25:894, 2002.

64. Kullo IJ, Bailey KR, Kardia SL, et al: Ethnic differences in peripheral arterial disease in the NHLBI Genetic Epidemiology Network of Arteriopathy (GENOA) study, *Vasc Med* 8:237, 2003.

65. Weitz JI, Byrne J, Clagett GP, et al: Diagnosis and treatment of chronic arterial insufficiency of the lower extremities: a critical review, *Circulation* 94:3026, 1996.

66. Ishii H, Kumada Y, Takahashi H, et al: Impact of diabetes and glycaemic control on peripheral artery disease in Japanese patients with end-stage renal disease: long-term follow-up study from the beginning of haemodialysis, *Diabetologia* 55:1304, 2012.

67. Barrett-Connor EL, Cohn BA, Wingard DL, et al: Why is diabetes mellitus a stronger risk factor for fatal ischemic heart disease in women than in men? The Rancho Bernardo Study, *JAMA* 265:627, 1991.

68. Wannamethee SG, Papacosta O, Lawlor DA, et al: Do women exhibit greater differences in established and novel risk factors between diabetes and non-diabetes than men? The British Regional Heart Study and British Women's Heart Health Study, *Diabetologia* 55:80, 2012.

69. Kanaya AM, Herrington D, Vittinghoff E, et al: Glycemic effects of postmenopausal hormone therapy: the Heart and Estrogen/progestin Replacement Study. A randomized, double-blind, placebo-controlled trial, *Ann Intern Med* 138:1, 2003.

70. Chlebowski RT, Anderson GL, Gass M, et al: Estrogen plus progestin and breast cancer incidence and mortality in postmenopausal women, *JAMA* 304:1684, 2010.

71. Gustafsson I, Brendorp B, Seibaek M, et al: Influence of diabetes and diabetes-gender interaction on the risk of death in patients hospitalized with congestive heart failure, *J Am Coll Cardiol* 43:771, 2004.

72. King H, Aubert RE, Herman WH: Global burden of diabetes, 1995–2025: prevalence, numerical estimates, and projections, *Diabetes Care* 21:1414, 1998.

73. Shaw JE, Sicree RA, Zimmet PZ: Global estimates of the prevalence of diabetes for 2010 and 2030, *Diabetes Res Clin Pract* 87:4, 2010.

TABLE 8-2 Plaque Characteristics in Patients with Type 1 Diabetes and Those with Type 2 Diabetes Versus Nondiabetic Patients from Sudden Coronary Death Registry

	TYPE 1 DM (n = 16)	TYPE 2 DM (n = 50)	NON-DM (n = 66)	P VALUE (TYPE 1 DM VERSUS NON-DM)	P VALUE (TYPE 2 DM VERSUS NON-DM)
Acute coronary thrombi	21%	42%	51%	0.03	0.2
Acute plaque rupture	6%	32%	27%	0.09	0.6
Plaque erosion	6%	12%	29%	0.02	0.04
Necrotic core area (%)*	12.0±5.7	11.6±8.4	9.4±9.3	0.05[†]	0.004[†]
Calcified matrix area (%)*	7.8±9.1	12.1±11.2	11.4±13.5	0.9[†]	0.05[†]
Fibroatheroma (n)	7.1±5.0	8.8±4.3	6.9±4.7	0.9	0.02
Thin-cap fibroatheroma (n)	1.0±1.3	0.8±0.8	0.7±0.8	0.5	0.8
Healed plaque rupture (n)	2.6±2.1	2.6±1.8	1.9±1.8	0.2	0.04
Total plaque burden (%)	275±129	358±114	232±128	0.04	0.0001
Distal plaque burden (%)	310±114	630±263	331±199	0.8	0.0001
Macrophage area (mm²)	0.15±0.02	0.13±0.03	0.10±0.02[‡]	0.03[†]	0.03[†]

Values are expressed as mean±standard deviation or percentage.
DM=diabetes mellitus.
*Divided by plaque area.
[†]P values calculated using log-normalized data.
[‡]P=0.006 versus type 1 and 2 diabetes combined.
Data from Burke AP, Kolodgie FD, Zieske A, et al: Morphologic findings of coronary atherosclerotic plaques in diabetics: a postmortem study, *Arterioscler Thromb Vasc Biol* 24:1266-1271, 2004.

TABLE 8-3 Relationship of Risk Factors, Including Diabetes, to Plaque Characteristics: A Multivariate Analysis

INDEPENDENT VARIABLES (RISK FACTORS)	% NECROTIC CORE AREA*		NUMBER OF FIBROATHEROMAS[†]		% MACROPHAGE AREA[‡]	
	T	P VALUE	T	P VALUE	T	P VALUE
Glycohemoglobin (%)	2.8	0.005	1.7	0.09	2.9	0.004
TC/HDL cholesterol	2.5	0.01	3.0	0.0003	1.3	0.19
Body mass index	3.5	0.006	0.57	0.57	1.5	0.14
Smoking	−0.4	0.7	−1.1	0.24	−0.6	0.5
Age	−1.2	0.2	−1.2	0.2	−5.4	0.0001

The population for this table is the 132 patients with three separate one-way analysis of variance (ANOVA) analyses correlating three dependent variables (mean % necrotic core area, mean % macrophage area).
*Mean percent necrotic core area (of the four arteries studies per patient).
[†]Mean number of fibroatheromas per heart.
[‡]Mean macrophage area (of the four arteries per patient).
Data from Burke AP, Kolodgie FD, Zieske A, et al: Morphologic findings of coronary atherosclerotic plaques in diabetics: a postmortem study, *Arterioscler Thromb Vasc Biol* 24:1266-1271, 2004.

autoimmune disease with a common genetic susceptibility to other disorders, like autoimmune thyroiditis, which may also be of pathophysiological significance in coronary plaque pathology.[13] There was a strong positive correlation between macrophage area and glycohemoglobin, independent of HDL-C, ratio of TC to HDL-C, age, smoking, and gender (T=2.9, P=0.004) (see **Table 8-3**). The combined effect of hypercholesterolemia and diabetes on macrophage infiltration and necrotic core size were further evaluated. The degree of macrophage infiltrate and necrotic core size as assessed by morphometry were significantly greater in diabetic patients with normal cholesterol or hyperlipidemia as compared to nondiabetic patients (**Fig. 8-6**).

Acute Coronary Thrombosis

The incidence of acute thrombi was significantly less in individuals with type 1 diabetes (21%) than in those without diabetes (51%, P=0.03) in sudden coronary death victims (see **Table 8-2**). Individuals with type 1 diabetes showed a trend toward lower incidence of acute plaque rupture than those without diabetes (6% versus 27%, P=0.09), and plaque erosion was significantly less frequent in individuals with type 1

and type 2 diabetes than in those without diabetes (6%, 12% versus 29%, P=0.02 and P=0.04). The incidence of acute thrombi in individuals with type 2 diabetes was lower than in those without diabetes, whereas stable severe coronary artery disease and chronic total occlusion were more frequently observed in individuals with type 2 diabetes than in those without diabetes (see **Fig. 8-3C**). The incidence of acute plaque rupture in individuals with type 2 diabetes (32%) was comparable to that in individuals without diabetes (27%).

Diffuse Coronary Atherosclerosis

In sudden death victims, approximately half of individuals with diabetes showed triple-vessel disease, whereas those without diabetes had a higher prevalence of single-vessel disease (see **Fig. 8-3D**). To further evaluate the extent of coronary atherosclerosis, plaque burden was calculated by adding the maximal percent cross-sectional area luminal narrowing in four main arterial beds—that is, the left main, left anterior descending, left circumflex, and right coronary arteries.[14] A similar number was obtained for distal arteries. Total plaque burden was significantly greater in individuals with type 2 diabetes than in those without diabetes

DIABETES AND ATHEROSCLEROSIS

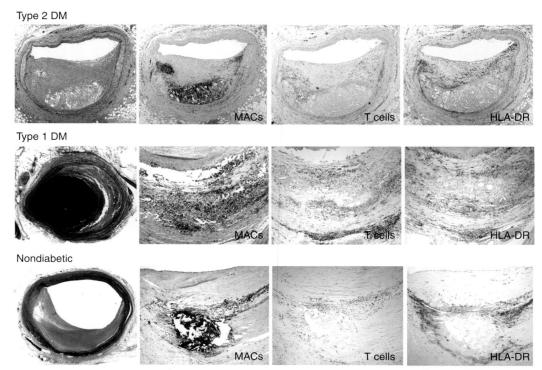

FIGURE 8-4 Inflammation in diabetic coronary arteries. Coronary fibroatheromas illustrating the extent of macrophages (CD68), T cells (CD45RO), and HLA-DR expression in patients with type 1 and 2 diabetes mellitus (DM) and nondiabetic patients. *(Modified from Burke AP, Kolodgie FD, Zieske A, et al: Morphologic findings of coronary atherosclerotic plaques in diabetics: a postmortem study,* Arterioscler Thromb Vasc Biol *24:1266-1271, 2004.)*

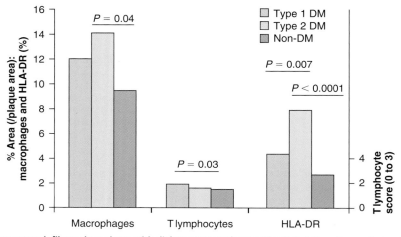

FIGURE 8-5 Comparison of inflammatory infiltrate in patients with diabetes versus those without diabetes. Bar graph showing quantitative and semiquantitative comparisons of the extent of macrophages, T lymphocytes, and HLA-DR expression in coronary arteries from patients with diabetes and those without diabetes. Plaque macrophages and HLA expression were greater in patients with diabetes (type 1 and 2) than in those without diabetes, whereas T-cell infiltration was maximal in patients with type 1 diabetes. *(Modified from Burke AP, Kolodgie FD, Zieske A, et al: Morphologic findings of coronary atherosclerotic plaques in diabetics: a postmortem study,* Arterioscler Thromb Vasc Biol *24:1266-1271, 2004.)*

(358 ± 114 versus 232 ± 128, $P=0.0001$), and distal plaque burden was also significantly greater in individuals with type 2 diabetes than in those without diabetes (630 ± 263 versus 331 ± 199, $P=0.0001$) (see **Table 8-2**). Individuals with type 1 diabetes showed greater total plaque burden (275 ± 129) than those without diabetes ($P=0.04$), whereas distal plaque burden in individuals with type 1 diabetes (310 ± 114) was comparable to that in individuals without diabetes ($P=0.8$). Thus, individuals with type 2 diabetes who died suddenly with severe coronary disease had extensive coronary atherosclerosis, including distal involvement, as compared with those without diabetes. Part of the reason

for increased plaque burden may be attributed to a higher rate of healed plaque ruptures, which may contribute to plaque progression.[15] The effect of diabetes on plaque burden has also been demonstrated by calcium imaging studies.[16] The implication of these findings is unclear, but a direct atherogenic effect of type 2 diabetes may be implicated, which is probably related to the development of lipid-rich cores. The known risk of diabetes for the late development of complications following coronary artery bypass graft surgery, which include acute myocardial infarction and graft failure,[17,18] may in part be attributable to distal disease, which may impair blood flow distal to graft anastomoses.

MACROPHAGE INFILTRATE

NECROTIC CORE SIZE

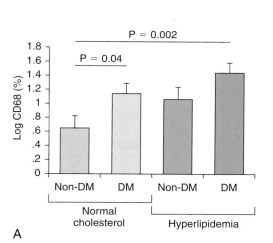

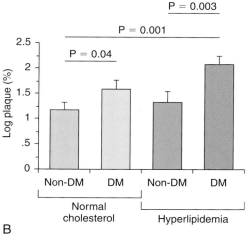

FIGURE 8-6 Combined effect of hyperlipidemia and diabetes on macrophage infiltration and necrotic core size. **A,** Combined effect on mean macrophage percent (log-normalized). **B,** Combined effect on mean necrotic core size (log-normalized). There is a significant difference between diabetic patients (DM) and nondiabetic patients (non-DM) when cases were separated by the presence or absence of hyperlipidemia. Hyperlipidemia was defined as TC over 200 mg/dL or ratio of TC to HDL-C exceeding 5. *(Modified from Burke AP, Kolodgie FD, Zieske A, et al: Morphologic findings of coronary atherosclerotic plaques in diabetics: a postmortem study,* Arterioscler Thromb Vasc Biol *24:1266-1271, 2004.)*

Coronary Arterial Remodeling

Coronary artery remodeling was first described by Glagov in 1987 in a landmark paper showing that vessels enlarge as atherosclerotic plaque burden increases.[19] Glagov showed that vessel lumen compromise is not observed until the vessel is greater than 40% narrowed in cross-sectional area by atherosclerotic plaque. In other words, the vessel is said to be positively remodeled—that is, there is vessel enlargement, and the internal elastic lamina (IEL) area is increased (**Fig. 8-7**).[20] A vessel is negatively remodeled when the lumen area is smaller than the expected lumen, including reduction that may occur from tapering of the vessel.[21]

We have shown that the IEL area, when adjusted for the distance from the coronary ostium, was greater in individuals with type 1 and 2 diabetes than in those without diabetes (18.2 ± 6.6 mm^2, 16.5 ± 4.4 mm^2, and 16.0 ± 4.5 mm^2, respectively). The mean IEL area was also significantly greater in individuals with type 1 ($P=0.001$) and type 2 diabetes ($P=0.01$). By multivariable analysis, there was a correlation between individuals with type 1 diabetes and IEL area independent of heart weight, plaque area, percent necrotic core, and percent plaque calcification ($P=0.0004$). In this analysis, percent necrotic core ($P=0.05$), plaque area ($P<0.0001$), and heart weight ($P=0.05$) also showed positive correlation with IEL area.

The findings of clinical studies in patients with diabetes have been ambiguous, with some patients showing positive remodeling and others showing negative remodeling.[22,23] Our studies involving sudden coronary death victims without a known history of coronary artery disease support the notion that individuals with diabetes are more likely to show positive remodeling. However, it is possible that those who survive will eventually undergo negative remodeling, but this will require long-term follow-up either by multislice computed tomography (MSCT) or intravascular ultrasound (IVUS) studies. Our laboratory has shown that the necrotic core and macrophage infiltrates are associated with expansion of the IEL independent of plaque size and independent

of diabetic status.[20] Therefore it is not surprising that sudden coronary death victims with type 1 and 2 diabetes show positive remodeling when they have greater macrophage and T-cell infiltration and larger necrotic cores as compared with those without diabetes.

Hemorrhage and Angiogenesis

Plaque hemorrhage has been shown to be associated with intraplaque angiogenesis. In type 2 diabetes, angiogenesis is increased and is associated with plaque hemorrhage and rupture.[24] Increasing intraplaque hemorrhage as assessed by glycophorin A staining of red cell membranes has been linked with plaque progression, enlarging necrotic core, greater macrophage infiltration, and iron deposition within coronary atherosclerotic plaques.[25] In type 2 diabetes, angiogenesis is increased and is associated with plaque hemorrhage and rupture.[24] Moreno and Fuster[24] showed that intraplaque hemorrhage and angiogenesis in abdominal or thoracic aorta were greater in individuals with type 2 diabetes than in those without diabetes. Intraplaque hemorrhage leads to the release of free Hb, in which iron is incorporated and acts as an oxidant, which stimulates inflammation (**Fig. 8-8**). The extent of neovascularization correlates with macrophage and T-call infiltration and plaque hemorrhage, which were greater in individuals with diabetes than in those without diabetes (**Fig. 8-9**).[26]

The untoward effects of free Hb are antagonized by Hp which binds free Hb and facilitates the uptake of Hb-Hp complexes by macrophages that have the receptors (CD163) which help remove free Hb.[27] The Hp gene has two alleles (1 and 2) giving rise to three genotypes—Hp2-2, Hp2-1, and Hp1-1—and individuals with Hp2-2 and diabetes have impaired clearance for Hb.[28] Individuals with diabetes and Hp2-2 had increased iron as compared to Hp1-1 or 2-1 (46% versus 12%). Among the nondiabetic patients with the Hp2-2 genotype, there was a nonsignificant trend toward higher prevalence of iron in plaques.[28]

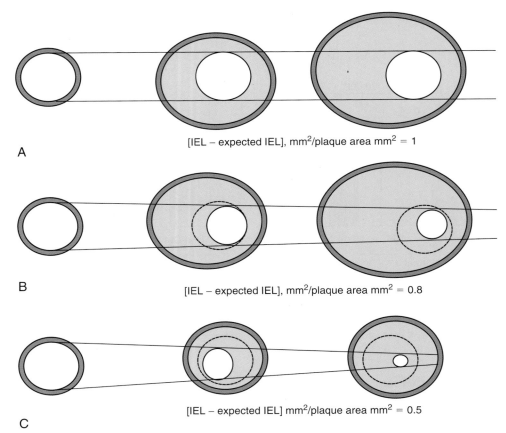

$$[\text{IEL} - \text{expected IEL}], \text{mm}^2/\text{plaque area mm}^2 = 1$$

A

$$[\text{IEL} - \text{expected IEL}], \text{mm}^2/\text{plaque area mm}^2 = 0.8$$

B

$$[\text{IEL} - \text{expected IEL}] \text{mm}^2/\text{plaque area mm}^2 = 0.5$$

C

FIGURE 8-7 Method of assessing positive remodeling. The left circles indicate normal reference segments without plaque, and the two right figures are two examples of positive remodeling with an equal remodeling score. Using the formula (IEL − Expected IEL)/Plaque area, remodeling that allows no reduction in lumen with increasing plaque size **(A)** would result in a value of 1. The increase in IEL area resulting from plaque expansion is equivalent to the total plaque area. Any lesser degree of remodeling results in eventual occlusion with increased plaque area. **B,** With a score of 0.8, the increase in IEL over the predicted value is greater than the plaque area bounded by the expected IEL by a ratio of 4:1. The dotted circle represents the predicted IEL based on the reference segment. In **C,** a score of 0.5 indicates that the increase in IEL increase over expected (IEL − expected IEL) is the same as the plaque area impinging into the lumen from the expected IEL; therefore the IEL expansion is one half the plaque area. IEL = Internal elastic lamina. *(Reproduced with permission from Burke AP, Kolodgie FD, Farb A, et al: Morphological predictors of arterial remodeling in coronary atherosclerosis,* Circulation *105:297-303, 2002.)*

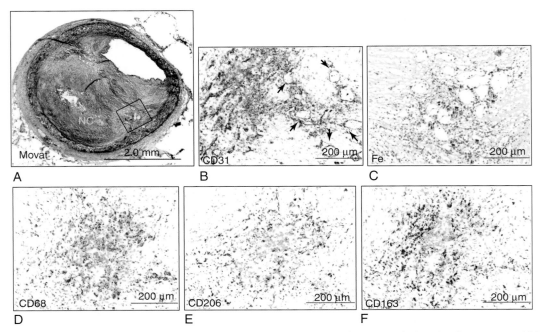

FIGURE 8-8 Angiogenesis, hemorrhage, iron deposition, and inflammation in diabetic coronary plaques. Histologic sections from a 48-year-old black man with history of hypertension and diabetes who died suddenly. **A,** A low-power image shows fibroatheroma with severe luminal narrowing and angiogenesis. **B** to **F,** High-power images of the black box in **A. B,** Note abundant CD31 (platelet endothelial cell adhesion molecule 1 [PECAM-1]) staining that indicates the presence of angiogenesis (arrows). **C,** The same area shows abundance of iron (blue), suggestive of hemorrhage. **D** to **F,** There are also abundant macrophages that are detected by CD68, CD206 (mannose receptor), and CD163 (Hb-haptoglobin receptor) staining.

9 Vascular Biology of Atherosclerosis in Patients with Diabetes

Hyperglycemia, Insulin Resistance, and Hyperinsulinemia

Ravichandran Ramasamy, Shi Fang Yan, and Ann Marie Schmidt

DIABETES AND ACCELERATED ATHEROSCLEROSIS

Scope and Complexity of the Problem

One of the most deadly complications of types 1 and 2 diabetes is accelerated atherosclerosis, the consequences of which include more frequent and more deadly heart attacks and strokes, as well as myocardial dysfunction. The latter occurs both secondary to myocardial infarctions and as a result of innate diabetes-mediated damage to the myocardium. With the worldwide rise in both types 1 and 2 diabetes, an epidemic of cardiovascular complications in diabetes is almost certainly on the horizon.[1] Together with the cost of affected individuals' productivity and the very high costs to already heavily burdened health care systems, the cardiovascular complications of diabetes have many potentially devastating consequences for personal well-being and global economies. Hence, it is essential to delineate the diabetes-specific mechanisms that accelerate cardiovascular disease to identify the optimal therapeutic regimens to combat these heterogeneous diseases.

Hyperglycemia is both defining and common to types 1 and 2 diabetes, yet there are common and distinct threads in these two syndromes. The potential underlying mechanisms linking diabetes and cardiovascular complications may differ, at least in part, between these two most common forms of diabetes. Specifically, insulin resistance is significantly more common in type 2 diabetes, but it may appear in later stages of type 1 diabetes as well. Furthermore, hyperinsulinemia is more associated with type 2 diabetes, because type 1 diabetes, at least in the absence of therapies, is caused by a reduction in naturally produced and circulating insulin. In this chapter we review the evidence supporting, or not, the roles of hyperglycemia, hyperinsulinemia, and insulin resistance in cardiovascular complications. Note that this chapter does not consider in depth the influences of dyslipidemia, inflammation, hypercoagulability, or endothelial dysfunction in diabetes; these are the focus of **Chapter 10**.

Diabetes and Atherosclerosis: What Is the Role of Hyperglycemia?

Long-term intervention studies have begun to answer the critical question of whether strict control of hyperglycemia imbues protection or at least reduction in cardiovascular consequences in diabetes. The answer to this question may depend on the cause of diabetes.

In type 1 diabetes, reviewed more extensively in **Chapter 11 by Dr. Maahs**, the results of the Diabetes Control and Complications Trial (DCCT) and Epidemiology of Diabetes Interventions and Complications (EDIC) study have provided clear answers. In the original DCCT study, type 1 diabetic subjects were adolescents versus young adults at the time of entry into the study. Specifically, of the adolescents, the mean age of subjects randomized to either arm of strict versus standard glycemic control was age 15 years (a total of 87 patients). Of the adults, the mean age of patients randomized to either arm of glycemic control was age 28 years (a total of 191 patients).[2] Strict control of hyperglycemia was shown early in the study to reduce microvascular complications of diabetes compared with standard regimens of glycemic control.[3] However, because of the delay in cardiovascular events in this population, most likely a result of the younger age at entry into the study, the answer to the question of cardiovascular complications was revealed years later and particularly in the follow-up study to the DCCT, the EDIC study. Both surrogate markers of atherosclerosis (carotid intima-media thickness) and myocardial infarction, stroke, and death from cardiovascular consequences were shown to be reduced in the group of patients treated with strict versus standard regiments of glucose control.[4,5] It is important to note that the reduced cardiovascular complications were evident years after the levels of glycosylated hemoglobin between both groups became indistinguishable, suggesting a "legacy" effect. The legacy effect—mechanisms and implications—is discussed later.

In type 2 diabetes, current epidemiologic data have identified that the overall risk of cardiovascular complications is twofold to fourfold greater than that observed in nondiabetic patients, even after accounting for the traditional risk factors. In type 2 diabetes, the heterogeneous nature of the concomitant ailments and exposures, such as hyperlipidemia, hypertension, obesity, smoking, and environmental pollutants, has rendered the question of the specific role of hyperglycemia more difficult to address unequivocally. The United Kingdom Prospective Diabetes Study (UKPDS) in type 2 diabetic patients was originally composed of 3867 patients randomized to strict versus standard glycemic control. After 10 years the study showed that levels of glycosylated hemoglobin were significantly lower in the strict control group versus standard (7.0% versus 7.9%, respectively). In parallel, the UKPDS reported a 16% reduction in risk of myocardial infarction, but the result did not achieve statistical significance.[6] Years later, however, in the post-trial monitoring program, even after glycosylated hemoglobin levels were indistinguishable from those in the former standard control group, the risk of myocardial infarction was significantly lower in the former strict glycemic control group.[7] As in the case of type 1 diabetes and the DCCT and EDIC trials, the results of the UKPDS suggested that a legacy effect might have imparted long-term cardiovascular benefit in the group previously treated with strict glycemic control.

It is noteworthy that a recent study, ACCORD (Action to Control Cardiovascular Risk in Diabetes), found that stricter control of glycemia versus standard regimens in type 2 diabetes was associated with higher cardiovascular mortality as well as higher all-cause mortality, leading to premature discontinuation of the glycemic control arms of the study for safety purposes, after a mean follow-up period of 3.5 years. There was, however, a non–statistically significant trend toward lower nonfatal myocardial infarction, nonfatal stroke, or death from cardiovascular causes in those in the glycemic control groups.[8] More recent analysis has suggested that the risk of hypoglycemia was greater in the glycemic control arms and might have contributed to the increased cardiovascular risk. From the multiple analyses of ACCORD and two other related studies—ADVANCE (Action in Diabetes and Vascular Disease: Preterax and Diamicron Modified Release Controlled Evaluation)[9] and VADT (Veterans Affairs Diabetes Trial)[10]—in which glycemic control arms in type 2 diabetes were associated with neither reduced nor higher cardiovascular events, refined recommendations for the implementation of glycemic control are emerging, because subgroup analyses may suggest reduction in cardiovascular disease in the glycemic control arms based on entry cardiovascular disease surrogate markers, such as coronary calcification scores. Hence, cardiovascular status at entry into the study may in fact define the groups most likely to benefit, and not be harmed, by glycemic control measures.

In addition to glycemic control measures, the Steno-2 trial showed that a broader approach to management, including glycemic control and control of lipid levels, blood pressure, and microalbuminuria in type 2 diabetic patients led to a 50% reduction in cardiovascular mortality.[11,12] The Steno-2 studies, however, did not identify the specific factor or combination of factors most responsible for cardiovascular benefit.

In the following sections we review the evidence that hyperglycemia and its consequences contribute to atherosclerosis in diabetes.

Polyol Pathway

The two major enzymes of the polyol pathway include aldose reductase (AR), the first and rate-limiting enzyme of this pathway, and sorbitol dehydrogenase (SDH). By the action of these enzymes, glucose is metabolized to sorbitol and fructose, respectively. In the process, as shown later, AR action results in the conversion of nicotinamide adenine dinucleotide phosphate, reduced form (NADPH) to nicotinamide adenine dinucleotide phosphate (NADP$^+$) and the action of SDH consumes nicotinamide adenine dinucleotide (NAD$^+$) to yield NADH.[13]

Compared with human or rat tissues, in the mouse the levels of AR are significantly lower; hence, a strategy to specifically test the role of AR in atherosclerosis used transgenic mice, which expressed human-relevant levels of AR on the major histocompatibility type 1 promoter, thereby exerting global overexpression of the enzyme. When these mice were bred with mice deficient in the low-density lipoprotein (LDL) receptor and made diabetic with streptozotocin, a significant increase in atherosclerosis, both by percentage of aortic arch lesion area and by en face analysis of the entire aorta, resulted after 6 weeks of a high-cholesterol diet, without a change in total cholesterol or triglyceride or in levels of very low-density lipoprotein cholesterol (VLDL-C), LDL-C, or high-density lipoprotein cholesterol (HDL-C) in the two groups of diabetic mice (those overexpressing or not transgenic for human AR [hAR]) (**Fig. 9-1**).[14] Similar roles for hAR in acceleration of atherosclerosis in diabetic LDL receptor null mice fed a high-cholesterol diet at 8 or 12 weeks were found, and when mice were fed a cholic acid–containing diet, atherosclerosis increased in the diabetic tg hAR animals versus the nondiabetic LDL receptor null mice.[14] Of note, there were no differences observed in nondiabetic mice overexpressing transgenic hAR or not in the LDL receptor null background, thereby suggesting that glucose flux via the polyol pathway was specific to the diabetic state in atherosclerosis. In parallel with increased atherosclerosis in the diabetic transgenic hAR-overexpressing mouse, macrophages retrieved from these animals revealed increased expression of inflammatory mediators and greater uptake of modified lipoproteins. In addition to these findings in mice, Gleissner and colleagues discovered increased expression and activity of AR in human monocyte-derived macrophages during foam cell formation stimulated by oxidized LDL (oxLDL), a process that was further exacerbated when macrophages were grown in hyperglycemic conditions (30 mM D-glucose) compared with osmotic control conditions.[15]

Recent studies by Vedantham and colleagues demonstrated that when tg hAR mice were bred into the apoE null background and rendered diabetic with streptozotocin, increased atherosclerosis ensued compared with the nontransgenic diabetic apoE null mice (see **Fig. 9-1A, B**). As in the case of LDL receptor null mice, there was no effect of transgenic hAR expression in the nondiabetic apoE null mice. Furthermore, they showed that administration of an AR inhibitor, zopolrestat, was effective in reducing accelerated atherosclerosis in the diabetic transgenic hAR mice in the apoE null background (see **Fig. 9-1C**). Important roles for endothelial cell hAR in diabetic atherosclerosis were demonstrated in that work. When tg Tie2-hAR mice in the apolipoprotein (apo) E null background were rendered diabetic with streptozotocin, atherosclerotic lesion size was increased, suggesting that endothelial cell AR contributes importantly to acceleration of atherosclerosis in diabetes.[16]

It is important to note that an earlier study suggested that distinct inhibitors of AR (ARIs; tolrestat and sorbinil) and genetic ablation of AR in diabetic apoE null mice increased early lesion formation as a result of increased levels of toxic aldehydes in the lipid particles.[17] Differences in the mouse models, specifically genetic overexpression of AR to human

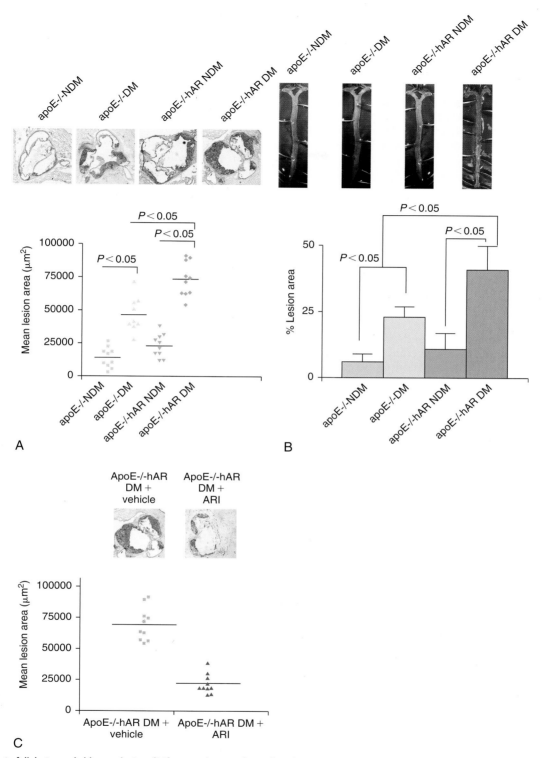

FIGURE 9-1 **Impact of diabetes and aldose reductase (AR) expression on atherosclerosis at 14 weeks after induction of diabetes.** Shown are representative images of aortic root sections stained with oil red O **(A)** and Sudan IV stained aortic enface **(B).** Hearts were retrieved from nondiabetic and diabetic apoE −/− (n = 10 and 9, respectively) mice, nondiabetic and diabetic apoE −/− hAR+(n = 10 in each group) mice, and diabetic apoE −/− hAR+mice treated with and without aldose reductase inhibitor (ARI) (n = 10 and 10, respectively) **(C)**, and mean atherosclerotic lesion areas were determined. *(Reprinted from Vedantham S, et al., 2012.[16])*

relevant levels or complete genetic deletion, as well as potential distinct off-target effects of the different ARIs may underlie these findings. In human patients with diabetes and neuropathy, however, 1 year of treatment with the ARI zopolrestat resulted in improved cardiac function, not worsened function, as measured by echocardiography.[18]

In contrast, the vehicle-treated diabetic patients continued to display reduction in their cardiac function. This study, which did not directly address diabetic atherosclerosis, did however suggest that pharmacologic inhibition of AR by zopolrestat did not worsen cardiovascular complications of diabetes. Hence, it is possible that more potent ARIs with less off-target effects may hold promise for the treatment of atherosclerosis in diabetes.

Finally, it is important to note that increased oxidative stress may result from the overactivity of the polyol pathway.[19] NADPH is a cofactor of glutathione production; consumption of glutathione by action of the polyol pathway may result in reduced availability of this antioxidant mechanism.[20] These considerations are consistent with the observations in mouse models and human macrophages that AR activity increases oxidative stress on high glucose and oxLDL exposure.

Hexosamine Pathway

When excess levels of glucose are shunted into the hexosamine biosynthetic pathway (HBP), products emerge that have been shown to cause endoplasmic reticulum stress and to alter transcriptional activity of key molecules implicated in atherosclerosis. In this pathway, fructose-6-phosphate is converted to glucosamine-6-phosphate and uridine diphosphate (UDP)–N-acetyl glucosamine via the actions of the rate-limiting enzyme of the hexosamine pathway, L-glutamine:D-fructose-6-phosphate amidotransferase (GFAT).[21]

Examples of how the HBP may contribute to conditions that exacerbate atherosclerosis in diabetes include the following. First, in a manner dependent on mitochondrial superoxide production, hyperglycemia increases hexosamine biosynthesis and O-glycosylation of the transcription factor Sp1 in bovine aortic endothelial cells. Consequences of increased modification of Sp1 include increased expression of plasminogen activator inhibitor type 1 (PAI-1) and transforming growth factor beta 1 (TGF-β1).[22] Second, findings similar to the effects of high glucose and the HBP on PAI-1 expression were also shown in adipose tissue.[23] Third, in bovine aortic endothelial cells, endothelial nitric oxide synthase (eNOS) activity was inhibited by HBP-mediated increases in O-linked N-acetylglucosamine modification of eNOS and a decrease in O-linked serine phosphorylation at residue 1177.[24] In the aortas of diabetic mice, similar changes in eNOS activity and these post-translational modifications were also observed. Because reduced eNOS activity is observed in diabetes and linked to endothelial dysfunction, HBP-mediated reductions in eNOS activity spurred by hyperglycemia may contribute to endothelial cell dysfunction, which presages accelerated atherosclerosis.

Protein Kinase C

Hyperglycemia stimulates the generation of diacylglycerol (DAG), which is an activator of at least certain isoforms of protein kinase C (PKC).[25] The PKC family of enzymes consists of at least 12 members.[26] PKCs are involved in a diverse array of cellular functions, many of which may be considered to play roles in diabetic atherosclerosis, such as cellular proliferation, signal transduction, cellular fate, and transcription factor modulation (e.g., Egr1, NF-κB, and Sp1), cytokine expression, and oxidative stress in cells such as endothelial cells, smooth muscle cells, and monocytes and macrophages, all of which contribute to atherosclerosis mechanisms.[27]

In atherosclerosis, isoforms of PKC have been implicated in the pathogenesis of this disorder. First, work by Harja and colleagues showed that global deletion of the PKCβ isoform resulted in significant reduction in atherosclerosis in apoE null mice, even without diabetes.[28] In parallel, these researchers showed that a chief mechanism by which deletion of this PKC isoform was protective was by reduction in

the vascular expression of the key transcription factor, Egr1. Egr1, previously shown to influence proinflammatory and prothrombotic genes in atherosclerosis, is regulated by PKCβ. Furthermore, treatment of the apoE null mice with the PKCβ inhibitor LY333531 (or ruboxistaurin) resulted in decreased atherosclerosis. This work, although not performed in diabetic animals, nevertheless may suggest that this PKC isoform may play key roles in diabetic atherosclerosis. Supportive of this conclusion is the report showing that administration of ruboxistaurin to type 2 diabetic patients improved brachial artery flow-mediated dilation compared with vehicle treatment.[29] In addition to PKCβ, possible protective roles for PKCδ in atherosclerosis have been suggested, particularly in smooth muscle cell survival. In a model of vein graft atherosclerosis in nondiabetic mice, deletion of PKCδ resulted in more severe atherosclerosis.[30] As in the case of PKCβ, further studies are essential to determine potential implications in diabetes.

Other studies have suggested that advanced glycation endproduct (AGE) pathways may contribute to activation of PKC isoforms—for example, studies reported in bovine retinal endothelial cells.[31]

Oxidative Stress

Studies testing samples retrieved from humans and animals with diabetes show increased levels of markers of oxidative stress such as plasma and urinary F2-isoprostanes and 8-hydroxydeoxyguanosine.[32,33] Such markers of increased oxidative stress have been linked to diabetic complications, and in aortic rings retrieved from type 1 or type 2 diabetic animals, oxidative stress appears to contribute to endothelial dysfunction.[34] Beyond endothelial dysfunction, specific roles for oxidative stress in diabetes were suggested by experiments in which heterozygous deletion of the lipoic acid synthase gene in streptozotocin-induced diabetic apoE null mice resulted in marked increases in atherosclerosis compared with diabetic mice expressing lipoic acid synthase.[35] In the atherosclerotic lesions of the mice with heterozygous deletion of lipoic acid synthase, more macrophages and greater degrees of cellular apoptosis were observed. In addition, oxidative stress and markers of inflammation such as interleukin 6 (IL-6) were observed. These studies directly suggested that oxidative stress was an important contributing mechanism to diabetes-associated accelerated atherosclerosis.

Although antioxidant therapies in the clinic have been generally disappointing, e.g. a large-scale study of the use of vitamin E (400 IU/day) in patients at high risk for cardiovascular disease (such as diabetic patients), it has been suggested that the potency and half-life of available antioxidants may not be consistent with the potential for longstanding protection against diabetic vascular dysfunction.[36] Furthermore, others have suggested that perhaps treatment of the most at-risk patients in terms of exaggerated oxidative stress might be useful, such as those bearing the haptoglobin (Hp) 2-2 genotype.[37] Given the multiple potential caveats regarding the specific antioxidant, dose, schedule, and vulnerable populations in exacting the greatest efficacy from this class of molecules, it is not surprising that the specific sources of oxidative stress in diabetes are a subject of intense investigation.

In diabetes, two major sources of oxidative stress have been suggested by experimental model systems. In the first case, it has been proposed that in endothelial cells, as well in other cell types, hyperglycemia results in overproduction of mitochondrial reactive oxygen species (ROSs) and that such increases in ROSs relay many adverse consequences in the vasculature, such as activation of PARP (poly [ADP-ribose] polymerase) and endothelial upregulation of an array of prothrombotic and proinflammatory molecules.[38,39] In this context, it has been suggested that such overproduction of mitochondrial ROSs might in fact underlie increased activity of other pathways implicated in diabetic cardiovascular disease, such as activation of the HBP pathway (discussed earlier) and PKC and glycation and activation of the receptor for AGE (RAGE) (see later). Although earlier efforts focused on the use of benfotiamine as a means to reduce the consequences of excess mitochondrial ROS production driven by high glucose,[40] more recent publications suggest that mitochondrially targeted antioxidants are under development to address the issue of availability and sustainability in pathophysiologic settings characterized by deleterious levels of oxidative stress.[41]

In addition to increased mitochondrial sources of ROSs in hyperglycemia and diabetes, ROSs derived from NADPH oxidase have been extensively studied.[42] There are multiple forms of Nox, and conserved among these six-transmembrane domain family members are binding sites for NADPH, flavin adenine dinucleotide (FAD), and two hemes.[43] Nox isoforms may be activated by hyperglycemia as well as by AGE and RAGE pathways.[44] Hence, multiple fuel forward mechanisms initiated by high levels of glucose may generate and sustain ROS production by this family of pro-oxidant molecules.

Using specific Nox-modified animals, it has been shown that deletion of p47phox subunit of the Nox1 and Nox2 complex in apoE null mice (without diabetes) resulted in decreased atherosclerosis in a manner independent of diet or serum lipid levels. Superoxide production in the vessel wall was reduced by this genetic approach, and smooth muscle proliferation was also suppressed.[45] Mice deficient in both Nox1 and apoE demonstrated reduced atherogenesis in parallel with decreased macrophage infiltration in the lesions.[46] Similar findings were observed in nondiabetic Nox2 null mice in the apoE null background fed a high-fat diet. Decreased aortic ROS production was observed in these animals compared with the Nox2-expressing counterpart apoE null mice.[47] Such findings may have implications for the pathogenesis of diabetes-accelerated atherosclerosis, although this has not been formally proved.

Other studies consistent with a key role for oxidative stress in atherosclerosis (nondiabetic) were performed in diabetic LDL receptor mice devoid of glutathione peroxidase. In these animals, increased atherosclerosis and inflammation resulted.[48] Of note, in tg hAR mice in the LDL receptor null background with streptozotocin-induced type 1 diabetes, levels of glutathione peroxidase in the aorta were significantly lower than those observed in the diabetic LDL receptor null mice not expressing hAR.[14] Taken together, these data indicate that loss of key antioxidant protective enzymes in atherosclerosis is deleterious.

Association studies in human aortas suggested that increased expression of Nox4 was found to be decreased in regions of the aorta with de-differentiated smooth muscle cells. In contrast, strong expression of Nox4 was observed in smooth muscle cells within the aorta that retained the contractile phenotype.[49] It is important to note that various classes of compounds are under development for isoform-specific inhibition of Noxes. These advances may need to be viewed with caution, because it is possible that isoform specificity of the inhibitors may not be feasible, and furthermore that ROS production has salutary effects in vivo, such as in responses to infectious challenges.[50] In this context, broad inhibition of Nox isoforms may be accompanied by side effects. Hence, a careful and isoform- and cell-specific strategy may be most beneficial. Until cell-specific deletion of various Nox isoforms in diabetic mice with atherosclerosis or subjected to infections challenge has been performed, the broad applicability of such inhibitors in chronic diseases such as diabetes is an untested concept.

Glycation: Receptor-Dependent and Independent Mechanisms in Diabetic Atherosclerosis

In addition to the multiple direct consequences of high levels of glucose, "indirect" consequences of this metabolic state include the nonenzymatic glycation and oxidation of proteins and lipids to form AGEs.[51] The critical "intermediates" in these pathways to AGE formation are the dicarbonyl compounds, such as methylglyoxal (MG), glyoxal, and 3-deoxyglucone (3-DG) (**Fig. 9-2**). There are multiple mechanisms implicated in the formation of AGEs: (1) reactions between the aldehydic group of reducing sugars with proteins or lipids, forming the Schiff bases and Amadori products; (2) glucose flux via the polyol pathway; and (3) lipid and sugar oxidation steps.[52] These dicarbonyl intermediate products may undergo further rearrangements to generate AGEs. AGEs are a heterogeneous group of compounds and include the highly cross-linked "brown" fluorescent AGEs such as pentosidine and crosslines; the nonfluorescent cross-linking AGEs such as arginine-lysine imidazole; and the non–cross-linking forms of AGEs such as carboxymethyl lysine (CML)–AGEs.[53]

AGEs also form in distinct settings that may exacerbate AGE complications in diabetic tissues. For example, natural aging may lead to AGE formation, particularly on long-lived proteins whose exposure to even normal levels of glucose may gradually lead to the formation of AGEs. Hypoxia and ischemia/reperfusion (I/R) may generate AGEs, thereby increasing AGE damage in settings such as myocardial infarction, stroke, or severe peripheral vascular disease.[54] Renal failure is a setting in which AGE formation is greatly accelerated; in patients with diabetes and severe nephropathy, the accelerated formation of AGEs atop basal diabetes-associated glycation may greatly increase the production and accumulation of these damaging species.[55] In other settings, the actions of the myeloperoxidase enzyme have been shown to generate CML-AGEs.[56] Hence, in infectious or inflamed milieus, the action of inflammatory cell myeloperoxidase in generation of AGEs may lead to further tissues stress, thereby, perhaps, impairing effective wound healing mechanisms.

It has been postulated that food-derived AGEs may form in high-temperature cooking conditions.[57] Other forms of AGE exposure have been suggested in environmental pollutants such as in fly ash particles.[58] Taken together, although AGEs may form in conditions beyond hyperglycemia, it is conceivable that AGE formation in associated conditions, such as those delineated previously, may in fact exacerbate AGE damaging pathways in the diabetic tissues.

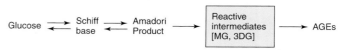

FIGURE 9-2 Mechanisms of hyperglycemia-induced AGE generation.

It is noteworthy that a chief detoxification mechanism for one class of the toxic AGE precursors, the MG dicarbonyl, is the glyoxalase enzyme system or Glo1. Glo1 blocks MG formation into AGEs, resulting in the production of lactate.[59] Glo1 is a glutathione-dependent enzyme. In RAGE-deficient mice, levels of Glo1 mRNA and protein are significantly higher in the kidneys compared with those found in diabetic wild-type RAGE-expressing mice.[60] This may result, in part, because of (1) decreased RAGE-dependent generation of ROSs (which depletes glutathione) and (2) RAGE-dependent transcriptional regulation of Glo1 (**Fig. 9-3**).

Receptor-Independent Pathways

One of the significant consequences of the cross-linking AGEs in particular is the formation of intermolecular bonds between extracellular matrix (ECM) elements. There are multiple potential consequences of such AGE formation in the vasculature such as arterial stiffness and trapping of molecules in the vascular tissues. Trapping of oxidized lipoproteins, for example, may contribute to early atherogenesis mechanisms in the diabetic macrovessels.[61] We and others have shown that oxLDL contains significant degrees of AGE.[62] Furthermore, AGE-induced modification of the ECM in the microvessels or macrovessels may result in increased vascular permeability, thereby facilitating the movement of inflammatory or other cells into the perturbed vessel wall.[63]

Receptor-Dependent Pathways

Given the heterogeneous nature of the AGEs, it is not surprising that multiple different AGE "receptors" have been identified, such as AGE-R1 (an anti-inflammatory AGE receptor),[64] members of the scavenger receptor families such as CD36,[65] and the macrophage scavenger receptor.[66] Among the AGE receptors, the receptor for AGEs (RAGE) is a well-characterized signal transduction receptor of the immunoglobulin superfamily.[67] RAGE binds AGEs such as CML-AGE and possibly hydroimidazolone AGEs.[68] Very likely, distinct AGEs may bind to RAGE as well.

RAGE is characterized by the presence of three extracellular domains led by an N-terminal V-type Ig domain. This is followed by two distinct C-type Ig domains.[69] A number of recent publications have implicated the V-C1 domain as a chief unit for ligand binding.[70] Two recent papers reporting on the structure of extracellular RAGE indicated that it is composed of a large hydrophobic patch and a large negative patch; these regions modulate the patterns of RAGE ligand binding profiles to this region.[71,72]

In addition to AGEs, RAGE also binds distinct ligands. RAGE is a signal transduction receptor for at least certain of the S100/calgranulin family members.[73] Although RAGE was first described as a receptor for S100A12, distinct work has shown that S100B, S100P, S100A8/A9, S100A4, and S100A6, as examples, may bind to and signal via RAGE.[70] Members of the S100 family exert multiple effects in the tissues, including induction and sustenance of inflammatory reactions, and in tumors, S100s are linked to tumor cell proliferation, migration, upregulation of matrix metalloproteinase expression and activity, and the regulation of cell survival.[74] RAGE is also a signal transducer for high-mobility group box 1 (HMGB1).[75] HMGB1, like many of the RAGE ligand families, is also promiscuous and is able to bind to not only RAGE but also certain members of the toll receptor signaling family.[76] Like S100/calgranulins, HMGB1 exerts both proinflammatory and protumor properties. In tumor cells, HMGB1 has been suggested to mediate, via RAGE, increased pancreatic tumor cell autophagy and decreased apoptosis, processes that together enhance tumor cell survival.[77] RAGE is also a receptor for amyloid-β peptide and other forms of amyloidogenic polypeptides.[78] Recent work has shown that RAGE binds complement-related factor C1q[79] and that RAGE is a signaling receptor for lysophosphatidic acid (LPA).[80] Hence, these considerations highlight the complexity of RAGE; RAGE is not simply a "one ligand–one disease" molecule. Rather, we speculate that multiple ligands of RAGE may converge in distinct settings and thereby contribute, perhaps at different time points, to the pathogenesis of chronic diseases such as diabetic atherosclerosis. Taken together, the multi-ligand nature of RAGE places this molecule in the midst of cellular milieus in which hyperglycemia, inflammation, and tumor propagation are key events. A plethora of evidence links these ligands to diabetes and atherosclerosis in humans and in animal models.

In that context, one of the first tests of RAGE in human diabetic atherosclerosis was its expression pattern in the affected tissues. Human atherosclerotic plaques subjected to immunohistochemical localization of RAGE demonstrated that RAGE was expressed in atherosclerotic plaques retrieved at carotid endarterectomy[81] and in coronary artery lesions[82] but to greater degrees in the lesions retrieved from the diabetic versus nondiabetic patients. In these settings, RAGE expression in the diabetic lesions was associated with greater degrees of inflammation (higher numbers of macrophages and T cells), increased activation of NF-κB and expression of COX-2/mPGES-1, increased expression and activity of matrix metalloproteinase (MMPs), higher numbers of apoptotic smooth muscle cells, and higher levels of the RAGE ligand S100A12. It is interesting to note that RAGE expression in the diabetic carotid plaques increased in parallel with the levels of glycosylated hemoglobin. Indeed, at the level of the RAGE (AGER) gene, RAGE ligands such as AGEs contribute to upregulation of RAGE itself, at least in part via NF-κB binding elements within the RAGE promoter.[83]

RAGE is expressed in multiple cell types linked to atherosclerosis, such as endothelial cells, monocytes and macrophages, smooth muscle cells, and T lymphocytes. In these cell types, RAGE ligands have been shown to mediate upregulation of inflammatory signals and key transcription factors such as NF-κB and Egr-1 that have been shown to contribute critically to atherosclerosis, including that in diabetes.[84]

In vivo studies have used a variety of approaches to test the role of RAGE in diabetic atherosclerosis in animal models. Mice deficient in apoE made type 1 diabetic with streptozotocin demonstrated increased atherosclerotic plaque area at the aortic sinus and increased vascular inflammation compared with vehicle-treated mice whose levels of glucose were within the normal range. The role of RAGE was initially tested

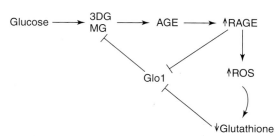

FIGURE 9-3 Methylglyoxal and glyoxalase1: influence of RAGE and ROSs.

with use of soluble RAGE (sRAGE), the extracellular ligand-binding domain of RAGE. Administration of sRAGE to diabetic apoE null mice resulted in a dose-dependent suppression of early acceleration of atherosclerosis and, in other studies, suppression of progression of accelerated diabetic atherosclerosis.[85,86] Of note, although levels of cholesterol were higher in the streptozotocin-treated mice, administration of sRAGE had no effect on levels of cholesterol in the diabetic animals. Rather, administration of sRAGE reduced inflammation in the aorta tissue—even tissue not directly affected by vascular lesions. Similar findings were observed in type 2 diabetic mice (db/db) in the apoE null background; administration of sRAGE reduced atherosclerosis.[87]

In additional approaches, mice globally devoid of RAGE or mice in which endothelial cell signaling was impaired by virtue of deletion of the RAGE cytoplasmic domain in endothelial cells (and other cell types in which pre-proendothelin-1 promoter might have been active) demonstrated significant reduction in atherosclerosis, including that in diabetes, in a manner independent of cholesterol or lipid levels.[62,88] Affymetrix gene array studies highlighted roles for the ROCK1 branch of the TGF-β signaling pathway in smooth muscle cells in regulation of migration and proliferation.[89]

Recent studies have uncovered that the cytoplasmic domain of RAGE binds to the formin family molecule diaphanous-1 (mDia1). The formins are a family of molecules that contribute to regulation of cellular signaling (effectors of Rho GTPase molecules) and to cellular migration and cytokinesis.[90] Studies to date in transformed cells, smooth muscle cells, and macrophages have illustrated that RAGE ligand-dependent signaling in these cell types is blocked in the presence of siRNA-knockdown of mDia1 or in mDia1 null cells.[91–93] In vivo, nondiabetic mice subjected to guidewire-induced femoral artery endothelial injury displayed significant upregulation of mDia1, especially in smooth muscle cells (**Fig. 9-4A-I**). Furthermore, mice devoid of mDia1 were protected from aberrant neointimal expansion (**Fig. 9-4J**). Consistent with the concept that mDia1 transduced RAGE signaling in the smooth muscle cells, mDia1 null injured vessels and isolated aortic smooth muscle displayed reduced oxidative stress, cell signaling via GSK-3β, and cellular migration compared with wild-type counterparts expressing mDia1 (**Fig. 9-5**).[92] Prompted by these findings, studies are under way to determine the impact of mDia1 in diabetic atherosclerosis.

Although RAGE antagonists have not yet been tested in humans with diabetic atherosclerosis, evidence is accruing linking RAGE to this disorder. Single-nucleotide polymorphisms (SNPs) of RAGE have been associated with human diabetic atherosclerosis.[94,95] Multiple reports have now described relationships between levels of sRAGE and diabetic cardiovascular disease in humans.[96,97] Hence, in addition to the potential of RAGE as a target for therapeutic intervention in diabetic atherosclerosis, RAGE may also present new biomarker opportunities to track the presence and/or extent of this complication.

It is important to note that RAGE-dependent roles in diabetic atherosclerosis are also accounted for by inflammatory mechanisms in addition to the effect of glycation. Given that multiple RAGE ligands are expressed in diabetic macrovessels and that they largely converge on this specific receptor, it is difficult to precisely discern the effects of individual ligand classes. Hence, targeting this pathway for clinical translation will depend on the identification of RAGE inhibitors. **Chapter 10** presents an in-depth discussion of the broader roles of inflammation in diabetic atherosclerosis.

Additional Mechanisms of Diabetic Atherosclerosis

Recent studies have suggested the certain microRNAs may contribute to regulation of inflammatory pathways in cell

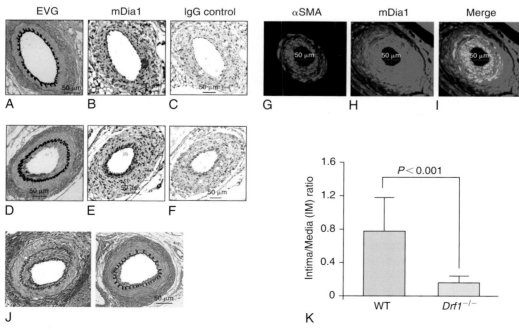

FIGURE 9-4 Increased expression and impact of mDia1 after endothelial denudation injury. Wild-type (WT), *Drf1*−/−, and *RAGE*−/− mice were subjected to femoral artery endothelial denudation or sham, and tissues analyzed at the indicated times. **A** and **D,** Assessment of neointimal expansion by elastic–van Gieson (E-VG) staining on day 21 after injury in WT mice (**A,** sham and **D,** injury). **B, C, E,** and **F,** Immunostaining for mDia1 or isotype IgG control in WT mice on day 21 after injury (**E** and **F**) or sham (**B** and **C**). **G** to **J,** Colocalization studies: sections of injured vessels were stained for mDia1 and α–smooth muscle cell actin (SMA). Immunofluorescence studies revealed a colocalization of the two molecules in the neointima on day 21. **K,** Intima/Media (I/M) ratio measurement based on morphometric analysis of the vessels of WT and aged-sex-matched *Drf1*−/− mice (n = 11/group) was performed 21 days after guidewire-induced femoral artery denudation. Representative images are shown. [92] *P* < 0.001. *(Reprinted from Toure, et al., 2012.)*

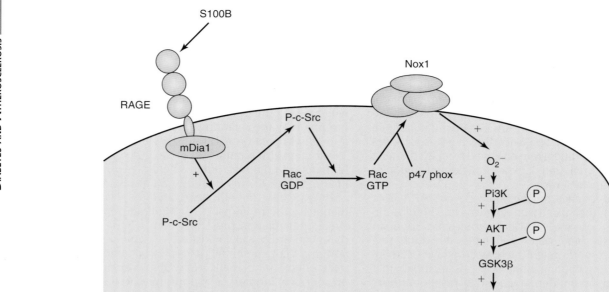

FIGURE 9-5 Proposed mechanism of the role of mDia1 in RAGE-induced redox signaling SMC migration and neointimal expansion. We propose that there is a critical role for mDia1 in transducing the effects of RAGE ligands on P-c-Src, Rac1, and Nox1 activation in consequent phosphorylation of AKT/GSK3β ser 9, processes essential for RAGE ligand-induced vascular SMC migration.[92] *(Reprinted from Toure, et al., 2012.)*

types that mediate diabetic atherosclerosis.[98] For example, miRNA (miR)-16 has been linked to RNA stability of cyclooxygenase (COX-2) in monocytes, and the RAGE ligand S100B downregulates miR-16 levels in these cells.[99] In vascular smooth muscle cells retrieved from type 2 diabetic db/db mice, miR-125 levels were higher than those in nondiabetic control animals. In those cells, higher levels of miR-125 were linked to increased expression of proinflammatory genes such as IL-6 and MCP-1, both key factors that are expressed early in diabetic atherosclerotic lesions in mouse models.[100] In these same smooth muscle cells, it has also been shown that miR-200b levels were higher in the diabetic versus nondiabetic cells and that miR-200b inhibited Zeb1, a factor that negatively regulates inflammatory genes.[101] How such differences in miRs may be directly implicated in diabetic atherosclerosis in vivo will be a key topic for study.

Chromatin-based epigenetic mechanisms have been implicated in the phenomenon of "metabolic memory." Metabolic memory has been suggested to contribute to the so-called "legacy effect" observed in human diabetic patients. As discussed earlier in this chapter, these legacy patients continued to experience benefit from microvascular and macrovascular complications through their earlier strict control of glycemia regimens compared with their counterparts' standard treatment regimens, even years after the original study was completed. Evidence is accruing to link diabetes-associated histone methylation and histone acetylation patterns to gene expression changes that may contribute to macrovascular disease.[102,103] In diabetic conditions, histone acetyltransferases (HATs) and histone deacetylases (HDACs) have been shown to play roles in regulation of inflammatory and oxidative stress genes, and in the NF-κB signaling pathway (another mechanism that has potential to broadly activate proinflammatory pathways). In the case of methylation, ChIP-on-chip studies showed that

when monocytes were cultured in high- (diabetes-relevant) versus low-glucose (non–diabetes-relevant) conditions, significant changes in H3K4me-2 activation marks and H3K9me2 repressive marks were observed, thereby suggesting that exposure of these inflammatory cells to high glucose might impart highly significant changes in gene expression programs that might influence diabetic vasculature.

Protective roles for SIRT1 (NAD-dependent histone deacetylase) have been shown in endothelial cells grown in high glucose. In high-glucose–exposed endothelial cells, expression of SIRT1 was found to be decreased. SIRT1 has been linked mechanistically to p53 levels; when levels of SIRT1 were decreased in endothelial cells by high glucose, the acetylation of p53 increased, thereby increasing its activity.[104] In this setting, evidence of high-glucose–induced endothelial senescence was observed but was prevented by overexpression of SIRT1 or by disruption of p53. Hence, as endothelial dysfunction is thought to critically underlie diabetic atherosclerosis, it is highly plausible that the effects of glucose in endothelial cells cause profound derangements in post-translational modifications, thereby providing a mechanism for inflammation, oxidative stress, and upregulation of proatherogenic pathways.

Taken together, multiple mechanisms converge in diabetic macrovessels to create an environment conducive to acceleration of atherosclerosis. Because there is a plethora of evidence that in nondiseased settings, cellular and metabolic pathways play important roles in ongoing vascular repair, it is logical to consider the situation in the diabetic tissues.

Diabetes and Impaired Regression of Atherosclerosis

As medical interventions in the treatment of atherosclerosis have improved, a critical question has been to what extent patients with diabetes display differences in response to treatments compared with nondiabetic individuals? In the COSMOS study (Coronary Atherosclerosis Study Measuring Effects of Rosuvastatin Using Intravascular Ultrasound in Japanese Subjects), plaque regression was significantly less in diabetic patients with glycosylated hemoglobin levels exceeding 6.5% compared with patients with more superior glycemic control—despite equivalent reductions in lipid levels.[105] Furthermore, the data analysis from COSMOS revealed that baseline levels of glycosylated hemoglobin were associated with the change in plaque volume. Such data suggest that lipid-related risk factors were not responsible for the differences in plaque responses, but, rather, that factors related to hyperglycemia and its consequences were more likely to reflect the diminished benefit observed in the diabetic patients.

Indeed, experiments in mouse models of atherosclerosis showed that when diabetic and nondiabetic mice were subjected to equivalent degrees of lipid lowering, diabetic animals displayed significantly less regression of established atherosclerosis.[106] When the atherosclerotic lesions of the diabetic mice after normalization of lipid levels were examined more closely, they revealed more macrophages per lesion area compared with the nondiabetic mice, suggesting that macrophage egress from the lesions was reduced. More oxidative stress and higher levels of macrophage M1 versus M2 polarization markers were observed in the diabetic versus nondiabetic lesions.

In addition to impaired regression of diabetic atherosclerosis, additional potential mechanisms linked to vascular injury in diabetes include impaired endothelial repair. Multiple studies have suggested that endothelial progenitor cells (EPCs) were reduced and/or defective in humans with type 1 and type 2 diabetes.[107] Similar findings were observed in diabetic animal models. In db/db mice, it was shown that EPCs were more sensitive to the effects of hypoxia and oxidative stress than nondiabetic control EPCs, in parallel with reduced ability to promote vascularization, diminished migration, and reduced expression of vascular endothelial growth factor (VEGF) and eNOS.[108] In streptozotocin-treated diabetic mice, EPCs were shown to display reduced mobilization and expression of eNOS, as well as reduced responses to stromal derived factor (SDF) and VEGF.[109]

Taken together, substantial evidence supports that multiple potential mechanisms contribute to accelerated diabetic atherosclerosis in humans. Furthermore, the contribution of defective repair mechanisms is important to consider, and endothelial progenitor dysfunction may contribute to the impaired regression of atherosclerosis observed in diabetes despite reduction in levels of lipids.

In the sections to follow, we consider the roles of insulin resistance and hyperinsulinemia on acceleration of atherosclerosis.

INSULIN RESISTANCE, HYPERINSULINEMIA, AND ACCELERATED ATHEROSCLEROSIS

Scope and Complexity of the Problem

Insulin resistance is a defining characteristic of type 2 diabetes, but it exists within a collection of associated disorders, such as hypertension, obesity, and dyslipidemia, each of which independently has been linked to cardiovascular disease.[110] As discussed earlier, a plethora of evidence links type 2 diabetes to cardiovascular complications. The San Antonio Heart Study showed that insulin resistance (as assessed in the patients by homeostatic model assessment, insulin resistance [HOMA-IR]) predicted future cardiovascular disease events.[111] Hence, efforts to understand the discrete role of insulin resistance in the acceleration of atherosclerosis have relied on both epidemiologic data and basic research experimentation. In the sections to follow, we detail the studies that sought to establish potential links among insulin resistance, hyperinsulinemia, and atherosclerosis. Of note, in the literature, "insulin resistance" may refer to the suppression of responsiveness to insulin action (signal transduction) and/or to the effects of hyperinsulinemia.

What Are the Roles of Insulin Resistance and Hyperinsulinemia in Atherosclerosis?

A review of the components of the insulin signaling suggests key roles for the PI3K/Akt signaling pathway as a central intermediary step that leads to the activation of downstream effectors.[112] These downstream effectors, such as phosphorylated FoxO and GSK-3β, may modulate the cellular responsiveness to insulin action and affect the vasculature.[113] The other "arm" of the insulin signaling pathway involves activation of MAP kinases; evidence suggests that in certain cell types insulin resistance selectively affects distinct arms of the pathways.[112] To test these concepts, particularly in the context of cell-specific contributions to insulin signaling and how this might affect organisms overall, insulin signaling in atherosclerosis has been addressed, to date, by the use of tissue-targeted knockout of the insulin receptor (IR) in mice with Cre-loxP technology and by bone marrow transplantation strategies.

Endothelial Cells and Insulin Receptor Signaling

First, we consider the effects of insulin signaling in endothelial cells. The floxed IR mouse has been one of the major tools used in these efforts. In endothelial cells, selective deletion of the IR in atherosclerosis-prone apoE null mice fed normal rodent chow for 24 or 52 weeks resulted in a significant increase in atherosclerosis compared with apoE null mice with IR expression in these cells.[114] There were no differences in levels of plasma glucose, lipids, or insulin or blood pressure in these mice, suggesting that innate, vessel-specific consequences of IR deletion in endothelial cells accounted for these findings. Insights into the potential mechanisms of increased atherosclerosis were deduced by reduced Ser1177 eNOS phosphorylation in the endothelial cell IR null mice together with increased adherence of leukocytes to these endothelial cells via intravital microscopy studies. Increased endothelial cell expression of vascular cell adhesion molecule 1 (VCAM-1) accompanied the deletion of IR in endothelial cells, thereby providing a well-established mechanism for the adherence of leukocytes to vascular structures, a key event in early atherogenesis.

Global deficiency of Akt1 in apoE null mice fed a high-fat Western type diet resulted in highly significant increases in atherosclerosis and more plaque vulnerability, with decreased Ser1177 eNOS phosphorylation in the lesions.[115] Of note, the specific effect of endothelial cell Akt1 in vivo was not discernible from these studies, given that the deletion of Akt1 was global in nature. However, endothelial cells retrieved from mice displayed reduced viability and proliferation. Taken together, these findings strongly support key adaptive roles for endothelial cell IR signaling in regulation of eNOS activity and suppression of vascular inflammation.

Vascular Smooth Muscle Cells and Insulin Receptor Signaling

In vascular smooth muscle cells, heterodimers of IRs and insulin-like growth factor receptors (IGF1Rs) are formed. Experimental evidence suggests that the IGF1 component mostly mediates the effects of insulin in this cell type.[116] IR null vascular smooth muscle cells were incubated with insulin; this resulted in reduced Akt phosphorylation and increased ERK1/2 phosphorylation. Functional responses included an increase in proliferation and migration, likely through the actions of IGF1R.[117] In the work of Fernandez Hernando referred to earlier, smooth muscle cells retrieved from the Akt null mice displayed reduced proliferation and migration, and higher degrees of apoptosis—features that, depending on the stage of atherosclerosis (early or late), might increase plaque vulnerability and atherosclerosis.[115]

Macrophages and Insulin Receptor Signaling

Studies have also been performed testing the role of macrophage IR with both LysM-cre recombinase mice (targeting macrophages, neutrophils, and to some degree monocytes) as well as bone marrow transplantation strategies. It is interesting to note that when these mice were bred with IR-floxed mice into the apoE null background and fed a high-cholesterol, cholate-containing diet, a 50% reduction in en face atherosclerosis resulted, without any differences in lipids or glucose levels.[118] In the macrophages from these animals, responses to LPS or IL-6 were decreased. These data suggested that macrophage IR signaling contributed to inflammation and insulin resistance.

In other studies in apoE null mice devoid of Akt1, more apoptotic macrophages in the lesions were found compared with their Akt1-expressing controls, with no apparent difference in atherosclerosis at the aortic root. The complexity of the implications of macrophage apoptosis in atherosclerotic lesions lies within the context that macrophage apoptosis in late-stage atherosclerotic plaques might contribute to plaque necrosis.[119] Overall, the full scope of implications of macrophage IR signaling in atherosclerosis is yet to be fully delineated for the following reasons related to study design, to date: the degree of macrophage apoptosis in the lesions, the timing of the sacrifice (early versus late atherosclerosis), the type of diet and the degree to which inflammatory substances might skew macrophage-dependent responses (such as the inclusion of cholate), the genetic background of the animals, and the study design (bone marrow transplantation versus LysM-cre recombinase animals). In the last case, the full range of target cells devoid of the IR differ slightly between the two strategies. Additional considerations include whether or not lethal irradiation was first imposed on the animals in the former strategy and the (unknown) extent to which IR signaling might contribute to survival and macrophage properties in that setting.

We may deduce from these data that IR signaling and its role in atherogenesis is dependent on cell type and time course. Finally, we address a recent study that directly tested the role of hyperinsulinemia in atherosclerosis.

The Effect of Hyperinsulinemia on Atherosclerosis

As discussed earlier, in experiments in which insulin resistance is assessed in the context of other distinct and atherosclerosis-stimulating factors, the specific effect of hyperinsulinemia itself on atherosclerosis is difficult to fully dissect. Toward that end, apoE null mice with a single allele deletion of the IR were studied, and the findings were compared with those in apoE null mice with both IR alleles intact. Plasma levels of insulin in the former group of mice were approximately 50% higher than those in the latter group in the fasted state, and 69% higher during a glucose tolerance test (overall, however, glucose tolerance was not different between the two groups of mice). Levels of C-peptide, insulin sensitivity, and postreceptor insulin signaling in muscle, liver, fat, and aorta did not differ between the two groups of animals, nor did levels of plasma lipids or glucose. At two different time courses in these mice fed a normal chow diet, aortic lesion area by en face analysis and at the aortic root did not differ at 24 and 52 weeks of age. Furthermore, cholesterol abundance in the brachiocephalic artery did not differ between the two groups of mice.[120] These data were the first to show that high levels of insulin, without concomitant associated factors that themselves are risk factors for atherosclerosis, exerted no differential effect on atherosclerosis. In that study, however, it is important to note that the animals within these colonies were largely in the C57BL/6 background. The authors reported in the manuscript that the study mice were 87.6% in the C57BL/6 background, as determined by an array that genotyped 377 SNPs in these animals. If and how such a consideration might have affected the conclusions is not possible to determine from the study as designed.

SUMMARY

The worldwide increase in types 1 and 2 diabetes suggests that complications from cardiovascular disease are likely to emerge as leading causes of disability and death in the years to come. Together with the lack of mechanism-based diabetes-specific therapies to combat the disorder, current approaches are limited to treating all of the confounding factors, such as hypertension, hyperlipidemia, and obesity. A number of key studies in type 2 diabetes have failed to show unequivocal benefit of strict glycemic control in reduction of myocardial infarction and death from cardiac events. In type 1 diabetes, the long-term results of DCCT and EDIC did show reduction in both surrogate markers of atherosclerosis, as well as myocardial infarction events and death, with institution of strict glycemic control measures years before the actual occurrence of the cardiac events.

Glucose and its direct and indirect consequences exert profound impact in the cell types highly implicated in atherosclerosis, such as endothelial cells, smooth muscle cells, and macrophages. Of note, the diabetes-specific mechanisms in these distinct cell types may vary according to the time course—that is, mechanisms underlying early lesion initiation may be somewhat different from mechanisms of late-stage lesion progression and plaque instability (**Fig. 9-6**). From this figure, it is apparent that multiple potential therapeutic targets have been identified, based on the results of many years of experimentation on the causes of diabetic accelerated atherosclerosis. We propose that what is needed is a multipronged approach that includes both treatment of comorbid risk factors and mechanism-based therapies that specifically target high glucose and its consequences. Identifying the optimal timing and duration of each therapeutic strategy in diabetic atherosclerosis may be the key to optimal success in treatment of this disorder.

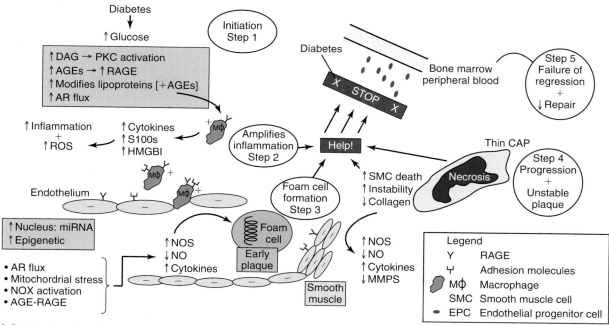

FIGURE 9-6 Mechanisms linked to early initiation versus late progression of diabetic atherosclerotic plaques. Diabetes is characterized by increased levels of glucose. Glucose has multiple consequences, such as increased generation of DAG and activation of PKCs; increased flux via the polyol pathway, which consumes NAD⁺, thereby leading to increased fructose, increased AGE precursors, and oxidative stress; increased activation of the hexosamine biosynthetic pathway and concomitant changes in gene expression; increased glycation and post-translational modifications of proteins and lipids that activate RAGE; and increased accumulation of modified lipoproteins, including modification by AGEs (*Initiation, Step 1*). In this highly proinflammatory environment, macrophages are activated; we predict that such activation of macrophages generates even further inflammation and oxidative stress, in part by release of cytokines, S100/calgranulins, and HMGB1 (*Amplifies inflammation, Step 2*). Once activated macrophages traverse the activated endothelial cell surface, upregulation of adhesion molecules and inflammatory species increases foam cell formation and the development of the early foam cell (*Foam cell formation, Step 3*). As smooth muscle cells begin to proliferate and migration, their role is to form stable fibrous caps that protect the plaque from rupture. In late-stage lesions, we hypothesize that smooth muscle cells are more prone to cell death; are more unstable, and produce less collagen and more MMPs (*Progression and unstable plaque, Step 4*). Finally, published data support that vascular repair mechanisms and atherosclerosis regression are impaired in diabetes. Such dysfunction of repair mechanisms likely forestalls normal vascular maintenance functions and perpetuating atherosclerosis (*Failure of regression and decreased repair, Step 5*).

References

1. Behn A, Ur E: The obesity epidemic and its cardiovascular consequences, *Curr Opin Cardiol* 21:353–360, 2006.
2. The Diabetes Control and Complications Trial (DCCT) Research Group: Results of the feasibility study. The DCCT Research Group, *Diabetes Care* 10:1–19, 1987.
3. The Diabetes Control and Complications Trial (DCCT) Research Group: The effect of intensive treatment of diabetes on the development and progression of long-term complications in insulin-dependent diabetes mellitus, *N Engl J Med* 329:977–986, 1993.
4. Nathan DM, Cleary PA, Backlund JY, et al: Intensive diabetes treatment and cardiovascular disease in type 1 diabetes, *N Engl J Med* 353:2643–2653, 2005.
5. Nathan DM, Lachin J, Cleary P, et al: Intensive diabetes therapy and carotid intima-media thickness in type 1 diabetes mellitus, *N Engl J Med* 348:2294–2303, 2003.
6. UK Prospective Diabetes Study (UKPDS) Group: Intensive blood-glucose control with sulphonylureas or insulin compared with conventional treatment and risk of complications in patients with type 2 diabetes (UKPDS 33), *Lancet* 352:837–853, 1998.
7. Holman RR, Paul SK, Bethel MA, et al: 10 year follow up of intensive glucose control in type 2 diabetes, *N Engl J Med* 359:1577–1589, 2008.
8. The ACCORD Study Group: Long-term effects of intensive glucose lowering on cardiovascular outcomes, *N Engl J Med* 364:818–828, 2011.
9. Patel A, MacMahon S, Chalmers J, et al: Intensive blood glucose control and vascular outcomes in patients with type 2 diabetes, *N Engl J Med* 358:2560–2572, 2008.
10. Duckworth W, Abraira C, Moritz T, et al: Glucose control and vascular complications in veterans with type 2 diabetes, *N Engl J Med* 360:129–139, 2009.
11. Gaede P, Lung-Anderson H, Parving HH, et al: Effect of a multifactorial intervention on mortality in type 2 diabetes, *N Engl J Med* 358:580–591, 2008.
12. Gaede P, Vedel P, Larsen N, et al: Multifactorial intervention and cardiovascular disease in patients with type 2 diabetes, *N Engl J Med* 348:383–393, 2003.
13. Ramasamy R: Aldose reductase: a novel strategy for cardioprotective interventions, *Curr Drug Targets* 4:625–632, 2003.
14. Vikramadithyan RK, Hu Y, Noh H-L, et al: Human aldose reductase expression accelerates diabetic atherosclerosis in transgenic mice, *J Clin Invest* 115:2434–2443, 2005.
15. Gleissner CA, Sanders JM, Nadler J, et al: Upregulation of aldose reductase during foam cell formation as possible link among diabetes, hyperlipidemia, and atherosclerosis, *Arterioscler Thromb Vasc Biol* 28:1137–1143, 2008.
16. Vedantham S, Noh H, Ananthakrishnan R, et al: Human aldose reductase expression accelerates atherosclerosis in diabetic apolipoprotein E−/− mice.
17. Srivastava S, Vladykovskaya E, Barski OA, et al: Aldose reductase protects against early atherosclerotic lesion formation in apolipoprotein E null mice, *Circ Res* 105:793–802, 2009.
18. Johnson BF, Nesto RW, Pfeifer MA, et al: Cardiac abnormalities in diabetic patients with neuropathy: effect of aldose reductase inhibitor administration, *Diabetes Care* 27:448–454, 2004.
19. Vedantham S, Ananthakrishnan R, Schmidt AM, et al: Aldose reductase, oxidative stress and cardiovascular complications, *Cardiovasc Hematol Agents Med Chem* 10:234–240, 2012.
20. Hothersall JS, Muirhead RP, Taylaur CE, et al: Anti-oxidant status in an in vitro model for hyperglycaemic lens cataract formation: competition for available nicotinamide adenine dinucleotide phosphate between glutathione reduction and the polyol pathway, *Biochem Int* 27:945–952, 1992.
21. Robinson KA, Weinstein ML, Lindenmayer GE, et al: Effects of diabetes and hyperglycemia on the hexosamine synthesis pathway in rat muscle and liver, *Diabetes* 44:1438–1446, 1995.
22. Du XL, Edelstein D, Rossetti L, et al: Hyperglycemia induced mitochondrial superoxide overproduction activates three pathways of hyperglycemic damage and induces plasminogen activator inhibitor-1 expression by increasing Sp1 glycosylation, *Proc Natl Acad Sci U S A* 97:12222–12226, 2000.
23. Gabriely I, Yang XM, Cases JA, et al: Hyperglycemia induces PAI-1 gene expression in adipose tissue by activation of the hexosamine biosynthetic pathway, *Atherosclerosis* 160:115–122, 2002.
24. Du XL, Edelstein D, Dimmeler S, et al: Hyperglycemia inhibits endothelial nitric oxide synthase activity by posttranslational modification at the Akt site, *J Clin Invest* 108:1341–1348, 2001.
25. Hoffmann JM, Ishizuka T, Farese RV: Interrelated effects of insulin and glucose on diacylglycerol-protein kinase C signaling in rat adipocytes and solei muscle in vitro and in vivo in diabetic rats, *Endocrinology* 128:2937–48, 1991.
26. Idris I, Gray S, Donnelly R: Protein kinase C activation: isozyme specific effects on metabolism and cardiovascular complications in diabetes, *Diabetologia* 44:659–673, 2001.
27. Geraldes P, King GL: Activation of protein kinase C isoforms and its impact on diabetic complications, *Circ Res* 106:1319–1331, 2010.
28. Harja E, Chang JS, Lu Y, et al: Mice deficient in PKCbeta and apolipoprotein E display decreased atherosclerosis, *FASEB J* 23:1081–1091, 2009.
29. Mehta NN, Sheetz M, Price K, et al: Selective PKC beta inhibition with ruboxistaurin and endothelial function in type 2 diabetes mellitus, *Cardiovasc Drugs Ther* 23:17–24, 2009.
30. Leitges M, Mayr M, Braun U, et al: Exacerbated vein graft atherosclerosis in protein kinase C delta null mice, *J Clin Invest* 108:1505–1512, 2001.
31. Mamputu JC, Renier G: Advanced glycation endproducts increase, through a protein kinase C dependent pathway, vascular endothelial growth factor expression in retinal endothelial cells. Inhibitory effect of gliclazide, *J Diabetes Complications* 16:284–293, 2002.
32. Deveraj S, Hirany SV, Burk RF, et al: Divergence between LDL oxidative susceptibility and urinary F(2) isoprostanes as measures of oxidative stress in type 2 diabetes, *Clin Chem* 47:1974–1979, 2001.
33. Wakabayashi Y, Usui Y, Shibauchi Y, et al: Increased levels of 8-hydroxydeoxyguanosine in the vitreous of patients with diabetic retinopathy, *Diabetes Res Clin Pract* 89:e59–e61, 2010.
34. Huang A, Yang YM, Feher A, et al: Exacerbation of endothelial dysfunction during the progression of diabetes: role of oxidative stress, *Am J Physiol Regul Integr Comp Physiol* 302:R674–R681, 2012.
35. Yi X, Xu L, Hiller S, et al: Reduced alpha lipoic acid synthase gene expression exacerbates atherosclerosis in diabetic apolipoprotein E deficient mice, *Atherosclerosis* 223:137–143, 2012.
36. Yusuf S, Dagenais G, Pogue J, et al: Vitamin E supplementation and cardiovascular events in high-risk patients. The Heart Outcomes Prevention Evaluation Study Investigators, *N Engl J Med* 342:154–160, 2000.
37. Levy Y, Blum S, Levy AP: Antioxidants in the prevention of atherosclerosis: the importance of proper patients selection, *Clin Nutr* 28:581–582, 2009.
38. Nishikawa T, Edelstein D, Du XL, et al: Normalizing mitochondrial superoxide production blocks three pathways of hyperglycemic damage, *Nature* 404:787–790, 2000.
39. Giacco F, Brownlee M: Oxidative stress and diabetic complications, *Circ Res* 107:1058–1070, 2010.
40. Hammes HP, Du X, Edelstein D, et al: Benfotiamine blocks three major pathways of hyperglycemic damage and prevents experimental diabetic retinopathy, *Nat Med* 9:294–299, 2003.
41. Mukhopadhyay P, Horváth B, Zsengellér Z, et al: Mitochondrially reactive oxygen species generation triggers inflammatory response and tissue injury associated with hepatic ischemia-reperfusion: therapeutic potential of mitochondrially targeted antioxidants, *Free Radic Biol Med* 53:1123–1138, 2012.
42. Sedeek M, Montezano AC, Hebert RL, et al: Oxidative stress, nox isoforms and complications of diabetes—potential targets for novel therapeutics, *J Cardiovasc Trans Res* 5:509–518, 2012.

43. Touyz RM, Briones AM, Sedeek M, et al: Nox isoforms and reactive oxygen species in vascular health, *Mol Interv* 11:27–35, 2011.

44. Wautier MP, Chappey O, Corda S, et al: Activation of NADPH oxidase by AGEs links oxidant stress to altered gene expression via RAGE, *Am J Physiol Endocrinol Metab* 280:E685–E694, 2001.

45. Barry-Lane PA, Patterson C, Van der Merwe M, et al: p47phox is required for atherosclerotic lesion progression in ApoE–/– mice, *J Clin Invest* 108:1513–1522, 2001.

46. Sheehan AL, Carrell S, Johnson B, et al: Role for Nox1 NADPH oxidase in atherosclerosis.

47. Judkins C, Diep H, Broughton BRS, et al: Direct evidence of a role for Nox2 in superoxide production, reduced nitric oxide bioavailability, and early atherosclerotic plaque formation in apoE–/– mice, *Am J Physiol Heart Circ Physiol* 298:H24–H32, 2010.

48. Lewis P, Stefanovic N, Pete J, et al: Lack of the antioxidant enzyme glutathione peroxidase-1 accelerates atherosclerosis in diabetic apolipoprotein E null mice, *Circ* 115:2178–2187, 2007.

49. Perrotta I, Sciangula A, Perrotta E, et al: Ultrastructural analysis and electron microscopic localization of Nox4 in healthy and atherosclerotic human aorta, *Ultrastruct Pathol* 35:1–6, 2011.

50. Rivera J, Sobey CG, Walduck AK, et al: Nox isoforms in vascular pathophysiology: insights from transgenic and knockout mouse models, *Redox Rep* 15:50–63, 2010.

51. Wells-Knecht KJ, Zyzak DV, Litchfield JE, et al: Mechanism of autooxidative glycosylation: identification of glyoxal and arabinose as intermediates in the autooxidative modification of proteins by glucose, *Biochemistry* 34:3702–3709, 1995.

52. Schalkwijk CG, Miyata T: Early and advanced non-enzymatic glycation in diabetic vascular complications: the search for therapeutics, *Amino Acids* 42:1193–1204, 2012.

53. Farboud B, Aotaki-Keen A, Miyata T, et al: Development of a polyclonal antibody with broad epitope specificity for advanced glycation endproducts and localization of these epitopes in Bruch's membrane of the aging eye, *Mol Vis* 5:11, 1999.

54. Chang JS, Wendt T, Qu W, et al: Oxygen deprivation triggers upregulation of early growth response1 by the receptor for advanced glycation endproducts, *Circ Res* 102:905–913, 2008.

55. Friedlander MA, Witko-Sarsat V, Nguyen AT, et al: The advanced glycation endproduct pentosidine and monocyte activation in uremia, *Clin Nephrol* 45:379–382, 1996.

56. Anderson MM, Requena JR, Crowley JR, et al: The myeloperoxidase system of human phagocytes generates Nepsilon-(carboxymethyl)lysine on proteins: a mechanism for producing advanced glycation endproducts at sites of inflammation, *J Clin Invest* 104:103–113, 1999.

57. Negrean M, Stirban A, Stratmann B, et al: Effects of low and high advanced glycation endproduct means on macro- and microvascular endothelial function and oxidative stress in patients with type 2 diabetes mellitus, *Am J Clin Nutr* 85:1236–1243, 2007.

58. Gursinsky T, Ruhs S, Friess U, et al: Air pollution associated fly ash particles induce fibrotic mechanisms in primary fibroblasts, *Biol Chem* 387:1411–1420, 2006.

59. McCann VJ, Davis RE, Welborn TA, et al: Glyoxalase phenotypes in patients with diabetes mellitus, *Aust N Z J Med* 11:380–382, 1981.

60. Reiniger N, Lau K, McCalla D, et al: Deletion of the receptor for advanced glycation endproducts reduces glomerulosclerosis and preserves renal function in the diabetic OVE26 mouse, *Diabetes* 59:2043–2054, 2010.

61. Schlondorff D: Cellular mechanisms of lipid injury in the glomerulus, *Am J Kidney Dis* 22:72–82, 1993.

62. Harja E, Bu DX, Hudson BI, et al: Vascular and inflammatory stresses mediate atherosclerosis via RAGE and its ligands in apoE–/– mice, *J Clin Invest* 118:183–194, 2008.

63. Boyd-White J, Williams JC Jr: Effect of cross-linking on matrix permeability. A model for AGE-modified basement membranes, *Diabetes* 45:348–353, 1996.

64. Stitt AW, Li YM, Gardiner TA, et al: Advanced glycation endproducts (AGEs) co-localize with AGE receptors in the retinal vasculature of diabetic and AGE-infused rats, *Am J Pathol* 150:523–531, 1997.

65. Ohgami N, Nagai R, Ikeomoto M, et al: CD36, a member of the class B scavenger receptor family, as a receptor for advanced glycation endproducts, *J Biol Chem* 276:3195–3202, 2001.

66. Araki N, Higashi T, Mori T, et al: Macrophage scavenger receptor mediates the endocytic uptake and degradation of advanced glycation endproducts of the Maillard reaction, *Eur J Biochem* 230:408–415, 1995.

67. Yan SF, Ramasamy R, Naka Y, et al: Glycation, inflammation and RAGE: a scaffold for the macrovascular complications of diabetes and beyond, *Circ Res* 93:1159–1169, 2003.

68. Kislinger T, Fu C, Huber B, et al: N(epsilon)-(carboxymethyl)lysine adducts of proteins are ligands for receptor for advanced glycation endproducts that activate cell signaling pathways and modulate gene expression, *J Biol Chem* 274:31740–31749, 1999.

69. Neeper M, Schmidt AM, Brett J, et al: Cloning and expression of a cell surface receptor for advanced glycosylation end products of proteins, *J Biol Chem* 267:4998–5004, 1992.

70. Leclerc E, Fritz G, Vetter SW, et al: Binding of S100 proteins to RAGE: an update, *Biochim Biophys Acta* 1793:993–1007, 2009.

71. Park H, Adsit FG, Boyington JC: The 1.5 Å crystal structure of human receptor for advanced glycation endproducts (RAGE) ectodomains reveal unique features determining ligand binding, *J Biol Chem* 285:40762–40770, 2010.

72. Koch M, Chitayat S, Dattilo BM, et al: Structural basis for ligand recognition and activation of RAGE, *Structure* 18:1342–1352, 2010.

73. Hofmann MA, Drury S, Fu C, et al: RAGE mediates a novel proinflammatory axis: a central cell surface receptor for S100/calgranulin polypeptides, *Cell* 97:889–901, 1999.

74. Hofmann Bowman MA, Schmidt AM: S100/calgranulins EN-RAGEing the blood vessels: implications for inflammatory responses and atherosclerosis, *Am J Cardiovasc Dis* 1:92–100, 2011.

75. Taguchi A, Blood DC, del Toro G, et al: Blockade of RAGE-amphoterin signaling suppresses tumour growth and metastases, *Nature* 405:354–360, 2000.

76. Rauvala H, Rouhiainen A: Physiological and pathophysiological outcomes of the interaction of HMGB1 with cell surface receptors, *Biochim Biophys Acta* 1799:164–170, 2010.

77. Kang R, Tang D, Schapiro N, et al: The receptor for advanced glycation endproducts (RAGE) sustains autophagy and limits apoptosis, promoting tumor cell survival, *Cell Death Differ* 17:666–676, 2010.

78. Yan SD, Chen X, Fu J, et al: RAGE and amyloid-beta peptide neurotoxicity in Alzheimer's disease, *Nature* 382:685–691, 1996.

79. Ma W, Rai V, Hudson BI, et al: RAGE binds C1q and enhances C1q mediated phagocytosis, *Cell Immunol* 274:72–82, 2012.

80. Rai V, Touré F, Chitayat S, et al: Lysophosphatidic acid targets vascular and oncogenic pathways via RAGE signaling, *J Exp Med* 209(13):2339–2350, 2012.

81. Cipollone F, Iezzi A, Fazia M, et al: The receptor RAGE as a progression factor amplifying arachidonate-dependent inflammatory and proteolytic response in human atherosclerotic plaques: role of glycemic control, *Circulation* 108:1070–1077, 2003.

82. Burke AP, Kolodgie FD, Zieske A, et al: Morphologic findings of coronary atherosclerotic plaques in diabetics: a postmortem study, *Arterioscler Thromb Vasc Biol* 24:1266–1271, 2004.

83. Li J, Schmidt AM: Characterization and functional analysis of the promoter of RAGE, the receptor for advanced glycation endproducts, *J Biol Chem* 272:16498–16506, 1997.

84. Goldin A, Beckman JA, Schmidt AM, et al: Advanced glycation endproducts: sparking the development of diabetic vascular injury, *Circulation* 114:597–605, 2006.

85. Bucciarelli L, Wendt T, Qu W, et al: RAGE blockade stabilizes established atherosclerosis in diabetic apolipoprotein E-null mice, *Circulation* 106:2827–2835, 2002.

86. Park L, Raman KG, Lee KJ, et al: Suppression of accelerated diabetic atherosclerosis by the receptor for advanced glycation endproducts, *Nat Med* 4:1025–1031, 1998.

87. Wendt T, Harja E, Bucciarelli L, et al: RAGE modulates vascular inflammation and atherosclerosis in a murine model of type 2 diabetes, *Atherosclerosis* 185:70–77, 2006.

88. Soro-Paavonen A, Watson AM, Li J, et al: Receptor for advanced glycation endproduct deficiency attenuates the development of atherosclerosis in diabetes, *Diabetes* 57:2461–2469, 2008.

89. Bu DX, Rai V, Shen X, et al: Activation of the ROCK1 branch of the transforming growth factor beta pathway contributes to RAGE-dependent acceleration of atherosclerosis in diabetic apoE null mice, *Circ Res* 106:1040–1051, 2010.

90. DeWard AD, Eisenmann KM, Matheson SF, et al: The role of formins in human disease, *Biochim Biophys Acta* 2010:226–233, 1803.

91. Hudson BI, Kalea AZ, Del Mar Arriero M, et al: Interaction of the RAGE cytoplasmic domain with diaphanous-1 is required for ligand-stimulated cellular migration through activation of Rac1 and Cdc42, *J Biol Chem* 283:4457–4468, 2008.

92. Touré F, Fritz G, Li Q, et al: Formin mDia1 mediates vascular remodeling via integration of oxidative and signal transduction pathways, *Circ Res* 110:1279–1293, 2012.

93. Xu Y, Toure F, Qu W, et al: Advanced glycation end product (AGE)-receptor for AGE (RAGE) signaling and upregulation of Egr-1 in hypoxic macrophages, *J Biol Chem* 285:23233–23240, 2010.

94. Engelen L, Ferreira I, Gaens KH, et al: The association between the -374 T/A polymorphism of the receptor for advanced glycation endproducts gene and blood pressure and arterial stiffness is modified by glucose metabolism status: the Hoorn and CoDAM studies, *J Hypertens* 28:285–293, 2010.

95. Gaens KH, van der Kallen CJ, van Greevenbroek MM, et al: Receptor for advanced glycation endproduct polymorphisms and type 2 diabetes: the CODAM study, *Ann N Y Acad Sci* 1126:162–165, 2008.

96. Katakami N, Matsuhisa M, Kaneto H, et al: Serum endogenous secretory RAGE level is an independent risk factor for the progression of carotid atherosclerosis in type 1 diabetes, *Atherosclerosis* 204:288–292, 2009.

97. Yang SJ, Kim S, Hwang SY, et al: Association between sRAGE, esRAGE levels and vascular inflammation: analysis with (18)F-fluorodeoxyglucose positron emission tomography, *Atherosclerosis* 220:402–406, 2012.

98. Natarajan R, Putta S, Kato M: MicroRNAs and diabetic complications, *J Cardiovasc Trans Res* 5:413–422, 2012.

99. Shanmugam N, Reddy MA, Natarajan R: Distinct roles of heterogeneous nuclear ribonuclear protein K and microRNA16 in cyclooxygenase-2 RNA stability induced by S100B, a ligand of the receptor for advanced glycation endproducts, *J Biol Chem* 283:36221–36233, 2008.

100. Villeneuve LM, Kato M, Reddy MA, et al: Enhanced levels of microRNA-125b in vascular smooth muscle cells of diabetic db/db mice lead to increased inflammatory gene expression by targeting the histone methyltransferase Suv39h1, *Diabetes* 59:294–295, 2010.

101. Reddy MA, Jin W, Villeneuve L, et al: Pro-inflammatory role of MicroRNA 200 in vascular smooth muscle cells from diabetic mice, *Arterioscler Thromb Vasc Biol* 32:721–729, 2012.

102. Keating ST, El-Osta A: Chromatin modifications associated with diabetes, *J Cardiovasc Transl Res* 5:399–412, 2012.

103. Villeneuve LM, Natarajan R: The role of epigenetics in the pathology of diabetic complications, *Am J Physiol Renal Physiol* 299:F14–F25, 2010.

104. Orimo M, Minamino T, Miyauchi H, et al: Protective role of SIRT1 in diabetic vascular dysfunction, *Arterioscler Thromb Vasc Biol* 29:889–894, 2009.

105. Daida H, Takayama T, Hiro T, et al: High HbA1c levels correlate with reduced plaque regression during statin treatment in patients with stable coronary artery disease: results of the coronary atherosclerosis study measuring effects of rosuvastatin using intravascular ultrasound in Japanese subjects (COSMOS), *Cardiovasc Diabetol* 11:87, 2012.

106. Parathath S, Grauer L, Huang LS, et al: Diabetes adversely affects macrophages during atherosclerotic plaque progression in mice, *Diabetes* 60:1759–1769, 2010.

107. Madonna R, De Caterina R: Cellular and molecular mechanisms of vascular injury in diabetes—Part II: cellular mechanisms and therapeutic targets, *Vasc Pharmacol* 54:75–79, 2011.

108. Galasso G, Schiekofer S, Sato K, et al: Impaired angiogenesis in glutathione peroxidase 1 deficient mice is associated with endothelial progenitor cell dysfunction, *Circ Res* 98:254–261, 2006.

109. Gallagher KA, Liu ZJ, Miao M, et al: Diabetic impairments in NO-mediated endothelial progenitor cell mobilization and homing are reversed by hyperoxia and SDF-1 alpha, *J Clin Invest* 117:1249–1259, 2007.

110. DeFronzo RA: Insulin resistance, type 2 diabetes, lipotoxicity and atherosclerosis: the missing links. The Claude Bernard Lecture, 2009, *Diabetologia* 53:1270–1287, 2010.

111. Hanley AJ, Williams K, Stern MP, et al: Homeostasis model assessment of insulin resistance in relation to the incidence of cardiovascular disease: the San Antonio Heart Study, *Diabetes Care* 25:1177–1184, 2002.

112. Jiang ZY, He Z, King BL, et al: Characterization of multiple signaling pathways of insulin in the regulation of vascular endothelial growth factor expression in vascular cells and angiogenesis, *J Biol Chem* 278:31964–31971, 2003.

113. Bornfeldt KE, Tabas I: Insulin resistance, hyperglycemia and atherosclerosis, *Cell Metab* 14:575–585, 2011.

114. Rask-Madsen C, Li Q, Freund B, et al: Loss of insulin signaling in vascular endothelial cells accelerates atherosclerosis in apolipoprotein E null mice, *Cell Metab* 11:39–389, 2010.

115. Fernandez Hernando C, Jozsef L, Jenkins D, et al: Absence of Akt reduces vascular smooth muscle cell migration and survival and induces features of plaque vulnerability and cardiac dysfunction during atherosclerosis, *Arterioscler Thromb Vasc Biol* 29:2033–2040, 2009.

116. Pfeifle B, Ditschuneit H: Receptors for insulin and insulin like growth factor in cultured arterial smooth muscle cells depend on their growth state, *J Endocrinol* 96:251–257, 1983.

117. Lightell DJ Jr, Moss SC, Woods TC: Loss of canonical insulin signaling accelerates vascular smooth muscle cell proliferation and migration through changes in p27Kip1 regulation, *Endocrinology* 152:651–658, 2011.

118. Baumgartl J, Baudler S, Scherner M, et al: Myeloid lineage cell restricted insulin resistance protects apolipoprotein E deficient mice against atherosclerosis, *Cell Metab* 3:247–256, 2006.

119. Selmon TA, Nadolski MJ, Liao X, et al: Atherogenic lipids and lipoproteins trigger CD36-TLR2-dependent apoptosis in macrophages undergoing endoplasmic reticulum stress, *Cell Metab* 12:467–482, 2010.

120. Rask-Madsen C, Buonomo E, Li Q, et al: Hyperinsulinemia does not change atherosclerosis development in apolipoprotein E null mice, *Arterioscler Thromb Vasc Biol* 32:1124–1131, 2012.

10 Vascular Biology of Atherosclerosis in Patients with Diabetes

Dyslipidemia, Hypercoagulability, Endothelial Dysfunction, and Inflammation

Jorge Plutzky, Barak Zafrir, and Jonathan D. Brown

OVERVIEW

The interaction between diabetes and atherosclerosis is complex and multifactorial. Despite unequivocal evidence for increased cardiovascular disease (CVD) risk in patients with diabetes; a well-documented epidemic of obesity and diabetes; intensive research efforts that include major preclinical scientific progress using unbiased "-omic" approaches; large cardiovascular (CV) outcome studies in diabetes; and new glucose-lowering therapies, the mechanisms that link diabetes to atherosclerosis remain murky. Indeed, challenges in this area begin with simple issues regarding definitions and expand quickly into problems of epistemology. Type 1 diabetes mellitus (T1DM) and type 2 diabetes mellitus (T2DM) differ fundamentally in their root causes, but share increased risk of micro-CVD and macro-CVD as compared with nondiabetic patients. Although these diseases are defined clinically by hyperglycemia, the pathologic picture of T2DM extends beyond glucose. Indeed, recent clinical trial data raise questions regarding whether glucose should be the primary therapeutic target for improving CVD outcomes. Such issues force consideration of other factors in the vascular biology of diabetic atherosclerosis that are outside the glucose-insulin axis discussed in Chapters 1–3.

Although it remains unlikely that one single pathway accounts for how diabetes promotes atherogenesis, atherosclerosis, and atherothrombotic complications, various mediators and pathogenic forces have been uncovered that help explain how the diabetic and even the prediabetic state modulate vascular biology, including specific responses in different cell types (**Fig. 10-1**). Aside from changes in glucose, diabetes is typically characterized by a dyslipidemia involving elevated triglycerides (TGs), lower high-density lipoprotein (HDL) levels, and a low-density lipoprotein (LDL) particle that is more atherogenic.[1–3] Diabetic atherosclerosis involves a prothrombotic state, suggesting basic changes in the coagulation system and its players. Although all cellular components of the arterial wall and

the inflammatory system appear involved in diabetic atherosclerosis, the endothelium and its functional roles have been especially implicated in the natural history of T2DM. Inflammation has arisen as a potential central driver in the pathogenesis of diabetes, atherosclerosis, and their intersection. The breadth of abnormalities, whether molecular or clinical, proposed to play a part in T2DM and atherosclerosis independent of glucose is impressive and beyond the scope of any one summary, especially given ongoing rapid evolution in this area. Here we review key concepts regarding how dyslipidemia, hypercoagulability, endothelial dysfunction, and inflammation alter cellular responses that promote atherosclerosis in the setting of diabetes, with an emphasis on emerging concepts, novel targets, and clinical relevance.

DIABETIC DYSLIPIDEMIA

Type 2 diabetes is characterized by a distinct lipid profile involving LDL cholesterol (LDL-C) levels that are often not particularly elevated, higher TG values, and lower HDL cholesterol (HDL-C) concentrations.[2] Also associated with diabetic dyslipidemia are elevated levels of circulating free fatty acids (FFAs). Often this constellation of lipid abnormalities arises early in T2DM including in prediabetic states, drawing further attention to diabetic dyslipidemia as a contributor to the pathogenesis of diabetic atherosclerosis and its complications.[4] Multiple inputs appear to foster diabetic dyslipidemia. Central adiposity may promote dyslipidemia, including the development of secondary factors such as increased inflammation within the fat, systemically, as well as through higher levels of FFAs.[4] The hypertriglyceridemia of diabetes involves changes in both production and combustion: the hepatic secretion of TG-rich lipoproteins such as very low-density lipoproteins (VLDLs) and altered hydrolysis of these and other TG-rich lipoproteins.[5,6] Yet another potential component of hypertriglyceridemia may

DIABETES AND ATHEROSCLEROSIS

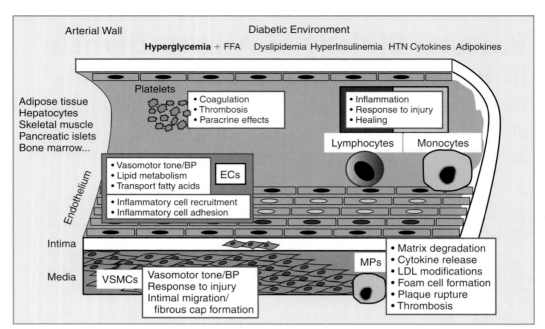

FIGURE 10-1 The arterial wall in diabetes. Although diabetes is defined by hyperglycemia, the key cellular players in the vasculature, such as endothelial cells (ECs) and vascular smooth muscle cells (VSMCs), as well as inflammatory cells including lymphocytes and monocytes and macrophages (MPs) encounter multiple pathogenic inputs in the patient with diabetes, including elevated free fatty acids (FFAs), dyslipidemia, hyperinsulinemia, hypertension (HTN), increased cytokines, and altered adipokine levels. As such, resolving whether diabetic atherosclerosis represents unique pathogenic mechanisms or similar proatherosclerotic responses amplified by these stimuli remains unclear. Central issues related to diabetic atherosclerosis focused on in this chapter are schematized here. The dyslipidemia of diabetes is characterized by elevated triglycerides, decreased high-density lipoprotein (HDL), and low-density lipoproteins (LDLs) that may be smaller, denser, and more pathogenic. Diabetes involves a fundamental shift to a more prothrombotic state, as evident in platelet biology. The endothelium is an integral player in vascular health; endothelial dysfunction often characterizes diabetes and involves both abnormal vasomotor function and also metabolic abnormalities. Inflammatory responses (highlighted in red) appear particularly involved in diabetic atherosclerosis, with inflammatory changes evident in the endothelium and in lymphocytes (T cells, B cells), monocytes, and monocyte-derived macrophages. In addition to these complexities, it is also important to note that atherosclerosis in diabetes is also influenced by "far-field" effects from other organs, including adipocytes and adipose tissue (e.g., adipokines, FFA release), hepatocytes (coagulation factor production, very low-density lipoprotein [VLDL] secretion), skeletal muscle (insulin resistance), pancreatic islets (insulin release), and bone marrow (progenitor cells). BP = Blood pressure.

be postprandial excursions in TG levels, which may be more predictive of CV risk than the fasting levels usually obtained in the clinic.[7-9]

Lipoprotein lipase (LPL), a key enzyme involved in hydrolyzing fatty acids from TGs and delivering these fatty acids to tissues, may be defective in T2DM. It is interesting to note that LPL-mediated hydrolysis of TGs has been shown to be a mechanism for generating natural ligands for the nuclear receptor known as peroxisome proliferator-activated receptor alpha (PPAR-α), which, when activated by ligands, controls the expression of multiple genes involved in lipid metabolism, inflammation, and fatty acid oxidation.[10-13] Fibrates, lipid-lowering agents used to treat hypertriglyceridemia, are thought to work as PPAR-α agonists.[14,15] Of note, other endogenous lipolytic pathways including adipose tissue TG lipase (ATGL) and hepatic lipase as well as fatty acid synthase can generate PPAR ligands in different physiologic contexts as well.[16-18] These lines of evidence suggest that in diabetes, loss of endogenous LPL action decreases activation of the PPAR-α–regulated gene cassette, which would be predicted to result in decreased expression of apolipoprotein (apo) A-I, which is involved in HDL function, and increased endothelial inflammation. It is important to note that fibrates, as synthetic PPAR-α agonists, may not faithfully replicate cellular responses to natural PPAR-α ligands. Of interest, the potential role of LPL has expanded to include other proteins involved in LPL action. For example, C-III is an endogenous inhibitor of LPL activity. Recent studies implicate apo C-III in promoting proatherogenic, proinflammatory responses,

which may occur through various mechanisms, including potential modulation of endogenous PPAR responses as outlined previously as well as other means.[19]

Given that HDL cholesterol levels are inversely associated with coronary heart disease (CHD) risk, significant effort has focused on the mechanisms underlying the low HDL commonly observed in patients with diabetes.[20] Both abnormal production of HDL and remodeling of this lipid by plasma enzymes may contribute to the low level of circulating HDL cholesterol observed in T2DM. Expression and activity of endothelial lipase (EL), a phospholipase that is synthesized in and expressed on the surface of vascular endothelium, catabolizes HDL, resulting in decreased levels of this putatively antiatherogenic lipoprotein. Elevated concentrations of EL protein are significantly correlated with coronary artery calcification score as well as other features of metabolic syndrome including waist circumference, blood pressure, TGs, HDL levels, and fasting glucose in individuals with a family history of premature CHD.[21] In addition, direct correlations have been observed between EL levels and circulating markers of inflammation including high-sensitivity C-reactive protein (hsCRP), interleukin 6 (IL-6), and soluble intercellular adhesion molecule. Low-dose endotoxemia in 20 subjects increased EL concentrations 12 to 16 hours after injection, and this increase in EL correlated with reductions in plasma HDL.[22-24] Collectively these data suggest that low-intensity inflammation, a common feature of T2DM, controls HDL through effects on EL, providing a possible mechanism for the low HDL in T2DM and the exaggerated CV risk associated with insulin-resistant states including metabolic syndrome and diabetes mellitus. Despite the clear epidemiologic inverse association between HDL and CV risk, the hypothesis that raising HDL can reduce CV events has not yet been proven. The recent failure of large randomized, placebo-controlled trials designed to test this hypothesis using cholesteryl ester transfer protein (CETP) inhibitors and niacin, which both raise HDL cholesterol levels, suggests that the biology of HDL's atheroprotective effects are likely very complex and cannot be ascribed exclusively to a single parameter such as HDL cholesterol quantity—the current lipid parameter measured in the clinic.[25,26]

Another input into diabetic dyslipidemia is hepatic dysregulation, itself a consequence of fatty liver, hyperinsulinemia, and hyperglycemia.[27] Hyperglycemia per se can alter the carefully controlled system of lipid metabolism, as, for example, through the glycation of proteins and lipoproteins. In addition to altering the normal function of these entities, the breakdown of glycated proteins and lipoproteins, known as advanced glycation endproducts (AGEs), activates specific receptors for AGEs (RAGEs), resulting in responses closely linked to atherosclerotic complications, such as increases in matrix metalloproteinases (MMPs) thought to promote plaque destabilization and rupture.[28–30]

Although total LDL-C levels are often average in patients with T2DM, LDL continues to appear as a significant predictor of CV risk in this patient population. As is usually seen with higher TG values, LDL particles in T2DM are considered more pathogenic as a result of their being smaller, more dense, and hence more prone to entry, oxidation, and retention in the arterial wall.[31] The notion that lipoprotein retention in the subendothelial space may contribute to atherosclerosis may be especially relevant in diabetes. Extensive evidence implicates the oxidation of LDL as a major player in atherosclerosis. Given that hyperglycemia and other aspects of diabetes may promote altered redox balance and increased oxidative stress, increased LDL oxidation in diabetes may be an additional factor in diabetic atherosclerosis. An intriguing newer direction for this field has been evidence that autoantibodies to oxidized LDL (oxLDL) may be involved in atherosclerosis and coronary calcification, which may extend to diabetes, including T1DM.[32]

Placing lipid metabolism into a broader context, lipoprotein particles can be reconsidered as circulating, biologically active entities whose very nature and function afford systemic pathologic effects. Lipoproteins in various forms exit the liver and interact with the vasculature. In their transit through the circulation, lipoproteins also encounter other factors in addition their interactions with vessel walls, including circulating cells and many other proteins. In this regard, one functional unit with which lipoproteins interact is the coagulation system, including both the relevant procoagulant and anticoagulant proteins as well as platelets. Consistent with this concept, studies have reported increased platelet reactivity and thrombogenicity in response to VLDL and TG-rich lipoproteins. Such interactions connect dysregulated lipid metabolism in diabetes to a potent force in atherosclerosis strongly suggested as being altered in the diabetic milieu, namely the coagulation system.

This brief preceding overview underscores the extent to which pathogenesis in diabetes, including alterations in lipid and cholesterol metabolism, are influenced by diverse, often overlapping issues.

DIABETES: A PROTHROMBOTIC STATE

T2DM is characterized by a prothrombotic and hypercoagulable state that is a significant contributor to the pathogenesis and progression of diabetic vascular complications. Multiple factors have been implicated in promoting the prothrombotic state in diabetes, including platelet hyperreactivity, increased coagulation, and impaired fibrinolysis. Although hyperglycemia itself may be a major factor in these pathways, as noted, other components of the clinical picture in diabetes, such as lipid abnormalities, obesity, and inflammation, as well as more specific pathogenic mechanisms such as oxidative stress may also contribute to the prothrombotic, procoagulant state found in those with diabetes, including changes in platelet function, changes in coagulation factors, and shifts in the fibrinolytic balance, as are considered here.

Altered Platelet Function

Platelets of patients with T2DM are characterized by dysregulation of several signaling pathways, leading to hyperreactive platelets with enhanced adhesion, aggregation, and activation (**Fig. 10-2**). Processes that define the diabetic state—hyperglycemia, insulin resistance, dyslipidemia, inflammation, and increased oxidation— are all implicated in platelet hyperactivity in diabetes. Hyperglycemia increases platelet reactivity by altering different biochemical pathways, including protein kinase C (PKC) activation, with subsequent increased platelet granule release and aggregation.[33,34] Glucose also has direct osmotic effects that can increase platelet reactivity.[35] In addition, by inducing nonenzymatic glycation of proteins on the surface of platelets, hyperglycemic states may decrease membrane fluidity while increasing adhesion and activation.[36] Consistent with these findings, acute hyperglycemia has been shown to increase markers of platelet activation such as P-selectin and CD40 ligand, whereas improved glycemic control may decrease platelet reactivity.[37,38]

Platelet aggregation is mediated by platelet surface receptors and adhesive proteins such as glycoproteins GPIIb/IIIa, GPIb, and P2Y12, each of which is altered in T2DM. Platelet turnover in patients with diabetes appears accelerated. Hyperglycemia increases the release of reticulated, larger, and thus more reactive platelets, including a higher capability of forming thromboxane—a potent vasoconstrictor and proaggregant. Diabetic platelets may also have altered signaling through the P2Y12 pathway, a key player in adhesion, aggregation, and procoagulant activity.[39] Increased levels of circulating microparticles, derived from platelets and various stimulated cell types, may also underlie the procoagulant potential in diabetes.[40] Microparticle size is larger in those with T2DM than in normal controls, and increases in microparticle number have been associated with an increased incidence of diabetic complications.[41]

Intracellular calcium is a central mechanism for regulating platelet function. Platelets in patients with diabetes contain lower cyclic adenosine monophosphate (cAMP) levels and higher intracellular calcium levels than in normal patients, which may contribute to hyperreactivity, increased aggregation and activation, and stimulation of thromboxane synthesis.[42] Altered calcium homeostasis may be in part attributable to changes in the activity of calcium ATPases, which are highly sensitive to oxidative damage.[43,44] Recent

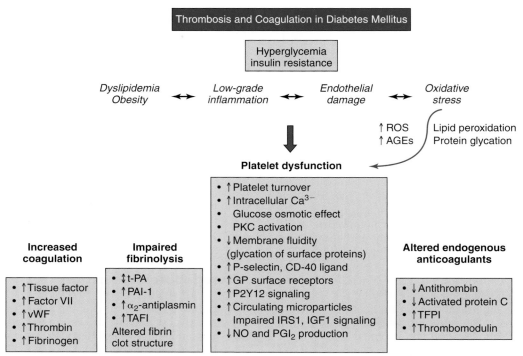

FIGURE 10-2 Abnormal thrombosis and coagulation in diabetes. Many pathologic inputs in diabetes contribute to platelet dysfunction and hypercoagulability, all of which drive a prothrombotic phenotype in patients with diabetes. Hyperglycemia and insulin resistance, a fundamental pathophysiologic feature of diabetes, drives inflammation, dyslipidemia, endothelial dysfunction, and oxidative stress. Each of these stimuli activates platelets by increasing expression of surface receptors for aggregation, increasing production of vasoactive molecules, reducing nitric oxide bioavailability. Simultaneously, production of coagulation factors by ECs including von Willebrand factor (vWF) and tissue factor, along with fibrinogen and factor VII from other sources, enhances coagulation. Lastly, a defect in endogenous fibrinolysis through increased PAI-1 expression tPA all conspire to heighten thrombosis in diabetes. AGEs = Advanced glycation end products; GP = glycoprotein; IGF-1, insulin-like growth factor 1; IRS-1 = insulin substrate receptor 1; NO = nitric oxide; PAI-1 = plasminogen activator inhibitor 1; PGI_2 = prostaglandin I_2; PKC = protein kinase C; ROSs = reactive oxygen species; TAFI = thrombin-activatable fibrinolysis inhibitor; TFPI = tissue factor pathway inhibitor; t-PA = tissue plasminogen activator.

research suggests that activity of calcium-activated proteases (calpains) is increased in platelets from diabetic patients, contributing to dysregulation of platelet calcium signaling and hyperreactivity of platelets.[45]

Insulin resistance and insulin deficiency can both alter platelet reactivity. Insulin opposes the effects of platelet agonists through activation of an inhibitory G protein by insulin receptor substrate 1 (IRS-1). During insulin resistance, impaired insulin receptor signaling attenuates insulin-mediated antagonism of platelet activation, thus increasing platelet reactivity. Insulin-like growth factor 1 (IGF-1), which is present in granules of platelets with IGF-1 receptors present on the platelet surface, stimulates tyrosine phosphorylation of IRS, potentiating platelet activation.[46,47] Reduced insulin sensitivity in platelets lowers cAMP levels and increases intracellular calcium levels, enhancing platelets degranulation and aggregation. In addition, platelets from insulin-resistant patients display diminished sensitivity to the actions of nitric oxide (NO) and prostacyclin while also manifesting significantly lower platelet NO-synthase activity.[48]

As noted, some of the systemic abnormalities often concomitant with diabetes can also alter platelet biology. Hypertriglyceridemia increases platelet reactivity, perhaps in part through apo E.[49] Glycation of LDL particles may also lead to impaired NO production and increased intraplatelet calcium concentration, with subsequent increased platelet hyperreactivity and microparticle formation in diabetic patients.[50] Central obesity appears to promote platelet dysfunction, with reduced platelet sensitivity to insulin, impaired platelet responses to nitrates and prostacyclin,

elevated platelet count and volume, increased cytosolic calcium concentration, and evidence for increased oxidative stress.[51] Furthermore, weight loss reverses some of these changes, reducing platelet activation.[52] Increased platelet reactivity has been tied to increased oxidative stress found in T2DM.[53,54] Superoxide and reactive oxygen species (ROSs) may increase platelet reactivity by enhancing postactivation intraplatelet activation calcium.[44] In addition, lipid peroxidation and protein glycation may affect platelet activation.[55] Inflammation may foster platelet reactivity by increasing expression of mediators of platelet activation, such as CD40 ligand, whose plasma-soluble levels are increased in T2DM. CD40L, found in activated platelets, has proinflammatory properties.[56]

Increased Coagulation Factors

The coagulation system involves a complex cascade of procoagulant proteins that ultimately result in thrombin generation and conversion of fibrinogen to fibrin, and formation of fibrin clots. Increased activation of prothrombotic coagulation factors has been reported in T2DM (see **Fig. 10-2**). For example, tissue factor, expressed by endothelial cells (ECs) and vascular smooth muscle cells (VSMCs), is a potent procoagulant that can initiate the thrombotic process. In healthy individuals, tissue factor synthesis was reported to be inhibited by insulin, with platelets from T2DM patients found to produce more tissue factor than platelets from matched controls.[57] The increased level of circulating tissue factor observed in T2DM has been associated with hyperglycemia and hyperinsulinemia in an additive manner.[58] AGEs, discussed earlier, can contribute to the activation of surface clotting factors.[28] AGEs and ROS can promote tissue factor expression by activating nuclear factor kappa B (NF-κB) transcription factors.

In addition to tissue factor, many other coagulant proteins are implicated in the prothrombotic state of T2DM. Factor VII, which has been associated with increased fatal cardiac events, is elevated in hyperglycemia, insulin resistance, and T2DM.[59,60] Factor VII activity levels in patients with diabetes was shown to be independently associated with hypertriglyceridemia.[61] Factor XIII, activated by thrombin, produces multiple cross-links in the fibrin clot, increasing resistance to lysis. Factor XIII subunit levels were shown to correlate with features of the metabolic syndrome and insulin resistance. In addition, there is some evidence for association between factor XIII polymorphisms and the risk of thrombotic vascular diseases.

Von Willebrand Factor and Fibrinogen

Von Willebrand factor (vWF), which promotes platelet adhesion by binding to the platelet glycoprotein GPIb receptor and is associated with EC damage, has been linked to atherosclerosis and future CV events.[62] vWF levels may be increased in insulin resistance and T2DM. Increased platelet thrombin, which converts fibrinogen to fibrin, has been found in association with hyperglycemia. Thrombin is increased in patients with diabetes, including as a function of glucose control.[37,63] Thus, improved glycemic control may reduce blood thrombogenicity.[64] Fibrinogen, an acute-phase protein that independently predicts future CV events, is elevated in diabetic patients and is associated with microvascular and macrovascular complications.[65-68] Glycemia and insulin resistance correlate with increased fibrinogen levels.[69] Mechanisms that may explain the increased fibrinogen levels observed in T2DM include enhanced fibrinogen production facilitated by hyperinsulinemia and the low-grade inflammation often found in T2DM.[70] IL-6 cytokine levels, which are elevated in T2DM, can stimulate hepatocytes to produce fibrinogen, connecting between inflammation and hypercoagulation. Despite these findings, evidence that improved glycemic control reduces fibrinogen levels remains to be established.[71]

Changes in Endogenous Anticoagulants

The prothrombotic state of T2DM involves not only increases in procoagulants, but also changes in endogenous anticoagulants, such as antithrombin, tissue factor pathway inhibitor (TFPI), protein C, and thrombomodulin, which help maintain the physiologic balance in coagulation. Antithrombin inhibits thrombin by forming a stable complex with thrombin and other coagulation factors, and inhibits factor VII bound to tissue factor. Diabetic patients reportedly have reduced antithrombin anticoagulant activity.[72] Hyperglycemia may also induce conformational changes to antithrombin, leading to its retention and aggregation.[73] Suggested mechanisms of the glucose effects on antithrombin are nonenzymatic glycation and endoplasmic reticulum (ER) stress induced by hyperglycemia.

The endogenous anticoagulant TFPI, produced mainly in ECs and associated with atherosclerosis, inhibits tissue factor–initiated coagulation by binding with activated factor X and modifying the activity of factor VII–tissue factor catalytic complex.[74,75] TFPI circulates primarily bound to lipoproteins in the plasma. Increased levels of atherogenic lipoproteins have been associated with a shift of the tissue factor–TFPI balance toward higher plaque thrombogenicity.[76] Increase in TFPI activity was also demonstrated in patients with T1DM, a hypothesized consequence of increased thrombin formation and altered binding of TFPI to glycosaminoglycans after vascular damage.[77] Other recently identified noncoagulant roles of TFPI, including action in inflammation, angiogenesis, and lipid metabolism, may be associated with vascular damage in diabetes.[78]

Activated protein C (APC), converted from protein C by the action of the thrombin-thrombomodulin complex present on ECs, functions as an anticoagulant by inactivating the coagulation factors V and VIII. APC may also have profibrinolytic activity by inactivating plasminogen activator inhibitor type 1 (PAI-1) in addition to having anti-inflammatory, antioxidant and cytoprotective properties.[79,80] A recent study suggested that low protein C levels are a risk factor for incident ischemic stroke but not CHD.[81] Decreased APC generation has been reported to be associated with progressive atherosclerosis in T2DM.[82]

As noted, thrombomodulin, a membrane protein synthesized predominantly by ECs, is a cofactor for thrombin-mediated activation of protein C, and also reduces procoagulant activities such as fibrinogen clotting, factor V, and platelet activation. Thrombomodulin also exerts important effects that modulate cellular proliferation, adhesion, and inflammation and may serve as a marker for endothelial damage.[83] However, the association between circulating levels of thrombomodulin and incident CHD is controversial.[84,85] In healthy individuals, researchers have demonstrated an inverse association between soluble thrombomodulin levels and risk for future T2DM.[86] However, in patients with T2DM, plasma thrombomodulin levels were increased and positively correlated with the metabolic syndrome.[87] Elevated plasma concentrations of soluble thrombomodulin in T2DM may reflect enhanced hypercoagulability and altered fibrinolysis.[88]

Impaired Fibrinolysis

The maintenance of blood flow involves a coordinated balance between clot formation and clot removal. Fibrinolysis, the process of clot dissolution and removal, involves a cascade of interacting proenzymes and enzymes. Inhibition of fibrinolytic pathways promotes clot formation; shifts in fibrinolytic balance have been strongly implicated in atherothrombosis. Impairment of fibrinolysis has been noted in T2DM, and hypofibrinolysis is a risk factor for the development of CV complications in patients with diabetes.

Changes in glucose concentrations can induce modifications in the fibrin network that promote thrombosis.[89] Fibrin clots in patients with diabetes are altered in structure, with a more compact structure, decreased pore size of the clot matrix itself, and resistance to fibrinolysis, resulting in longer time to clot lysis as compared with healthy controls.[90] Furthermore, improving glycemic control in T2DM has been suggested to result in a more benign clot structure.[91]

The balance between clot formation and dissolution involves important offsetting action between tissue plasminogen activator (t-PA) and PAI-1. t-PA, produced by ECs, mediates the conversion of plasminogen to plasmin and is the main factor responsible for initiating the fibrinolytic process. PAI-1 regulates fibrinolysis by binding to t-PA, blocking the conversion of plasminogen into active plasmin, and thus inhibiting fibrinolysis. It is interesting to note that PAI-1 is also produced by adipocytes, making it of obvious significance as a potential link between diabetic adiposity and CVD. In general, both t-PA and PAI-1 are linked to increased risk of CV events as well as a worse postevent prognosis,[92,93] although this issue is not without controversy.[94] PAI-1 is elevated in insulin-resistant states, correlates strongly with components of the metabolic syndrome, and may predict future T2DM.[95,96] Hyperglycemia and hyperinsulinemia, by increasing expression and activation of proinflammatory forces such as the transcription factor NF-κB as well as PAI-1, reduce the activity of t-PA and shift fibrinolytic balance toward thrombosis. Glucose-lowering effects have been reported to reduce PAI-1 levels.[97]

Although t-PA, and its relationship with PAI-1 are critically important to the thrombotic state, other endogenous anticoagulants have also been suggested as contributing to increased atherothrombosis in diabetes. For example, thrombin-activatable fibrinolysis inhibitor (TAFI) is a proenzyme activated by the thrombin-thrombomodulin complex. TAFI inhibits fibrinolysis by cleaving lysine residues on fibrin, thus preventing t-PA and plasminogen binding. Increased plasma TAFI levels were reported in insulin resistance and T2DM patients.[98,99] However, studies report inconsistent results regarding the role of TAFI levels and activation in thrombosis, especially in coronary artery disease.[100] Alpha$_2$-antiplasmin is the main physiologic inhibitor of plasmin. Elevated alpha$_2$-antiplasmin levels may correlate with the risk of myocardial infarction (MI).[101] Moreover, generation of plasmin–alpha$_2$-antiplasmin complex, which reflects reactive fibrinolysis, was shown to be associated with subclinical atherosclerosis and incidence of coronary disease in small studies.[102–104] Nevertheless, the role of alpha$_2$-antiplasmin in the risk of arterial thrombosis remains unresolved. Limited studies suggest the possibility of changes in alpha$_2$-antiplasmin in T2DM. In general, global assessment of whole plasma fibrinolytic potential may provide stronger evidence linking fibrinolysis to arterial thrombosis than separate evaluation of individual fibrinolytic factors, with further such studies needed in T2DM[105] (**Table 10-1**).

ENDOTHELIAL FUNCTION AND DYSFUNCTION IN DIABETES

It is worthwhile noting that the processes of coagulation and lipid metabolism discussed here, with their elaborate, carefully controlled steps that are altered in T2DM, are carried out to a significant extent on the endothelial surface. A central tenet of our evolved view of the vasculature and atherosclerosis is that the endothelium is not a simple platform but rather a dynamic, reactive organ engaged in endocrine, paracrine, and autocrine function. Given its anatomic position in the vasculature, the single-cell-thick endothelium, which lines the entire vascular tree, can be understood as a transducer of components of the circulation, including circulating mediators of risk such as glucose, FFAs, and pathogenic lipoproteins. As the physical barrier separating flowing blood from the vessel wall, the endothelium is uniquely positioned to control homeostatic processes including blood pressure, hemostasis, and homing of immune cells to sites of inflammation. When dysregulated, all of these processes can contribute to the development of atherosclerosis and have been especially implicated in diabetic atherosclerosis (**Table 10-2**). In this context, it is especially significant to note studies that suggest abnormal endothelial responses among the earliest precursor abnormalities found in seemingly healthy individuals ultimately destined to develop diabetes. For example, in one clinical study, flow-mediated endothelium-dependent vasodilation (EDV) was 38% lower in patients with a family history of T2DM in both parents (+FH) versus those with no family history of diabetes.[106] Of importance, the +FH group did not carry a diagnosis of diabetes, although fasting blood sugar was somewhat higher (5.3 versus 4.9 mmol/L).

The control of vascular resistance by the endothelium is essential for maintaining mean arterial pressure and for autoregulating flow regionally to different tissues depending on metabolic demands. ECs synthesize NO from L-arginine by the action of the Ca^{2+}-dependent, endothelial-specific nitric oxide synthase isoform (eNOS) in response to changes in blood flow.[107] Once formed, NO activates soluble guanylate cyclase located in adjacent VSMCs, leading to increased cyclic guanosine monophosphate (cGMP) levels, smooth muscle cell (SMC) relaxation, and functional vasodilation. This process is dependent on intact vascular endothelium and is a defining feature of normal endothelial function (**Fig. 10-3**).[108,109] As discussed later, endothelial dysfunction, among the earliest features of atherosclerosis and especially diabetic atherosclerosis, manifests as loss of flow-mediated vasodilation, which can be measured noninvasively by brachial artery ultrasound. ECs produce other important vasoactive mediators, including prostacyclin and endothelium-derived hyperpolarizing factor (EDHF), that couple tissue blood flow to metabolic demands. In response to stimuli including proinflammatory cytokines, the vascular endothelium also elaborates vasoconstrictors including endothelin-1, angiotensin II, thromboxane A$_2$, and isoprostanes that increase vascular tone, permeability, hemostasis, and inflammation. The balance of these vasodilator and vasoconstrictor factors is pivotal for maintaining arteriolar resistance and establishing mean arterial blood

TABLE 10-1 Impaired Fibrinolysis in Diabetes

FIBRINOLYTIC FACTORS	FUNCTION	IMPAIRMENT IN DIABETES	POSSIBLE UNDERLYING MECHANISMS FOR IMPAIRED FIBRINOLYSIS
t-PA	Clot lysis (converts plasminogen to plasmin)	↓	Endothelial cell dysfunction (t-PA)
PAI-1	Inhibition of clot lysis (binding to t-PA, blocking the conversion of plasminogen into plasmin)	↑	Inflammatory response Protein glycation (plasminogen)
TAFI	Cleaves lysine residues on fibrin, preventing t-PA and plasminogen binding	↑	Hyperglycemia and insulin resistance
Alpha$_2$-antiplasmin	Physiologic inhibitor of plasmin	↑	Increased secretion by adipocytes (PAI-1) Altered clot structure, ↓ pore size, ↑ clot-lysis time

TABLE 10-2 Resident Vascular Cells, Cells of Innate and Adaptive Immunity, and the Pathways and Mediators Dysregulated in the Diabetic State

VASCULAR CELL	PATHWAYS	MEDIATORS	REFERENCES
Endothelium	Leukocyte trafficking Vascular reactivity Inflammation Metabolism Redox signaling Biomechanical forces Apoptosis Thrombosis and fibrinolysis	E-selectin P-selectin VCAM-1 ICAM-1 NF-κB eNOS, nitric oxide EDHF FoxO PPAR-γ, PPAR-α SOD PAI-1, t-PA Thrombomodulin vWF Tissue factor	107, 111, 119, 124, 125, 136, 144, 190
VSMCs	Inflammation Vascular reactivity Matrix remodeling Proliferation and migration	iNOS, nitric oxide MCP-1 IL-6 TGF-β Collagen MMPs PDGF	169–171, 191, 192
Monocyte/Mφ	Inflammation NLRP3 inflammasome Matrix remodeling Autophagy ER stress, UPR Lipid transport	IL-6 TNF-α IL-1β MMP COX-2 Toll-like receptors CHOP/caspase/JNK PPAR-α, PPAR-γ, PPAR-δ FABPs	156, 161, 164, 189, 193, 194
Lymphocyte	Inflammation T and B cell proliferation Autoimmunity	IFN-γ IL-17 LDL autoantibodies	32, 130
Platelet	Thrombosis Microparticles	Nitric oxide Thromboxane A_2 IGF-1 Calpains P-selectin Protein kinase C P2Y12	39, 47, 49, 56, 57, 68, 85, 195

Endothelial dysfunction, a seminal event in diabetic atherogenesis, involves loss of nitric oxide and proinflammatory gene expression including adhesion molecule expression that promotes leukocyte homing to nascent plaque. Activation of master transcription factors including NF-κB, PPAR-γ, and Forkheads (FoxO) by glucose, lipoproteins, FFAs, and insulin drive this phenotypic change that encompasses endothelial dysfunction. Vascular smooth muscle cells proliferate and secrete matrix proteins in response to the same stimuli in diabetes, enlarging the neointima. Monocyte recruitment through chemokines such as MCP-1 leads to macrophage foam cell formation in the growing plaque. Emerging literature has demonstrated an important role for autophagy and ER stress responses in regulating macrophage inflammation, apoptosis, and plaque stability in atherosclerosis. Finally, lymphocytes are primed to produce autoantibodies and secrete proinflammatory cytokines including IFN-γ that worsen plaque inflammation. Patients with diabetes also have higher thrombosis risk. Platelet dysfunction occurs through activation of multiple pathways including calpains, PKC, IGF-1 and enhanced production of vasoconstrictor lipids such as thromboxane. CHOP = C/EBP homologous protein; COX-2 = cyclooxygenase 2; EDHF = endothelium-derived hyperpolarizing factor; eNOS = endothelial isoform of nitric oxide synthase; ER = endoplastic reticulum; FABPs = fatty acid binding proteins; ICAM-1 = intercellular adhesion molecule-1; IFN-γ = interferon gamma; iNOS = inducible macrophage-type nitric oxide synthase; JNF = c-Jun N-terminal kinase; MCP-1 = monocyte chemoattractant protein 1; NLRP3 = Nod-like receptor protein 3; PDGF = platelet derived growth factor; SOD = superoxide dismutase; TGF-β, transforming growth factor beta; TNF-α = tumor necrosis factor alpha; UPR = unfolded protein response; VCAM-1 = vascular adhesion molecule-1; VSMCs = vascular smooth muscle cells.

pressure. NO also reduces platelet aggregation and leukocyte adhesion, thereby suppressing endogenous thrombus formation, maintaining blood rheology, and suppressing leukocyte accumulation in the vessel wall. As discussed further later, extensive evidence implicates shifts in all these components of normal endothelial function in the setting of diabetes and its associated abnormalities.

In addition to helping control vascular homeostasis, the endothelium also plays a part in host response to inflammation by regulating leukocyte trafficking to sites of injury. Proinflammatory signals including interleukin 1-beta (IL-1β), tumor necrosis factor α (TNF-α), and oxLDL induce EC expression of genes involved in leukocyte homing and diapedesis, a multistep and orchestrated process collectively known as the *leukocyte adhesion cascade*. The induction of specific endothelial gene networks, composed of key mediators of leukocyte adhesion such as E-selectin, P-selectin, vascular adhesion molecule-1 (VCAM-1), and intercellular adhesion molecule-1 (ICAM-1), along with chemoattractants such as IL-8 and monocyte chemoattractant protein 1 (MCP-1), coordinate each aspect of leukocyte rolling, firm adhesion to ECs, and transmigration into the vessel wall.[110] The ability of neutrophils, monocytes, and lymphocytes to home to local areas of inflammation is vital to host defense during acute inflammatory responses. However, this endothelial activation becomes maladaptive in chronic states of inflammation, such as encountered in atherosclerosis and in particular perhaps diabetic atherosclerosis, enabling monocytes or other immune cells to accumulate within the vessel wall and propagate

AORTIC RING PREPARATION

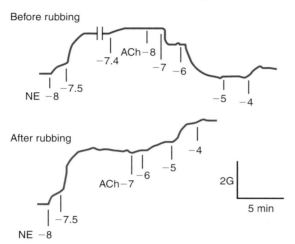

FIGURE 10-3 Endothelial-dependent vasodilation and the importance of endothelial function. Pioneering work by Furchgott and colleagues identified the critical importance of endothelial cells, the single-cell-thick layer lining the vascular tree, in maintenance of vasomotor tone. Serendipitously, these investigators discovered that acetylcholine treatment of isolated aortic rings isolated from rabbit induced vasodilation or vasoconstriction depending on whether the intimal cell layer was intact or accidentally rubbed off during the tissue preparation. This observation identified a novel role for endothelium, at the time considered only a passive cell layer, and also ushered in a new era in vascular biology and led to the eventual discovery of nitric oxide—a key regulator of vascular homeostasis. Now, the vascular endothelium is understood to be a dynamic organ that regulates (1) vascular tone, (2) inflammatory responses through recruitment of leukocytes to sites of injury including in atherosclerosis, (3) nutrient availability for metabolically active tissues such as fat and muscle, (4) resident vascular cell proliferation, and (5) thrombosis and platelet aggregation. Endothelial dysfunction is one of the earliest features of diabetic (and nondiabetic) atherosclerosis and can be measured noninvasively with brachial artery ultrasound, or invasively with acetylcholine (Ach) infusion during coronary artery angiography. Normal endothelial function results in vasodilation after Ach, whereas endothelial dysfunction results in paradoxical vasoconstriction. More recent work suggests that endothelial function may more broadly encompass regulation of systemic metabolic responses including fatty acid transport and adiposity. NE = Norepinephrine. *(From Furchgott RF, Zawadzki JV: The obligatory role of endothelial cells in the relaxation of arterial smooth muscle by acetylcholine,* Nature *288:373-376, 1980.)*

atherosclerotic plaque as well as plaque rupture. Most of the abnormalities associated with T2DM—hyperglycemia, elevated FFAs, hypertriglyceridemia, hypertension—have all been linked to an activated endothelial state.

A major factor promoting insight into the role of the endothelium in atherosclerosis as well as diabetic atherosclerosis has been the ability to measure endothelial function, either invasively in the cardiac catheterization laboratory or noninvasively with techniques such as brachial artery ultrasound. These techniques build on the seminal observations that after removal of just the endothelium in arterial preparations, the normal vasodilatory response to substances such as acetylcholine became paradoxical, resulting in vasoconstriction.[108] Quantitative coronary angiography can document the change in vascular diameter in response to acetylcholine (or bradykinin, substance P, or serotonin). In patients with endothelial dysfunction, the vasodilator response to acetylcholine is blunted, or results in paradoxical vasoconstriction. In brachial artery ultrasound, forearm blood flow is occluded for 5 minutes with use of a sphygmomanometer, maintained at constant pressure. After release of the cuff, reactive hyperemia ensues, leading to endothelium-dependent, flow-mediated NO production and vasodilation, measured by an increase in artery diameter on ultrasound. In patients with endothelial dysfunction, these responses are severely blunted.

Endothelial dysfunction is a defining feature of early atherosclerosis in diabetic patients and also occurs in the presence of other traditional CV risk factors such as hypertension and hyperlipidemia.[111,112] Mechanistically, endothelial dysfunction results from a loss of NO bioavailability, which can occur through impaired production by eNOS or increased degradation. As a consequence, the atheroprotective effects of NO including vasodilation, inhibition of thrombosis or aggregation, and suppression of leukocyte adhesion to the vessel wall are lost. There are multiple metabolic derangements common to T2DM and metabolic syndrome including insulin resistance, hyperglycemia, high circulating FFA levels, and elevated levels of ROSs that all contribute to loss of NO and endothelial dysfunction in patients with diabetes.[113,114] The specific role of hyperglycemia and insulin resistance in vascular function is discussed elsewhere. The infusion of FFAs reduces EDV in animal models and in humans.[115] FFAs activate PKC, driving signal transduction pathways that reduce NO production by eNOS.[116] The accumulation of lipids in tissues and cells including FFAs, fatty acyl-coenzyme As, and others such as diacylglycerols is termed *lipotoxicity* because of the effect these lipid mediators have on intracellular signal transduction pathways including insulin. Another major cause of reduced NO bioavailability is the formation of peroxynitrite (ONOO−) through the reaction of NO with superoxide anion. High intracellular FFAs result in uncoupling of fatty acid oxidation, which increases levels of free radicals such as superoxide anion (O_2^-). Normally, superoxide is rapidly removed by scavenging enzymes such as superoxide dismutase. When superoxide anion levels rise, as occurs in patients with diabetes in response to elevated FFAs and hyperglycemia, peroxynitrite is formed nonenzymatically at high levels. Other enzymes that increase superoxide, including nicotinamide adenine dinucleotide phosphate, reduced form (NADPH) oxidases and xanthine oxidase, can also indirectly promote formation of peroxynitrite in the setting of diabetes. Once generated, peroxynitrite fosters endothelial dysfunction and vascular disease in several postulated ways.[117–119] Peroxynitrite can trigger apoptosis and cell death in ECs and VSMCs, induce endothelial adhesion molecule expression, and disrupt the endothelial glycocalyx. In addition, peroxynitrite-dependent oxidation of tetrahydrobiopterin, a critical cofactor for eNOS function, uncouples eNOS, leading to production of superoxide instead of NO.[120,121] Lastly, ROSs can enhance proinflammatory gene expression leading to endothelial activation (**Fig. 10-4**).

Alterations in NO bioavailability and the increased nitrosative stress in the form of greater peroxynitrite production and protein nitrosylation contribute to macrovascular disease in diabetes.[122] Increased nitrotyrosine levels are detectable in the plasma of diabetic patients.[123] Levels of nitrotyrosine correlate with cell death in ECs. Neutralization of peroxynitrite improves endothelial dysfunction in murine models of diabetes.

Recent preclinical work also provides another perspective on endothelial dysfunction, namely that this dysfunction may extend beyond altered vasomotor function to also include changes in metabolism. Several recent studies have reported pathways that when altered result in changes in glucose and FFA handling. For example, a loss of PPAR-γ in the endothelium changes lipid metabolism, FFA levels, and adiposity with concomitant changes in diabetes.[124] Other work finds that regulation of insulin receptor adaptor

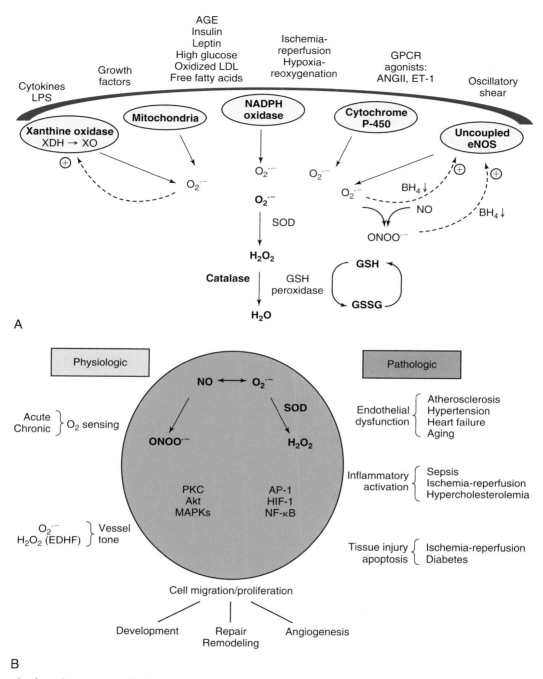

FIGURE 10-4 The role of reactive oxygen species in endothelial dysfunction. **A,** Multiple inputs including proinflammatory cytokines, growth factors, and metabolites elevated in T2D including free fatty acids and glucose can lead to production of superoxide anion ($O_2^{\cdot-}$). **B,** Superoxide anion reacts with nitric oxide (NO), reducing NO bioavailability and leading to alterations in vascular tone, endothelial adhesion, angiogenesis, and cell viability. ANGII = Angiotensin II; AP-1 = Activator protein 1; ET-1 = endothelin 1; GPCR = g-protein coupled receptor; GSH peroxidase = monomeric glutathione; GSSG = glutathione disulfide; HIF-1 = hypoxia-induced factor-1; LPS = lipopolysaccharide; MAPKs = mitogen activated protein kinase; XDH = xanthine dehydrogenase; XO = xanthine oxidase. *(From Li and Shah; AJP Regulatory, Integrative and Comparative Physiology 287:R1014-R1030, 2004.)*

proteins in the endothelium (IRS1 and IRS2) by the Forkhead box proteins (FoxO), a family of DNA binding transcription factors that regulate expression of genes involved in growth, proliferation, and metabolism, can mediate atherogenesis. In these studies, deletion of the three genes encoding FoxO isoforms conditionally in the endothelium protects against atherosclerosis while also promoting hepatic insulin resistance.[125,126] These and other studies, by establishing a role for ECs directly in metabolism, force a broader definition of what endothelial dysfunction might represent. Furthermore, these observations link to clinical studies identifying changes in the endothelium as an early and important part of diabetes and not just diabetic atherosclerosis.

Endothelial Adhesion and Inflammation

Endothelial dysfunction is also associated with increased adhesiveness of the endothelium. Indeed, the induction of vascular cell adhesion molecule 1 (VCAM1) messenger RNA (mRNA) and VCAM-1 protein in vascular ECs is one of the earliest molecular events in experimental models of atherosclerosis such as the Watanabe heritable hyperlipidemic rabbit.[127,128] In humans, adhesion molecule expression can also be detected in atherosclerotic plaque, and circulating levels of soluble adhesion molecules such as VCAM-1 and ICAM-1 positively predict future risk of CVD, as also suggested in T2DM.[129] Aortic endothelium from genetic models of hyperlipidemia such as the LDL receptor null mouse supports greater leukocyte rolling and firm adhesion of leukocytes as determined by mononuclear cell adhesion assays versus aortas from animals with normal lipid levels.[130] Diabetes is associated with activation of the vascular endothelium resulting in enhanced leukocyte adhesion.[131] In diabetes, this activation of the endothelium occurs as a result of many forces including reduced NO bioavailability and the chronic proinflammatory state within the vasculature. Recent work identifies Toll-like receptors (TLRs) as proteins on the surface of ECs and macrophages that bind circulating FFAs and propagate signal transduction cascades that promote proinflammatory gene expression.[132–134] The master transcription factor, NF-κB, mediates multiple proinflammatory responses including those in the endothelium, enhancing expression of adhesion molecules and chemoattractant cytokines, or chemokines, that call monocytes to sites of injury.[135,136] Chemokines such as MCP-1 have been strongly implicated as integral signals in atherosclerosis and diabetic atherosclerosis. Thus, one can understand endothelial activation as enabling a series of steps in response to injury—whether as a result of hyperglycemia, elevated FFAs, hypertension, smoking, or other noxious stimuli—that promote multiple steps of leukocyte trafficking into the vessel wall.[136] In other settings, such responses are integral to host defenses and healing; in the setting of atherosclerosis, such important responses may ultimately prove maladaptive. The influx of leukocytes including monocytes and lymphocytes increases plaque cellularity. Lipid-laden macrophages, termed *foam cells*, phagocytose necrotic cells and free cholesterol in the vessel wall, forming the characteristic atherosclerotic plaque and promoting plaque disruption.[137] Aside from these classic models of atherogenesis, loss of the ECs, known as *superficial erosion*, has been identified as another pathologic mechanism that can also lead to atherosclerotic plaque formation and its complications.[138,139]

Hemodynamic Forces

Early atherosclerotic lesions, known as "fatty streaks," typically form at branch points in the aorta. These regions are characterized by a disturbed blood flow profile that is distinct from the physiologic laminar shear stress in other regions of the aorta. Silver staining of aortic endothelium has revealed that the ECs at these branch points appear irregular in shape, whereas ECs from other regions align in the direction of blood flow. Pioneering research using flow models to study vascular endothelium in vitro has revealed that shear stress forces not only alter EC shape, but also modulate EC gene expression, with the identification of gene regulatory regions modulated in response to distinct patterns of flow.[140] Exposure of static monolayers of cultured ECs to physiologic levels of shear stress results in dynamic induction of genes known to suppress atherogenesis including eNOS, superoxide dismutase, catalase, and TGF-β signaling molecules.[141,142] ECs exposed to disturbed, nonlaminar shear stress fail to express these atheroprotective gene

programs. In addition to regulating NO bioavailability by eNOS and the enzymes involved in reducing ROS generation (superoxide dismutase aka SOD, catalase), shear stress also alters NF-κB tissue levels and activation. Confocal microscopy has demonstrated that lesion-prone regions of the aorta, including branch points, are associated with higher levels of nuclear localized, active NF-κB in the endothelium.[143] In addition, the NF-κB–dependent transcriptional responses at these branch points are significantly higher when stimulated by low-level, proinflammatory stimuli, including factors common in patients with diabetes.[143] Enhanced inflammatory signaling through altered NF-κB activation and loss of NO results in heightened endothelial activation and contributes to the endothelial dysfunction observed in early diabetic atherosclerosis. Collectively, these studies reveal that hemodynamic forces have broad effects on endothelial function and inflammation that contribute to the early atherosclerotic plaque formation. Given the frequency of hypertension in T2DM, many of these mechanisms are activated, if not augmented, in patients with diabetes.

INFLAMMATION: A UNIFYING HYPOTHESIS OF DIABETES AND ATHEROSCLEROSIS?

Although early epidemiologic studies identified risk factors associated with CVD (now considered "traditional"), the mechanisms by which hypertension, cigarette smoking, hypercholesterolemia, and T2DM directly promote atherosclerosis remain intensively investigated.[144] By some estimates, 35% of patients may have clinically significant atherosclerosis in the absence of traditional risk factors.[145] Furthermore, despite treatment with maximal medical therapy, patients recovering from an acute coronary syndrome have substantial residual risk of recurrent events.[146] These and other similar observations have stimulated interest in identifying common as well as additional mechanisms driving atherosclerosis in general as well as in the setting of diabetes.

Considerable evidence now points to chronic, low-grade inflammation as a factor in initiating and perpetuating atherothrombosis as well as diabetes itself. For example, in the Physicians' Health Study (N = 22,000 men) and the Women's Health Study (N = 38,000), the relative risk of future MI, stroke, and CV death in these otherwise healthy individuals at baseline was linearly associated with hsCRP across the normal range of hsCRP values (≤3 mg/L).[147,148] Furthermore, this relationship was evident even after other risk factors were controlled for. Similar findings have since been validated in other large cohorts, with only a few controversial exceptions. Other circulating inflammatory biomarkers including IL-6, MMP-9, pentraxin-3, and lipoprotein-associated phospholipase A_2 (Lp-PLA$_2$) and soluble adhesion molecules have demonstrated similar results for predicting CVD risk, albeit with different magnitudes and variable usefulness as clinical tools.[129,149] These results suggest that the clinical observations regarding hsCRP may reflect inflammatory responses in the vasculature. Important to our focus here, hsCRP has also been suggested to be associated with future risk of diabetes. Inflammatory changes have been found in adipose tissue and pancreatic beta cells as well as in other settings that may relate to insulin resistance and beta cell failure.[150]

Notably, infiltration of visceral adipose tissue by macrophages and other leukocytes has been shown to contribute to the systemic proinflammatory state observed in diabetes. Moreover, studies with salicylates, thiazolidinediones, and other agents have raised the question regarding whether treating inflammation can improve the course of diabetes itself.[151] This convergence between diabetes and atherosclerosis around inflammation suggests this as a potentially central component of the common soil long proposed to link diabetes with atherosclerosis and a mechanism worthy of further attention.

Multiple lines of evidence have demonstrated that inflammatory signaling is relevant for the pathobiology of atherosclerosis in T2DM. In a cross-sectional study of 48 patients with T1DM and 66 nondiabetic patients from the Diabetes Control and Complications Trial (DCCT), higher levels of acute-phase proteins including alpha$_1$-acid glycoprotein (53.5 versus 40.0 mg/dL) and hsCRP (0.23 versus 0.14 mg/dL) were found in those with diabetes.[152] No correlation was found between the acute-phase proteins and other demographic, clinical, or laboratory variables including blood cholesterol. The proinflammatory markers such as soluble ICAM-1 and soluble TNF-α receptors (sTNF-α-Rs) are elevated in T2DM. Inflammatory biomarkers measured in DCCT including soluble intercellular adhesion molecule-1 (sICAM-1) sICAM-1 and sVCAM-1 were also found to decrease after intensive glycemic control over a 3-year period.[153] In the case of hsCRP, there was a more complex effect based on change in body weight during the study, suggesting that the effects of glycemic control on inflammation are complex and can be influenced by body weight. Ultimately, from the perspective of vascular biology, the evidence for inflammation as a force contributing to diabetic atherosclerosis can be pursued in terms of specific responses among relevant cellular players including monocytes and macrophages, lymphocytes, VSMCs, and ECs (discussed earlier). The importance of statin therapy in diabetic vascular disease risk reduction is reflected in the most recent ACC/AHA guidelines that identify individuals aged 40–75 with diabetes mellitus and LDL cholesterol between 70–189 mg/dL, but without clinical manifestations of atherosclerotic vascular disease as candidates for treatment with at least moderate if not high intensity (if calculated 10 year risk is greater than or equal to 7.5%) statin. This issue will be addressed in more detail in subsequent chapters.[153a]

Monocyte and Macrophages

Endothelial dysfunction and low-grade inflammation drive the recruitment of monocytes into the vessel wall.[136] Monocyte differentiation into macrophages enables these phagocytes to begin engulfing cholesterol, forming foam cells and the characteristic fatty streak. Formation of foam cells leads to further inflammation within the vessel wall that amplifies initial proatherogenic signals emanating from ECs, circulating monocytes, and lesional macrophages. Notably, the presence of diabetes has been shown to increase peripheral blood monocyte count.[154] Furthermore, in humans with T1DM, circulating levels of monocyte-derived, proinflammatory cytokines are elevated. For example, as compared with controls, TNF-α, IL-6, IL-1β, and IL-1α serum levels have all been shown to be increased.[155] Other proinflammatory biomarkers including hsCRP, sICAM-1, sE-selectin, and sP-selectin are also

elevated. Monocytes isolated from human patients with T1DM spontaneously secrete the proinflammatory cytokines IL-1β, IL-6, and TNF-α, which corresponds to increases in gene expression of these molecules.[156] Monocytes isolated from those with diabetes and co-cultured with lymphocytes induced greater levels of IL-17–positive lymphocytes, a population of proinflammatory cells involved in vascular inflammation.[156] Monocytes from patients with diabetes also secrete greater levels of inflammatory cytokines such as IL-6 in response to model stimuli such as lipopolysaccharide (LPS). In this cohort, there was no correlation of levels of CRP, adhesion molecules, and monocyte function with body mass index (BMI) or glycemic control, as measured by hemoglobin A1c or plasma glucose level.

Although monocytes typically constitute only 5% to 10% of circulating leukocytes, they are considered critical determinants of atherosclerosis. Moreover, there exists significant phenotypic heterogeneity within this cell population.[154] In humans, classically activated monocytes (M1 cells) are positive for the surface marker CD14 and negative for CD16 (also known as FcγRIII). M1 cells represent 90% of the entire monocyte pool. Alternatively, activated macrophages (M2 cells) are both CD14 and CD16 positive and serve a posited anti-inflammatory role in tissue patrolling and inflammation resolution. These two monocyte populations also differ in chemokine receptor expression. The CD14+/CD16− express high levels of C-C motif chemokine receptor 2 (CCR2), the receptor for MCP-1, whereas the CD16+ monocytes express low levels of CCR2, high levels of CCR5, and high levels of the fractalkine receptor CX3CR1. Analogous populations of mouse monocytes have been defined based on the level of the cell surface marker Ly6C. Ly-6Chigh cells correspond to CD14+/CD16− monocytes, whereas Ly-6Clow cells correspond to human CD14+/CD16+ monocytes. Notably, in murine models of atherosclerosis, such as the apo E–deficient mouse, exposure to a high-cholesterol diet over time results in expansion of the proinflammatory Ly-6Chigh monocyte pool.[157] These monocytes preferentially expand in number and home to atherosclerotic plaque. In terms of diabetes, Ly-6Chigh monocytosis is also associated with obesity-induced adipose tissue infiltration of Ly-6Chigh macrophages, which may contribute to the proinflammatory state associated with metabolic syndrome and diabetes. Direct connections among diabetic-associated vascular dysfunction, atherosclerosis, and monocyte-subsets in these animal models have not yet been made. However, in humans with diabetes and known vascular complications, the circulating levels of CD16+ monocytes are reduced. The importance of this finding is unclear as it relates to atherosclerosis pathogenesis in diabetes but continues to be pursued.

The role of specific monocyte subsets in diabetic macrovascular disease remains an active area of study. In murine models of T1DM, peritoneal macrophages elicited in response to thioglycolate injections demonstrate increased mRNA expression of proinflammatory mediators including TNF-α, IL-1β, prostaglandin- endoperoxide synthase 2 (TPGS2), and cyclooxygenase 2 (COX-2).[158,159] The effect on PTGS2 implicates long-chain fatty acids, and eicosanoids in particular, as potentially important sources of immunomodulation of monocytes and other vascular cells. Indeed, an important relationship between fatty acid signaling and monocyte activation exists in diabetes. TLRs, primitive pattern recognition receptors that activate proinflammatory signal transduction cascades through NF-κB, can be activated by long-chain fatty acids. There is a twofold induction of cell surface TLR expression in peritoneal macrophages 6 weeks after induction of diabetes in mice, with lesser effects on TLR4 expression.[134] These peritoneal macrophages also demonstrate greater activation of NF-κB. Knockout of TLR2 abrogates almost all the augmentation in NF-κB activity. Similarly, levels of proinflammatory cytokines IL-1β, IL-6, MCP-1, and TNF-α are elevated in diabetic macrophages compared with nondiabetic cells, and TLR2 knockout significantly attenuates this induction. Altered PTGS2 expression along with the enzyme long-chain acyl-CoA synthetase (ACSL1) from mouse monocytes with T1DM correlates with increased levels of prostaglandin E_2 (PGE_2). In addition, $CD14^+$ monocytes from human patients with T1DM also demonstrated elevated levels of ACSL1 mRNA.[155] In M1 activated murine macrophages derived from bone marrow–derived monocytes, or human monocyte–derived macrophages (induced with LPS and interferon gamma [IFN-γ]), *ACSL1* gene expression is significantly induced as well. Notably, ACSL1 deficiency reduced the release of proinflammatory cytokines from LPS-stimulated macrophages isolated from diabetic mice.[158] ACSL1 deficiency in bone marrow reduced diabetes-associated atherosclerosis and monocyte accumulation in the vessel wall in low-density lipoprotein receptor (LDLr) deficient mice, suggesting that ACSL1 plays a specific role in monocyte recruitment and activation in experimental diabetic atherosclerosis. Whether this effect relates to altered PGE_2 production has not been proven, but it suggests that alterations in eicosanoid handling can influence diabetic atherosclerosis through changes in monocyte inflammatory activation.

Other drivers of inflammation and atherosclerosis relevant to diabetes are also under study. The activity of plasma and cell-surface enzymes, including Lp-PLA$_2$, can generate proinflammatory metabolites derived from oxidized phospholipids, a phenomenon that is being exploited as a candidate therapeutic target in prospective clinical trials.[160] Oxidatively modified lipoproteins and oxidized lipid constituents, and their impact on monocyte-macrophage biology and circulating antibodies, continue to received attention in general and also with regard to diabetes.[32] Autophagy—the process through which cells engulf and consumes themselves—has been invoked as a novel inflammatory mechanism in macrophages, influencing issues such as monocyte subtypes.[137,161] It is interesting to note that autophagy has also been raised as an important pathway in myocyte and cardiac myocyte biology. Another mechanism that has received increasing attention as a potential factor underlying diabetes and atherosclerosis is the notion of ER stress.[162–164] The ER is integral to the metabolism of proteins, lipids, and glucose, playing a part in lipoprotein secretion and other basic cellular processes. As such, the data identifying a role for ER stress in diabetes and atherosclerosis, with changes in apoptosis, inflammation, hepatic dysfunction, and other relevant settings, seem quite plausible and exciting, offering a new perspective on these complex issues.

Lymphocytes

Both B and T lymphocytes have been implicated in atherogenesis in both the absence and presence of diabetes. By immunohistochemistry, most lymphocytes in atherosclerotic plaque are $CD4^+$ cells, which have the capacity to differentiate along Th1 or Th2 lineages. Factors in the vessel wall including cytokine production by other lymphocytes, ECs, and macrophages dictate the differentiation fate of these cells. Lymphocyte differentiation has important effects on atherosclerotic plaque biology. Disruption of Th1 lineage reduces atherosclerosis in murine models of disease and has been generally associated with proatherosclerotic responses.[165,166] The role of Th2 cells is more controversial. In addition, smaller subsets of T cells including T regulatory cells (Tregs) and Th17 lymphocytes exert local control on plaque inflammation and plaque expansion. In diabetic patients, a lymphocytosis has been observed with expansion of a rare, proatherogenic $CD4^+$ CD28null T lymphocyte.[167] In patients with overt coronary syndromes and T2DM, the frequency of this lymphocyte population was 12.7% versus 3.8% in patients with acute coronary syndrome without T2DM. This effect was independently associated with glycosylated hemoglobin levels. Recent data demonstrate that the expansion of visceral fat is associated with a loss of local Treg cells. This highlights emerging data connecting changes in inflammatory cells and cardiometabolic issues.[168] The specific role of diabetes in lymphocyte activation during atherosclerosis lesion formation remains an active area of research.

Vascular Smooth Muscle

During the atherosclerotic process, VSMCs proliferate in the media and also migrate out of the media to the subintimal space, thereby enlarging the neointimal lesion. In human diabetes, VSMC reactivity is enhanced in isolated arteries exposed to norepinephrine or phenylephrine.[169] This effect correlates with reduced subplasmalemmal Ca^{2+}, which controls K^+ channels that regulate VSMC relaxation. VSMCs grown in culture medium supplemented with high glucose proliferate, migrate, hypertrophy, and produce extracellular matrix to a greater degree than cells grown in low-glucose media.[170,171] VSMCs isolated from the aortas of db/db mice—an established model of aggressive T2DM—demonstrate increased proinflammatory gene expression including MCP-1 and IL-6.[172,173] VSMCs from db/db animals migrated in response to platelet-derived growth factor (PDGF) to a significantly greater degree than VSMCs isolated from control, nondiabetic mice. These observations suggest that the diabetic environment "preactivates" VSMCs and predisposes these cells to invade the intima and further inflame the vessel wall.

Inflammation as a Therapeutic Target in Diabetic Atherosclerosis?

Although cell biologic approaches and animal models have provided key scientific insights into atherogenesis, ongoing efforts are directed toward translating these findings to human disease. The identification of stable, circulating biomarkers of inflammation has allowed investigators to test prospectively how indices of inflammation relate to atherosclerosis disease burden and clinical events, including responses to current agents and therapies under development.

PPARs have been extensively explored as therapeutic targets for improving both T2DM and diabetic atherosclerosis and provide an interesting example of the challenges in extending scientific advances to clinical benefit.[14,15] PPARs, members of the nuclear hormone receptor family, are ligand-activated transcription factors that control metabolic gene expression in multiple tissues including adipose tissue, skeletal muscle, and liver. PPARs consist of PPAR-α, PPAR-γ, and PPAR-β/δ, different isotypes with unique profiles. The drugs constituting the class of thiazolidinediones (rosiglitazone, pioglitazone) were found to be potent insulin sensitizers by activating PPAR-γ, whereas fibrates lower hypertriglyceridemia and increase HDL by activating PPAR-α. It is interesting to note that these drugs were in clinical use before it was realized that these receptors were also expressed in vascular and immune cells. Subsequent studies established that PPARs were expressed in vascular and inflammatory cells, with a fairly extensive database demonstrating in general that PPAR activation limits inflammatory gene expression in ECs, VSMCs, and macrophages in vitro.[174–176] In vivo treatment of hypercholesterolemic mice with PPAR-α and PPAR-γ ligands also suppressed lesion formation in different models with and without diabetes.[177] PPAR effects correlated with alterations in macrophage foam cell formation in vitro. PPAR-δ has also been studied and implicated in these processes, although no PPAR-δ agonist has ever reached clinical approval.[178] Surrogate marker studies revealed that PPAR-γ and PPAR-α agonists could reduce hsCRP and decrease carotid intima-media thickness.[179] However, extending this relatively robust dataset to humans has yielded mixed results, as discussed elsewhere. Briefly, a meta-analysis of smaller studies with rosiglitazone suggested increased CV events.[180] A prospective, placebo-controlled study with pioglitazone— PRoACTIVE (Prospective Pioglitazone Clinical Trial in Macrovascular Events)—did demonstrate a 20% reduction in the secondary endpoint of major CV events in patients with diabetes.[181] A potentially misguided primary combined endpoint, which included typically unresponsive endpoints such as peripheral vascular disease intervention, was null, rendering this result more difficult to interpret. Important, pioglitazone did not seem to have higher risk of adverse events in this study. Similarly, fibrates as PPAR-α agonists have shown reduced CV events when used alone (gemfibrozil, Veterans Administration-HDL Intervention Trial "VA-HIT"), but there has been less definitive evidence in combination with statins, with perhaps the subgroup of patients with higher TG and lower HDL levels being the ones most likely to benefit.[182,183]

In terms of the vascular biology of diabetes, the PPAR experience offers potential insights and cautionary points. Prior data and studies that continue to emerge identify PPARs as critical regulators at the intersection of metabolism, inflammation, and atherosclerosis. A necessary distinction must be maintained between the biologic target and the therapeutic agent(s). Indeed, along these lines, some efforts continue to identify better approaches to modulating PPAR activity, including a dual PPAR-α–PPAR-γ agonist that is in a large, late-stage clinical trial in patients with acute coronary syndromes.[184] PPAR biology establishes several rationales for how different PPAR interacting agents might exert different biologic responses. If rosiglitazone does increase CV risk, one might also question the validity of surrogate markers, given the improvements observed with rosiglitazone. Perhaps the broader conclusion is that to appropriately evaluate agents with the potential to decrease CV events, definitive randomized clinical trials are needed. The experience with pioglitazone underscores the need for those trials to be carefully thought out, given that reversal of the primary and secondary endpoints in this trial, and a

longer duration, may well have had a profound effect on the diabetes therapeutic landscape. Incretins (glucagon-like peptide-1 analogs), a new therapeutic modality for diabetes, also have direct effects on the vasculature.[185,186] Incretins are gastrointestinal hormones that increase insulin release from the pancreatic beta cell. As in the case of PPAR biology, the effects of incretins on CV outcomes remain an important issue of study.

In contrast to the complexities of the clinical experience with PPAR agents, HMG-CoA reductase inhibitors (statins) have been shown to clearly decrease CV risk in general as well as in patients with diabetes.[187] Several lines of evidence suggest that the benefits of statins may derive from anti-inflammatory effects, including some that may be independent of LDL lowering. Statins lower circulating hsCRP levels, as seen in the randomized, prospective primary and secondary CVD outcomes trials. Notably, in the Pravastatin or Atorvastatin Evaluation and Infection Therapy— Thrombolysis in Myocardial Infarction 22 (PROVE IT–TIMI 22) trial, the patients who benefited the most from high-dose atorvastatin therapy after acute coronary syndrome events were those individuals who achieved an LDL cholesterol level below 70 mg/dL and hsCRP level below 2.0 mg/L.[146] These clinical findings suggest that statins possess anti-inflammatory properties. In JUPITER (Justification for the Use of Statins in Prevention: an Intervention Trial Evaluating Rosuvastatin), 17,802 individuals without known CVD with average LDL cholesterol levels (<130 mg/dL, median 108 mg/dL) but hsCRP levels of 2 mg/L or higher were randomized to either placebo or rosuvastatin.[188] The study was terminated after only 3 years when the interim analysis revealed a 44% reduction in the primary CV end point. The treatment group had significant reductions in hsCRP (37%), but also reductions in LDL cholesterol (50%), making a definitive conclusion that the benefit derived from decreased inflammation difficult. Preclinical studies continue to suggest various mechanisms through which statins may decrease inflammation independent of LDL lowering, including changes in modification of proteins, induction of other targets such as the kruppel-like factor (KLF) transcription factors, and changes in mRNA stability, as reported for eNOS.

Given that statins appear to decrease both inflammation and LDL, interest has arisen in other therapies that might decrease inflammation in an LDL-neutral manner. Two large clinical trials are under way that will directly test the inflammation hypothesis: the Cardiovascular Inflammation Reduction Trial (CIRT; ClinicalTrials.gov identifier NCT01594333) and the Cardiovascular Risk Reduction Trial (CANTOS; ClinicalTrials.gov identifier NCT01327846).

The CIRT study, sponsored by the National Institutes of Health, is a multicenter, placebo-controlled trial in which patients with stable CAD on standard care (including statins) *and* metabolic syndrome or T2DM (n = 7000) who will be randomized to very low-dose methotrexate (15 to 20 mg weekly) with folate supplementation. Methotrexate was chosen because this U.S. Food and Drug Administration (FDA)–approved medication lowers hsCRP without affecting lipid levels, has an excellent safety profile, is well tolerated, and is inexpensive. Seven nonrandomized observational studies of patients with rheumatoid arthritis or psoriatic arthritis have demonstrated significant CV event reduction among individuals taking low-dose methotrexate. Notably, patients with chronic inflammatory conditions such as lupus, rheumatoid arthritis, or inflammatory bowel disease are excluded from the trial. This study will directly test whether lowering inflammation can reduce recurrent CVD in patients with diabetes. Enrollment was scheduled to begin in October, 2012.

The CANTOS trial is a randomized, double-blind placebo-controlled, event-driven trial that will test whether quarterly, subcutaneous canakinumab, a human monoclonal anti-body that neutralizes IL-1β action, can reduce the rates of recurrent MI, stroke, and CVD death. The fact that intracellular cholesterol crystals activate the Nod-like receptor protein 3 (NLRP3) inflammasome, a signaling pathway that generates the active form of IL-1β, along with other data, provided the rationale to study IL-1β inhibition in CVD.[189] IL-1β has been directly implicated in atherosclerosis and thrombosis. The study will enroll patients at least 30 days after MI with hsCRP levels of 2 mg/L or higher. Canakinumab has been shown to reduce inflammatory biomarkers including hsCRP. The results of both CIRT and CANTOS will provide crucial clinical trial data regarding whether targeting inflammation itself can alter the natural history of CVD in patients with metabolic disease or T2DM.

SUMMARY

Diabetes is a complex condition with a pathogenesis, like atherosclerosis, that involves multiple different inputs and likely represents distinct forms even beyond designations such as type 1 and type 2. The intricacies of this picture are evident in attempts to deconvolute the nature of the vascular biology of diabetic atherosclerosis—the factors that drive the disorder, determine outcomes, and, it is hoped, offer openings for interrupting the natural history. The challenges in understanding the molecular basis of the intersection of diabetes and atherosclerosis are legion, given overlapping issues between these two diseases: very long subclinical phases, a frequency in the population that sets up multiple confounding variables, shared mechanistic underpinnings, and cellular players such as adipocytes and macrophages with many similar characteristics. All of these issues combine with clinical experience to frame a fundamental question in this field: To what extent is diabetic atherosclerosis unique and distinct from atherosclerosis, or is it simply the same disease accelerated in the context of hyperglycemia and other factors? It is amazing that, despite intense efforts by many groups using different approaches over many years, this question remains unresolved. Clearly the issues considered here are important in diabetic atherosclerosis independent of whether they are unique to diabetes or not. Diabetic dyslipidemia is a central part of the diabetic picture, with all the key components of the arterial wall and the inflammatory system altered by interaction with the altered lipid metabolism of diabetes. Increased thrombogenicity clearly contributes to CV outcomes in patients with diabetes; the extent to which all aspects of coagulation are shifted in diabetes is impressive. Endothelial dysfunction is an early part of the disease even before diabetes or cardiovascular complications become apparent. Ultimately, the inflammatory responses generated by core elements of diabetes, such as hyperglycemia, elevated FFAs, and increased ROSs, may be pointing us in the direction we must head if we are to understand better diabetic atherosclerosis, identify the problems earlier, and further improve outcomes.

References

1. Eckel RH: Diabetic dyslipidemia and cardiovascular risk, *Curr Diab Rep* 8:421–423, 2008.
2. Mooradian AD: Dyslipidemia in type 2 diabetes mellitus, *Nat Clin Pract Endocrinol Metab* 5:150–159, 2009.
3. Renard CB, Kramer F, Johansson F, et al: Diabetes and diabetes-associated lipid abnormalities have distinct effects on initiation and progression of atherosclerotic lesions, *J Clin Invest* 114:659–668, 2004.
4. Neeland IJ, Turer AT, Ayers CR, et al: Dysfunctional adiposity and the risk of prediabetes and type 2 diabetes in obese adults, *JAMA* 308:1150–1159, 2012.
5. Adiels M, Borén J, Caslake MJ, et al: Overproduction of VLDL1 driven by hyperglycemia is a dominant feature of diabetic dyslipidemia, *Arterioscler Thromb Vasc Biol* 25:1697–1703, 2005.
6. Adiels M, Olofsson SO, Taskinen MR, et al: Overproduction of very low-density lipoproteins is the hallmark of the dyslipidemia in the metabolic syndrome, *Arterioscler Thromb Vasc Biol* 28:1225–1236, 2008.
7. Chan DC, Pang J, Romic G, et al: Postprandial hypertriglyceridemia and cardiovascular disease: current and future therapies, *Curr Atheroscler Rep* 15:309, 2013.
8. Pang J, Chan DC, Barrett PH, et al: Postprandial dyslipidaemia and diabetes: mechanistic and therapeutic aspects, *Curr Opin Lipidol* 23:303–309, 2012.
9. Teno S, Uto Y, Nagashima H, et al: Association of postprandial hypertriglyceridemia and carotid intima-media thickness in patients with type 2 diabetes, *Diabetes Care* 23:1401–1406, 2000.
10. Ruby MA, Goldenson B, Orasanu G, et al: VLDL hydrolysis by LPL activates PPAR-alpha through generation of unbound fatty acids, *J Lipid Res* 51:2275–2281, 2010.
11. Ziouzenkova O, Perrey S, Asatryan L, et al: Lipolysis of triglyceride-rich lipoproteins generates PPAR ligands: evidence for an antiinflammatory role for lipoprotein lipase, *Proc Natl Acad Sci U S A* 100:2730–2735, 2003.
12. Augustus A, Yagyu H, Haemmerle G, et al: Cardiac-specific knock-out of lipoprotein lipase alters plasma lipoprotein triglyceride metabolism and cardiac gene expression, *J Biol Chem* 279:25050–25057, 2004.
13. Chawla A, Lee CH, Barak Y, et al: PPARdelta is a very low-density lipoprotein sensor in macrophages, *Proc Natl Acad Sci U S A* 100:1268–1273, 2003.
14. Brown JD, Plutzky J: Peroxisome proliferator-activated receptors as transcriptional nodal points and therapeutic targets, *Circulation* 115:518–533, 2007.
15. Rosenson RS, Wright RS, Farkouh M, et al: Modulating peroxisome proliferator-activated receptors for therapeutic benefit? Biology, clinical experience, and future prospects, *Am Heart J* 164:672–680, 2012.
16. Chakravarthy MV, Lodhi IJ, Yin L, et al: Identification of a physiologically relevant endogenous ligand for PPARalpha in liver, *Cell* 138:476–488, 2009.
17. Haemmerle G, Moustafa T, Woelkart G, et al: ATGL-mediated fat catabolism regulates cardiac mitochondrial function via PPAR-alpha and PGC-1, *Nat Med* 17:1076–1085, 2011.
18. Brown JD, Oligino E, Rader DJ, et al: VLDL hydrolysis by hepatic lipase regulates PPARdelta transcriptional responses, *PLoS One* 6:e21209, 2011.
19. Zheng C, Azcutia V, Aikawa E, et al: Statins suppress apolipoprotein CIII-induced vascular endothelial cell activation and monocyte adhesion, *Eur Heart J*, 2012.
20. Asztalos BF, Demissie S, Cupples LA, et al: LpA-I, LpA-I:A-II HDL and CHD-risk: the Framingham Offspring Study and the Veterans Affairs HDL Intervention Trial, *Atherosclerosis* 188:59–67, 2006.
21. Badellino KO, Wolfe ML, Reilly MP, et al: Endothelial lipase concentrations are increased in metabolic syndrome and associated with coronary atherosclerosis, *PLoS Med* 3:e22, 2006.
22. Paradis ME, Badellino KO, Rader DJ, et al: Visceral adiposity and endothelial lipase, *J Clin Endocrinol Metab* 91:3538–3543, 2006.
23. Paradis ME, Badellino KO, Rader DJ, et al: Endothelial lipase is associated with inflammation in humans, *J Lipid Res* 47:2808–2813, 2006.
24. Badellino KO, Wolfe ML, Reilly MP, et al: Endothelial lipase is increased in vivo by inflammation in humans, *Circulation* 117:678–685, 2008.
25. Li C, Zhang W, Zhou F, et al: Cholesteryl ester transfer protein inhibitors in the treatment of dyslipidemia: a systematic review and meta-analysis, *PLoS One* 8:e77049, 2013.
26. AIM-HIGH Investigators, Boden WE, Probstfield JL, et al: Niacin in patients with low HDL cholesterol levels receiving intensive statin therapy, *N Engl J Med* 365:2255–2267, 2011.
27. Adiels M, Taskinen MR, Boren J: Fatty liver, insulin resistance, and dyslipidemia, *Curr Diab Rep* 8:60–64, 2008.
28. Barlovic DP, Soro-Paavonen A, Jandeleit-Dahm KA: RAGE biology, atherosclerosis and diabetes, *Clin Sci (Lond)* 121:43–55, 2011.
29. Harja E, Bu DX, Hudson BI, et al: Vascular and inflammatory stresses mediate atherosclerosis via RAGE and its ligands in apoE−/− mice, *J Clin Invest* 118:183–194, 2008.
30. Yan SF, Barile GR, D'Agati V, et al: The biology of RAGE and its ligands: uncovering mechanisms at the heart of diabetes and its complications, *Curr Diab Rep* 7:146–153, 2007.
31. Hirayama S, Soda S, Ito Y, et al: Circadian change of serum concentration of small dense LDL-cholesterol in type 2 diabetic patients, *Clin Chim Acta* 411:253–257, 2009.
32. Lichtman AH, Binder CJ, Tsimikas S, et al: Adaptive immunity in atherogenesis: new insights and therapeutic approaches, *J Clin Invest* 123:27–36, 2013.
33. Assert R, Scherk G, Bumbure A, et al: Regulation of protein kinase C by short term hyperglycaemia in human platelets in vivo and in vitro, *Diabetologia* 44:188–195, 2001.
34. Lemkes BA, Hermanides J, Devries JH, et al: Hyperglycemia: a prothrombotic factor? *J Thromb Haemost* 8:1663–1669, 2010.
35. Keating FK, Sobel BE, Schneider DJ: Effects of increased concentrations of glucose on platelet reactivity in healthy subjects and in patients without and with diabetes mellitus, *Am J Cardiol* 92:1362–1365, 2003.
36. Yamagishi S, Matsui T, Ueda S, et al: Advanced glycation end products (AGEs) and cardiovascular disease (CVD) in diabetes, *Cardiovasc Hematol Agents Med Chem* 5:236–240, 2007.
37. Undas A, Wiek I, Stepien E, et al: Hyperglycemia is associated with enhanced thrombin formation, platelet activation, and fibrin clot resistance to lysis in patients with acute coronary syndrome, *Diabetes Care* 31:1590–1595, 2008.
38. Yngen M, Ostenson CG, Li N, et al: Acute hyperglycemia increases soluble P-selectin in male patients with mild diabetes mellitus, *Blood Coagul Fibrinolysis* 12:109–116, 2001.
39. Ueno M, Ferreiro JL, Tomasello SD, et al: Functional profile of the platelet P2Y(1)(2) receptor signalling pathway in patients with type 2 diabetes mellitus and coronary artery disease, *Thromb Haemost* 105:730–732, 2011.
40. Morel O, Kessler L, Ohlmann P, et al: Diabetes and the platelet: toward new therapeutic paradigms for diabetic atherothrombosis, *Atherosclerosis* 212:367–376, 2010.
41. Tsimerman G, Roguin A, Bachar A, et al: Involvement of microparticles in diabetic vascular complications, *Thromb Haemost* 106:310–321, 2011.
42. Li Y, Woo V, Bose R: Platelet hyperactivity and abnormal Ca(2+) homeostasis in diabetes mellitus, *Am J Physiol Heart Circ Physiol* 280:H1480–H1489, 2001.
43. Dean WL, Chen D, Brandt PC, et al: Regulation of platelet plasma membrane Ca2+-ATPase by cAMP-dependent and tyrosine phosphorylation, *J Biol Chem* 272:15113–15119, 1997.
44. Schaeffer G, Wascher TC, Kostner GM, et al: Alterations in platelet Ca2+ signalling in diabetic patients is due to increased formation of superoxide anions and reduced nitric oxide production, *Diabetologia* 42:167–176, 1999.

45. Randriamboavonjy V, Isaak J, Elgheznawy A, et al: Calpain inhibition stabilizes the platelet proteome and reactivity in diabetes, *Blood* 120:415–423, 2012.
46. Ferreira IA, Mocking AI, Feijge MA, et al: Platelet inhibition by insulin is absent in type 2 diabetes mellitus, *Arterioscler Thromb Vasc Biol* 26:417–422, 2006.
47. Hers I: Insulin-like growth factor-1 potentiates platelet activation via the IRS/PI3Kalpha pathway, *Blood* 110:4243–4252, 2007.
48. Anfossi G, Mularoni EM, Burzacca S, et al: Platelet resistance to nitrates in obesity and obese NIDDM, and normal platelet sensitivity to both insulin and nitrates in lean NIDDM, *Diabetes Care* 21:121–126, 1998.
49. Pedreno J, Hurt-Camejo E, Wiklund O, et al: Platelet function in patients with familial hypertriglyceridemia: evidence that platelet reactivity is modulated by apolipoprotein E content of very-low-density lipoprotein particles, *Metabolism* 49:942–949, 2000.
50. Ferretti G, Rabini RA, Bacchetti T, et al: Glycated low density lipoproteins modify platelet properties: a compositional and functional study, *J Clin Endocrinol Metab* 87:2180–2184, 2002.
51. Anfossi G, Russo I, Trovati M: Platelet dysfunction in central obesity, *Nutr Metab Cardiovasc Dis* 19:440–449, 2009.
52. Russo I, Traversa M, Bonomo K, et al: In central obesity, weight loss restores platelet sensitivity to nitric oxide and prostacyclin, *Obesity (Silver Spring)* 18:788–797, 2009.
53. Freedman JE: Oxidative stress and platelets, *Arterioscler Thromb Vasc Biol* 28:s11–s16, 2008.
54. Schneider DJ: Factors contributing to increased platelet reactivity in people with diabetes, *Diabetes Care* 32:525–527, 2009.
55. De Cristofaro R, Rocca B, Vitacolonna E, et al: Lipid and protein oxidation contribute to a prothrombotic state in patients with type 2 diabetes mellitus, *J Thromb Haemost* 1:250–256, 2003.
56. Lim HS, Blann AD, Lip GY: Soluble CD40 ligand, soluble P-selectin, interleukin-6, and tissue factor in diabetes mellitus: relationships to cardiovascular disease and risk factor intervention, *Circulation* 109:2524–2528, 2004.
57. Gerrits AJ, Koekman CA, van Haeften TW, et al: Platelet tissue factor synthesis in type 2 diabetic patients is resistant to inhibition by insulin, *Diabetes* 59:1487–1495, 2010.
58. Boden G, Rao AK: Effects of hyperglycemia and hyperinsulinemia on the tissue factor pathway of blood coagulation, *Curr Diab Rep* 7:223–227, 2007.
59. Heywood DM, Mansfield MW, Grant PJ: Factor VII gene polymorphisms, factor VII:C levels and features of insulin resistance in non-insulin-dependent diabetes mellitus, *Thromb Haemost* 75:401–406, 1996.
60. Meade TW, Ruddock V, Stirling Y, et al: Fibrinolytic activity, clotting factors, and long-term incidence of ischaemic heart disease in the Northwick Park Heart Study, *Lancet* 342:1076–1079, 1993.
61. Karatela RA, Sainani GS: Interrelationship between coagulation factor VII and obesity in diabetes mellitus (type 2), *Diabetes Res Clin Pract* 84:e41–e44, 2009.
62. Grant PJ: Diabetes mellitus as a prothrombotic condition, *J Intern Med* 262:157–172, 2007.
63. Aoki I, Shimoyama K, Aoki N, et al: Platelet-dependent thrombin generation in patients with diabetes mellitus: effects of glycemic control on coagulability in diabetes, *J Am Coll Cardiol* 27:560–566, 1996.
64. Osende JI, Badimon JJ, Fuster V, et al: Blood thrombogenicity in type 2 diabetes mellitus patients is associated with glycemic control, *J Am Coll Cardiol* 38:1307–1312, 2001.
65. Guardado-Mendoza R, Jimenez-Ceja L, Pacheco-Carrasco MF, et al: Fibrinogen is associated with silent myocardial ischaemia in type 2 diabetes mellitus, *Acta Cardiol* 64:523–530, 2009.
66. Koenig W: Fibrin(ogen) in cardiovascular disease: an update, *Thromb Haemost* 89:601–609, 2003.
67. Le DS, Miles R, Savage PJ, et al: The association of plasma fibrinogen concentration with diabetic microvascular complications in young adults with early-onset of type 2 diabetes, *Diabetes Res Clin Pract* 82:317–323, 2008.
68. Rodrigues TC, Snell-Bergeon JK, Maahs DM, et al: Higher fibrinogen levels predict progression of coronary artery calcification in adults with type 1 diabetes, *Atherosclerosis* 210:671–673, 2010.
69. Raynaud E, Pérez-Martin A, Brun J, et al: Relationships between fibrinogen and insulin resistance, *Atherosclerosis* 150:365–370, 2000.
70. Barazzoni R, Kiwanuka E, Zanetti M, et al: Insulin acutely increases fibrinogen production in individuals with type 2 diabetes but not in individuals without diabetes, *Diabetes* 52:1851–1856, 2003.
71. Kakafika AI, Liberopoulos EN, Mikhailidis DP: Fibrinogen: a predictor of vascular disease, *Curr Pharm Des* 13:1647–1659, 2007.
72. Sobel BE, Schneider DJ: Platelet function, coagulopathy, and impaired fibrinolysis in diabetes, *Cardiol Clin* 22:511–526, 2004.
73. Hernández-Espinosa D, Ordóñez A, Miñano A, et al: Hyperglycaemia impairs antithrombin secretion: possible contribution to the thrombotic risk of diabetes, *Thromb Res* 124:483–489, 2009.
74. Falciani M, Gori AM, Fedi S, et al: Elevated tissue factor and tissue factor pathway inhibitor circulating levels in ischaemic heart disease patients, *Thromb Haemost* 79:495–499, 1998.
75. Mitchell CT, Kamineni A, Palmas W, et al: Tissue factor pathway inhibitor, vascular risk factors and subclinical atherosclerosis: the Multi-Ethnic Study of Atherosclerosis, *Atherosclerosis* 207:277–283, 2009.
76. Zawadzki C, Susen S, Richard F, et al: Dyslipidemia shifts the tissue factor/tissue factor pathway inhibitor balance toward increased thrombogenicity in atherosclerotic plaques: evidence for a corrective effect of statins, *Atherosclerosis* 195:e117–e125, 2007.
77. Leurs PB, van Oerle R, Wolffenbuttel BH, et al: Increased tissue factor pathway inhibitor (TFPI) and coagulation in patients with insulin-dependent diabetes mellitus, *Thromb Haemost* 77:472–476, 1997.
78. Holroyd EW, Simari RD: Interdependent biological systems, multi-functional molecules: the evolving role of tissue factor pathway inhibitor beyond anti-coagulation, *Thromb Res* 125 (Suppl 1):S57–S59, 2010.
79. Dahlback B, Villoutreix BO: The anticoagulant protein C pathway, *FEBS Lett* 579:3310–3316, 2005.
80. Yamaji K, Wang Y, Liu Y, et al: Activated protein C, a natural anticoagulant protein, has antioxidant properties and inhibits lipid peroxidation and advanced glycation end products formation, *Thromb Res* 115:319–325, 2005.
81. Folsom AR, Ohira T, Yamagishi K, et al: Low protein C and incidence of ischemic stroke and coronary heart disease: the Atherosclerosis Risk in Communities (ARIC) Study, *J Thromb Haemost* 7:1774–1778, 2009.
82. Matsumoto K, Yano Y, Gabazza EC, et al: Inverse correlation between activated protein C generation and carotid atherosclerosis in Type 2 diabetic patients, *Diabet Med* 24:1322–1328, 2007.
83. Li YH, Shi GY, Wu HL: The role of thrombomodulin in atherosclerosis: from bench to bedside, *Cardiovasc Hematol Agents Med Chem* 4:183–187, 2006.
84. Karakas M, Baumert J, Herder C, et al: Soluble thrombomodulin in coronary heart disease: lack of an association in the MONICA/KORA case-cohort study, *J Thromb Haemost* 9:1078–1080, 2011.
85. Salomaa V, Wu KK: Soluble thrombomodulin as predictor of incident coronary heart disease, *Lancet* 354:1646–1647, 1999.
86. Thorand B, Baumert J, Herder C, et al: Soluble thrombomodulin as a predictor of type 2 diabetes: results from the MONICA/KORA Augsburg case-cohort study, 1984–1998, *Diabetologia* 50:545–548, 2007.
87. Aso Y, Fujiwara Y, Tayama K, et al: Relationship between plasma soluble thrombomodulin levels and insulin resistance syndrome in type 2 diabetes: a comparison with von Willebrand factor, *Exp Clin Endocrinol Diabetes* 109:210–216, 2001.
88. Aso Y, Fujiwara Y, Tayama K, et al: Relationship between soluble thrombomodulin in plasma and coagulation or fibrinolysis in type 2 diabetes, *Clin Chim Acta* 301:135–145, 2000.
89. Dunn EJ, Ariens RA, Grant PJ: The influence of type 2 diabetes on fibrin structure and function, *Diabetologia* 48:1198–1206, 2005.
90. Dunn EJ, Philippou H, Ariens RA, et al: Molecular mechanisms involved in the resistance of fibrin to clot lysis by plasmin in subjects with type 2 diabetes mellitus, *Diabetologia* 49:1071–1080, 2006.
91. Pieters M, Covic N, van der Westhuizen FH, et al: Glycaemic control improves fibrin network characteristics in type 2 diabetes - a purified fibrinogen model, *Thromb Haemost* 99:691–700, 2008.
92. Carter AM, Catto AJ, Grant PJ: Determinants of tPA antigen and associations with coronary artery disease and acute cerebrovascular disease, *Thromb Haemost* 80:632–636, 1998.
93. Hoekstra T, Geleijnse JM, Schouten EG, et al: Plasminogen activator inhibitor-type 1: its plasma determinants and relation with cardiovascular risk, *Thromb Haemost* 91:861–872, 2004.
94. Ajjan R, Grant PJ: Coagulation and atherothrombotic disease, *Atherosclerosis* 186:240–259, 2006.
95. Alessi MC, Juhan-Vague I: PAI-1 and the metabolic syndrome: links, causes, and consequences, *Arterioscler Thromb Vasc Biol* 26:2200–2207, 2006.
96. Festa A, Williams K, Tracy RP, et al: Progression of plasminogen activator inhibitor-1 and fibrinogen levels in relation to incident type 2 diabetes, *Circulation* 113:1753–1759, 2006.
97. Cefalu WT, Schneider DJ, Carlson HE, et al: Effect of combination glipizide GITS/metformin on fibrinolytic and metabolic parameters in poorly controlled type 2 diabetic subjects, *Diabetes Care* 25:2123–2128, 2002.
98. Hori Y, Gabazza EC, Yano Y, et al: Insulin resistance is associated with increased circulating level of thrombin-activatable fibrinolysis inhibitor in type 2 diabetic patients, *J Clin Endocrinol Metab* 87:660–665, 2002.
99. Yano Y, Kitagawa N, Gabazza EC, et al: Increased plasma thrombin-activatable fibrinolysis inhibitor levels in normotensive type 2 diabetic patients with microalbuminuria, *J Clin Endocrinol Metab* 88:736–741, 2003.
100. Colucci M, D'Aprile AM, Italia A, et al: Thrombin activatable fibrinolysis inhibitor (TAFI) does not inhibit in vitro thrombolysis by pharmacological concentrations of t-PA, *Thromb Haemost* 85:661–666, 2001.
101. Meltzer ME, Doggen CJ, de Groot PG, et al: Plasma levels of fibrinolytic proteins and the risk of myocardial infarction in men, *Blood* 116:529–536, 2010.
102. Bayés-Genís A, Guindo J, Oliver A, et al: Elevated levels of plasmin-alpha2 antiplasmin complexes in unstable angina, *Thromb Haemost* 81:865–868, 1999.
103. Cushman M, Lemaitre RN, Kuller LH, et al: Fibrinolytic activation markers predict myocardial infarction in the elderly. The Cardiovascular Health Study, *Arterioscler Thromb Vasc Biol* 19:493–498, 1999.
104. Sakkinen PA, Cushman M, Psaty BM, et al: Relationship of plasmin generation to cardiovascular disease risk factors in elderly men and women, *Arterioscler Thromb Vasc Biol* 19:499–504, 1999.
105. Guimarães AH, de Bruijne EL, Lisman T, et al: Hypofibrinolysis is a risk factor for arterial thrombosis at young age, *Br J Haematol* 145:115–120, 2009.
106. Goldfine AB, Beckman JA, Betensky RA, et al: Family history of diabetes is a major determinant of endothelial function, *J Am Coll Cardiol* 47:2456–2461, 2006.
107. Moncada S, Higgs A: The L-arginine-nitric oxide pathway, *N Engl J Med* 329:2002–2012, 1993.
108. Kinlay S, Libby P, Ganz P: Endothelial function and coronary artery disease, *Curr Opin Lipidol* 12:383–389, 2001.
109. Furchgott RF, Zawadzki JV: The obligatory role of endothelial cells in the relaxation of arterial smooth muscle by acetylcholine, *Nature* 288:373–376, 1980.
110. Gerszten RE, Garcia-Zepeda EA, Lim YC, et al: MCP-1 and IL-8 trigger firm adhesion of monocytes to vascular endothelium under flow conditions, *Nature* 398:718–723, 1999.
111. Johnstone MT, Creager SJ, Scales KM, et al: Impaired endothelium-dependent vasodilation in patients with insulin-dependent diabetes mellitus, *Circulation* 88:2510–2516, 1993.
112. Williams SB, Cusco JA, Roddy MA, et al: Impaired nitric oxide-mediated vasodilation in patients with non-insulin-dependent diabetes mellitus, *J Am Coll Cardiol* 27:567–574, 1996.
113. Takaya T, Hirata K, Yamashita T, et al: A specific role for eNOS-derived reactive oxygen species in atherosclerosis progression, *Arterioscler Thromb Vasc Biol* 27:1632–1637, 2007.
114. Hayashi T, Sumi D, Juliet PA, et al: Gene transfer of endothelial NO synthase, but not eNOS plus inducible NOS, regressed atherosclerosis in rabbits, *Cardiovasc Res* 61:339–351, 2004.
115. Steinberg HO, Tarshoby M, Monestel R, et al: Elevated circulating free fatty acid levels impair endothelium-dependent vasodilation, *J Clin Invest* 100:1230–1239, 1997.
116. Griffin ME, Marcucci MJ, Cline GW, et al: Free fatty acid-induced insulin resistance is associated with activation of protein kinase C theta and alterations in the insulin signaling cascade, *Diabetes* 48:1270–1274, 1999.
117. Paixao J, Dinis TC, Almeida LM: Dietary anthocyanins protect endothelial cells against peroxynitrite-induced mitochondrial apoptosis pathway and Bax nuclear translocation: an in vitro approach, *Apoptosis* 16:976–989, 2011.
118. Dickhout JG, Hossain GS, Pozza LM, et al: Peroxynitrite causes endoplasmic reticulum stress and apoptosis in human vascular endothelium: implications in atherogenesis, *Arterioscler Thromb Vasc Biol* 25:2623–2629, 2005.
119. Zou MH, Shi C, Cohen RA: High glucose via peroxynitrite causes tyrosine nitration and inactivation of prostacyclin synthase that is associated with thromboxane/prostaglandin H(2) receptor-mediated apoptosis and adhesion molecule expression in cultured human aortic endothelial cells, *Diabetes* 51:198–203, 2002.
120. Bauersachs J, Schafer A: Tetrahydrobiopterin and eNOS dimer/monomer ratio–a clue to eNOS uncoupling in diabetes? *Cardiovasc Res* 65:768–769, 2005.
121. Kar S, Bhandar B, Kavdia M: Impact of SOD in eNOS uncoupling: a two-edged sword between hydrogen peroxide and peroxynitrite, *Free Radic Res* 46:1496–1513, 2012.
122. Gow AJ, Farkouh CR, Munson DA, et al: Biological significance of nitric oxide-mediated protein modifications, *Am J Physiol Lung Cell Mol Physiol* 287:L262–L268, 2004.
123. Ceriello A, Mercuri F, Quagliaro L, et al: Detection of nitrotyrosine in the diabetic plasma: evidence of oxidative stress, *Diabetologia* 44:834–838, 2001.
124. Kanda T, Brown JD, Orasanu G, et al: PPARgamma in the endothelium regulates metabolic responses to high-fat diet in mice, *J Clin Invest* 119:110–124, 2009.
125. Tsuchiya K, Tanaka J, Shuiqing Y, et al: FoxOs integrate pleiotropic actions of insulin in vascular endothelium to protect mice from atherosclerosis, *Cell Metab* 15:372–381, 2012.
126. Qiang L, Tsuchiya K, Kim-Muller JY, et al: Increased atherosclerosis and endothelial dysfunction in mice bearing constitutively deacetylated alleles of Foxo1 gene, *J Biol Chem* 287:13944–13951, 2012.
127. Li H, Cybulsky MI, Gimbrone MA Jr, et al: An atherogenic diet rapidly induces VCAM-1, a cytokine-regulatable mononuclear leukocyte adhesion molecule, in rabbit aortic endothelium, *Arterioscler Thromb* 13:197–204, 1993.
128. Cybulsky MI, Gimbrone MA Jr: Endothelial expression of a mononuclear leukocyte adhesion molecule during atherogenesis, *Science* 251:788–791, 1991.
129. de Lemos JA, Hennekens CH, Ridker PM: Plasma concentration of soluble vascular cell adhesion molecule-1 and subsequent cardiovascular risk, *J Am Coll Cardiol* 36:423–426, 2000.
130. Maganto-Garcia E, Tarrio ML, Grabie N, et al: Dynamic changes in regulatory T cells are linked to levels of diet-induced hypercholesterolemia, *Circulation* 124:185–195, 2011.
131. Hernandez-Mijares A, Rocha M, Rovira-Llopis S, et al: Human leukocyte/endothelial cell interactions and mitochondrial dysfunction in type 2 diabetic patients and their association with silent myocardial ischemia, *Diabetes Care,* 2013.

132. Devaraj S, Jialal I, Yun JM, et al: Demonstration of increased toll-like receptor 2 and toll-like receptor 4 expression in monocytes of type 1 diabetes mellitus patients with microvascular complications, *Metabolism* 60:256–259, 2010.
133. Devaraj S, Tobias P, Jialal I: Knockout of toll-like receptor-4 attenuates the pro-inflammatory state of diabetes, *Cytokine* 55:441–445, 2011.
134. Devaraj S, Tobias P, Kasinath BS, et al: Knockout of toll-like receptor-2 attenuates both the pro-inflammatory state of diabetes and incipient diabetic nephropathy, *Arterioscler Thromb Vasc Biol* 31:1796–1804.
135. Fullard N, Wilson CL, Oakley F: Roles of c-Rel signalling in inflammation and disease, *Int J Biochem Cell Biol* 44:851–860, 2012.
136. Ley K, Laudanna C, Cybulsky MI, et al: Getting to the site of inflammation: the leukocyte adhesion cascade updated, *Nat Rev Immunol* 7:678–689, 2007.
137. Tabas I: Consequences and therapeutic implications of macrophage apoptosis in atherosclerosis: the importance of lesion stage and phagocytic efficiency, *Arterioscler Thromb Vasc Biol* 25:2255–2264, 2005.
138. Arbustini E, Dal Bello B, Morbini P, et al: Plaque erosion is a major substrate for coronary thrombosis in acute myocardial infarction, *Heart* 82:269–272, 1999.
139. Farb A, Burke AP, Tang AL, et al: Coronary plaque erosion without rupture into a lipid core. A frequent cause of coronary thrombosis in sudden coronary death, *Circulation* 93:1354–1363, 1996.
140. Gimbrone MA Jr, Topper JN, Nagel T, et al: Endothelial dysfunction, hemodynamic forces, and atherogenesis, *Ann N Y Acad Sci* 902:230–239, 2000, discussion 239–240.
141. Topper JN, Cai J, Qiu Y, et al: Vascular MADs: two novel MAD-related genes selectively inducible by flow in human vascular endothelium, *Proc Natl Acad Sci U S A* 94:9314–9319, 1997.
142. Topper JN, Wasserman SM, Anderson KR, et al: Expression of the bumetanide-sensitive Na-K-Cl cotransporter BSC2 is differentially regulated by fluid mechanical and inflammatory cytokine stimuli in vascular endothelium, *J Clin Invest* 99:2941–2949, 1997.
143. Hajra L, Evans AI, Chen M, et al: The NF-kappa B signal transduction pathway in aortic endothelial cells is primed for activation in regions predisposed to atherosclerotic lesion formation, *Proc Natl Acad Sci U S A* 97:9052–9057, 2000.
144. Libby P, Ridker PM, Hansson GK: Progress and challenges in translating the biology of atherosclerosis, *Nature* 473:317–325, 2011.
145. Castelli WP: Lipids, risk factors and ischaemic heart disease, *Atherosclerosis* 124(Suppl):S1–S9, 1996.
146. Cannon CP, Braunwald E, McCabe CH, et al: Intensive versus moderate lipid lowering with statins after acute coronary syndromes, *N Engl J Med* 350:1495–1504, 2004.
147. Ridker PM, Buring JE, Shih J, et al: Prospective study of C-reactive protein and the risk of future cardiovascular events among apparently healthy women, *Circulation* 98:731–733, 1998.
148. Ridker PM, Cushman M, Stampfer MJ, et al: Inflammation, aspirin, and the risk of cardiovascular disease in apparently healthy men, *N Engl J Med* 336:973–979, 1997.
149. Ridker PM, MacFadyen JG, Wolfert RL, et al: Relationship of lipoprotein-associated phospholipase A(2) mass and activity with incident vascular events among primary prevention patients allocated to placebo or to statin therapy: an analysis from the JUPITER trial, *Clin Chem* 58:877–886, 2012.
150. Despres JP: Abdominal obesity and cardiovascular disease: is inflammation the missing link? *Can J Cardiol* 28:642–652, 2012.
151. Goldfine AB, Silver R, Aldhahi W, et al: Use of salsalate to target inflammation in the treatment of insulin resistance and type 2 diabetes, *Clin Transl Sci* 1:36–43, 2008.
152. Gomes MB, Piccirillo LJ, Nogueira VG, et al: Acute-phase proteins among patients with type 1 diabetes, *Diabetes Metab* 29:405–411, 2003.
153. Schaumberg DA, Glynn RJ, Jenkins AJ, et al: Effect of intensive glycemic control on levels of markers of inflammation in type 1 diabetes mellitus in the diabetes control and complications trial, *Circulation* 111:2446–2453, 2005.
153a. Stone NJ, Robinson J, Lichtenstein AH, et al: 2013 ACC/AHA Guideline on the Treatment of Blood Cholesterol to Reduce Atherosclerotic Cardiovascular Risk in Adults: A Report of the American College of Cardiology/American Heart Association Task Force on Practice Guidelines, *Circulation* 2013 Nov 12 epub ahead of print.
154. Hilgendorf I, Swirski FK: Making a difference: monocyte heterogeneity in cardiovascular disease, *Curr Atheroscler Rep* 14:450–459, 2012.
155. Kanter JE, Bornfeldt KE: Inflammation and diabetes-accelerated atherosclerosis: myeloid cell mediators, *Trends Endocrinol Metab,* 2012.
156. Bradshaw EM, Raddassi K, Elyaman W, et al: Monocytes from patients with type 1 diabetes spontaneously secrete proinflammatory cytokines inducing Th17 cells, *J Immunol* 183:4432–4439, 2009.
157. Swirski FK, Libby P, Aikawa E, et al: Ly-6Chi monocytes dominate hypercholesterolemia-associated monocytosis and give rise to macrophages in atheromata, *J Clin Invest* 117:195–205, 2007.
158. Kanter JE, Kramer F, Barnhart S, et al: Diabetes promotes an inflammatory macrophage phenotype and atherosclerosis through acyl-CoA synthetase 1, *Proc Natl Acad Sci U S A* 109: E715–E724.
159. Brown AL, Zhu X, Rong S, et al: Omega-3 fatty acids ameliorate atherosclerosis by favorably altering monocyte subsets and limiting monocyte recruitment to aortic lesions, *Arterioscler Thromb Vasc Biol* 32:2122–2130, 2012.
160. Ryu SK, Mallat Z, Benessiano J, et al: Phospholipase A2 enzymes, high-dose atorvastatin, and prediction of ischemic events after acute coronary syndromes, *Circulation* 125:757–766, 2012.
161. Liao X, Sluimer JC, Wang Y, et al: Macrophage autophagy plays a protective role in advanced atherosclerosis, *Cell Metab* 15:545–553, 2012.
162. Furuhashi M, Tuncman G, Görgün CZ, et al: Treatment of diabetes and atherosclerosis by inhibiting fatty-acid-binding protein aP2, *Nature* 447:959–965, 2007.
163. Hotamisligil GS: Endoplasmic reticulum stress and atherosclerosis, *Nat Med* 16:396–399, 2010.
164. Ozcan U, Yilmaz E, Ozcan L, et al: Chemical chaperones reduce ER stress and restore glucose homeostasis in a mouse model of type 2 diabetes, *Science* 313:1137–1140, 2006.
165. Lichtman AH: Adaptive immunity and atherosclerosis: mouse tales in the AJP, *Am J Pathol* 182:5–9, 2012.
166. Hansson GK, Jonasson L: The discovery of cellular immunity in the atherosclerotic plaque, *Arterioscler Thromb Vasc Biol* 29:1714–1717, 2009.
167. Giubilato S, Liuzzo G, Brugaletta S, et al: Expansion of CD4+CD28null T-lymphocytes in diabetic patients: exploring new pathogenetic mechanisms of increased cardiovascular risk in diabetes mellitus, *Eur Heart J* 32:1214–1226, 2011.
168. Deiuliis J, Shah Z, Shah N, et al: Visceral adipose inflammation in obesity is associated with critical alterations in tregulatory cell numbers, *PLoS One* 6:e16376, 2011.
169. Fleischhacker E, Esenabhalu VE, Spitaler M, et al: Human diabetes is associated with hyperreactivity of vascular smooth muscle cells due to altered subcellular Ca2+ distribution, *Diabetes* 48:1323–1330, 1999.
170. Sun J, Xu Y, Dai Z, et al: Intermittent high glucose enhances proliferation of vascular smooth muscle cells by upregulating osteopontin, *Mol Cell Endocrinol* 313:64–69, 2009.
171. Christopher J, Velarde V, Zhang D, et al: Regulation of B(2)-kinin receptors by glucose in vascular smooth muscle cells, *Am J Physiol Heart Circ Physiol* 280:H1537–H1546, 2001.
172. Li SL, Reddy MA, Cai Q, et al: Enhanced proatherogenic responses in macrophages and vascular smooth muscle cells derived from diabetic db/db mice, *Diabetes* 55:2611–2619, 2006.
173. Reddy MA, Jin W, Villeneuve L, et al: Pro-inflammatory role of microrna-200 in vascular smooth muscle cells from diabetic mice, *Arterioscler Thromb Vasc Biol* 32:721–729, 2012.
174. Glass CK, Ogawa S: Combinatorial roles of nuclear receptors in inflammation and immunity, *Nat Rev Immunol* 6:44–55, 2006.
175. Marx N, Mach F, Sauty A, et al: Peroxisome proliferator-activated receptor-gamma activators inhibit IFN-gamma-induced expression of the T cell-active CXC chemokines IP-10, Mig, and I-TAC in human endothelial cells, *J Immunol* 164:6503–6508, 2000.
176. Marx N, Schonbeck U, Lazar MA, et al: Peroxisome proliferator-activated receptor gamma activators inhibit gene expression and migration in human vascular smooth muscle cells, *Circ Res* 83:1097–1103, 1998.
177. Li AC, Binder CJ, Gutierrez A, et al: Differential inhibition of macrophage foam-cell formation and atherosclerosis in mice by PPARalpha, beta/delta, and gamma, *J Clin Invest* 114:1564–1576, 2004.
178. Lee CH, Chawla A, Urbiztondo N, et al: Transcriptional repression of atherogenic inflammation: modulation by PPARdelta, *Science* 302:453–457, 2003.
179. Cariou B, Charbonnel B, Staels B: Thiazolidinediones and PPARgamma agonists: time for a reassessment, *Trends Endocrinol Metab* 23:205–215, 2012.
180. Nissen SE, Wolski K: Effect of rosiglitazone on the risk of myocardial infarction and death from cardiovascular causes, *N Engl J Med* 356:2457–2471, 2007.
181. Dormandy JA, Charbonnel B, Eckland DJ, et al: Secondary prevention of macrovascular events in patients with type 2 diabetes in the PROactive Study (PROspective pioglitAzone Clinical Trial In macroVascular Events): a randomised controlled trial, *Lancet* 366:1279–1289, 2005.
182. ACCORD Study Group, Ginsberg HN, Elam MB, et al: Effects of combination lipid therapy in type 2 diabetes mellitus, *N Engl J Med* 362:1563–1574, 2010.
183. Rubins HB, Robins SJ, Collins D, et al: Gemfibrozil for the secondary prevention of coronary heart disease in men with low levels of high-density lipoprotein cholesterol. Veterans Affairs High-Density Lipoprotein Cholesterol Intervention Trial Study Group, *N Engl J Med* 341:410–418, 1999.
184. Cavender MA, Lincoff AM: Therapeutic potential of aleglitazar, a new dual PPAR-alpha/gamma agonist: implications for cardiovascular disease in patients with diabetes mellitus, *Am J Cardiovasc Drugs* 10:209–216, 2010.
185. Watts GF, Chan DC: Novel insights into the regulation of postprandial lipemia by glucagon-like peptides: significance for diabetes, *Diabetes* 62:336–338, 2013.
186. Simsek S, de Galan BE: Cardiovascular protective properties of incretin-based therapies in type 2 diabetes, *Curr Opin Lipidol* 23:540–547, 2012.
187. Brugts JJ, Yetgin T, Hoeks SE, et al: The benefits of statins in people without established cardiovascular disease but with cardiovascular risk factors: meta-analysis of randomised controlled trials, *BMJ* 338:b2376, 2009.
188. Ridker PM, Danielson E, Fonseca FA, et al: Rosuvastatin to prevent vascular events in men and women with elevated C-reactive protein, *N Engl J Med* 359:2195–2207, 2008.
189. Duewell P, Kono H, Rayner KJ, et al: NLRP3 inflammasomes are required for atherogenesis and activated by cholesterol crystals, *Nature* 464:1357–1361, 2010.
190. Plutzky J: Peroxisome proliferator-activated receptors in vascular biology and atherosclerosis: emerging insights for evolving paradigms, *Curr Atheroscler Rep* 2:327–335, 2000.
191. Di Pietro N, Di Tomo P, Di Silvestre S, et al: Increased iNOS activity in vascular smooth muscle cells from diabetic rats: potential role of Ca(2+)/calmodulin-dependent protein kinase II delta 2 (CaMKIIδ(2)), *Atherosclerosis* 226:88–94, 2012.
192. Gomez D, Owens GK: Smooth muscle cell phenotypic switching in atherosclerosis, *Cardiovasc Res* 95:156–164.
193. Devaraj S, Glaser N, Griffen S, et al: Increased monocytic activity and biomarkers of inflammation in patients with type 1 diabetes, *Diabetes* 55:774–779, 2006.
194. Scull CM, Tabas I: Mechanisms of ER stress-induced apoptosis in atherosclerosis, *Arterioscler Thromb Vasc Biol* 31:2792–2797, 2011.
195. Yngen M, Ostenson CG, Hu H, et al: Enhanced P-selectin expression and increased soluble CD40 ligand in patients with type 1 diabetes mellitus and microangiopathy: evidence for platelet hyperactivity and chronic inflammation, *Diabetologia* 47:537–540, 2004.

11 Type 1 Diabetes and Associated Cardiovascular Risk and Disease

David M. Maahs and Robert H. Eckel

Type 1 diabetes (T1D) is an autoimmune disease that causes destruction of the pancreatic beta cells, leading to absolute insulin deficiency (see also Chapter 3).[1] Type 2 diabetes (T2D), in contrast, is associated with obesity and is characterized by insulin resistance accompanied by an insufficient compensatory insulin secretory response (see also Chapter 1). T1D is not a rare condition; it affects an estimated 1.5 million people in the United States and 30 million worldwide.[2] T1D is the most common type of diabetes in youth, and by 18 years of age, 1/300 youth in the United States has T1D. However, T1D can also be diagnosed in adulthood; this accounts for 5% to 10% of all cases of diabetes worldwide.[3] The underlying differences in pathophysiology (autoimmune beta cell destruction in T1D compared with obesity accompanied by insulin resistance and beta cell dysfunction in T2D) are important considerations in the context of cardiovascular disease (CVD), cardiovascular mortality, and CVD risk factors in T1D as compared with T2D (see also Chapter 7). Another important consideration is that many people with T1D are under the age of 21 years, and the screening and treatment of CVD and its risk factors in children and adolescents with T1D are different from those in adults and less evidence based. (*Note:* The abbreviation *CVD* is used throughout the chapter unless a specific research study uses a different term.) In this chapter, the history, the scope of the problem of CVD in T1D including rates of disease, pathophysiology, risk factors, and treatment, and the outlook for CVD risk factors in T1D are reviewed. A recent consensus statement by the American Diabetes Association (ADA) and the American Heart Association (AHA) states that current recommendations for primary prevention of CVD in T2D appear appropriate for patients with T1D.[4] In addition, the ADA and AHA have recently published a joint scientific statement on T1D and CVD.[5]

HISTORY

T1D was a uniformly fatal disease before the discovery of insulin by Banting and Best in 1921.[6] The discovery of insulin and advances in care have transformed T1D from a subacute and fatal disease to a chronic disease with a high burden of daily individual care and serious acute (severe hypoglycemia and diabetic ketoacidosis [DKA]) and chronic (retinopathy, neuropathy, nephropathy, and CVD) complications. Achieving near-normal glucose control continues to be challenging because of limitations in compliance, medical care, and risk of hypoglycemia. In the past, patients with T1D were characterized by underinsulinization and a thin body habitus. However, increased emphasis has been placed on achieving near-normal glucose levels to prevent long-term microvascular and macrovascular complications since the publication of the findings from the Diabetes Control and Complications Trial (DCCT) in 1993 demonstrated the beneficial effects of intensive diabetes management on reduction of microvascular complications,[7] and then in 2005 the Epidemiology of Diabetes Interventions and Complications (EDIC) findings regarding macrovascular disease.[8] Diabetes care continues to improve based on such studies and advances in technology[9] including self-monitoring of blood glucose with home glucose meters and continuous glucose monitors,[10] continuous subcutaneous insulin infusions (insulin pumps),[11] insulin analogues with pharmacokinetic properties for basal and bolus administration,[12] and emerging artificial pancreas technology.[13–15]

MAGNITUDE OF THE CLINICAL PROBLEM OF CARDIOVASCULAR DISEASE IN TYPE 1 DIABETES

Epidemiology of Type 1 Diabetes

Numerous multicenter epidemiologic studies such as the SEARCH for Diabetes in Youth study,[16,17] the EURODIAB study,[18,19] and the DIAMOND Project (World Health Organization Multinational Project for Childhood Diabetes)[20,21] report increases in T1D of 2% to 5% annually worldwide. The prevalence of T1D in youth younger than 20 years of age in the United States was estimated in the SEARCH study to be 2.28/1000 or over 150,000 youth with diabetes in the United States in 2001, the majority with T1D.[16] Worldwide rates of T1D vary as expected because of variation in autoimmune system genetics, exposure to environmental triggers, and differences in survival from diagnosis of T1D and lifespan postdiagnosis as a result of differences in health care systems. These rapid and sustained increases suggest a cause that is environmental or related to a gene-environment interaction instead of genetic shifts. Multiple ongoing studies are investigating the cause of T1D to identify targets for prevention.[22,23] Such studies are likely long-term projects, barring dramatic scientific breakthroughs, highlighting the need to improve cardiovascular health for people with T1D. (See also Chapter 3.)

Despite progress in clinical care and outcomes for patients with T1D, improvements in outcomes are urgently needed.[24,25] EURODIAB followed 28,887 children in 12 European countries and found a standardized mortality rate of 2.0.[26] CVD was emphasized as the predominant cause for premature mortality in people with T1D in a report from the United Kingdom with a hazard ratio of 3.7 for annual mortality for people with T1D compared with the general population (8.0 versus 2.4/100,000 person-years).[27] These data highlight the need for improved CVD health in patients with T1D; however, there is reason to believe that health outcomes for people more recently diagnosed with T1D will be superior, given that these data are based on historic outcomes before the widespread adoption of many of the current methods of care for T1D. For example, the Pittsburgh Epidemiology of Diabetes Complications (EDC) study findings reported that life expectancy for people with T1D diagnosed from 1965 to 1980 was 15 years longer than for those diagnosed from 1950 to 1964.[28] The life expectancy of patients with T1D continues to improve[29,30]; however, the average life expectancy remains reduced by approximately 20 years relative to the general population.[31]

Rates of Cardiovascular Disease in Type 1 Diabetes

Increased rates of coronary heart disease (CHD) and death from CHD in T1D were reported in the 1970s.[32,33] The Pittsburgh Insulin-Dependent Diabetes Mellitus (IDDM) Morbidity and Mortality study reported a 10-fold higher rate of CHD mortality associated with type 1 diabetes mellitus (T1DM) as compared with individuals without diabetes in the United States,[34] similar to a study from the Joslin Diabetes Clinic that reported a six-times higher rate of CHD by 55 years of age in people with T1D as compared with controls with use of Framingham study data.[35] Among people diagnosed with diabetes who were younger than 30 years of age, the Wisconsin Epidemiologic Study of Diabetic Retinopathy (WESDR) reported a standardized mortality rate of 9.1 for men and 13.5 for women.[36] More recent data from 23,751 people with insulin-treated diabetes diagnosed before 30 years of age continue to show increased standardized mortality rates for ischemic heart disease, with a markedly increased rate in women, who had rates of death from heart disease that were similar to those in men younger than 40 years with diabetes.[37] The Pittsburgh EDC study has followed people with T1D (diagnosed from 1950 to 1980) for incidence of coronary artery disease (CAD) and has not detected decreases in CAD over time (stratified for T1D durations of 20, 25, and 30 years) despite decreases in mortality, neuropathy, and renal failure.[38] Data from the large (N = 21,789) population-based Scottish Registry Linkage Study reported that the age-adjusted incidence rate ratio for CVD and mortality in patients with T1D compared with those without diabetes was 3.0 (95% confidence interval [CI] 2.4-3.8) for women and 2.3 (95% CI 2.0-2.7) for men. Moreover, the incidence rate ratio for all-cause mortality was elevated similarly for both women 2.7 (95% CI 2.2-3.4) and men 2.6 (95% CI 2.2-3.0).[39] The authors concluded that despite improvement in risks for CVD and mortality for people with T1D, these rates continue to be higher than in the nondiabetic population and that CVD risk factor management needs to be improved, especially methods to achieve better glucose control.

Multiple risk factors for CVD in T1D exist, with glucose control considered to be the most likely factor accounting for increased risk as compared with nondiabetic controls. Despite a relatively small number of events compared with studies in patients with T2D, the DCCT and EDIC trials reported a 57% reduction in CVD in the intensively managed as compared with the conventional arm after 17 years of follow-up.[8] Similarly, the Coronary Artery Calcification in Type 1 Diabetes (CACTI) study, a longitudinal study of atherosclerosis in 1416 young adults with and without T1D, reported an association of HbA1c with progression of coronary artery calcification (CAC), an intermediate marker of coronary atherosclerosis.[40] However, data from epidemiologic studies on glucose control in T1D and CVD are inconclusive and have been the subject of review.[41] The ADA recommends an ABC approach to CVD: In addition to glucose control (HbA1c or A), blood pressure (B) and cholesterol (C) are emphasized.[42] Other modifiable CVD risk factors for people with T1D include kidney disease, obesity, insulin resistance, inflammation, and lifestyle factors such as smoking, diet, and exercise. Nonmodifiable CVD risk factors include genetics and family history and T1D duration. These are reviewed later in the chapter.

Specific Considerations for Cardiovascular Disease in Type 1 Diabetes: Age and Comparison with Type 2 Diabetes

T1D is frequently diagnosed in childhood, which includes the challenges associated with the physiologic changes of puberty. It has been well established by studies such as the Bogalusa Heart Study,[43] the Muscatine study,[44] the Pathobiological Determinants of Atherosclerosis in Youth (PDAY) study,[45] and the Young Finns Study[46] that atherosclerosis begins in youth and that the extent of atherosclerosis is associated with the presence and extent of CVD risk factors. These studies also demonstrate tracking of CVD risk factors from childhood into adulthood and argue for earlier attention to CVD risk.[47] Therefore, primary prevention of CVD and attention to CVD risk factors has gained increased attention in the past decade. For example, the ADA,[48] the AHA,[49] the American Academy of Pediatrics (AAP),[50] and the International Society for Pediatric and Adolescent Diabetes (ISPAD)[51] have all published guidelines for CVD health in youth with T1D; **Figure 11-1** shows the AHA guidelines for risk stratification and treatment. One such example of these includes thresholds for pharmacologic treatment of dyslipidemia and goals for lipids, although these are not based on randomized trials assessing CVD outcomes. Age- and gender-specific normal and abnormal values linked to the National Cholesterol Education Program—Adult Treatment Panel III (NCEP-ATP III) lipoprotein thresholds have also been calculated using National Health and Nutrition Examination Survey (NHANES) data[52] that recognize physiologic variations seen with pubertal development. Additional considerations for CVD risk factors in the pediatric diabetes population that have raised concerns about treatment include costs, lack of outcome data, potential life-long treatment, and adverse effects. Arguments for treatment include the tracking of CVD risk factors levels from childhood into adulthood, extensive data in adults on the benefits of lowering CVD risk factors to prevent CVD in adults with T1D, and the association of CVD risk factors with intermediate markers of atherosclerosis (**Table 11-1**).[53]

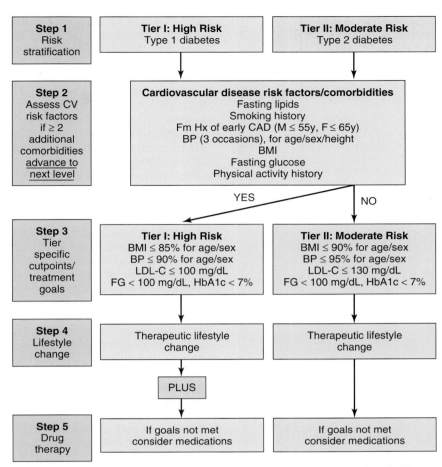

FIGURE 11-1 American Heart Association guidelines for risk stratification and treatment in youth with diabetes. *(Modified from Maahs DM, Wadwa RP, Bishop F, et al: Dyslipidemia in youth with diabetes: to treat or not to treat? J Pediatr 153:458-465, 2008.)*

In adults, recommendations for CVD risk modification in T1D continue to evolve. For adults, NCEP-ATP III considers diabetes to be a CHD risk equivalent and therefore uses goals for low-density lipoprotein cholesterol (LDL-C) and non–high-density lipoprotein cholesterol (HDL-C) of below 100 mg/dL (optional <70) and below 130 mg/dL (optional <100), respectively. The most recent joint position statement from the ADA and AHA does not distinguish CVD risk between T1D and T2D, citing a lack of evidence to do so.[4] As additional data accumulate, specific recommendations for adults with T1D will evolve. The recent ADA-AHA Scientific Statement on CVD in T1D summarizes the relative association of specific CVD risk factors and CVD events in T1D versus T2D (**Table 11-2**),[5] including that women with T1D are equally affected as men with T1D, unlike in T2D, in which men have increased rates of CVD.

Cardiovascular Disease Pathophysiology in Type 1 Diabetes

The recent ADA-AHA Scientific Statement calls for additional research into the differences in the atherosclerotic process between T1D and T2D,[5] although a summary of available data follows. A small study found similar CAC scores in T1D and T2D patients, but more obstructive lesions, more noncalcified lesions, and more lesions in general in T2D compared with T1D patients.[54] An earlier small study reported less atherosclerosis in T1D versus T2D patients.[55] Angiographic studies suggest more severe stenoses and more extensive involvement in people with T1D compared

with those without diabetes,[56] and another reported more severe distal disease with an approximately four times higher burden of atherosclerosis.[57] An autopsy study in T1D reported plaques were soft and fibrous with a more concentric location.[58] These studies were generally small and may not be representative of the T1D population. The nature of plaque in T1D is less well studied than in T2D, but the plaque may be more calcified and fibrotic and contain less lipid. More studies using techniques such as intravascular ultrasound and postmortem studies are needed.

CARDIOVASCULAR DISEASE RISK FACTORS IN TYPE 1 DIABETES

Modifiable Risk Factors: ABCs

A: A1c (or Hemoglobin A1c and Glucose Control)

As reviewed earlier, outcomes in T1D continue to improve as care for T1D improves. Although data suggest that the mean hemoglobin A1c (HbA1c) level has improved post-DCCT, these improvements are not as rapid as clinicians or patients wish. For example, the Diabetes Patienten Verlaufsdokumentation (DPV) study in children and adolescents with T1D in Germany and Austria (N = 30,708) reported a decrease in HbA1c of 0.038%/year from 8.7% in 1995 to 8.1% in 2009.[59] Although encouraging, at this pace of improvement mean HbA1c will not reach the adolescent goal of 7.5% for many years to come. Similarly, large studies from Australia,[60,61] Norway,[62] and Denmark[63] support improvement in HbA1c in the past decades. In the United States, the Type 1 Diabetes Exchange

TABLE 11-1 Pros and Cons of Pharmacologic Treatment of Cardiovascular Disease (CVD) Risk Factors in Patients with Type 1 Diabetes

PROS	CONS
CVD risk factors extend into adulthood and likely will remain abnormal.	Wait until adulthood to treat CVD risk factors for the following reasons: The 10-year risk of a CVD event is unknown at the present time. Refer patient to an adulthood endocrinologist once the patient is 18 years old for treatment at that time.
Adolescent risk factors predict surrogate markers of cardiovascular disease (CIMT) in adults (Young Finns, Bogalusa).	Some data suggest that regression, or at least slowing of progression, of atherosclerosis with aggressive treatment is possible in adults.
CVD risk factors are associated with atherosclerosis in childhood.	There are no data that treatment in youth will reduce long-term CVD complications.
CVD risk factors are an important microvascular and macrovascular risk factors.	*Primum non nocere:* There are potential adverse events from pharmacologic treatment. There is potential teratogenicity for adolescent girls.
Type 1 diabetes (T1D) is considered a CVD risk factor equivalent in adults.	Cost: The number needed to treat to prevent CVD events cannot be calculated. Many years of treatment are required, with potential for life-time treatment.
Earlier T1D onset results in a longer T1D disease burden and potential adverse "vasculo-metabolic memory" and an increased "area under the curve" for CVD risk factors.	There is some measurement variability with regression to the mean of CVD risk factors, although they tend to track as high or normal.
There is a long-term elevated risk of CVD in youth with CVD risk factors (PDAY, Young Finns, Bogalusa).	There are no outcome data and no safety data in youth with T1D.
There is a preponderance of data regarding lowering CVD risk in adults; why wait?	

CIMT = Carotid intima-media thickness; PDAY = Pathobiological Determinants of Atherosclerosis in Youth study.
Data from Maahs DM, Wadwa RP, Bishop F, et al: Dyslipidemia in youth with diabetes: to treat or not to treat? *J Pediatr* 153:458-465, 2008.)

TABLE 11-2 Relative Association between Specific Cardiovascular Risk Factors and CVD Events in T1D versus T2D (Range 0 To +++)

	T1DM	T2DM
Hypertension	+++	++
Cigarette smoke	++	++
Inflammation	+	++
High LDL-C	+	++
Low HDL-C	0,+	++
TG	No data	++
Microalbuminuria	+++	+++
Insulin resistance	+	+++
Poor glycemic control	++	+++

TG = Triglyceride(s); + = strong association; ++ = stronger association; +++ = strongest association.
Data from de Ferranti SD: Type 1 diabetes mellitus and cardiovascular disease, *Circulation.* In press.

reported only 27% of children younger than 13 years and 23% of 13- to 20-year-olds met the ISPAD HbA1c target of 7.5%.[64] In adults with T1D, the EDC study reported decreases in HbA1c from 9.0% to 8.5% to 8.3% from the mid-1980s to the mid-2000s (**Table 11-3**). The Type 1 Diabetes Exchange reported that the mean HbA1c level in T1D exceeds the ADA goal in all age groups (**Fig. 11-2**). These data on HbA1c are important because, as mentioned previously, the DCCT-EDIC study demonstrated that intensive diabetes management (with resultant HbA1c contrast of 7.3% in the intensive arm versus 9.1% in the conventional arm) resulted in a 57% reduction in CVD events,[8] although there were relatively few events. Similarly, a meta-analysis found a lower relative risk for macrovascular events (0.38, 95% CI 0.26-0.56) for intensive versus conventional therapy.[65] These data are consistent with other DCCT-EDIC data on intensive management (and lower HbA1c), with more favorable effects on intermediate markers of CVD such as carotid intima-media wall thickness (CIMT)[66] and CAC.[67] However, perhaps because of methodologic issues, HbA1c has not consistently been associated with CVD in epidemiologic studies.[41] For example, the EURODIAB study did not find an association of HbA1c with CHD,[68] nor did the Pittsburgh EDC study in earlier investigations,[69,70] but did in a later study in which glucose control was more strongly associated with CAD mortality than morbidity.[71] Similarly, in the WESDR study, HbA1c was associated with CVD mortality but not myocardial infarction.[72,73] A large Swedish database (N = 7454) reported a 30% increased hazard ratio for CAD per 1% increase in HbA1c.[74]

With improved glucose control, there is a concern that this will lead not only to increases in hypoglycemia and weight, but an altered lipoprotein profile as seen in a subset of patients in the DCCT.[75] There are data to suggest that properly focused intensification of glucose control can be achieved without increases in weight,[76] and such efforts are important to avoid the unwanted effects of weight gain on insulin resistance and lipids.

B: Blood Pressure or Hypertension
Hypertension is a strong risk factor for CVD. In T1D, hypertension is related to increased risk of both microvascular[77–79] and macrovascular disease.[70,80] In both youth and adults, the prevalence of hypertension is higher in people with T1D as compared with those without diabetes. Data from the Pittsburgh EDC study on the predictors of major outcomes in T1D showed that the importance of glucose control on outcomes diminished over time (perhaps because of improved control), but hypertension continued to be a strong predictor of CVD, suggesting the importance of blood pressure control on outcomes in T1D.[81] Few findings from pharmacologic intervention trials regarding the ideal threshold for blood pressure in T1D have been published, and angiotensin-converting enzyme (ACE) inhibitors and angiotensin receptor blockers (ARBs) are most commonly used,[82] consistent with professional society recommendations.[42] In a small randomized clinical trial (N = 54), no difference was reported in blood pressure lowering or glomerular filtration rate (GFR) between the enalapril or nifedipine arms.[83]

One important consideration in youth is that hypertension is defined based on age and gender percentiles. In youth with T1D, estimates of hypertension prevalence range from 4% to 8%.[84–87] Predictors of blood pressure in youth with diabetes include glucose control,[88] obesity,[89] and diet.[90] Of note, treatment of hypertension in youth with diabetes is reported to be low, with only 1.5% and 2.1% of youth reporting treatment

TABLE 11-3 Clinical Characteristics of the DCCT/EDIC and EDC Cohorts

| | Conventional | | | | | | Intensive | | |
| | DCCT | | EDIC | EDC | | | DCCT | | EDIC |
Characteristic	Baseline (1983-1989) (N = 730)	Closeout (1993) (N = 723)	Year 12 (2005) (N = 606)	Baseline (1986-1988) (N = 161)	Year 10 (1996) (N = 105)	Year 18 (2006) (N = 88)	Baseline (1983-1989) (N = 711)	Closeout (1993) (N = 698)	Year 12 (2005) (N = 620)
Age, mean (SD), years	27 (7)	33 (7)	46 (7)	20 (4)	31 (4)	40 (4)	27 (7)	34 (7)	46 (7)
Duration, mean (SD), years	5 (4)	12 (5)	24 (5)	11 (2)	21 (2)	30 (2)	6 (4)	12 (5)	25 (5)
BMI, mean (SD)	24 (3)	25 (3)	28 (5)	24 (3)	26 (4)	28 (5)	23 (3)	27 (4)	28 (5)
BMI ≥30, %	2	6	28	3	1	27	1	19	31
Current smoker, %	18	20	12	20	17	15	19	20	15
HbAtc % (SD)	8.9 (1.6)	9.1 (1.5)	7.7 (1.2)	9.0 (1.7)	8.5 (1.4)	8.3 (1.8)	8.9 (1.6)	7.4 (1.1)	7.8 (1.2)

BMI = Body mass index; SD = standard deviation.
Data from Diabetes Control and Complications Trial/Epidemiology of Diabetes Interventions and Complications (DCCT/EDIC) Research Group; Nathan DM, Zinman B, Cleary PA, et al: Modern-day clinical course of type 1 diabetes mellitus after 30 years' duration: the Diabetes Control and Complications Trial/Epidemiology of Diabetes Interventions and Complications and Pittsburgh Epidemiology of Diabetes Complications experience (1983-2005), *Arch Intern Med* 169:1307-1316, 2009.

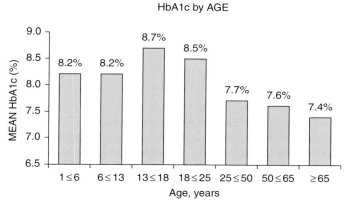

FIGURE 11-2 Mean HbA1c in T1D Exchange by age.

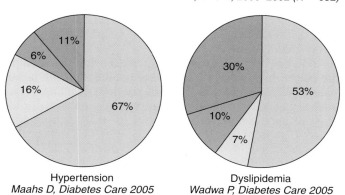

FIGURE 11-3 Hypertension and dyslipidemia remain poorly controlled in patients with T1D, CACTI, 2000-2002 (N = 652). *(Data from Maahs DM, Kinney GL, Wadwa P, et al: Hypertension prevalence, awareness, treatment, and control in an adult type 1 diabetes population and a comparable general population, Diabetes Care 28:301-306, 2005; and Wadwa RP, Kinney GL, Maahs DM, et al: Awareness and treatment of dyslipidemia in young adults with type 1 diabetes, Diabetes Care 28:1051-1056, 2005.)*

with blood pressure–lowering medications in the SEARCH[86] and DPV[87] studies, despite 5.9% and 8.1% prevalence of hypertension in the T1D subjects in each study. In addition to measurement of blood pressure during office visits, 24-hour ambulatory blood pressure has been used to detect reduced nocturnal dipping, which has been associated with development of microalbuminuria.[91]

In adults, the CACTI study reported higher rates of hypertension prevalence (43% versus 15%, $P < 0.0001$), awareness of hypertension, treatment, and control in adults with T1D than in those without diabetes (**Fig. 11-3**).[82] These observations suggest that adults with T1D are more likely to be hypertensive than individuals without diabetes, but also to be more aware of the diagnosis and to be treated, although only 42% of the T1D adults achieved the JNC 7 goal of below 130/80 mm Hg.[92] Similarly, the EURODIAB study reported that less than 50% of T1D adults with hypertension were treated to goal.[93] The most recent ADA recommendations suggest that blood pressure should be measured routinely at each visit and that patients with hypertension should be treated to a goal of less than 140/80 mm Hg, although lower targets may be appropriate.[42] Patients with a blood pressure exceeding 120/80 mm Hg are recommended to make healthy lifestyle changes including weight loss, dietary changes (such as use of the DASH diet [Dietary Approaches to Stop Hypertension]), moderation of alcohol intake, and increased physical activity. ACE inhibitors or ARBs are recommended as first-line pharmacologic treatment, and multiple medications are often required to achieve control.

C: Cholesterol (Dyslipidemia)

Data from the DCCT[94] and others such as the CACTI study[95] indicate that adults with well-controlled T1D have fasting lipid profiles similar to or even less atherogenic than nondiabetic controls. As in the nondiabetic population, dyslipidemia is considered an important risk factor for CVD in T1D, although the frequency of dyslipidemia does not explain the increased rates of CVD in T1D. Data from the EDC study suggest that LDL-C levels below 100 mg/dL are associated with increased CVD risk[96] and that the usual inverse association of HDL-C to CVD risk is seen in men but not in women, who had little association between HDL-C levels above the 50- to 60-mg/dL range and CVD risk.[97] In addition, rates of statin treatment have increased in adults with T1D over time. For example, the CACTI study reported statin use increased from 17% to 32% to 46% of the cohort over three study visits from 2000 to 2006.[98] Longitudinal data from the DCCT-EDIC, the EDC, and the Scottish Care Information–Diabetes Collaboration database studies also show a similar increase in the use of statins.[39,99] However, despite this increase in statin use, 39% of people with T1D who were older than 40 years in the Scottish study were not treated with a statin. Moreover, the trials with statins have included too few patients with T1D to be definitive, but the outcomes suggest benefit with regard to major CVD events.[100] One of the potential effects of more intensive glucose control is increased weight gain with associated deleterious effects on the lipid panel[75,101]; however, the increased use of statins in T1D may explain improved lipid profiles over time.

Risk factors for elevated lipids in T1D include male gender, older age, increased waist circumference and visceral fat, and higher HbA1c[98] as well as renal disease (proteinuria and decreased GFR) and autoimmune thyroid disease. In longitudinal analyses of epidemiologic data in both children and adults, change in HbA1c was associated with change in lipids; however, these associations are relatively modest—for example, a 4-mg/dL change in LDL-C for every 1% change in HbA1c[98,102]—a much weaker effect than would be expected from a statin. This suggests that although glucose control is the cornerstone of care, it may be insufficient to achieve lipid targets in most people with T1D (**Fig. 11-4**).

Excellent reviews of the pathophysiology of lipid disorders in T1D have been published historically[103] and more recently by Verges.[104] In general, abnormalities of lipoproteins in T1D can be classified in the context of the underlying glucose control, which is a function of matching exogenous insulin delivery to maintain near euglycemia (or the failure to do so) and how this alters normal lipid and lipoprotein physiology. T1D lipid pathophysiology can be considered in the categories of untreated T1D with extreme insulin deficiency such as seen in DKA in contrast to treated T1D with varying degrees of glucose control and insulin resistance.

Since publication of the 2003 ADA statement on Management of Dyslipidemia in Children and Adolescents with

Diabetes,[105] data have accumulated indicating dyslipidemia is common in youth with T1D. A retrospective cross-sectional analysis of 682 youth with T1D younger than 21 years revealed that 18.6% had total cholesterol (TC) exceeding 200 mg/dL or HDL-C below 35 mg/dL,[106] with longitudinal analysis in the same cohort indicating sustained abnormalities over time with only 6% being treated with a lipid-lowering medication.[107] The DPV study (N = 27,358) in Germany and Austria reported dyslipidemia (defined as TC above 200 mg/dL, LDL-C above 130 mg/dL, or HDL-C below 35 mg/dL) in 29% of the participants younger than 26 years with increasing rates in older age categories.[87] Similarly, only 0.4% in this study received lipid-lowering medications. In the SEARCH study of youth with T1D (N = 2165), the prevalence of LDL-C above 160, above 130, and above 100 mg/dL was 3%, 14%, and 48%, respectively.[108] Among these participants, only 1% were on lipid-lowering medications, indicating that in the years after the 2003 ADA statement,[105] few pediatric endocrinologists or primary care providers were treating elevated LDL-C pharmacologically as recommended by the ADA. However, these data may not reflect more current practice in pediatrics. More recently, data from the Type 1 Diabetes Exchange report similar rates of dyslipidemia among participants with available data; 95% and 86% met ADA (HDL-C of 35 mg/dL or higher) and ISPAD (HDL-C above 1.1 mmol/L or 41 mg/dL) HDL-C targets, and 35% and 10% exceeded LDL-C (100 mg/dL) and TG (150 mg/dL) targets.[64]

The ADA recommends screening for dyslipidemia in children with T1D after glucose control has been established in children older than 2 years if there is a family history of hypercholesterolemia or a CVD event before age 55 years or if the history is unknown (**Table 11-4**). If family history is not a concern, then screening is recommended at puberty; if findings are normal, then screening is repeated every 5 years,[42] similar to the AHA guidelines (see **Fig. 11-1**).[110] In children with diabetes, goals for lipids include LDL-C below 100 mg/dL, HDL-C above 35 mg/dL, and TG below 150 mg/dL. Similar cut points are used for AHA[110] and ISPAD.[51] For adults, NCEP-ATP III considers diabetes (without distinction between T1D or T2D) to be a CHD risk equivalent and therefore uses goals for LDL-C and non–HDL-C of below 100 (optional <70) and below 130 (optional <100) mg/dL, respectively.

Additional considerations in a patient with T1D include the risk of hypoglycemia while the patient is in the fasted state, when fasting for the purpose of lipid profiling. It has been suggested that a nonfasting sample for analysis of lipids may be an effective screening tool for most people with T1D.[53] Data from the DPV registry (N = 29,979) suggest that fasting status had a minimal effect on TC, LDL-C, and HDL-C.[111] Therefore it seems reasonable to screen for dyslipidemia in people with T1D with a nonfasting sample, with the caveat that a repeat evaluation may be required to better delineate lipid health.

An additional factor in treatment of dyslipidemia as with other CVD risk factors in T1D will be continued advances in pharmacologic therapy. Statins have been introduced, and the accumulation of safety and efficacy data as well as a decrease in price have led to their increased use. Data on the use of lipid-lowering medications in T1D are more limited than in T2D; specifically, the Cholesterol Treatment Trialists' Collaborators reported a 21% proportional reduction in major vascular events per mmol/L reduction

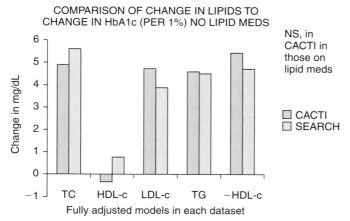

FIGURE 11-4 Association of change in lipids/1% change in HbA1c in CACTI and SEARCH. (*Data from Maahs DM, Ogden LG, Dabelea D, et al: Association of glycaemia with lipids in adults with type 1 diabetes: modification by dyslipidaemia medication, Diabetologia 53:2518-2525, 2010; and Maahs DM, Dabelea D, D'Agostino RB Jr, et al: Glucose control predicts 2-year change in lipid profile in youth with type 1 diabetes, J Pediatr 162:101-107, 2013.*)

TABLE 11-4 ADA Recommendations for Lipid Screening and Management in Youth with Diabetes

	TID	T2D
Initial screening age (after glycemic control has been achieved)	Over 2 years at diagnosis if unknown or with a positive family history; otherwise at 12 years (puberty)	At diagnosis
Rescreening if lipid levels are normal	5 years	2 years
Optimal concentrations	LDL-C: <100 mg/dL	LDL-C: <100 mg/dL
	HDL-C: >35 mg/dL	HDL-C: >35 mg/dL
	Triglycerides: <150 mg/dL	Triglycerides: <150 mg/dL
	Goal LDL-C: <100 mg/dL	Goal LDL-C: <100 mg/dL
Management of Elevated LDL-C		
Initial therapy	Glycemic control, MNT, physical activity, weight control, tobacco cessation	Glycemic control, MNT, physical activity, weight control, tobacco cessation
After 3 to 6 months	LDL-C >160 mg/dL: begin medication	LDL-C >160 mg/dL: begin medication
	LDL-C 130-159 mg/dL: recommended after MNT failure based on other CVD risk factors	LDL-C 130-159 mg/dL: recommended after MNT failure based on other CVD risk factors
	Pregnancy counseling if statin is started	Pregnancy counseling if statin is started

MNT = Medical nutritional therapy.
Data from Maahs DM, Wadwa RP, Bishop F, et al: Dyslipidemia in youth with diabetes: to treat or not to treat? *J Pediatr* 153:458-465; 2008.

(38.6 mg/dL reduction) in LDL-C in people with T1D (n = 1466 in a meta-analysis from 14 randomized statin trials).[100] However, there is some concern that adequate documentation of T1D was lacking.

For initial treatment of dyslipidemia, the ADA recommends optimization of glucose control and medical nutritional therapy (MNT), basically a diet that includes multiple servings of fruits and vegetables, whole grains, lean poultry, and fish and contains limited amounts of saturated fat. Statin therapy is recommended for patients with LDL-C above 160 mg/dL, or above 130 mg/dL in the presence of one or more CVD risk factors after MNT and lifestyle changes in patients with T1D younger than 10 years.[42] Presently, the ADA considers an adult T1D patient statin eligible unless he or she has LDL-C below 100 mg/dL and/or is pregnant, nursing, or attempting to conceive.[42] At what age the statin should be started or given to T1D patients who have LDL-C below 100 mg/dL remains an uncertainty.[53]

Other Cardiovascular Disease Risk Factors
Kidney Disease

With advances in clinical care, people with T1D are living longer and healthier lives, which highlights the need for refinement of care for chronic comorbidities such as CVD and its risk factors. Historically in the 1970s and 1980s, diabetic renal disease (most commonly with proteinuria) was associated with rapid progression to death, frequently as a result of CVD.[112,113] With advances in diabetes care including improved glucose and blood pressure control, patients with T1D without baseline diabetic kidney disease (either estimated glomerular filtration rate [eGFR] <60 mL/min/1.73 m^2 or microalbuminuria) had similar mortality outcomes to those of nondiabetic patients over 7 years in the Finnish Diabetic Nephropathy Study (FinnDiane)[114] and over 20 years in the Pittsburgh EDC study.[115] The CACTI study found increased CAC progression in a stepwise manner with increasing albumin-to-creatinine ratios (ACR) and decreasing eGFRs (**Fig. 11-5A, B**). In contrast, even in the absence of early diabetic kidney disease, people with T1D had increased odds of progression of CAC over 6 years compared with those without diabetes.[116] Whether increases in CAC predict an earlier development of CVD events and/or related mortality in people with T1D remains to be shown.

Given the well-established association of kidney disease to CVD and mortality in T1D, screening for elevated urinary ACR is recommended annually in adolescents and adults and eGFR is recommended in adults with T1D.[42] Rates of microalbuminuria in research studies in youth with T1D have ranged from 5% to 10% in recent decades,[117–119] with reports of the clinical diagnosis of microalbuminuria of 4.3% and 3.8% from the large DPV study[120] (n = 27,805) and the Type 1 Diabetes Exchange (N = 6784),[121] respectively. Of note, in the Type 1 Diabetes Exchange, only 41% of adolescents with the diagnosis of microalbuminuria reported ACE inhibitor or ARB treatment. Prevention and treatment of early diabetic kidney disease remains a clinical challenge in T1D with important implications for CVD prevention.

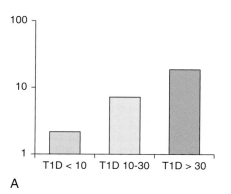

A

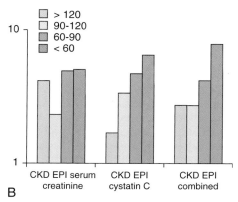

B

FIGURE 11-5 Odds ratio for CAC progression (CACp) by ACR and eGFR status. A, Odds ratio for CACp by ACR status. **B,** Odds ratio for CACp by eGFR category (patients without diabetes are reference group with odds ratio of 1) in CACTI. *(Modified from Maahs D, Jalal D, Chonchol M, et al: Impaired renal function further increases odds of 6 year coronary artery calcification progression in adults with type 1 diabetes: the CACTI Study,* Diabetes Care *36:2607-2614, 2013.)*

Obesity and Insulin Resistance

Rates of obesity in people with T1D in the United States are now similar to the increased rates of obesity in the U.S. general population. The average body mass index (BMI) has increased in the past two decades in the DCCT-EDIC and the Pittsburgh EDC studies, likely because of aging of the patients, more intensive glucose control, and the increasing prevalence of obesity in the United States in general (see **Table 11-3**). Similarly, in children with diabetes, an increased prevalence of obesity has been reported over the past decade.[122] The SEARCH study found either overweight or obesity in 37% of female patients and 32% of male patients with T1D.[123] Increased weight gain with intensive glucose control can be an impediment to reaching HbA1c goals and could worsen some CVD risk factors. Obesity also increases insulin resistance both in people without diabetes[124,125] and in those with T1D, both historically[126,127] and in the post-DCCT era with achievement of tighter glucose control.[128,129]

In addition to poor glucose control, insulin resistance caused by increasing adiposity and associated peripheral hyperinsulinemia can result in a lipid profile similar to that seen in the metabolic syndrome or T2D with elevated TG and decreased HDL-C. Studies have evaluated the addition of metformin to insulin to improve insulin resistance in people with T1D with mixed effects on HbA1c but some improvement in lipids.[130] The role of insulin sensitizers in T1D and the potential benefits with regard to CVD risk factors require further evaluation.[131] Recent data from the DCCT-EDIC study indicate that excess weight gain in DCCT was associated with sustained increases in central obesity, insulin resistance, dyslipidemia, and blood pressure and more atherosclerosis as measured by CAC and CIMT.[132]

With current methods of intensive glucose control, insulin is delivered subcutaneously and leads to peripheral hyperinsulinemia,[133] but research is ongoing regarding intraperitoneal insulin infusion with implantable insulin pumps that more closely mimic physiologic insulin delivery. Such devices have the potential to achieve more physiologic control of T1D and may have beneficial effects on CVD risk factors.[134,135]

Inflammation

Inflammation is a fundamental factor in the cause of atherosclerosis (see also Chapter 10)[136] and is implicated in the pathophysiologic process of the development of T1D (see also Chapter 3).[137,138] Higher levels of interleukin 6 (IL-6) and fibrinogen were reported in children and adolescents with T1D as compared with normal-weight controls in the SEARCH for Diabetes in Youth study.[139] Also, C-reactive protein (CRP) was higher in the top quartiles of HbA1c, and inflammation was associated with dyslipidemia. Wadwa and colleagues have reported that soluble IL-2 receptor, a marker of T cell activation, was associated with progression of CAC in people with (and without) T1D in the CACTI study.[140] In addition, subjects with T1D exhibit elevated levels of inflammatory endothelial markers such as sICAM, sVCAM, sE-selectin, suggesting endothelial dysfunction.[141] More recently, Alman and colleagues reported that a broad panel of inflammatory markers (with sTNFR2, sIL-2R, IL-18, sIL-1RA, and tumor necrosis factor α [TNF-α] being the most strongly loaded in the principal component analysis) was associated with progression of CAC in the CACTI cohort.[142] In addition, recent data suggest that a postinfarction autoimmune syndrome (myocarditis) may contribute to worse postmyocardial infarction outcomes in people with T1D.[143,144]

Additional data are required on the mechanisms of inflammation in CVD in T1D, whether it differs from findings in individuals without diabetes, and what therapeutic targets exist to reduce CVD.

Lifestyle Modification: Smoking, Diet, and Exercise

Smoking prevention, healthy diet, and increasing exercise are standard lifestyle modifications for people with T1D with well-documented health benefits including CVD health.[42] Cigarette smoking is one of the leading preventable causes of CVD (and other diseases) in the United States, and its prevention has been the focus of extensive public health efforts. In adults with T1D, smoking was associated with progression of CIMT in the DCCT-EDIC study[145] and arterial stiffness in the EDC study.[146] Use of tobacco was reported in 2.7% of 10- to 14-year-olds, 17.1% of 15- to 19-year-olds), and 34.0% of individuals older than 20 years in the SEARCH study and was associated with higher TG and physical inactivity.[147] Schwab and colleagues have reported that in adolescents with T1D, smoking contributes to CVD via worsening glucose control, dyslipidemia, and endothelial function.[148] The SEARCH study also reported that less than 50% of 10- to 14-year-old participants with diabetes reported being counseled by their health care provider to not smoke or to stop smoking.[147] Smoking increases CVD risk factors, including deterioration of glucose control, lipids, and endothelial function[148] in T1D, and increases the risk of nephropathy, retinopathy, and neuropathy.[149]

The role of nutrition in CVD is well established,[150-152] and MNT improves CVD risk factors in adults with T2D.[152,153] ADA guidelines for MNT recommend adequate calories be provided for growth and development in children and adolescents and that the combination of carbohydrates, protein, and fat be adjusted to meet glucose, blood pressure, and lipid goals.[42] Adults with T1D in the CACTI study reported higher than recommended intake of fat and saturated fat that was associated with worse glucose control, CVD risk factors, and CAC.[154] Most studies indicate that youth with diabetes fail to meet recommended nutritional intake of fruits, vegetables, and whole grains but exceed recommended intake of fat.[155-159] The SEARCH study reported that adherence to the DASH diet was associated with lower blood pressure, a better HDL/LDL ratio, and lower HbA1c level in youth with T1D.[161] Of interest, both sugar-sweetened beverage and diet beverage intake were also associated with a higher HbA1c level, higher blood pressure, and higher lipids.[162] Healthy diet has an important—and complex—role in T1D management both for glucose control and for CVD risk reduction. For example, the standard of care for meal-time insulin dosage is based on concurrent blood glucose and carbohydrate intake; however, protein and fat intake (as well as dietary fiber) can influence blood glucose levels,[163,164] with potential effects on dietary choices and CVD risk.

Physical activity is recommended as an integral part of T1D management.[42] Adults with diabetes are advised to exercise for more than 150 min/wk, and it is recommended by the AAP that youth engage in 60 minutes of moderate-to-vigorous physical activity daily. Several studies suggest that youth with T1D are more sedentary and less fit than nondiabetic youth.[165-167] One study in adults reported no difference in physical activity between adults with and without T1D and that physical inactivity and smoking were both associated with CAC.[168] The EDC study found a beneficial association between physical activity and CVD and mortality.[169]

PART III

MANAGEMENT OF CORONARY HEART DISEASE RISK AND DISEASE IN PATIENTS WITH DIABETES

12 Effect of Lifestyle Interventions on Coronary Heart Disease Risk in Patients with Diabetes

Barry A. Franklin, Wendy M. Miller, and Tracy R. Juliao

In the United States, the prevalence of high cholesterol, hypertension, and cigarette smoking together with age-adjusted cardiovascular deaths has declined over the last several decades.[1] On the other hand, the prevalence of diabetes has risen steadily, largely because of an epidemic of obesity and adiposity and our increasingly inactive lifestyle (see also Chapters 1 and 5).[2] These trends will likely mitigate further reductions in cardiovascular mortality and even reverse the decline in cardiovascular disease (CVD) incidence.[3]

Using 2010 as the baseline, the estimated direct and indirect costs of CVD are expected to triple by the year 2030, making this a critical medical and societal issue.[4,5] These sobering projections and other recent data[6,7] suggest that effective preventive strategies are needed if we are to limit the growing burden of CVD (see also Chapters 5 and 6). The current reactive-based health care model, in which patients are seen when they become ill, typically during outpatient visits or hospitalizations, often fails to proactively improve health, because so many health outcomes are explained by individual behaviors and the lifestyle choices people make on a daily basis.[6,8]

Unfortunately, many patients as well as individuals in the medical community continue to rely on costly coronary revascularization procedures and/or cardioprotective medications as a first-line strategy to stabilize or favorably modify established risk factors and the course of coronary heart disease (CHD). However, these therapies do not address the root of the problem, that is, the most proximal risk factors for CHD, including poor dietary practices, physical inactivity, and cigarette smoking, as shown in **Figure 12-1**.[3] Unhealthy lifestyle habits strongly influence not only conventional risk factors (e.g., blood pressure, lipid and lipoprotein levels, glucose-insulin homeostasis) but also novel or emerging risk factors such as endothelial function, inflammation (e.g., C-reactive protein), thrombosis and coagulation, arrhythmias, and other disease modulators (e.g., psychosocial stressors),[3] even among users of lipid-lowering and antihypertensive medications.[9] Collectively, these data suggest it is time to change our emphasis from disease management to disease prevention, focusing on the foundational causes of CVD by reengineering prevention into the U.S. health care system.[7]

This chapter emphasizes the role of lifestyle interventions in the prevention and treatment of CVD in patients with diabetes, with specific reference to weight management and energy balance, dietary intake and cardiometabolic risk, smoking cessation, exercise and physical activity, cardiorespiratory fitness, and research-based psychosocial

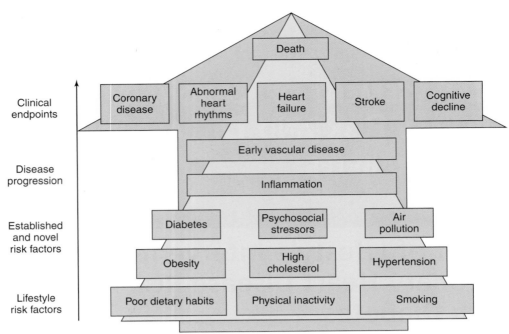

FIGURE 12-1 Unhealthy lifestyle habits lead to coronary risk factors, the progression of cardiovascular disease, and ultimately adverse outcomes or clinical endpoints. Thus the first-line strategy to prevent coronary heart disease (or recurrent cardiac events) is to favorably modify poor lifestyle habits or practices, including suboptimal dietary habits, physical inactivity, and cigarette smoking. *(Modified from Mozaffarian D and colleagues.[3])*

interventions (e.g., readiness for changes, motivational interviewing, counseling strategies) to support cardioprotective lifestyle change in this at-risk patient subset (see also Chapter 5).

WEIGHT MANAGEMENT AND ENERGY BALANCE

Obesity is an independent risk factor for hypertension, dyslipidemia, and CVD, increasing the risk of cardiovascular events and mortality in patients with type 2 diabetes.[10-12] Distribution of body fat also plays a role in cardiometabolic risk; individuals with central adiposity, as evidenced by increased waist measurement or "apple" body shape, have higher risk.[13] Elevated waist circumference is defined as greater than 100 cm (40 inches) for North American men and greater than 88 cm (35 inches) for North American women.[14] The proposed Diabetes Federation cut points for other geographical areas and countries are somewhat lower.[15] Most individuals with type 2 diabetes are overweight or obese and/or have an elevated waist circumference. Therefore weight reduction is commonly indicated for patients with type 2 diabetes.

Increased waist measurement is a surrogate marker for visceral adiposity, which is fat tissue within the peritoneal cavity surrounding the intra-abdominal organs. Visceral adiposity is metabolically active, secreting a number of cytokine-like factors, referred to as *adipokines*. Adipokines promote inflammation and a prothrombotic state and are associated with development of atherogenic dyslipidemia (hypertriglyceridemia, low high-density lipoprotein [HDL] cholesterol [HDL-C] level, and an elevated subfraction of small, dense low-density lipoprotein [LDL] cholesterol [LDL-C] level), insulin resistance, dysglycemia and elevated blood pressure.[16] Inflammation, as measured by serum level

of high-sensitivity C-reactive protein, is also associated with type 2 diabetes and CVD.[17] Modest weight reduction of 5% total body weight in individuals with type 2 diabetes is associated with decreased visceral adiposity and improvement in serum lipid concentrations, insulin action, and fasting blood glucose, as well as reductions in blood pressure, serum markers of inflammation, and the need for diabetes medication(s).[18] In some patients, substantial weight loss can lead to clinical resolution of type 2 diabetes (see also Chapters 2, 9, and 10).[19]

Weight loss occurs when energy intake is lower than energy expenditure. An energy deficit of 500 to 1000 kcal/day (3500 to 7000 kcal/wk) usually results in a weight loss of 1 to 2 lb/wk. Rate of weight loss can vary, however, depending on genetic factors, age, fidgeting, amount of lean body mass, and habitual physical activity. Older individuals tend to lose weight more slowly than younger persons because metabolic rate declines by approximately 2% each decade.[20] A higher lean body mass is associated with greater energy expenditure and therefore a higher rate of weight loss. Most overweight or obese adults will lose weight if they comply with a diet of 1000 to 1200 kcal/day for women or 1200 to 1600 kcal/day for men.[14] An alternative approach to determining prescribed calorie content is based on current total body weight and is divided into five weight categories (**Table 12-1**).[21]

Investigators have attempted to define the dietary macronutrient composition that is optimal for weight reduction, improvement in cardiometabolic risk factors, and long-term weight maintenance in overweight and obese individuals, as well as patients with type 2 diabetes (see also Chapter 5). Overall, it appears that lower-carbohydrate diets (<40% of total calories) may result in greater short-term weight loss, improvement in hypertriglyceridemia, and possibly improvement in insulin resistance and glycosylated hemoglobin, but degree of weight loss and improvement in cardiometabolic

TABLE 12-1 Determining Prescribed Calorie Content

PRESCRIBED CALORIE CONTENT (KCAL/DAY)	CURRENT TOTAL BODY WEIGHT (POUNDS)
1000–1200	150–199
1200–1500	200–249
1500–1800	250–299
1800–2000	300–349
2000	300 or higher

risk factors is similar to that seen with low-fat or high-protein diets at 1 to 2 years.[22] Of note, however, is that many participants have difficulty maintaining the macronutrient composition of their assigned diet after 6 to 12 months, so the true impact of differing macronutrient composition dietary intake in the long term is not known. It is likely that the optimal macronutrient composition varies for different individuals with regard to long-term compliance. Therefore, dietary guidance should be individualized to the patient's lifestyle, preferences, and culture. According to the American Diabetes Association (ADA) 2013 Position Statement,[23] the mix of carbohydrate, protein, and fat may be adjusted to meet the metabolic goals and individual preferences of the person with diabetes.

The ADA, the Obesity Society, and the American Society for Nutrition recommend a 500- to 1000-kcal/day deficit through a diet that meets guidelines for reducing risk of comorbidities with obesity.[18] Specifically, these organizations recommend that the dietary macronutrient content and nutritional quality be based on guidelines from the ADA,[24] the American Heart Association (AHA),[25] and the National Cholesterol Education Program—Adult Treatment Panel (**Box 12-1**).[26] These are evidence-based dietary interventions that have been shown to improve selected cardiovascular risk factors, including hypertension and LDL-cholesterol level, and therefore are appropriate for patients with type 2 diabetes. According to the 2013 ADA Position Statement,[23] individuals who have prediabetes or diabetes should receive individualized medical nutritional therapy (MNT) as needed to achieve treatment goals, preferably provided by a registered dietitian familiar with the components of diabetes MNT. The ADA statement recognizes that for weight loss, low-carbohydrate, low-fat, calorie-restricted, or Mediterranean diets may be effective in

BOX 12-1 Dietary Guidelines Associated with Cardiovascular Risk Reduction

Eat a variety of fruits, vegetables, whole grains, legumes, and low-fat or nonfat dairy products.

Choose lean meats and poultry without skin, and prepare them without added saturated and trans fat.

Consume two or more servings of fish per week (with the exception of commercially fried fish fillets).

Limit saturated fat to less than 7% of total calories.

Minimize intake of *trans* fat by greatly limiting foods containing partially hydrogenated vegetable oil.

Limit dietary cholesterol intake to less than 200 mg/day.

Consume 20 to 30 g of fiber daily.

Greatly limit foods and beverages with added sugars.

Choose and prepare foods with little or no salt. Limit sodium intake to 2300 mg/day or less, according to ADA guidelines (or less than 1500 mg/day per AHA guidelines).

Limit alcohol intake to ≤ two drinks per day for men and ≤ one drink per day for women.

Data from the ADA,[24] the AHA,[25] and the National Cholesterol Education Program Expert Panel.[26]

the short term (up to 2 years). However, for patients on low-carbohydrate diets, it is recommended to monitor lipid profiles, renal function, and protein intake (for those with nephropathy) and adjust hypoglycemic pharmacotherapy as needed.

Prepackaged meal replacements in the form of liquid shakes, bars, and entrees are a useful tool to simplify a prescribed diet and minimize errors with portion control and high-caloric-density food choices. Meal replacement diets can enhance weight loss, improve cardiovascular risk factors, and have shown durable weight loss for periods of 4 to 5 years.[27–32] A meal replacement weight loss diet typically consists of replacing two food meals and two snacks with four approximately 110- to 200-kcal shakes or bars, plus one food meal consisting of lean protein, low-starch vegetables, a fruit serving, and a starch serving. Total daily caloric intake often ranges from 900 to 1300 kcal/day. For weight maintenance, individuals typically have two food meals and replace a third meal and one to two snacks per day with a shakes and/or bars. In a study of 119 patients with type 2 diabetes, use of prepackaged meal replacements, compared with calorie-equivalent usual-care diet, resulted in greater weight loss (-3.0 ± 5.4 kg versus -1.0 ± 3.8 kg), improved glycemic control with lower hemoglobin A1c (HbA1c) levels, improved quality of life, and better compliance with dietary recommendations after 1 year.[27] Another study found that the use of liquid meal replacements for 12 weeks in patients with type 2 diabetes resulted in significantly greater weight losses and reductions in fasting blood sugar compared with a conventional diet with the same calorie goal.[33]

With the prescription of a meal replacement diet, care must be taken to lower or discontinue medications that can lead to significant hypoglycemia, such as sulfonylureas, insulin secretagogues, and insulin. Required medication adjustments are based on the patient's current glycemic control, the prescribed dietary carbohydrate content, and the anticipated rate of weight loss based on calorie deficit. Patients should monitor blood glucose on a scheduled basis, and assessment for further medication adjustments should be completed daily to weekly for the first 3 to 4 weeks on the diet and then at intervals of 2 to 4 weeks during weight loss.

Recently, the Look AHEAD (Action for Health in Diabetes) study[34] examined whether cardiovascular morbidity and mortality in persons with type 2 diabetes were reduced through an intensive lifestyle intervention aimed at achieving and maintaining at least a 10% loss of body weight over 4 years. This large randomized controlled trial of 5145 participants included moderate-intensity exercise with a goal of 200 min/wk, a healthy diet that included portion-controlled foods, and behavior modification, versus a usual-care control group (diabetes support and education). The primary outcome was a composite of death from cardiovascular causes, or hospitalization for angina pectoris for up to 13.5 years. One-year results showed an average 8.6% weight loss, significant reduction of glycosylated hemoglobin, and reduction in several cardiovascular risk factors in the intervention group. Other important health benefits included improvement in obstructive sleep apnea, reduction in diabetes medications, maintenance of physical mobility, and improvement in quality of life. However, despite these numerous health improvements, the intensive lifestyle intervention did not reduce the rate of cardiovascular events and the trial was halted early.

Dietary Intake and Cardiometabolic Risk

The ADA MNT goals include achieving and maintaining blood glucose levels in the normal range or as close to normal as safely possible, a lipid and lipoprotein profile that reduces the risk for CVD, and blood pressure levels in the normal range or as close to normal as possible.[24] In type 2 diabetes, there is evidence that more intensive treatment of glycemia, particularly in newly diagnosed diabetes, may reduce long-term CVD events. The glycosylated hemoglobin goal according to ADA guidelines is below 7.0% but should be individualized based on factors such as age and life expectancy, comorbid conditions, and hypoglycemia unawareness. MNT has been shown to reduce glycosylated hemoglobin levels by 1% to 2% in type 2 diabetes, depending on duration of diabetes.[35,36] Lowering of LDL-C to a target of less than 100 mg/dL has been shown to decrease cardiovascular risk in type 2 diabetes; and for high-risk individuals with overt CVD, an LDL-C goal of below 70 mg/dL is recommended.[37] There is also evidence that lowering blood pressure to below 140 mm Hg systolic and below 80 mm Hg diastolic in individuals with type 2 diabetes reduces cardiovascular events.[38,39] Accordingly, the ADA guidelines recommend a systolic blood pressure target of below 140 mm Hg and a diastolic blood pressure target of below 80 mm Hg.

Dietary carbohydrate intake is the major determinant of postprandial blood glucose levels, which in turn have a significant impact on overall diabetes control and glycosylated hemoglobin level. Therefore the impact of carbohydrate intake on blood sugars with regard to carbohydrate amount, type, glycemic index, and glycemic load has been the focus of several investigations. Glycemic index is a measure that compares postprandial blood glucose responses to constant amounts of different carbohydrate-containing foods.[40] Glycemic load is calculated by multiplying the glycemic index of the food by the amount of carbohydrate. Fiber, lactose, fructose, and fat tend to lower glycemic index. Examples of carbohydrate foods with a lower glycemic index include oats, barley, bulgur, lentils, apples, oranges, milk, and yogurt. High–glycemic index foods include items such as white bread, most white rice, potato, pretzels, corn flakes, and extruded breakfast cereals. A meta-analysis of the effects of low–glycemic index diets on blood sugar control found a 0.4% reduction in glycosylated hemoglobin in comparison with high–glycemic index diets.[41] In addition to the modest benefit of low–glycemic index diets on glycosylated hemoglobin, many low–glycemic index foods have higher nutritional quality with regard to fiber, vitamins, and minerals. The ADA recommends a diet that includes carbohydrates from fruits, vegetables, whole grains, legumes, and low-fat milk, which are lower–glycemic index foods.

The total amount of carbohydrate in a meal also affects postprandial glucose levels. The recommended daily allowance for carbohydrate intake is 130 g/day, which is the average minimum requirement.[42] There are no large randomized long-term trials that evaluate outcomes of low-carbohydrate diets specifically in individuals with diabetes. One small weight loss trial reported improvement in fasting glucose among a subset with diabetes after 1 year on a lower-carbohydrate diet (120 g/day) compared with a higher-carbohydrate diet (230 g/day), but no significant change in glycosylated hemoglobin.[43] Because of lack of long-term data on the safety of low-carbohydrate diets in patients with diabetes as well as minimal evidence of benefit, it is recommended that clinicians focus on the nutritional quality of carbohydrates rather than the quantity of carbohydrates. Therefore, counseling diabetic patients to consume most or all of their carbohydrates from fruits, vegetables, whole grains, legumes, and low-fat milk is preferred.

Dietary strategies associated with reducing blood pressure in individuals with diabetes include the DASH (Dietary Approaches to Stop Hypertension) diet and moderation of alcohol intake. The DASH diet is high in fruit and vegetables, moderate in low-fat dairy products, and low in animal protein and includes a substantial intake of plant protein from legumes and nuts. This diet, which is promoted by the National Heart, Lung and Blood Institute for the prevention and treatment of hypertension, substantially reduces both systolic and diastolic blood pressure.[44] Additional sodium restriction in combination with DASH results in even greater blood pressure lowering.[45] The ADA recommends a reduced-sodium diet (e.g., 2300 mg/day) for normotensive and hypertensive individuals with diabetes. The DASH diet has also been shown to reduce LDL-C.[46] A large prospective cohort study from the Nurses' Health Study found that adherence to the DASH-style diet was associated with a lower risk of CHD and stroke among middle-aged women during 24 years of follow-up.[47]

Chronic excessive alcohol intake is associated with increased risk of hypertension, whereas light-to-moderate alcohol intake is associated with reductions in blood pressure.[38] Therefore it is recommended that adults with diabetes who choose to drink alcohol should limit consumption to a moderate amount, defined as 1 drink or less per day for women and 2 drinks or less per day for men, ideally with meals.

Findings from large trials on dietary fat intake and cardiovascular outcomes in individuals with diabetes are not available. Because patients with diabetes have similar cardiovascular risk as those with preexisting CVD, the same dietary goals are recommended. These include limiting saturated fat intake to less than 7% of total calories, minimizing *trans* fatty acids, and limiting cholesterol intake to less than 200 mg daily. Saturated and *trans* fatty acids are the main dietary determinants of LDL-C, and reduction of dietary intake of these fats has been shown to decrease plasma total cholesterol and LDL-C. Dietary n-3 polyunsaturated fatty acids appear to have beneficial effects on plasma lipid concentrations, lowering plasma triglycerides in individuals with hypertriglyceridemia and type 2 diabetes. Both fish and fish oil supplements contain n-3 polyunsaturated fatty acids, and consumption from either source may reduce adverse CVD outcomes.[48] Other recent analyses, however, have reported no additional cardioprotective benefit from omega-3 fatty acid supplementation.[49,50] The ADA guidelines recommend two or more servings of fish per week (with the exception of commercially fried fish filets).

Smoking Cessation

Smoking is an independent risk factor for all-cause mortality in patients with diabetes, mainly because of CVD.[51] There is also a higher risk of stroke in diabetic patients who smoke compared with those who do not smoke.[52] The Nurses' Health Study found there is a higher relative risk of CVD among women who smoke a higher number of cigarettes per day as well as an increased relative risk based on pack-years.[53] However, this study also found that quitting smoking for 10 or more years virtually eliminated excess mortality risk.

Smoking is associated with cardiovascular risk factors including elevated serum total cholesterol and LDL-C levels, low serum HDL-C levels, and insulin resistance.[54] In addition, smoking is associated with poorer glycemic control.[55,56] In patients with type 1 diabetes, smokers have higher levels of intracellular adhesion molecule-1, which is a marker of endothelial dysfunction, compared with nonsmokers.[57]

Given the greatly increased cardiovascular risk associated with smoking in those with diabetes as well as the near elimination of increased risk 10 years after quitting, smoking cessation is an important lifestyle change target for cardiovascular risk reduction in individuals with diabetes. The ADA recommends including smoking cessation counseling and other forms of treatment as routine components of diabetes care.[24] A number of large randomized controlled trials demonstrate that even brief counseling on smoking cessation, including the use of quit dates, can be efficacious and cost-effective. For the patient who is motivated to quit, pharmacologic therapy in addition to counseling is more effective than either treatment alone.[58] There is also evidence that smoking cessation programs are cost-effective and successful in patients with diabetes. One proposed strategy for clinicians managing smoking in diabetic patients is the five As strategy[59]:

1. Ask every patient about tobacco use.
2. Advise the patient about the importance of smoking cessation at every visit, in a brief, clear, and unambiguous manner.
3. Assess the patient's willingness to quit smoking within the next 30 days.
4. Assist the patient who is interested in quitting by offering self-help material, setting a quit date, offering referral to a local support group, and considering nicotine replacement therapy.
5. Arrange follow-up with those patients who are ready to quit, and give positive reinforcement during the first year after cessation.

EXERCISE AND PHYSICAL ACTIVITY IN THE PREVENTION AND TREATMENT OF TYPE 2 DIABETES MELLITUS

There is a pathophysiologic cascade by which physical inactivity predisposes to a cluster of cardiometabolic diseases, including type 2 diabetes mellitus. With an increasingly inactive lifestyle, skeletal muscle downregulates its capacity to convert nutritional substrates to adenosine triphosphate. Inactive skeletal muscle's impaired ability to oxidize glucose and fatty acids is presumably mediated by several mechanisms, including decreased mitochondrial concentration and oxidative enzymes; a reduced ability to remove glucose from blood because of fewer capillaries and diminished glucose transporter; and an attenuated capacity to hydrolyze blood triglycerides to free fatty acids, secondary to decreased lipoprotein lipase activity.[60] Collectively, these metabolic perturbations reduce the somatic capacity to burn fuel, resulting in hyperinsulinemia, insulin resistance, and hypertriglyceridemia, and ultimately increased cardiovascular risk. On the other hand, regular moderate-to-vigorous leisure-time physical activity, structured aerobic exercise, or both, can often reverse these adverse sequelae. A significant increase in physical activity and daily energy expenditure also improves insulin action in obesity, with or without a concomitant reduction in body weight and fat stores.[61] This is an important (and often overlooked) salutary effect, suggesting that physical activity is as efficacious in preventing insulin resistance as losing body weight.

Several recent randomized controlled trials in patients with type 2 diabetes have investigated the effects of moderate-to-vigorous aerobic exercise and resistance training on cardiorespiratory fitness, modifiable cardiovascular risk factors, and arterial stiffness, with specific reference to changes in body weight and fat stores.[62–64] Compared with the control group and/or counseling alone, supervised exercise produced significant improvements in cardiorespiratory fitness, upper and lower body strength, HbA1c, systolic and diastolic blood pressure, total serum cholesterol, HDL-C and LDL-C, body mass index (BMI), waist circumference, insulin resistance, inflammation (high-sensitivity C-reactive protein), leptin, and CHD risk scores, independent of body weight losses. Structured exercise durations exceeding 150 min/wk were associated with greater HbA1c declines than those of 150 min/wk or less (0.89% and 0.36% reductions, respectively).[65] On the other hand, large-artery elasticity, assessed by measuring pulse wave velocity, did not improve.[62] A systematic review and meta-analysis of the relevant literature from 1970 to 2009 revealed that combined aerobic exercise and resistance training, as well as aerobic exercise alone, were related to statistically significant declines in HbA1c, triglyceride levels, waist circumference, and systolic blood pressure among individuals with type 2 diabetes.[66] In contrast, the meta-analysis found little support for the benefits of resistance training alone on cardiovascular risk factors, including changes in HbA1c or resting systolic blood pressure, in patients with diabetes. Others, however, have reported that resistance training alone is associated with reductions in HbA1c as compared with a control group of patients with type 2 diabetes.[65]

Compared with overweight and obese individuals, those with a normal weight at the time of diabetes diagnosis have higher mortality rates, even after adjustment for potential confounding variables.[67] Because these data extend the "obesity paradox" to patients with diabetes, other potential modulators of survival, including body composition, fat distribution, regular physical activity, and cardiorespiratory fitness, beyond the measurement of BMI, may help the medical community clarify the relationships among obesity, morbidity, and mortality in adults with diabetes.[68]

Numerous investigations and systematic reviews have examined the relationships among habitual physical activity, cardiorespiratory fitness, diabetes, BMI, and mortality. The risk for all-cause and/or cardiovascular mortality is lower among overweight and obese individuals with good aerobic fitness than in individuals with normal BMI and low fitness.[69,70] This finding has also been reported in a study of African American and Caucasian veterans with diabetes, in whom the obesity paradox was observed along with an independent association between poor exercise capacity and mortality within BMI categories.[71] Others have reported that higher levels of cardiorespiratory fitness are associated with a substantial reduction in health risk for a given level of visceral and subcutaneous fat,[72] and that increased physical activity and/or cardiorespiratory fitness is inversely associated with all-cause and cardiovascular mortality in persons with diabetes.[68,73–75] Collectively, these data and other recent reports[76,77] strongly support the role of structured exercise, regular moderate-to-vigorous physical activity, or both, in interventions designed to prevent and treat type 2 diabetes, regardless of the patient's BMI.

Walking: "Exercise is Medicine" for Patients with Diabetes

Epidemiologic studies and clinical trials have consistently demonstrated the survival benefits of regular exercise, especially walking, in the prevention and treatment of type 2 diabetes mellitus (see also Chapter 5). In epidemiologic studies, brisk walking for at least 30 min/day has been associated with a 30% to 40% reduction in the risk of developing type 2 diabetes in women.[78] Two clinical trials demonstrated that regular walking or other moderate exercise in conjunction with dietary changes and modest weight losses resulted in a 58% reduction in the development of diabetes in overweight patients with impaired fasting glucose, as compared with usual-care control groups.[79,80] In the Diabetes Prevention Program, drug therapy with metformin reduced the risk by only 31%.

In a nationally representative sample (n = 2896) of Americans with diabetes aged 18 years or older, regular walking was associated with significant reductions in all-cause and cardiovascular mortality, up to 39% and 54% for walking at least 2 hr/wk and 3 to 4 hr/wk, respectively.[81] The inverse association held in multivariable analyses after potential confounding variables (e.g., risk factors, BMI, comorbid conditions) were controlled for. Walking at moderate-intensity levels was associated with the greatest reduction in mortality rates. The authors concluded that "1 death per year may be preventable for every 61 people who could be persuaded to walk at least 2 hours [per] week." These findings are consistent with previous studies conducted among younger and healthier populations with diabetes. In the Nurses' Health Study, in which baseline CVD and cancer patients were eliminated, moderate and vigorous levels of physical activity were associated with reduced rates of overall cardiovascular events among diabetic women aged 30 to 55 years.[82] Similarly, the Aerobics Center Longitudinal Study reported that men with type 2 diabetes who had a low fitness level and were physically inactive had higher mortality rates during follow-up than did their counterparts who were active and fit.[73] The clinical and public health implications of these data are enormous, because the survival benefits of moderate- to vigorous-intensity exercise, often achieved by brisk walking alone, may be even greater than those achieved by contemporary pharmacologic therapies to manage diabetes.[83]

Cardioprotective Effects of Regular Exercise

Two meta-analyses[84,85] have now shown that regular exercise participation can decrease the overall risk of cardiovascular events by up to 50%, presumably from multiple mechanisms, including antiatherosclerotic, anti-ischemic, antiarrhythmic, antithrombotic, and psychological effects (**Fig. 12-2**). As noted earlier, aerobic exercise, with and without resistance training, has favorable effects on the diabetic patient's cardiovascular risk factor profile, as well as on coagulability, fibrinolysis, and coronary endothelial function. Because more than 40% of the risk reduction associated with exercise training cannot be explained by changes in conventional risk factors, a cardioprotective "vascular conditioning" effect, including enhanced nitric oxide vasodilator function, improved vascular reactivity, altered vascular structure, or combinations thereof, has been proposed.[86] Decreased vulnerability to threatening arrhythmias and increased resistance to ventricular fibrillation have also been postulated to reflect exercise-related adaptations in autonomic control. As a result of endurance training, sympathetic drive at rest is reduced and vagal tone and heart rate variability are increased. Moreover, ischemic preconditioning before coronary occlusion, at least in animal models, can reduce subsequent infarct size and/or the potential for malignant ventricular arrhythmias.[87,88]

PHYSICAL ACTIVITY, EXERCISE PROGRAMMING, AND PRESCRIPTION

In many patients with type 2 diabetes, adequate glycemic control can often be achieved by dietary changes, regular physical activity, structured exercise, and weight reduction. The exercise program should generally follow contemporary guidelines for the treatment of excessive body weight and fat stores,[89] and other risk factors associated with this common metabolic condition (i.e., dyslipidemia, hypertension, inflammatory markers, fibrinolytic factors, waist circumference). Overall, individuals with type 2 diabetes have an increased risk of morbidity and mortality from CVD as compared with their age- and gender-matched counterparts without this comorbidity. Accordingly, a physical examination and a careful preliminary cardiovascular assessment, including peak or symptom-limited exercise testing, with estimated or directly measured peak oxygen consumption ($\dot{V}O_2$ peak), should be considered before beginning a vigorous ($\geq 60\%$ $\dot{V}O_2$ reserve) exercise training program, where

$$\dot{V}O_2 \text{ reserve} = \% \text{ intensity} \times (\dot{V}O_2 \text{ peak} - \dot{V}O_2 \text{ rest})$$
$$+ \dot{V}O_2 \text{ rest}$$

With this formula, $\dot{V}O_2$ is generally expressed in mL O_2/kg/min or in metabolic equivalents (METs), where 1 MET = 3.5 mL O_2/kg/min. Both the AHA[90] and the American College of Sports Medicine (ACSM) guidelines for exercise testing and prescription[91] recommend that peak or symptom-limited exercise testing be considered before initiation of vigorous exercise training in individuals with known or suspected CVD, including patients with diabetes mellitus.[92]

Type of Exercise

Aerobic (or endurance) exercise has been the most frequently studied mode of physical conditioning, and the resultant increases in cardiorespiratory fitness in patients with type 2 diabetes have been consistently associated with improvements in modifiable cardiovascular risk factors, independent of weight loss.[64] The most effective exercises for the endurance phase use large muscle groups, are maintained continuously, and are rhythmic in nature, such as walking, jogging, elliptical training, stationary or outdoor cycling, swimming, rowing, stair climbing, and combined arm-leg ergometry. Other exercise modalities commonly used in structured exercise training programs for patients with type 2 diabetes include calisthenics, particularly those involving sustained total-body movement, recreational activities (e.g., golf, doubles tennis, pickleball), and resistance training.[93] The last is a particularly important option, because traditional aerobic-conditioning regimens often fail to accommodate participants who require improved muscle strength or endurance to perform occupational or leisure-time activities. Moreover, studies have now shown that muscular strength is inversely associated with all-cause mortality, independent of cardiorespiratory fitness levels.[94]

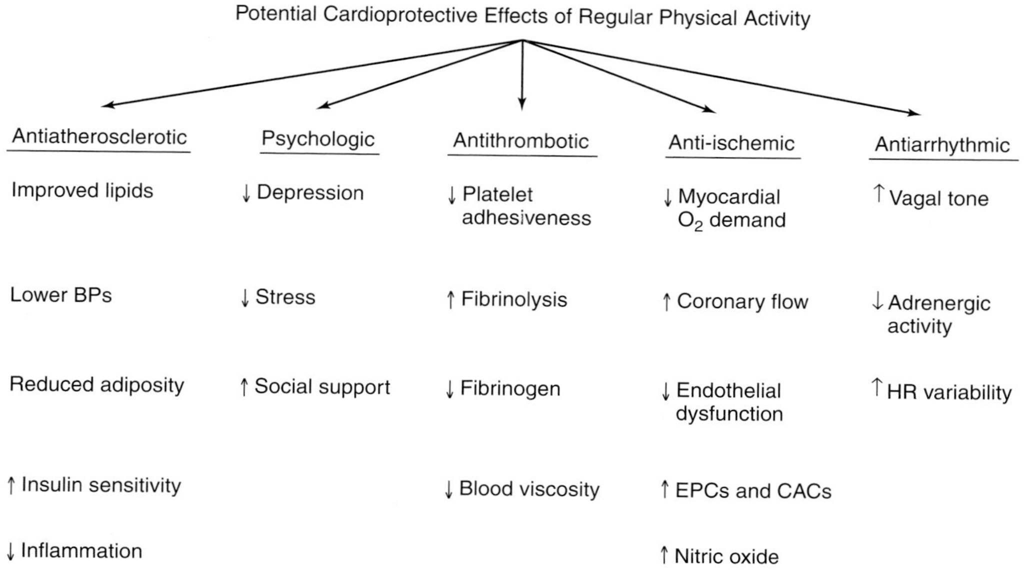

Potential Cardioprotective Effects of Regular Physical Activity

Antiatherosclerotic	Psychologic	Antithrombotic	Anti-ischemic	Antiarrhythmic
Improved lipids	↓ Depression	↓ Platelet adhesiveness	↓ Myocardial O$_2$ demand	↑ Vagal tone
Lower BPs	↓ Stress	↑ Fibrinolysis	↑ Coronary flow	↓ Adrenergic activity
Reduced adiposity	↑ Social support	↓ Fibrinogen	↓ Endothelial dysfunction	↑ HR variability
↑ Insulin sensitivity		↓ Blood viscosity	↑ EPCs and CACs	
↓ Inflammation			↑ Nitric oxide	

FIGURE 12-2 A structured endurance exercise program, increased lifestyle physical activity, or both, sufficient to maintain and enhance cardiorespiratory fitness may provide multiple mechanisms to reduce nonfatal and fatal cardiovascular events in "at-risk" patients with diabetes. BP = Blood pressure; CACs = cultured angiogenic cells; EPCs = endothelial progenitor cells; HR = heart rate; O$_2$ = oxygen; ↑ = increased; ↓ = decreased.

Because of the high prevalence of underlying ischemic heart disease, and the heightened risk for exertion-related cardiovascular events and orthopedic injuries, adoption of a moderate intensity (e.g., walking), rather than a vigorous physical activity program (e.g., jogging, running) may be more appropriate for diabetic patients, especially those who are middle-aged and older.[83] Walking has several advantages over other forms of exercise during the initial phase of a physical conditioning program, including inherent neuromuscular limitations on the speed of walking (and therefore the rate of energy expenditure). Brisk walking programs can significantly increase aerobic capacity and reduce body weight and fat stores, particularly when the walking duration exceeds 30 minutes.[95] Additional advantages of a walking program include accessibility, social companionship, lack of special equipment (other than a pair of well-fitted athletic shoes), an easily tolerable exercise intensity, and fewer musculoskeletal and orthopedic problems of the legs, knees, and feet than with jogging or running. Walking in water,[96] with a backpack, or with a weighted vest[97] are options for those who seek to progressively increase the exercise intensity and associated energy expenditure.

The Rule of 2 and 3 Miles per Hour (mph)

Because most diabetic patients, many of whom are overweight or obese, prefer to walk at moderate intensities, it is helpful to recognize that walking on level ground at 2 and 3 mph approximates 2 and 3 METs, respectively. For patients who prefer the slower walking pace (2 mph; 3.2 km/h), each 3.5% increase in treadmill grade adds approximately 1 MET to the gross energy cost. Therefore, patients who desire to walk at a 2-mph pace, but require a 4-MET workload for training, would be advised to add 7.0% grade to this speed. For patients who can negotiate the faster walking speed (3 mph; 4.8 km/h), each 2.5% increase in treadmill grade adds an additional 1 MET to the gross energy expenditure. Accordingly, a workload of 3 mph, 7.5% grade, would approximate an aerobic requirement of 6 METs. Use of this practical rule can be helpful to clinicians in prescribing treadmill exercise workloads for their diabetic patients, without the need for consulting tables, nomograms, or metabolic formulas or calculations.[98]

Resistance Training

Although resistance exercise has generally been considered to be less effective in preventing and treating type 2 diabetes, some reviews suggest that it provides independent and additive benefits to an aerobic exercise program for virtually the entire cluster of associated cardiovascular risk factors.[99] For example, numerous studies show that resistance training improves insulin sensitivity, significantly decreases HbA1c and blood pressure in diabetic and hypertensive adults, respectively, and reduces body fat stores and visceral adipose tissue in both men and women. In addition, the maintenance or enhancement of lean body mass from chronic resistance training is associated with a modest increase in basal metabolic rate, which over time may facilitate greater reductions in body weight than can be achieved with increased physical activity and/or structured exercise. Weight-training–induced attenuation of the hemodynamic response to lifting standardized loads has also been reported, which may decrease cardiac demands during daily activities such as carrying packages or lifting moderate to heavy objects.[100] There are also intriguing data to suggest that strength training can increase endurance capacity without an accompanying increase in cardiorespiratory fitness.[101]

Although the traditional weight-training prescription has involved performing each exercise three times (e.g., three sets of 10 to 15 repetitions per set), it appears that one set provides similar improvements in muscular strength and endurance, at least for the novice exerciser.[102] Consequently, single-set programs performed at least two times a week are recommended rather than multiset programs, because they are highly effective, less time-consuming, and less likely to cause musculoskeletal injury or soreness. Such regimens should include 8 to 10 different exercises involving the trunk and upper and lower extremities at loads that permit 8 to 15 repetitions per set. At least 60 minutes of resistance training should be completed each week (e.g., two 30-minute sessions).

Lifestyle Physical Activity

Despite contemporary exercise guidelines and the much-heralded Surgeon General's report,[103] the traditional model for getting people to be more physically active (i.e., a regimented or structured exercise program) has been only marginally effective. Randomized clinical trials have now shown that a lifestyle approach to physical activity among previously sedentary adults has similar effects on cardiorespiratory fitness, body composition, and coronary risk factors as a structured exercise program.[104,105] These findings have important implications for public health, suggesting an alternative approach to sedentary people who, for one reason or another, are not ready to integrate a formal exercise commitment into their daily schedule.[106] The skyrocketing prevalence of overweight and obesity and related sequelae (e.g., type 2 diabetes, metabolic syndrome) suggests the need for "real world" interventions designed to circumvent and attenuate barriers to achieving an adequate daily energy expenditure.[107] Accordingly, physicians and allied health professionals should counsel patients to integrate multiple short bouts of physical activity into their lives.[108] Nonexercise activity thermogenesis—the spontaneous physical activities of daily living (e.g., fidgeting while sitting, standing while reading, moving the lower extremities while working at the computer)—represents another source of energy expenditure.[109] Standing also elevates lipoprotein lipase, an enzyme that improves fat metabolism while reducing insulin resistance.[110,111] Thus, energy expenditure during nonexercise time may be as critical for preventative health as structured exercise time. Pedometers can be helpful in this regard, as can programs that use them (e.g., America on the Move) to enhance awareness of physical activity by progressively increasing daily step totals. According to one systematic review, pedometer users significantly increased their physical activity by an average of 2491 steps per day more than their control counterparts.[112] The Activity Pyramid (**Fig. 12-3**) has also been suggested as a model to combat America's increasingly hypokinetic environment.[113] This schematic presents a tiered set of weekly goals to promote improved cardiorespiratory fitness and health, building on a base that emphasizes the importance of accumulating at least 30 minutes of moderate-intensity activity on 5 or more days per week.

Intensity and Duration

There is some controversy regarding the most appropriate exercise intensity and duration that are needed to optimally physically condition patients with insulin resistance syndrome.[114] Different risk factors associated with this condition may respond more favorably to different exercise dosages and intensities. For example, a randomized, controlled trial of previously inactive, overweight men and women with abnormal lipoprotein profiles compared the effectiveness of three different exercise regimens versus controls: high-amount, high-intensity exercise; low-amount, high-intensity exercise; and low-amount, moderate-intensity exercise.[115] Although all exercise groups demonstrated improved responses on a variety of lipid and lipoprotein variables as compared with the control group, the most beneficial changes were noted in the high-amount, high-intensity exercise regimen. Because type 2 diabetes has been associated with increased body weight and fat stores, a sedentary lifestyle, and a low level of cardiorespiratory fitness, the initial exercise intensity should approximate at least 40% of the $\dot{V}O_2$ or heart rate reserve or 55% of the maximal heart rate, at a rating of perceived exertion (6 to 20 category scale) of 11 (fairly light) or higher, for a minimum accumulated duration of 30 min/day.[116,117] Over time, in the absence of adverse signs and symptoms, the exercise intensity should be gradually increased, generally corresponding to a rating of perceived exertion up to 14 (somewhat hard to hard), to provide the stimulus to improve cardiorespiratory fitness

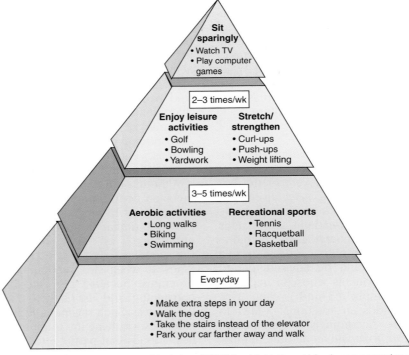

FIGURE 12-3 The Activity Pyramid, analogous to the U.S. Department of Agriculture (USDA) Food Guide Pyramid, has been suggested as a model to facilitate public and patient education for adoption of a progressively more active lifestyle. *(Copyright ©1996 Park Nicollet Health-source Institute for Research and Education. Reprinted with permission).*

overwhelming. When multiple changes may be necessary to reach an identified health goal (e.g., control of diabetes signs and symptoms, weight loss), it often helps if patients determine which behavior to focus on first.[127,131,140]

Principles of Motivational Interviewing
Express Empathy
It is important to be able to express understanding in a manner that enables patients to feel heard and understood, in a nonjudgmental manner that reflects the viewpoints and experiences of the patient.[127,131,134,140,141]

Support Self-Efficacy
Motivational interviewing is a strengths-based approach that operates from the perspective that patients have within themselves the capability to change behaviors successfully. Healthcare providers support self-efficacy by focusing on previous successes and highlighting skills and strengths that patients already possess. To this end, healthcare providers can suggest skills and strengths that can be used or built on, as change is being considered, planned, and implemented. In addition, allowing patients to set their own agenda for change will support self-efficacy. For example, when considering multiple lifestyle changes that might be necessary for successful management of diabetes (e.g., self-monitoring of glucose levels, changing eating habits, increasing physical activity, reducing stress), allowing patients to determine which change to make first empowers them and increases the likelihood of the behavior change being sustained over time.[127,131,140–142]

Roll with Resistance
Resistance is not a part of the personality or character of patients. Instead, it is a manifestation of the process going on between providers and patients, as well as the ambivalence that is felt or experienced by patients when they contemplate making behavioral changes. When patients argue against, challenge, or discount information presented by providers or interrupt and/or talk over providers, they are likely demonstrating resistance to hearing or truly accepting the need for change. Resistance also presents itself in the form of denial, when patients deny they have lifestyle deficits, blame others for the problem, or minimize the potential negative impact of the habit at hand. Finally, resistance may occur when patients overtly ignore what providers say, do not respond, or sidetrack, discussing issues unrelated to what providers have just articulated. Rather than engaging in a head-to-head confrontation, or meeting force with force, rolling with resistance involves use of techniques that allow the scenario to dissipate. Some of the techniques that enable this to occur are described later.[127,131,140,141]

Develop Discrepancy
When discussing change possibilities, helping to develop differences among the beliefs of patients regarding their health, current behaviors, and desired goal(s) may assist them to move along the readiness to change continuum. If an agenda is set and self-efficacy is supported, discrepancies among patients' understanding, beliefs, and goals often come to light. Essentially, motivation for change occurs when individuals perceive a discrepancy between where they are and where they want to be. Once discrepancies are identified and reflected back to patients, carefully crafted questions can be asked to help the patients understand the mismatch and empower them to move toward behavior change.[127,131,140,142]

Interviewing Skills and Strategies
Motivational interviewing uses varied interviewing skills and strategies that are taught as basic communication skills for developing strong healthcare provider–patient relationships. The acronym OARS can cue healthcare providers to implement the most commonly used skills and strategies, including open-ended questions, affirmations, reflections, and summaries.[140]

- *Open-ended questions:* Asking questions that cannot be answered easily with a "yes/no" or limited response can lead to obtaining useful information from patients that allows healthcare providers to develop a better understanding of their concerns and perspectives. Open-ended questions encourage patients to talk and provide personal viewpoints. These types of questions often begin with what, how, why, or could.[131,140,141]
- *Affirmations:* Statements that highlight patient strengths can be a useful tool to support behavior change. Pointing out positive traits or characteristics to patients empowers them to build on existing skills and strengths. Affirmations may include complimenting effort, acknowledging small successes, or stating appreciation.[131,140,141]
- *Reflections:* Reflective listening involves recognizing key words or feelings expressed by patients and using them to paraphrase what was heard. The main ideas or concepts reflected back to patients should represent their point of view, not those of the healthcare provider. Reflective listening accomplishes two goals: first, it enables providers to express empathy and demonstrate understanding of patients' perspectives; second, healthcare providers can use reflective listening to identity ambivalence regarding behavior change and guide patients toward resolving their uncertainty.[131,140,141]
- *Summaries:* Recapping what has occurred in healthcare provider–patient interactions communicates interest and understanding and can lead to movement away from previous unhealthy behaviors.[131,140,141]

In addition to OARS, other skills are also useful within the context of motivational interviewing. Establishing structure, or setting an agenda for the visit, helps providers to focus on readiness for change and appropriate behavior change processes.[127] The recommended structure is to ask a question that determines readiness for change, listen to patients' responses, and provide information that might help patients move along the change continuum. Once healthcare providers have shared information with patients, they can then ask patients to share their understanding or interpretation of the information that was provided.[131]

Other important strategies when engaged in motivational interviewing include assessing the importance of the change being discussed, along with the confidence level of patients in their ability to make the change, and finally attempting to increase patients' motivation for change.[127,135] Readiness to change is influenced by how important individuals perceive change to be, as well as how confident they are that they can make the change.

For healthcare providers, assessing importance and confidence regarding a mutually agreeable change goal are necessary. For example, "On a scale of 1 to 10, with 10 being the highest, how important is it for you to keep your blood sugar level within the normal range each day?" In

TABLE 12-4 Stages of Readiness to Change with Sample Motivational Interviewing Questions to Favorably Modify Patient's Behaviors (e.g., Weight Reduction)

STAGE OF CHANGE	PATIENT STATEMENT OR BELIEF	HEALTHCARE PROVIDER INTERVENTION
Precontemplation	I am comfortable at my current weight.	I am worried about the effect that your weight is having on other health factors, and although you aren't ready to discuss weight loss strategies today, I would like to discuss this issue the next time we meet, okay?
Contemplation	I would like to lose weight, but I don't know where to begin.	What do you like least about your current habits? Which habit can you see yourself changing first? How might you set things up in your life to be able to do so?
Preparation	I am going to buy a gym membership next month so that I can start exercising 3 days per week.	It sounds like you have decided that physical activity is the most important thing to change right now. What can you do now to help ensure that you will be able to go to the gym 3 days per week like you stated you want to do?
Action	I have gotten all of the junk food out of the house so that I can focus on eating healthier foods without any temptations.	That's wonderful. What are some other barriers that you find get in the way of making healthy eating choices on a consistent basis?
Maintenance	I have been going to the gym 3-5 times weekly and am no longer eating fast food. I have been able to sustain these behaviors for the past 6 months.	It sounds like you have been able to maintain positive changes with your eating habits and physical activity for quite a long time. Do you worry about particular triggers that might tempt you to engage in old, unhealthy behaviors? If so, have you thought about how to combat the triggers if they arise?
Relapse	Things got so busy at work that I started stopping for fast food on my way home from work and I have regained some of the weight I lost this past year.	It sounds like you were able to identify the trigger that led you off target. What are some things you can do to balance work demands while continuing to engage in the healthier new behaviors you have been working toward creating as habits that you would like to last for life?
Exit	I have maintained my current weight for the past 2 years and I don't see myself ever going back to my old ways.	If you were giving someone else advice regarding how to maintain consistent healthy choices, what would you tell him or her?

assessing the level of importance for making a change, it is common for resistance to arise. If a patient rates the level of importance below 7, it suggests that the healthcare provider may be moving too quickly in the approach.

Once an importance level has been established, it is also possible to use the rating to increase the patient's motivation level to engage in change by asking him or her to elaborate on why he or she rated the importance at the particular level that was chosen. Whether the rating is higher or lower in the range, questions can be asked to solidify or shift the rating upward. For example, "Although you indicated that you want to pay closer attention to the fluctuation in your blood sugar throughout the day, when I asked you to rate the importance of monitoring your blood sugars daily, you rated the importance as 6. What would it take to increase the importance level to a 7 or 8?"

Similar methods can be used to determine patients' confidence level for making a behavioral change. Once again, a confidence rating below 7 suggests the need to determine what would be necessary to increase the level of confidence that change can be made successfully. Without a higher confidence level, patients are likely to fail in their effort to change behaviors.

Using Change Talk in Motivational Interviewing

Change talk includes statements made by patients that suggest consideration of change, motivation for change, or commitment to change. The acronym DARN CAT can help healthcare providers to remember the different types of statements and their meanings. The first four types of change talk, represented by *DARN*, reflect precommitment to change (desire, ability, reason, need). There may be conflict or ambivalence noted between statement types, which are often paired together with the connector word *but*. For example, "I want to [desire], *but* I can't [ability]".[140,141] The last three types of change talk, represented by *CAT*, reflect commitment to change (commitment, activation, taking steps).

In summary, motivational interviewing offers healthcare providers a therapeutic approach to health-related behavior change issues that allows for increased mutual understanding regarding patients' perceptions and experience, as well as methods to increase importance, confidence, and motivation regarding making behavioral changes and developing an action plan to achieve long-term success.

Table 12-4 combines the transtheoretical model of stages of change and motivational interviewing strategies to illustrate how the two models can be used in conjunction with each other.[143] Weight loss goals are used as examples for interventions for all stages.

Evidenced-Based Mind-Body Therapies

Research demonstrates reduction in risk for both cardiovascular events and mortality when stress reduction techniques are used by patients.[125] Yet traditional medicine often falls short in offering integrative approaches for stress reduction. Healthcare providers can recommend options such as meditation, yoga, mindfulness-based stress reduction, pet ownership, guided imagery, biofeedback, and tai chi, or combinations thereof, all of which are associated with significant reductions in stress and stress-related illnesses.[125,142] Many of these methods can be taught by healthcare providers, learned in settings identified by healthcare providers, and offered to patients at risk, including those with diabetes.

SUMMARY

The treatment of CVD has evolved from simple lifestyle modifications in the 1960s, largely focused on a "prudent diet" and regular exercise, to an array of costly medical and revascularization interventions that too often fail to address the underlying causes—poor dietary habits, physical inactivity, and cigarette smoking. The INTERHEART study examined the risk factors associated with first acute myocardial infarction in 52 countries, including 15,152 patients and 14,820 controls.[144] Five risk factors (abnormal lipids, smoking, hypertension, diabetes mellitus, abdominal obesity) accounted for approximately 80% of the population attributable risk in men and women. Similarly, Khot and colleagues[145] and Greenland and colleagues[146] examined data from 14 randomized clinical trials and three prospective cohort studies and reported that more than 80% of patients who developed CHD and 87% or more of patients who experienced a fatal coronary event had antecedent exposure to at least one of the four conventional cardiovascular risk factors (cigarette smoking, dyslipidemia, hypertension, diabetes mellitus). Collectively, these data and other recent reports[147,148] suggest that a more rigorous focus on these risk factors and the lifestyle behaviors that promote them has great potential to reduce the burden of atherosclerotic CVD. Added benefits include a reduction in angina symptoms, decreases in exercise-induced signs or symptoms of myocardial ischemia, fewer recurrent cardiac events, an improved quality of life, and diminished need for coronary revascularization.

The issue is not information but methods, motivation, and behavioral changes.[149] Accordingly, patients with diabetes should be directed toward comprehensive programs designed to change behavior and facilitate cardiovascular risk reduction, with use of individually tailored interventions to circumvent or attenuate barriers to participation and adherence. The challenge is yours!

References

1. Thom T, Haase N, Rosamond W, et al: Heart disease and stroke statistics—2006 update: a report from the American Heart Association Statistics Committee and Stroke Statistics Subcommittee, *Circulation* 113(6):e85–e151, 2006.
2. Gregg EW, Cheng YJ, Cadwell BL, et al: Secular trends in cardiovascular disease risk factors according to body mass index in US adults, *JAMA* 293(15):1868–1874, 2005.
3. Mozaffarian D, Wilson PW, Kannel WB: Beyond established and novel risk factors: lifestyle risk factors for cardiovascular disease, *Circulation* 117(23):3031–3038, 2008.
4. Heidenreich PA, Trogdon JG, Khavjou OA, et al: Forecasting the future of cardiovascular disease in the United States: a policy statement from the American Heart Association, *Circulation* 123 (8):933–944, 2011.
5. Weintraub WS, Daniels SR, Burke LE, et al: Value of primordial and primary prevention for cardiovascular disease: a policy statement from the American Heart Association, *Circulation* 124 (8):967–990, 2011.
6. Asch DA, Muller RW, Volpp KG: Automated hovering in health care—watching over the 5000 hours, *N Engl J Med* 367(1):1–3, 2012.
7. Marvasti FF, Stafford RS: From sick care to health care—reengineering prevention into the U.S. system, *N Engl J Med* 367(10):889–891, 2012.
8. Schroeder SA: Shattuck lecture. We can do better—improving the health of the American people, *N Engl J Med* 357(12):1221–1228, 2007.
9. Chiuve SE, McCullough ML, Sacks FM, et al: Healthy lifestyle factors in the primary prevention of coronary heart disease among men: benefits among users and nonusers of lipid-lowering and antihypertensive medications, *Circulation* 114(2):160–167, 2006.
10. Krauss RM, Winston M, Fletcher BJ, et al: Obesity: impact on cardiovascular disease, *Circulation* 98(14):1472–1476, 1998.
11. Wilson PW, D'Agostino RB, Sullivan L, et al: Overweight and obesity as determinants of cardiovascular risk: the Framingham experience, *Arch Intern Med* 162(16):1867–1872, 2002.
12. Lew EA, Garfinkel L: Variations in mortality by weight among 750,000 men and women, *J Chronic Dis* 32(8):563–576, 1979.
13. Balkau B, Deanfield JE, Després JP, et al: International Day for the Evaluation of Abdominal Obesity (IDEA): a study of waist circumference, cardiovascular disease, and diabetes mellitus in 168,000 primary care patients in 63 countries, *Circulation* 116(17):1942–1951, 2007.
14. National Heart, Lung and Blood Institute: Clinical guidelines on the identification, evaluation and treatment of overweight and obesity in adults. The evidence report, NIH Publication No. 98-4083 Bethesda, MD, September 1998, National Institutes of Health.
15. Alberti KG, Zimmet P, Shaw J: Metabolic syndrome—a new world-wide definition. A consensus statement from the International Diabetes Federation, *Diabet Med* 23(5):469–480, 2006.
16. Bray GA, Clearfield MB, Fintel DJ, et al: Overweight and obesity: the pathogenesis of cardiometabolic risk, *Clin Cornerstone* 9(4):30–40, 2009, discussion 41–2.
17. Kaptoge S, Di Angelantonio E, Lowe G, et al, for the Emerging Risk Factors Collaboration: C-reactive protein concentration and risk of coronary heart disease, stroke, and mortality: an individual participant meta-analysis, *Lancet* 375(9709):132–140, 2010.
18. Klein S, Sheard NF, Pi-Sunyer X, et al: Weight management through lifestyle modification for the prevention and management of type 2 diabetes: rationale and strategies: a statement of the American Diabetes Association, the North American Association for the Study of Obesity, and the American Society for Clinical Nutrition, *Diabetes Care* 27(8):2067–2073, 2004.
19. Janosz KE, Zalesin KC, Miller WM, et al: Impact of surgical and nonsurgical weight loss on diabetes resolution and cardiovascular risk reduction, *Curr Diab Rep* 9(3):223–228, 2009.
20. Goldstein DJ: Beneficial health effects of modest weight loss, *Int J Obes Relat Metab Disord* 16 (6):397–415, 1992.
21. Klein S, Wadden T, Sugerman HJ: AGA technical review on obesity, *Gastroenterology* 123:882–932, 2002.
22. Sacks FM, Bray GA, Carey VJ, et al: Comparison of weight-loss diets with different compositions of fat, protein, and carbohydrates, *N Engl J Med* 360(9):859–873, 2009.
23. American Diabetes Association: Standards of medical care in diabetes—2013, *Diabetes Care* 36 (Suppl 1):S11–S66, 2013.
24. American Diabetes Association, Bantle JP, Wylie-Rosett J, Albright AL, et al: Nutrition recommendations and interventions for diabetes: a position statement of the American Diabetes Association, *Diabetes Care* 31(Suppl 1):S61–S78, 2008.
25. Krauss RM, Eckel RH, Howard B, et al: AHA dietary guidelines: revision 2000: A statement for healthcare professionals from the Nutrition Committee of the American Heart Association, *Circulation* 102(18):2284–2299, 2000.
26. Executive summary of the third report of the National Cholesterol Education Program (NCEP) Expert Panel on Detection, Evaluation, and Treatment of High Blood Cholesterol in Adults (Adult treatment panel III), *JAMA* 285(19):2486–2497, 2001.
27. Metz JA, Stern JS, Kris-Etherton P, et al: A randomized trial of improved weight loss with a prepared meal plan in overweight and obese patients: impact on cardiovascular risk reduction, *Arch Intern Med* 160(14):2150–2158, 2000.
28. Haynes RB, Kris-Etherton P, McCarron DA, et al: Nutritionally complete prepared meal plan to reduce cardiovascular risk factors: a randomized clinical trial, *J Am Diet Assoc* 99(9):1077–1083, 1999.
29. Pi-Sunyer FX, Maggio CA, McCarron DA, et al: Multicenter randomized trial of a comprehensive prepared meal program in type 2 diabetes, *Diabetes Care* 22(2):191–197, 1999.
30. Quinn Rothacker D: Five-year self-management of weight using meal replacements: comparison with matched controls in rural Wisconsin, *Nutrition* 16(5):344–348, 2000.
31. Ditschuneit HH, Flechtner-Mors M, Johnson TD, et al: Metabolic and weight-loss effects of a long-term dietary intervention in obese patients, *Am J Clin Nutr* 69(2):198–204, 1999.
32. Flechtner-Mors M, Ditschuneit HH, Johnson TD, et al: Metabolic and weight loss effects of long-term dietary intervention in obese patients: four-year results, *Obes Res* 8(5):399–402, 2000.
33. Yip I, Go VL, DeShields S, et al: Liquid meal replacements and glycemic control in obese type 2 diabetes patients, *Obes Res* 9(Suppl 4):341S–347S, 2001.
34. The Look AHEAD Research Group: Cardiovascular effects of intensive lifestyle intervention in type 2 diabetes, *N Engl J Med* 369(2):145–154, 2013.
35. Pastors JG, Warshaw H, Daly A, et al: The evidence for the effectiveness of medical nutrition therapy in diabetes management, *Diabetes Care* 25(3):608–613, 2002.
36. Pastors JG, Franz MJ, Warshaw H, et al: How effective is medical nutrition therapy in diabetes care? *J Am Diet Assoc* 103(7):827–831, 2003.
37. Smith SC Jr., Benjamin EJ, Bonow RO, et al: AHA/ACCF secondary prevention and risk reduction therapy for patients with coronary and other atherosclerotic vascular disease: 2011 update; a guideline from the American Heart Association and American College of Cardiology Foundation, *Circulation* 124(22):2458–2473, 2011.
38. Chobanian AV, Bakris GL, Black HR, et al: The seventh report of the Joint National Committee on Prevention, Detection, Evaluation, and Treatment of High Blood Pressure: the JNC 7 report, *JAMA* 289(19):2560–2572, 2003.
39. Adler AI, Stratton IM, Neil HA, et al: Association of systolic blood pressure with macrovascular and microvascular complications of type 2 diabetes (UKPDS 36): prospective observational study, *BMJ* 321(7258):412–419, 2000.
40. Jenkins DJ, Wolever TM, Taylor RH, et al: Glycemic index of foods: a physiological basis for carbohydrate exchange, *Am J Clin Nutr* 34(3):362–366, 1981.
41. Brand-Miller J, Hayne S, Petocz P, et al: Low-glycemic index diets in the management of diabetes: a meta-analysis of randomized controlled trials, *Diabetes Care* 26(8):2261–2267, 2003.
42. Trumbo P, Schlicker S, Yates AA, et al: Food and Nutrition Board of the Institute of Medicine: The National Academies. Dietary reference intakes for energy, carbohydrate, fiber, fat, fatty acids, cholesterol, protein and amino acids, *J Am Diet Assoc* 102(11):1621–1630, 2002.
43. Stern L, Iqbal N, Seshadri P, et al: The effects of low-carbohydrate versus conventional weight loss diets in severely obese adults: one-year follow-up of a randomized trial, *Ann Intern Med* 140 (10):778–785, 2004.
44. Appel LJ, Moore TJ, Obarzanek E, et al: A clinical trial of the effects of dietary patterns on blood pressure. DASH Collaborative Research Group, *N Engl J Med* 336(16):1117–1124, 1997.
45. Sacks FM, Svetkey LP, Vollmer WM, et al: Effects on blood pressure of reduced dietary sodium and the Dietary Approaches to Stop Hypertension (DASH) diet. DASH-Sodium Collaborative Research Group, *N Engl J Med* 344(1):3–10, 2001.
46. Obarzanek E, Sacks FM, Vollmer WM, et al: Effects on blood lipids of a blood pressure-lowering diet: the Dietary Approaches to Stop Hypertension (DASH) Trial, *Am J Clin Nutr* 74(1):80–89, 2001.
47. Fung TT, Chiuve SE, McCullough ML, et al: Adherence to a DASH-style diet and risk of coronary heart disease and stroke in women, *Arch Intern Med* 168(7):713–720, 2008.
48. Wang C, Harris WS, Chung M, et al: n-3 Fatty acids from fish or fish-oil supplements, but not alpha-linolenic acid, benefit cardiovascular disease outcomes in primary- and secondary-prevention studies: a systematic review, *Am J Clin Nutr* 84(1):5–17, 2006.
49. Rizos EC, Ntzani EE, Bika E, et al: Association between omega-3 fatty acid supplementation and risk of major cardiovascular disease events: a systematic review and meta-analysis, *JAMA* 308 (10):1024–1033, 2012.
50. Roncaglioni MC, Tombesi M, Avanzini F, et al, for the Risk and Prevention Study Collaborative Group: N-3 fatty acids in patients with multiple cardiovascular risk factors, *N Engl J Med* 368 (19):1800–1808, 2013.
51. Moy CS, LaPorte RE, Dorman JS, et al: Insulin-dependent diabetes mellitus mortality. The risk of cigarette smoking, *Circulation* 82(1):37–43, 1990.
52. Mulnier HE, Seaman HE, Raleigh VS, et al: Risk of stroke in people with type 2 diabetes in the UK: a study using the General Practice Research Database, *Diabetologia* 49(12):2859–2865, 2006.
53. Al-Delaimy WK, Willett WC, Manson JE, et al: Smoking and mortality among women with type 2 diabetes: the Nurses' Health Study cohort, *Diabetes Care* 24(12):2043–2048, 2001.
54. Facchini FS, Hollenbeck CB, Jeppesen J, et al: Insulin resistance and cigarette smoking, *Lancet* 339(8802):1128–1130, 1992.
55. Lundman BM, Asplund K, Norberg A: Smoking and metabolic control in patients with insulin-dependent diabetes mellitus, *J Intern Med* 227(2):101–106, 1990.
56. Hofer SE, Rosenbauer J, Grulich-Henn J, et al: DPV-Wiss Study Group: Smoking and metabolic control in adolescents with type 1 diabetes, *J Pediatr* 154(1):20–23 e1, 2009.
57. Zoppini G, Targher G, Cacciatori V, et al: Chronic cigarette smoking is associated with increased plasma circulating intercellular adhesion molecule 1 levels in young type 1 diabetic patients, *Diabetes Care* 22(11):1871–1874, 1999.
58. Ranney L, Melvin C, Lux L, et al: Systematic review: smoking cessation intervention strategies for adults and adults in special populations, *Ann Intern Med* 145(11):845–856, 2006.
59. Fiore MC, Jaen CR: A clinical blueprint to accelerate the elimination of tobacco use, *JAMA* 299 (17):2083–2085, 2008.
60. Chakravarthy MV, Booth FW: Hot topics: exercise, Philadelphia, 2003, Hanley and Belfus (Elsevier).
61. Kelley DE, Goodpaster BH: Effects of physical activity on insulin action and glucose tolerance in obesity, *Med Sci Sports Exerc* 31(11 Suppl):S619–S623, 1999.
62. Loimaala A, Groundstroem K, Rinne M, et al: Effect of long-term endurance and strength training on metabolic control and arterial elasticity in patients with type 2 diabetes mellitus, *Am J Cardiol* 103(7):972–977, 2009.

63. Balducci S, Zanuso S, Nicolucci A, et al: Effect of an intensive exercise intervention strategy on modifiable cardiovascular risk factors in subjects with type 2 diabetes mellitus: a randomized controlled trial: the Italian Diabetes and Exercise Study (EDES), *Arch Intern Med* 170 (20):1794–1803, 2010.
64. Balducci S, Zanuso S, Cardelli P, et al: Changes in physical fitness predict improvements in modifiable cardiovascular risk factors independently of body weight loss in subjects with type 2 diabetes participating in the Italian Diabetes and Exercise Study (IDES), *Diabetes Care* 35 (6):1347–1354, 2012.
65. Umpierre D, Ribeiro PA, Kramer CK, et al: Physical activity advice only or structured exercise training and association with HbA1c levels in type 2 diabetes: a systematic review and meta-analysis, *JAMA* 305(17):1790–1799, 2011.
66. Chudyk A, Petrella RJ: Effects of exercise on cardiovascular risk factors in type 2 diabetes: a meta-analysis, *Diabetes Care* 34(5):1228–1237, 2011.
67. Carnethon MR, De Chavez PJ, Biggs ML, et al: Association of weight status with mortality in adults with incident diabetes, *JAMA* 308(6):581–590, 2012.
68. Florez H, Castillo-Florez S: Beyond the obesity paradox in diabetes: fitness, fatness, and mortality, *JAMA* 308(6):619–620, 2012.
69. Wei M, Kampert JB, Barlow CE, et al: Relationship between low cardiorespiratory fitness and mortality in normal-weight, overweight, and obese men, *JAMA* 282(16):1547–1553, 1999.
70. Fogelholm M: Physical activity, fitness and fatness: relations to mortality, morbidity and disease risk factors. A systematic review, *Obes Rev* 11(3):202–221, 2010.
71. Kokkinos P, Myers J, Faselis C, et al: BMI-mortality paradox and fitness in African American and Caucasian men with type 2 diabetes, *Diabetes Care* 35(5):1021–1027, 2012.
72. Lee S, Kuk JL, Katzmarzyk PT, et al: Cardiorespiratory fitness attenuates metabolic risk independent of abdominal subcutaneous and visceral fat in men, *Diabetes Care* 28(4):895–901, 2005.
73. Wei M, Gibbons LW, Kampert JB, et al: Low cardiorespiratory fitness and physical inactivity as predictors of mortality in men with type 2 diabetes, *Ann Intern Med* 132(8):605–611, 2000.
74. Church TS, LaMonte MJ, Barlow CE, et al: Cardiorespiratory fitness and body mass index as predictors of cardiovascular disease mortality among men with diabetes, *Arch Intern Med* 165 (18):2114–2120, 2005.
75. Sluik D, Buijsse B, Muckelbauer R, et al: Physical activity and mortality in individuals with diabetes mellitus: a prospective study and meta-analysis, *Arch Intern Med* 172(17):1285–1295, 2012.
76. Lyerly GW, Sui X, Lavie CJ, et al: The association between cardiorespiratory fitness and risk of all-cause mortality among women with impaired fasting glucose or undiagnosed diabetes mellitus, *Mayo Clin Proc* 84(9):780–786, 2009.
77. Rejeski WJ, Ip EH, Bertoni AG, et al: Lifestyle change and mobility in obese adults with type 2 diabetes, *N Engl J Med* 366(13):1209–1217, 2012.
78. Hu FB, Sigal RJ, Rich-Edwards JW, et al: Walking compared with vigorous physical activity and risk of type 2 diabetes in women: a prospective study, *JAMA* 282(15):1433–1439, 1999.
79. Tuomilehto J, Lindström J, Eriksson JG, et al: Prevention of type 2 diabetes mellitus by changes in lifestyle among subjects with impaired glucose tolerance, *N Engl J Med* 344(18):1343–1350, 2001.
80. Knowler WC, Barrett-Connor E, Fowler SE, et al: Reduction in the incidence of type 2 diabetes with lifestyle intervention or metformin, *N Engl J Med* 346(6):393–403, 2002.
81. Gregg EW, Gerzoff RB, Caspersen CJ, et al: Relationship of walking to mortality among US adults with diabetes, *Arch Intern Med* 163(12):1440–1447, 2003.
82. Hu FB, Stampfer MJ, Solomon C, et al: Physical activity and risk for cardiovascular events in diabetic women, *Ann Intern Med* 134(2):96–105, 2001.
83. Hu FB, Manson JE: Walking: the best medicine for diabetes? *Arch Intern Med* 163(12):1397–1398, 2003.
84. Powell KE, Thompson PD, Caspersen CJ, et al: Physical activity and the incidence of coronary heart disease, *Annu Rev Public Health* 8:253–287, 1987.
85. Berlin JA, Colditz GA: A meta-analysis of physical activity in the prevention of coronary heart disease, *Am J Epidemiol* 132(4):612–628, 1990.
86. Green DJ, O'Driscoll G, Joyner MJ, et al: Exercise and cardiovascular risk reduction: time to update the rationale for exercise? *J Appl Physiol* 105(2):766–768, 2008.
87. Billman GE, Schwartz PJ, Stone HL: The effects of daily exercise on susceptibility to sudden cardiac death, *Circulation* 69(6):1182–1189, 1984.
88. Hull SS Jr., Vanoli E, Adamson PB, et al: Exercise training confers anticipatory protection from sudden death during acute myocardial ischemia, *Circulation* 89(2):548–552, 1994.
89. Donnelly JE, Blair SN, Jakicic JM, et al: Appropriate physical activity intervention strategies for weight loss and prevention of weight regain for adults, *Med Sci Sports Exerc* 41(2):459–471, 2009.
90. Fletcher GF, Ades PA, Kligfield P, et al: Exercise standards for testing and training: a scientific statement from the American Heart Association, *Circulation* http://dx.doi.org/10.1161/CIR.0b013e31829b5b44 2013 [Epub ahead of print].
91. American College of Sports Medicine: *ACSM's guidelines for exercise testing and prescription*, ed 8, Philadelphia, 2010, Wolters Kluwer/Lippincott Williams & Wilkins pp. 233–234.
92. Thompson PD, Franklin BA, Balady GJ, et al: Exercise and acute cardiovascular events: placing the risks into perspective: a scientific statement from the American Heart Association Council on Nutrition, Physical Activity, and Metabolism; American Heart Association Council on Clinical Cardiology; American College of Sports Medicine, *Circulation* 115(17):2358–2368, 2007.
93. Williams MA, Haskell WL, Ades PA, et al: Resistance exercise in individuals with and without cardiovascular disease: 2007 update: a scientific statement from the American Heart Association Council on Clinical Cardiology and Council on Nutrition, Physical Activity, and Metabolism, *Circulation* 116(5):572–584, 2007.
94. FitzGerald SJ, Barlow CE, Kampert JB, et al: Muscular fitness and all-cause mortality: prospective observations, *J Phys Act Health* 1(1):7–18, 2004.
95. Pollock ML, Miller HS Jr., Janeway R, et al: Effects of walking on body composition and cardiovascular function of middle-aged man, *J Appl Physiol* 30(1):126–130, 1971.
96. Evans BW, Cureton KJ, Purvis JW: Metabolic and circulatory responses to walking and jogging in water, *Res Q* 49(4):442–449, 1978.
97. Shoenfeld Y, Keren G, Shimoni T, et al: Walking. A method for rapid improvement of physical fitness, *JAMA* 243(20):2062–2063, 1980.
98. Franklin BA, Gordon NF, editors: Contemporary diagnosis and management in cardiovascular exercise, Newtown, PA, 2009, Handbooks in Health Care Co.
99. Braith RW, Stewart KJ: Resistance exercise training: its role in the prevention of cardiovascular disease, *Circulation* 113(22):2642–2650, 2006.
100. McCartney N, McKelvie RS, Martin J, et al: Weight-training-induced attenuation of the circulatory response of older males to weight lifting, *J Appl Physiol* 74(3):1056–1060, 1993.
101. Hickson RC, Rosenkoetter MA, Brown MM: Strength training effects on aerobic power and short-term endurance, *Med Sci Sports Exerc* 12(5):336–339, 1980.
102. Feigenbaum MS, Pollock ML: Strength training: rationale for current guidelines for adult fitness programs, *Phys Sportsmed* 25(2):44–63, 1997.
103. United States Department of Health and Human Services: Physical activity and health: a report of the surgeon general, Atlanta, GA, 1996, US Department of Health and Human Services, Centers for Disease Control and Prevention, National Center for Chronic Disease and Health Promotion.
104. Dunn AL, Marcus BH, Kampert JB, et al: Comparison of lifestyle and structured interventions to increase physical activity and cardiorespiratory fitness: a randomized trial, *JAMA* 281 (4):327–334, Jan 27, 1999.
105. Andersen RE, Wadden TA, Bartlett SJ, et al: Effects of lifestyle activity vs structured aerobic exercise in obese women: a randomized trial, *JAMA* 281(4):335–340, 1999.
106. Dunn AL, Andersen RE, Jakicic JM: Lifestyle physical activity interventions. History, short- and long-term effects, and recommendations, *Am J Prev Med* 15(4):398–412, 1998.
107. Pratt M: Benefits of lifestyle activity vs structured exercise, *JAMA* 281(94):375–376, 1999.
108. Gordon NF, Kohl HW III, Blair SN: Life style exercise: a new strategy to promote physical activity for adults, *J Cardiopulm Rehabil* 13(3):161–163, 1993.
109. Levine JA: Nonexercise activity thermogenesis—liberating the life-force, *J Intern Med* 262 (3):273–287, 2007.
110. Bey L, Hamilton MT: Suppression of skeletal muscle lipoprotein lipase activity during physical inactivity: a molecular reason to maintain daily low-intensity activity, *J Physiol* 551(Pt 2):673–682, 2003.
111. Levine JA, Lanningham-Foster LM, McCrady SK, et al: Interindividual variation in posture allocation: possible role in human obesity, *Science* 307(5709):584–586, 2005.
112. Bravata DM, Smith-Spangler C, Sundaram V, et al: Using pedometers to increase physical activity and improve health: a systematic review, *JAMA* 298(19):2296–2304, 2007.
113. Leon AS, Norstrom J: Evidence of the role of physical activity and cardiorespiratory fitness in the prevention of coronary heart disease, *Quest* 47(3):311–319, 1995.
114. Shahid SK, Schneider SH: Effects of exercise on insulin resistance syndrome, *Coron Artery Dis* 11 (2):103–109, 2000.
115. Kraus WE, Houmard JA, Duscha BD, et al: Effects of the amount and intensity of exercise on plasma lipoproteins, *N Engl J Med* 347(19):1483–1492, 2002.
116. Marwick TH, Hordern MD, Miller T, et al: Exercise training for type 2 diabetes mellitus: impact on cardiovascular risk: a scientific statement from the American Heart Association, *Circulation* 119 (25):3244–3262, 2009.
117. Hordern MD, Dunstan DW, Prin JB, et al: Exercise prescription for patients with type 2 diabetes and pre-diabetes: a position statement from Exercise and Sport Science Australia, *J Sci Med Sport* 15(1):25–31, 2012.
118. Garber CE, Blissmer B, Deschenes MR, et al: American College of Sports Medicine position stand. Quantity and quality of exercise for developing and maintaining cardiorespiratory, musculoskeletal, and neuromotor fitness in apparently healthy adults: guidance for prescribing exercise, *Med Sci Sports Exerc* 43(7):1334–1359, 2011.
119. Colberg SR, Albright AL, Blissmer BJ, et al: Exercise and type 2 diabetes: American College of Sports Medicine and the American Diabetes Association: joint position statement. Exercise and type 2 diabetes, *Med Sci Sports Exerc* 42(12):2282–2303, 2010.
120. Borghouts LB, Keizer HA: Exercise and insulin sensitivity: a review, *Int J Sports Med* 21(1):1–12, 2000.
121. Blair SN, Kohl HW 3rd., Paffenbarger RS Jr., et al: Physical fitness and all-cause mortality. A prospective study of healthy men and women, *JAMA* 262(17):2395–2401, 1989.
122. Martin BJ, Arena R, Haykowsky M, et al: Cardiovascular fitness and mortality after contemporary cardiac rehabilitation, *Mayo Clin Proc* 88(5):455–463, 2013.
123. Barnard RJ, MacAlpin R, Kattus AA, et al: Ischemic response to sudden strenuous exercise in healthy men, *Circulation* 48(5):936–942, 1973.
124. Dimsdale JE, Hartley LH, Guiney T, et al: Postexercise peril. Plasma catecholamines and exercise, *JAMA* 251(5):630–632, 1984.
125. Guarneri M, Mercado N, Suhar C: Integrative approaches for cardiovascular disease, *Nutr Clin Pract* 24(6):701–708, 2009.
126. Salmela S, Poskiparta M, Kasila K, et al: Transtheoretical model-based dietary interventions in primary care: a review of the evidence in diabetes, *Health Educ Res* 24(2):237–252, 2009.
127. Van Nes M, Sawatzky JA: Improving cardiovascular health with motivational interviewing: a nurse practitioner perspective, *J Am Acad Nurse Pract* 22(12):654–660, 2010.
128. Angermayr L, Melchart D, Linde K: Multifactorial lifestyle interventions in the primary and secondary prevention of cardiovascular disease and type 2 diabetes mellitus-a systematic review of randomized controlled trials, *Ann Behav Med* 40(1):49–64, 2012.
129. Hardcastle S, Taylor A, Bailey M, et al: A randomised controlled trial on the effectiveness of a primary health care based counselling intervention on physical activity, diet and CHD risk factors, *Patient Educ Couns* 70(1):31–39, 2008.
130. Prochaska JO, DiClemente CC: The transtheoretical approach: crossing traditional boundaries of therapy, Homewood, IL, 1984, Dow Jones-Irwin.
131. Rollnick S, Mason P, Butler C: Health behavior change: a guide for practitioners, Edinburgh, 1999, Churchill Livingstone.
132. Armstrong MJ, Mottershead TA, Ronksley PE, et al: Motivational interviewing to improve weight loss in overweight and/or obese patients: a systematic review and meta-analysis of randomized controlled trials, *Obes Rev* 12(9):709–723, 2011.
133. Thompson DR, Chair SY, Chan SW, et al: Motivational interviewing: a useful approach to improving cardiovascular health? *J Clin Nurs* 20(9–10):1236–1244, 2011.
134. Antiss T: Motivational interviewing in primary care, *J Clin Psychol Med Settings* 16(1):87–93, 2009.
135. Greaves C, Sheppard K, Evans P: Motivational interviewing for lifestyle change, *Diabetes Prim Care* 12(3):178–182, 2010.
136. Burke LE, Fair J: Promoting prevention: skill sets and attributes of health care providers who deliver behavioral interventions, *J Cardiovasc Nurs* 18(4):256–266, 2003.
137. Sonntag U, Wiesner J, Fahrenkrog S, et al: Motivational interviewing and shared decision making in primary care, *Patient Educ Couns* 87(1):62–66, 2012.
138. Miller WR, Rollnick S: Motivational interviewing: preparing people for change, ed 2, New York, 2002, Guilford Press.
139. Miller WR, Rollnick S: Ten things that motivational interviewing is not, *Behav Cogn Psychother* 37 (2):129–140, 2009.
140. Rollnick S, Miller WR, Butler CC: Motivational interviewing in health care: helping patients change behavior, New York, 2008, The Guilford Press.
141. Levensky ER, Forcehimes A, O'Donohue WT, et al: Motivational interviewing: an evidence-based approach to counseling helps patients follow treatment recommendations, *Am J Nurs* 107 (10):50–58, 2007.
142. Lorig K, Holman H, Sobel D, et al: Living a healthy life with chronic conditions: self-management of heart disease, arthritis, diabetes, asthma, bronchitis, emphysema and others, ed 3, Boulder, CO, 2006, Bull Publishing Company.
143. Steinberg M: Clinical perspectives on motivational interviewing in diabetes care, *Diabetes Spectrum* 24(3):179–181, 2011.
144. Yusuf S, Hawken S, Ôunpuu S, et al: Effect of potentially modifiable risk factors associated with myocardial infarction in 52 countries (the INTERHEART study): case-controlled study, *Lancet* 364(9438):937–952, 2004.
145. Khot UN, Khot MB, Bajzer CT, et al: Prevalence of conventional risk factors in patients with coronary heart disease, *JAMA* 290(7):898–904, 2003.
146. Greenland P, Knoll MD, Stamler J, et al: Major risk factors as antecedents of fatal and nonfatal coronary heart disease events, *JAMA* 290(7):891–897, 2003.
147. Canto JG, Iskandrian AE: Major risk factors for cardiovascular disease: debunking the "only 50%" myth, *JAMA* 290(7):947–949, 2003.
148. Kannel WB, Vasan RS: Adverse consequences of the 50% misconception, *Am J Cardiol* 103 (3):426–427, 2009.
149. Franklin BA, Vanhecke TE: Counseling patients to make cardioprotective lifestyle changes: strategies for success, *Prev Cardiol* 11(1):50–55, 2008.

13 Effect of Glucose Management on Coronary Heart Disease Risk in Patients with Diabetes

Kasia J. Lipska and Silvio E. Inzucchi

Coronary heart disease (CHD) is the most common vascular complication of diabetes. Because elevated glucose defines diabetes and because diabetes is a well-recognized risk factor for CHD, strategies that lower glucose should theoretically reduce the risk of CHD events in diabetes. In reality, the relationship between glucose-lowering strategies and cardiovascular outcomes is complex and suggests that the impact of interventions on patient outcomes cannot be easily predicted from the effects of interventions on surrogate measures (such as glucose or hemoglobin A1c, HbA1c). Indeed, CHD can precede the development of diabetes, and some have suggested that both conditions (CHD and diabetes) have common genetic and environmental roots and spring from a "common soil" (**Fig. 13-1**) (see also Chapters 2, 8, and 9).[1] This chapter describes the epidemiologic relationship between glucose and CHD, reviews clinical trial evidence of the effects of glucose lowering on CHD outcomes, discusses the benefits and risks of glucose lowering with specific medications and in specific patient populations, and concludes with implications for clinical practice.

CHANGING EPIDEMIOLOGY OF DIABETES AND CORONARY HEART DISEASE

The general incidence and prevalence of CHD have declined in the United States in the last several decades, and this decline has been accompanied by a decline in CHD-related mortality.[2] These trends have been attributed to better cardiovascular risk factor control and treatment during and after acute coronary syndromes over time, primarily with the use of statin medications, blood pressure management, and anti-platelet therapies. In contrast to CHD trends, the incidence and prevalence of diabetes have been steadily increasing over time, with the disease now affecting close to a third of older U.S. adults (65 years or older) (see also Chapter 1).[3,4] In addition, adults with diabetes are living longer.[5] As a result, the burden of CHD attributable to diabetes is increasing (see also Chapter 7).[6] These

changes in the epidemiology of diabetes and CHD have important implications. First, strategies that mitigate the risk of CHD in diabetes patients will be of growing importance because heart disease is increasingly a complication of diabetes. Second, these strategies will be applied to an aging population with a high comorbidity burden and at higher risk for adverse effects of therapy.

EPIDEMIOLOGIC RELATIONSHIP OF GLUCOSE WITH CORONARY HEART DISEASE

Multiple studies have assessed the relationship between various glucose parameters—fasting glucose, 2-hour glucose during an oral glucose tolerance test, or HbA1c levels—and the risk of CHD in populations with and without diabetes. Most of this work suggests a continuous relationship between measures of glycemia and CHD risk.

Several studies and a metaregression analysis have shown that in nondiabetic populations, there is a graded relationship between initial fasting and postprandial glucose levels and subsequent occurrence of cardiovascular events over 12 years of follow-up.[7] The association is apparent even at levels below the diabetic thresholds. However, because HbA1c is the preferred test for monitoring blood glucose control during the chronic management of diabetes, data summarized here will be predominantly based on this glycemic parameter.

In the large prospective population study of Norfolk, in the United Kingdom, HbA1c and cardiovascular risk factors were assessed from 1995 to 1997, and cardiovascular disease events and mortality were examined during the next 6 to 8 years of follow-up.[8] The relationship between HbA1c and cardiovascular disease and total mortality was continuous and apparent even among persons without diabetes. The risk was lowest among persons with HbA1c below 5% and increased thereafter throughout the range of nondiabetic HbA1c levels up to 6.9%. Each one percentage point increase in HbA1c above 5% was associated with a 20% to

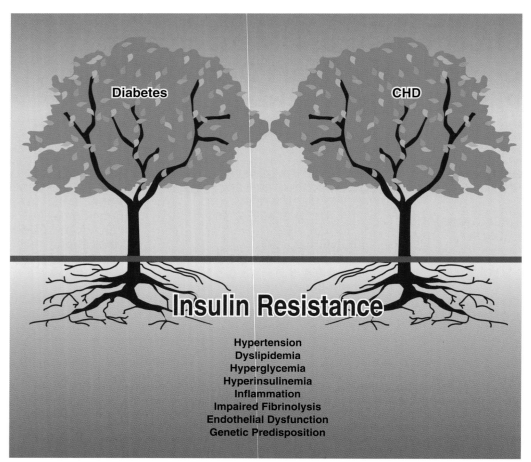

FIGURE 13-1 The "common soil" hypothesis of diabetes and coronary heart disease (CHD).

25% increase in the relative risk for CHD among men and women in age- and risk-factor adjusted models. Moreover, when known diabetes status and HbA1c concentration were included in the same model, diabetes was no longer a significant independent predictor of CHD, suggesting that the increased risk of CHD in dysglycemic states is mediated through hyperglycemia itself.

The prognostic value of HbA1c was also assessed in the Atherosclerosis Risk in Communities (ARIC) study of U.S. adults without a prior history of diabetes or cardiovascular disease and with up to 15 years of follow-up.[9] Similar to the observations from the Norfolk study, the risk for CHD increased with higher HbA1c values in a continuous fashion independent of classic cardiovascular risk factors. When compared with study participants with HbA1c of 5% to less than 5.5% (the reference range), the hazard ratio (HR) for CHD was increased 23% in those with HbA1c of 5.5% to less than 6%, 78% for HbA1c of 6% to less than 6.5%, and 95% for HbA1c of 6.5% or higher. Although, clearly, the causal role of glucose in the development of CHD could not be evaluated in this epidemiologic study, the findings suggest that HbA1c, even in the nondiabetic range, can be a useful independent marker of cardiovascular risk.

Although the association between HbA1c level and CHD may be prognostically important in nondiabetic individuals, to understand the effect of glucose lowering on CHD risk we must examine data in patients with diabetes. A prospective observational study of type 2 diabetes patients enrolled in the United Kingdom Prospective Diabetes Study (UKPDS)

examined the relationship between HbA1c and cardiovascular complications. They found that each 1% increase in the updated HbA1c was associated with a 14% relative risk increase for myocardial infarction (MI; **Fig. 13-2**).[10] A meta-analysis of 13 prospective cohort studies of HbA1c and cardiovascular disease in persons with diabetes (type 1 or 2) suggested that chronic hyperglycemia is associated with an increased risk for cardiovascular disease. The pooled relative risk for cardiovascular disease associated with a 1% increase in HbA1c was 1.18. In a subgroup of six studies conducted in patients with type 2 diabetes, a 1% increase in HbA1c was associated with a 13% increased relative risk for CHD.[11] The inclusion criteria for the meta-analysis did not specify pharmacologic treatment for diabetes; rather, these were observational studies involving patients on both medication and diet therapy. These results suggest a moderate increase in cardiovascular risk with increasing HbA1c in diabetic adults. However, the meta-analysis relied on small studies with some suggestion of heterogeneity of effects that could not be explored in detail.

One large analysis examined data from the U.K. General Practice Research Database (GPRD) on 27,965 patients with type 2 diabetes whose oral monotherapy was intensified to oral combination therapy, and 20,005 whose oral therapy was intensified to include insulin.[12] The primary and secondary outcomes for the two cohorts were all-cause mortality and major cardiovascular events, respectively, over the mean follow-up of 4.5 years. HbA1c in the study was based on the mean of any values recorded between the therapeutic

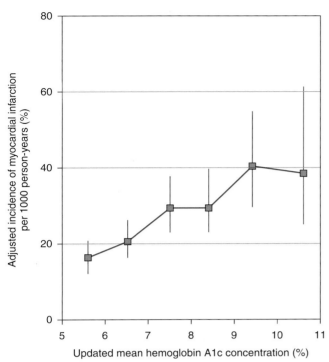

FIGURE 13-2 Epidemiologic relationship between hemoglobin A1c and cardiovascular events. *(Modified from Stratton et al. BMJ 2000.[16])*

switch and death or date of censor. In combined cohort analysis, the HbA1c decile with a median value of 7.5% (interquartile range 7.5% to 7.6%) was associated with the lowest mortality and the lowest progression to large-vessel disease among those without prior history of cardiovascular events. Higher and lower HbA1c values were associated with an increased risk, and the pattern of risk was U shaped. In the oral combination therapy group, a wider range of HbA1c values was safe with respect to mortality risk (median HbA1c 6.9% to 8.9%), whereas this range was narrower for patients on insulin (median HbA1c 7.5% to 8.1%). In addition, the use of insulin was associated with an approximately 50% higher hazard of mortality compared with the use of oral agents. Although no evidence supports a direct cardiotoxic effect of insulin in type 2 diabetes, it is certainly possible that age, comorbidities, and diabetes duration may be related to the decision to initiate insulin as well as to the higher mortality risk. The findings from this study differ significantly from the graded, continuous epidemiologic relationships between HbA1c and cardiovascular outcomes in individuals without diabetes. In nondiabetic populations, lower HbA1c values predict better outcomes without a clear threshold, but the data from treated patients with diabetes suggest that there may be a risk associated with achieving near-normal glycemia.

Another retrospective cohort study, this time performed in the United States, confirmed the results of the GPRD analysis. Here, data from 71,092 patients with type 2 diabetes age 60 years or older within the Kaiser Permanente Northern California system were analyzed to examine the association between baseline HbA1c level and subsequent nonfatal complications (metabolic, microvascular, and cardiovascular events) and mortality.[13] The authors found a similar U-shaped relationship between HbA1c level and mortality, with higher risk in those with HbA1c below 6% and 10%

or higher in the adjusted models. In contrast, however, the relationship between HbA1c and cardiovascular events was continuous with increasing risk above HbA1c of 6%. Integrating all of the outcomes together, the "optimal" HbA1c range identified by this study lay somewhere in the 6% to 7.9% range. As in the GPRD study, the analysis added important information about optimal glycemic targets in diabetes, suggesting that achievement of low glycemic levels may provide benefits (such as lower risk of CHD), but that very low levels of glycemia may be associated with harm (e.g., higher mortality risk). A third study, this involving all adults with type 2 diabetes drawn from the Kaiser Permanente Southern California system, showed a U-shaped relationship between HbA1c and cardiovascular events, with HbA1c levels of 6% or lower and greater than 8% associated with an increased risk of cardiovascular events.[14] Whether or not low HbA1c levels are a marker of sicker patients or a mediator of harm remains highly debatable. Moreover, whether this phenomenon is actually directly attributable to lower than desirable glycemia or to adverse effects of the medications clinicians use to achieve this range is not clear. Randomized clinical trials can test the effects of interventions directly on patient outcomes and may be able to provide greater insight into the effect of glucose lowering on CHD events.

TRIALS OF GLUCOSE-LOWERING INTERVENTIONS

The landmark trial in type 2 diabetes that investigated the effect of intensive glucose lowering on microvascular and macrovascular outcomes was the UKPDS. The trial was begun in 1977 and the results were published in 1998. In this trial, 3867 patients with newly diagnosed type 2 diabetes (median age 54) were randomized to intensive treatment with sulfonylureas (chlorpropamide, glibenclamide (glyburide in the U.S.), or glipizide) or with insulin, versus conventional therapy with diet alone.[15] The median HbA1c level in the intensive group during the course of the trial was 7%, versus 7.9% in the conventional arm. Three separate aggregate endpoints were studied over the 10 years of follow-up. The risk in the intensive group was 12% lower for any diabetes-related endpoint ($P=0.03$), which included both macrovascular and microvascular events as well as metabolic complications; not significantly lower for any diabetes-related death (-10%, $P=0.34$); and not significantly lower for mortality (-6%, $P=0.44$), compared with patients treated with diet only. The reduction in diabetes-related endpoints was driven by a 25% risk reduction in microvascular events, and the reduction in MI did not reach statistical significance (-16%, $P=0.052$). A subgroup of UKPDS patients who were overweight ($>120\%$ ideal body weight) were randomized either to intensive therapy with metformin (n=342, median HbA1c 7.4%) or conventional diet therapy (n=411, median HbA1c 8%).[16] In this subset of patients, treatment with metformin was associated with a 32% reduction in any diabetes-related endpoint ($P=0.002$), 42% reduction in diabetes-related death ($P=0.017$), and 36% reduction in mortality ($P=0.011$). In this cohort of patients treated with metformin, there was a significant 39% reduction in MI ($P=0.01$) (**Fig. 13-3**). In summary, the UKPDS trial established that intensive glucose control reduces the risk of microvascular complications in patients with newly

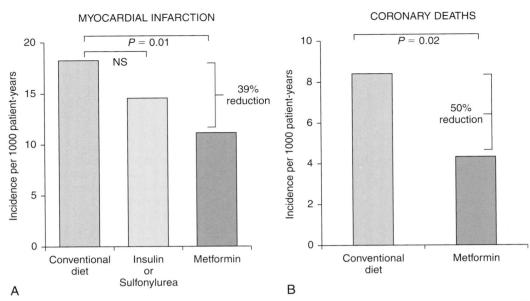

FIGURE 13-3 Results of the UKPDS trial with respect to myocardial infarction and coronary deaths. NS = Non significant. *(Modified from Effect of intensive blood-glucose control with metformin on complications in overweight patients with type 2 diabetes [UKPDS 34]. UK Prospective Diabetes Study [UKPDS] Group, Lancet 352:854, 1998).*

diagnosed type 2 diabetes, but suggested that macrovascular benefits may be confined to overweight patients treated with metformin therapy.

After the UKPDS trial was completed, study participants and their clinicians were advised to lower levels of blood glucose as much as possible, and patients returned to community or hospital-based diabetes care according to their clinical needs without any attempts to maintain previously randomized therapies. In the 10-year post-trial monitoring study of patients who survived to the end of the UKDPS trial, HbA1c levels were no longer different between the original intensive and conventional arms (approximately 8% at the end of the post-trial monitoring period).[17] In the sulfonylurea-insulin group, relative risk reductions for diabetes-related endpoints persisted, whereas significant risk reductions for MI (15%, $P=0.010$) and mortality (13%, $P=0.007$) emerged over time. In the metformin group, relative risk reductions persisted for any diabetes-related endpoint, MI (33%, $P=0.005$), and mortality (27%, $P=0.002$). These observations suggest a modest but sustained effect of intensive glucose lowering on cardiovascular events, but only after many years of follow-up. Whether the effect is confined to patients with newly diagnosed type 2 diabetes or whether it reflects the long period of time required to significantly affect subsequent atherosclerotic outcomes is not entirely clear.

Even before the cardiovascular benefits of intensive glucose therapy emerged in the long-term follow-up of the UKPDS trial, guidelines recommended a target HbA1c level of 7% or less in most patients. This was primarily driven by the expectation of microvascular benefits, albeit with uncertainty over the effects on macrovascular events. To settle the questions about the role of intensive glucose therapy in type 2 diabetes, three randomized controlled trials were specifically designed to examine the impact of targeting near-normal glycemia on cardiovascular risk. The HbA1c targets were set low because of the continuous epidemiologic relationship of glucose with cardiovascular risk, suggesting that perhaps much lower glucose levels need to be achieved for a significant benefit to emerge. The three trials all recruited

participants with type 2 diabetes who had either a history of or multiple risk factors for cardiovascular disease, thus ensuring adequate event rates to study the effects of the interventions. Participants were therefore quite distinct from patients in the UKPDS trial—they were older, had a longer duration of diabetes, and had a greater comorbidity burden.

The Action to Control Cardiovascular Risk in Diabetes (ACCORD) trial enrolled 10,251 patients (mean age 62, median baseline HbA1c 8.1%, 35% with history of prior cardiovascular event) to intensive glucose therapy (targeting HbA1c <6%, median achieved HbA1c 6.4%) versus conventional therapy (targeting HbA1c 7% to 7.9%, median achieved HbA1c 7.5%).[18] This trial was stopped prematurely after a mean follow-up of 3.5 years because of a higher mortality rate in the intensive therapy group compared with the control arm (HR 1.22, $P=0.04$). The primary endpoint of the trial, major cardiovascular events, was not significantly reduced (HR 0.90, $P=0.16$), although the rate of nonfatal MI was lower in the intensive therapy group (HR 0.76, $P=0.004$). To date, analyses have not identified any clear explanation for the higher mortality risk associated with the intensive glucose-lowering strategy. In the intensive therapy group, a median HbA1c level of 6.4% was rapidly achieved and maintained, but subsequent post hoc analyses implicated factors associated with persistently higher HbA1c, rather than low HbA1c, as likely contributors to the increased mortality risk.[19] In addition, rates of serious hypoglycemia requiring medical assistance were threefold higher in the intensive group than during standard therapy (10.5% versus 3.5%, $P<0.001$). Subsequent retrospective epidemiologic analyses of ACCORD have suggested, however, that severe hypoglycemia may not, in fact, account for the difference in mortality between the two study arms.[20] Although hypoglycemia was associated with increased mortality within each randomized group, the risk of death was actually lower in participants experiencing hypoglycemia in the intensive arm than in participants with hypoglycemia in the standard arm. Other explanations, such as the particular medication combinations or undetected medication

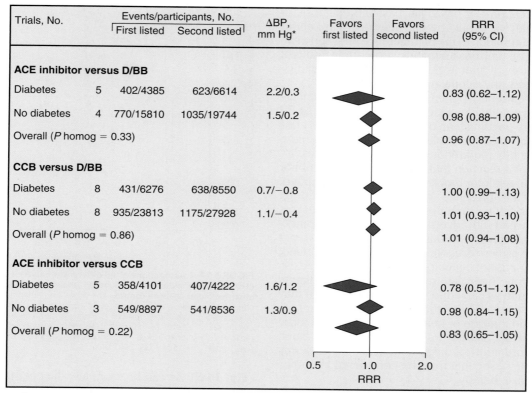

Trials, No.		Events/participants, No.		ΔBP, mm Hg*	Favors first listed	Favors second listed	RRR (95% CI)
		First listed	Second listed				
ACE inhibitor versus D/BB							
Diabetes	5	402/4385	623/6614	2.2/0.3			0.83 (0.62–1.12)
No diabetes	4	770/15810	1035/19744	1.5/0.2			0.98 (0.88–1.09)
Overall (P homog = 0.33)							0.96 (0.87–1.07)
CCB versus D/BB							
Diabetes	8	431/6276	638/8550	0.7/−0.8			1.00 (0.99–1.13)
No diabetes	8	935/23813	1175/27928	1.1/−0.4			1.01 (0.93–1.10)
Overall (P homog = 0.86)							1.01 (0.94–1.08)
ACE inhibitor versus CCB							
Diabetes	5	358/4101	407/4222	1.6/1.2			0.78 (0.51–1.12)
No diabetes	3	549/8897	541/8536	1.3/0.9			0.98 (0.84–1.15)
Overall (P homog = 0.22)							0.83 (0.65–1.05)

FIGURE 14-3 Effects of BP-lowering regimens based on different medication classes on the risk of CHD in patients with and without diabetes mellitus. Conventions as per Figure 14-2. D/BB = Diuretic/beta blocker (Modified from Turnbull F, Neal B, Algert C, et al: Effects of different blood pressure lowering regimens on major cardiovascular events in individuals with and without diabetes mellitus: results of prospectively designed overviews of randomized trials, Arch Intern Med 165:1410-1419, 2005.)

combinations of atenolol with a thiazide diuretic versus amlodipine with perindopril on the primary outcome of fatal and nonfatal CHD events.[25] The trial involved 19,257 participants, 27% of whom had diabetes at study entry. The point estimate of treatment effect favored the amlodipine-perindopril combination for the primary outcome, but this was not statistically significant. However, there were significant reductions in all secondary outcomes associated with the amlodipine-perindopril combination, ranging from a relative risk reduction of 11% to 24%, and including all-cause mortality (which led to early termination of the trial), all coronary events, and non-fatal MI and fatal CHD. However, it should be noted that despite a goal of achieving similar BP levels in both treatment arms, the amlodipine-based regimen was associated with a significant 2.7/1.9 mm Hg lower BP over the duration of follow-up. There was no evidence of heterogeneity of the treatment effect by the presence or absence of diabetes, evaluated on the basis of total cardiovascular outcomes.

The Ongoing Telmisartan Alone and in Combination with Ramipril Global Endpoint Trial (ONTARGET) included 25,620 patients at increased risk for cardiovascular disease.[26] Approximately 40% of study participants had diabetes at study entry. Patients were randomized to ramipril alone, to telmisartan alone, or to both drugs. The mean BP level at study entry was 142/82 mm Hg. Over the course of follow-up, BP was 2.4/1.4 mm Hg lower in the combination therapy group compared with the ramipril-alone group. The incidence of the primary outcome (cardiovascular death, non-fatal MI, nonfatal stroke, or hospitalized heart failure) did not differ between the ramipril-alone group and each of the other randomized groups. As expected, participants

allocated to telmisartan alone experienced less cough and angioedema than those who were randomized to ramipril. However, symptoms of hypotension occurred more frequently in the telmisartan group (2.7%) and in the combination group (4.8%) compared with the ramipril-alone group (1.7%). Renal dysfunction was observed most often in the combination group. It is important to note that there was no heterogeneity in treatment effects by diabetes status for the primary outcome. In summary, the results of ONTARGET confirmed comparable efficacy of the ACE inhibitor and the ARB, but provided no evidence of additional benefit from combination therapy.

The Avoiding Cardiovascular Events through Combination Therapy to Patients Living with Systolic Hypertension (ACCOMPLISH) trial is also relevant to populations with diabetes.[27] Approximately 60% of the 11,506 high-risk patients with hypertension included in this study had an additional diagnosis of diabetes at study entry. Participants were randomly allocated to receive one of two combination drug regimens—the ACE inhibitor benazepril plus the calcium channel blocker amlodipine, or benazepril with the diuretic hydrochlorothiazide (HCT). The mean baseline BP level was 145/80 mm Hg. Over the duration of follow-up, a 0.9/1.1-mm Hg lower BP was observed in the benazepril-amlodipine group compared with the benazepril-HCT group. This study was stopped prematurely after a mean follow-up period of 3 years because of an observed statistically significant 20% reduction in the primary outcome (cardiovascular death, nonfatal MI, nonfatal stroke, hospitalization for angina, resuscitation after cardiac arrest, and coronary revascularization) in the benazepril-amlodipine group compared with the benazepril-HCT group. As with ONTARGET, there was no

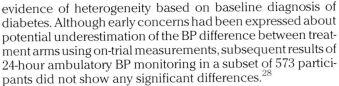

evidence of heterogeneity based on baseline diagnosis of diabetes. Although early concerns had been expressed about potential underestimation of the BP difference between treatment arms using on-trial measurements, subsequent results of 24-hour ambulatory BP monitoring in a subset of 573 participants did not show any significant differences.[28]

By and large, current hypertension and diabetes management guidelines worldwide acknowledge that achieving BP reduction is more pressing than decisions about which class of drug should be used, particularly given that two or more agents are frequently required in patients with diabetes.[8–13] In general, use of a regimen that includes an ACE-inhibitor or an angiotensin receptor blocker (ARB) is recommended, particularly in the presence of albuminuria. Although thiazide or thiazide-like diuretics as well as beta blockers have been associated with adverse effects on glucose homeostasis, the clinical relevance of this is doubtful and it does not preclude the use of these drugs in people with T2DM. Indeed, the indications for use of beta blockers in patients with existing CHD or systolic heart failure (particularly vasodilating beta blockers, such as carvedilol and nebivolol, which may also have more favorable metabolic effects than older beta blockers[29,30]) and thiazide or thiazide-like diuretics in those with cerebrovascular disease are compelling.[31,32] For much of the world, affordability of different classes of BP-lowering drugs is also a key issue that must be considered in choice of antihypertensive therapy.

More versus Less Blood Pressure Lowering and Target Blood Pressure Levels

Although acknowledging limitations of available randomized evidence, most guidelines worldwide currently recommend more aggressive management of hypertension (mostly, a target of 130/80 mm Hg or lower) among people with diabetes compared with those without diabetes.[8–13] In 1998, the UKPDS was the landmark trial that first compared more intensive BP lowering (with an ACE inhibitor or a beta blocker–based regimen) with less intensive control among newly diagnosed patients with T2DM and hypertension. The target BP levels for the randomized groups were below 150/85 mm Hg versus below 180/105 mm Hg, respectively. Achieved mean final BP levels were 144/82 mm Hg in the more intensive BP-lowering arm and 154/87 mm Hg in the less intensive BP-lowering arm. Compared with less tight control, more intensive BP lowering resulted in significant reductions in all "diabetes-related endpoints," as well as cerebrovascular events and microvascular disease.[33] For the secondary outcome of MI (fatal or nonfatal MI or sudden death), however, the observed relative risk reduction was not statistically significant (21% [95% CI −7% to 41%]). The second cycle of BPLTTC also addressed the question of whether more versus less BP reduction confers additional advantages, and for the outcome of CHD alone, the result was inconclusive.[20] However, the weighted mean BP differences among randomized groups within each trial appeared to correlate well with the magnitude of reduction of CHD risk (**Fig. 14-4**). Furthermore, there was no evidence of statistical heterogeneity between those with and without diabetes.[21]

Before the most recent evidence provided by the ADVANCE trial and the Action to Control Cardiovascular Risk in Diabetes (ACCORD) trial, Mancia and Grassi summarized the effects of BP-lowering drugs in patients with diabetes, focusing on entry and on-treatment BP levels

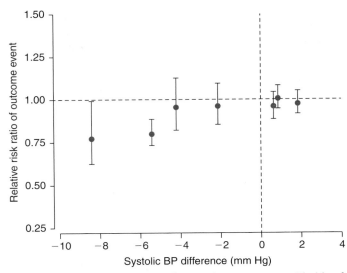

FIGURE 14-4 Associations of BP differences between groups with risks of CHD in seven published randomized trials comparing more versus less intensive blood pressure control. The circles are plotted at the point estimate of effect for the relative risk for every event type and the mean follow-up BP among randomized groups. *(From Turnbull F; Blood Pressure Lowering Treatment Trialists' Collaboration: Effects of different blood-pressure-lowering regimens on major cardiovascular events: results of prospectively-designed overviews of randomised trials, Lancet 362:1527-1535, 2003.)*

(**Fig. 14-5**). As can be seen, few data existed in relation to achieved SBP levels below 135 mm Hg, despite prevailing guideline recommendations.

The ACCORD trial was specifically designed to address a question of appropriate target BP levels in people with T2DM. This was a factorially randomized trial of 10,251 individuals with T2DM from 77 centers in North America.[34–36] Participants with a hemoglobin A1c (HbA1c) of 7.5% or more and aged 40 years or older with cardiovascular disease or 55 years or older with anatomic evidence of significant atherosclerosis, albuminuria, left ventricular hypertrophy, or at least two additional risk factors for cardiovascular disease (dyslipidemia, hypertension, smoking, or obesity) were randomized to intensive glucose control (aiming for HbA1c levels ≤6.0%) or standard control (aiming for HbA1c levels of 7.0% to 7.9%) (see also Chapter 13). Subsets of participants were also included in a factorially randomized evaluation of a BP-lowering intervention (n = 4733) or a lipid management intervention (n = 5518). The objective of the BP-lowering component of the study was to specifically examine the effects of targeting different SBP levels (an SBP target of 120 mm Hg or less, compared with 140 mm Hg or less). Participants who had SBP between 130 and 180 mm Hg on three or fewer antihypertensive medications and with no evidence of greater than 1.0 g of proteinuria per day or the equivalent were included. The BP-lowering regimen was at the physician's discretion but included any class of drug therapy known to produce cardiovascular benefits (ACE inhibitors, ARBs, diuretics, calcium channel blockers, or beta blockers). The primary outcome was a composite of major cardiovascular events defined as nonfatal MI, nonfatal stroke, and cardiovascular death. Secondary outcomes included all coronary events, all stroke events, and all-cause death, considered separately.

The mean baseline BP in ACCORD was 139/76 mm Hg, and at study entry, 87% of participants were already taking some form of antihypertensive therapy. Over a mean follow-up of 4.7 years, intensive therapy achieved an SBP

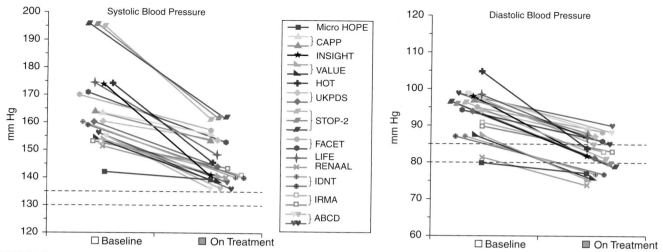

FIGURE 14-5 Effects of BP-lowering treatment on systolic and diastolic BP in patients with diabetes and hypertension in a number of trials before the ADVANCE and ACCORD trials. Values at trial entry and during treatment are shown for each trial. Dashed horizontal lines refer to goal BP values indicated by contemporary guidelines to be achieved during treatment. *(Reproduced with permission from Mancia G, Grassi G: Systolic and diastolic blood pressure control in antihypertensive drug trials,* J Hypertens 20:1461-1464, 2002.)

of 119 mm Hg compared with 134 mm Hg in the standard therapy group, resulting in a mean between-group difference of 14.2 mm Hg. Despite this difference in SBP, intensive therapy did not result in a statistically significant reduction in major cardiovascular events (relative risk reduction [RRR] 12%; 95% CI −6 to 27%; $P = 0.20$) (**Fig. 14-6**). When the components of the composite outcome were considered separately, intensive therapy did not reduce major coronary events (which included unstable angina) or cardiovascular death, but significantly reduced major strokes by 41% (95% CI 11%-61%). There was no statistically significant effect of intensive BP therapy on all-cause mortality or heart failure. There was no evidence of heterogeneity in treatment effect in subgroups of participants defined by age, sex baseline history of cardiovascular disease, and use of BP-lowering therapy at study entry.

Many have interpreted the ACCORD trial as being "negative" with respect to the BP-lowering component, stimulating discussion that the current target of 130/80 mm Hg or lower promulgated by many guidelines may not be justified. However, notwithstanding the clear benefits of a more aggressive approach to BP lowering for stroke well below this threshold, the 95% CIs around the estimates of effect size for other cardiovascular events, including CHD, do not exclude substantial and clinically important beneficial effects (approximately one-quarter reduction, which would be broadly consistent with a 14-mm Hg difference in SBP based on epidemiologic data). It is important to note that with the event rates in the control arm of ACCORD being approximately one half those anticipated, the trial was ultimately substantially underpowered. Intensive BP lowering in ACCORD was associated with an increased number of serious adverse events attributed to BP-lowering drugs, compared with the standard therapy group; however, overall rates over an average period of almost 5 years of follow-up were low (3.3% versus 1.3%). Particular concerns have been raised about higher levels of serum creatinine and lower levels of estimated glomerular filtration rate postrandomization among intensive–BP treatment participants. This did not translate to differences in end-stage renal disease (2.5% versus 2.4%), and intensive BP-lowering therapy was

associated with the development of numerically fewer cases of microalbuminuria and macroalbuminuria, the latter being significantly lower than the rates observed in the standard therapy group.

Legacy Effects of Blood Pressure Lowering

In 2008, the UKPDS study reported data from post-trial annual follow-up for an additional 6 years undertaken for all study participants, without attempts to maintain therapies based on the original randomization.[37,38] Long-term post-trial observational follow-up of the blood glucose–lowering arm demonstrated sustained, and in some cases newly emerged, reductions in clinical events associated with original randomization to intensive glucose control.[38] (See also Chapter 13.) These benefits were observed despite convergence of HbA1c values within a year of post-trial monitoring. Similarly, the BP difference achieved between randomized arms during the trial was no longer apparent within 2 years of the longer-term follow-up.[37] However, unlike the blood glucose intervention, the significant reductions in clinical events were lost during the additional observational period, without the emergence of any new benefits. A reasonable interpretation of these findings is that BP reduction needs to be maintained for the long-term benefits of such treatment to continue.

New Drugs

In addition to relatively recent approvals of the direct renin inhibitor aliskiren and the angiotensin II type 1 receptor (AT1R) blocker azilsartan, a number of novel BP-lowering compounds are currently in clinical testing.[39] These include dual-action AT1R inhibitors that also block either neutral endopeptidase or the endothelin A receptor; a dual inhibitor of neutral endopeptidase and endothelin-converting enzyme; an aldosterone synthase inhibitor; an antagonist of natriuretic peptide receptor A; and a soluble epoxide hydrolase inhibitor. As clinical data accumulate, the efficacy and comparative efficacy of the molecules that proceed to approval may be examined in the specific context of T2DM.

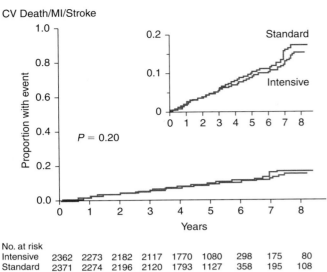

A

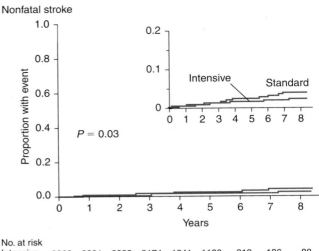

B

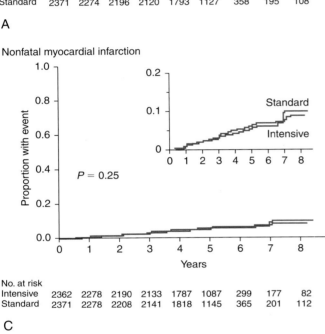

C

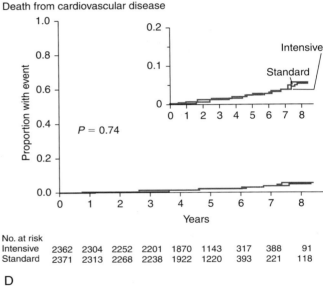

D

FIGURE 14-6 Kaplan-Meier curves for the primary composite outcome and its individual components in the ACCORD study. The insets show close-up versions of the graphs in each panel. CV = Cardiovascular; MI = myocardial infarction *(From ACCORD Study Group; Cushman WC, Evans GW, Byington RP, et al: Effects of intensive blood-pressure control in type 2 diabetes mellitus,* N Engl J Med *362:1575-1585, 2010.)*

EFFICACY AND SAFETY OF RENAL SYMPATHETIC DENERVATION

A recently developed therapeutic approach for the treatment of hypertension is endovascular catheter technology that allows selective sympathetic denervation of the kidney by transluminal radiofrequency ablation.[40] To date, the evaluation of efficacy and safety of this approach has been limited to populations with "resistant" primary hypertension, with persistently high levels of BP despite comprehensive combination drug therapy. The Symplicity HTN-2 trial is the first and only randomized study reported to date, including 106 patients (approximately 30% with T2DM) with baseline SBP levels of 160 mm Hg or greater ($\geq$150 mm Hg in the presence of diabetes), despite the use of at least three BP-lowering agents. The between-group difference in the primary outcome of office-measured BP level at 6 months was large and highly statistically significant (33/11 mm Hg,

$P < 0.0001$).[41] No separate analyses were performed in the subgroup with T2DM. No serious safety concerns were identified in this small study, but larger studies are under way and new studies in patients with milder forms of hypertension are being planned. Such studies may include a focus on patients with T2DM; in the meantime, renal sympathetic denervation is best described as a highly promising intervention requiring more reliable data on long-term efficacy and safety. Its applicability to the vast majority of patients with diabetes and hypertension globally, who have limited access to basic drugs, is a broader debate that will also take place.

SUMMARY

Available evidence about the effect of BP management on CHD risk in patients with T2DM can be reasonably summarized in the following way.

Lifestyle interventions (targeting physical activity and dietary modification) in people with T2DM can favorably affect BP levels, and trials powered to assess effects on clinical outcomes are ongoing. However, effective implementation strategies to enact sustained positive lifestyle changes—including for dietary sodium restriction, which is likely to be particularly important—are generally lacking.

Placebo-controlled trials provide clear evidence that BP lowering among individuals with diabetes and hypertension results in a reduction in CHD incidence. The findings of the most recent and largest of these trials suggest that routine provision of BP-lowering therapy to patients with T2DM, regardless of initial BP level, is an effective strategy for reducing CHD risk.

Debate about comparative efficacy of BP-lowering drugs for the prevention of CHD in patients with diabetes continues. Although not unequivocal, there are some data to support additional benefits of ACE inhibitor–based regimens over others for the outcome of CHD.

Specifically for the outcome of CHD, trial evidence of the benefits of more intensive versus less intensive BP lowering is consistently suggestive, but not definitive to date. The ACCORD trial failed to show clear benefits on CHD of aggressive management to a SBP target of below 120 mm Hg, compared with an SBP target of 140 mm Hg or lower, but this comparison was underpowered to exclude sizeable, clinically important effects.

These conclusions, however, should be considered in the context of a number of important points. First, recommendations about BP-lowering treatment must take into account the known or likely effects on all relevant health outcomes and not just CHD. For example, the evidence that more intensive versus less intensive BP lowering provides greater protection against stroke in patients with or without diabetes is unequivocal, including large beneficial effects in preventing stroke observed in the ACCORD trial. Similarly, calcium channel blocker or thiazide-based regimens may be more important for the prevention of stroke, whereas ACE-inhibitor or ARB-based regimens are more protective against the microvascular renal complications of diabetes. The use of beta blockers might be regarded as essential in patients with prior myocardial infarction or systolic heart failure. Thus, consideration of a number of individual patient characteristics that may be relevant to a broad range of clinical outcomes would be appropriate in making choices about the use of particular BP-lowering drug regimens in patients with T2DM.

Second, and related to this, is an understanding of the general paradigm of using an assessment of an individual's projected absolute risk of developing CHD (or stroke, or any cardiovascular disease) to help guide therapy. In the context of T2DM, this might be most relevant where uncertainty exists about the balance of potential risks and benefits in relation to the intensity of BP lowering in an individual patient. There are a number of clinical tools available to estimate CHD or CVD risk in people with T2DM, derived either from general populations or from specific populations with diabetes.[42-45] All have potential limitations including in relation to generalizability; nonetheless, these remain useful for clinical practice.[46,47]

Finally, any ongoing uncertainty about the relative efficacy of therapeutic regimens or appropriate targets for BP reduction in people with T2DM closer to the "normotensive" range is dwarfed by the lack of knowledge about effective strategies to ensure that people with T2DM receive any BP-lowering therapy in the first place, let alone what might be considered ideal regimens or acceptable levels of BP control. The "practice gaps" are very large, particularly in the low- and middle-income countries that have the highest numbers of people with T2DM, but also in countries with rich economies.[48-54] From a global perspective, these issues will not be addressed by new clinical trials establishing the efficacy of new drugs or new combinations of drugs. Rather, the development, implementation, and rigorous evaluation of interventions at the level of policy, systems, and services will be crucial to ensure maximal gains in human health from what we already know about the treatment of BP in people with T2DM.

References

1. Hypertension in Diabetes Study (HDS): Prevalence of hypertension in newly presenting type 2 diabetic patients and the association with risk factors for cardiovascular and diabetic complications, J Hypertens 11:309–317, 1993.
2. Pechere-Bertschi A, Greminger P, Hess L, et al: Swiss Hypertension and Risk Factor Program (SHARP): cardiovascular risk factors management in patients with type 2 diabetes in Switzerland, Blood Press 14:337–344, 2005.
3. Prospective Studies Collaboration: Age-specific relevance of usual blood pressure to vascular mortality: a meta-analysis of individual data for one million adults in 61 prospective studies, Lancet 360:1903–1913, 2002.
4. Asia Pacific Cohort Studies Collaboration, Kengne AP, Patel A, Barzi F, et al: Systolic blood pressure, diabetes and the risk of cardiovascular diseases in the Asia-Pacific region, J Hypertens 25:205–213, 2007.
5. Stamler J, Vaccaro O, Neaton JD, Wentworth D: Diabetes, other risk factors, and 12-yr cardiovascular mortality for men screened in the multiple risk factor intervention trial, Diabetes Care 16:343–344, 1993.
6. Adler AI, Stratton IM, Neil HA, et al: Association of the systolic blood pressure with macrovascular and microvascular complications of type 2 diabetes (UKPDS 36): prospective observational study, BMJ 321:412–419, 2000.
7. Cooper-DeHoff RM, Gong Y, Handberg EM, et al: Tight blood pressure control and cardiovascular outcomes among hypertensive patients with diabetes and coronary artery disease, JAMA 304:61–68, 2010.
8. National Heart Lung and Blood Institute, National Institutes of Health, U.S. Department of Health and Human Services: The seventh report of the Joint National Committee on Prevention, Detection, Evaluation, and Treatment of High Blood Pressure—complete report, 2004.www.nhlbi.nih.gov/guidelines/hypertension/jnc7full.htm(Accessed September 26, 2012).
9. American Diabetes Association. Standards of medical care in diabetes—2012. http://care.diabetesjournals.org/content/35/Supplement_1/S11.full. (Accessed September 26, 2012).
10. Ryden L, Standl E, Bartnik M, et al: Guidelines on diabetes, pre-diabetes, and cardiovascular diseases: full text, Eur Heart J Suppl 9(Suppl C):C3–C74, 2007.
11. Mancia G, De Backer G, Dominiczak A, et al: 2007 Guidelines for the management of arterial hypertension, Eur Heart J 28:1462–1536, 2007.
12. International Diabetes Federation: Global guideline for type 2 diabetes, 2005.www.idf.org/guidelines/type-2-diabetes(Accessed September 26, 2012).
13. World Health Organization, International Society of Hypertension Working Group: 2003 World Health Organization (WHO) / International Society of Hypertension (ISH) statement on management of hypertension, J Hypertens 21:1983–1992, 2003.
14. Wing RW, Bahnson JL, Bray GA, et al: Long-term effects of a lifestyle intervention on weight and cardiovascular risk factors in individuals with type 2 diabetes mellitus, Arch Intern Med 170:1566–1575, 2010.
15. Appel LJ, Moore T, Obarzanek E, et al: A clinical trial of the effects of dietary patterns on blood pressure, N Engl J Med 336:1117–1124, 1997.
16. Sacks FM, Svetkey LP, Vollmer WM, et al: Effects on blood pressure of reduced dietary sodium and the Dietary Approaches to Stop Hypertension (DASH) diet, N Engl J Med 344:3–10, 2001.
17. Graudal NA, Hubeck-Graudal T, Jurgens G: Effects of low sodium diet versus high sodium diet on blood pressure, renin, aldosterone, catecholamines, cholesterol, and triglyceride, Cochrane Database Syst Rev 2011.
18. World Health Organization: Reducing salt intake in populations: report of a WHO forum and technical meeting, 2006.www.who.int/dietphysicalactivity/Salt_Report_VC_april07.pdf(Accessed September 26, 2012).
19. Taylor RS, Ashton KE, Moxham T, et al: Reduced dietary salt for the prevention of cardiovascular disease, Cochrane Database Syst Rev (7):2011, http://dx.doi.org/10.1002/14651858.CD009217, Art. No.: CD009217.
20. Turnbull F, Neal B, Algert C, et al: Effects of different blood-pressure-lowering regimens on major cardiovascular events: results of prospectively-designed overviews of randomised trials, Lancet 362:1527–1535, 2003.
21. Turnbull F, Neal B, Algert C, et al: Effects of different blood pressure lowering regimens on major cardiovascular events in individuals with and without diabetes mellitus: results of prospectively designed overviews of randomized trials, Arch Intern Med 165:1410–1419, 2005.
22. Patel A, MacMahon S, Chalmers J, et al: Effects of a fixed combination of perindopril and indapamide on macrovascular and microvascular outcomes in patients with type 2 diabetes mellitus (the ADVANCE trial): a randomised controlled trial, Lancet 370:829–840, 2007.
23. Zoungas S, De Galan BE, Ninomiya T, et al: Combined effects of routine blood pressure lowering and intensive glucose control on macrovascular and microvascular outcomes in patients with type 2 diabetes, Diabetes Care 32:2068–2074, 2009.
24. Turnbull F, Neal B, Pfeffer M, et al: Blood pressure-dependent and independent effects of agents that inhibit the renin-angiotensin system, J Hypertens 25:951–958, 2007.
25. Dahlof B, Sever PS, Poulter NR, et al: Prevention of cardiovascular events with an antihypertensive regimen of amlodipine adding perindopril as required versus atenolol adding bendroflumethiazide as required, in the Anglo-Scandinavian Cardiac Outcomes Trial-Blood Pressure Lowering Arm (ASCOT-BPLA): a multicentre randomised controlled trial, Lancet 366:895–906, 2005.
26. Yusuf S, Diener H-C, Sacco RL, et al: Telmisartan to prevent recurrent stroke and cardiovascular events, N Engl J Med 359:1225–1237, 2008.
27. Jamerson K, Weber MA, Bakris GL, et al: Benazepril plus amlodipine or hydrochlorothiazide for hypertension in high-risk patients, N Engl J Med 359:2417–2428, 2008.

28. Jamerson KA, Devereux R, Bakris GL, et al: Efficacy and duration of benazepril plus amlodipine or hydrochlorthiazide on 24 hour ambulatory systolic blood pressure control, *Hypertension* 57:174–179, 2011.

29. Bakris GL, Fonseca V, Katholi RE, et al: Metabolic effects of carvedilol vs metoprolol in patients with type 2 diabetes mellitus and hypertension: a randomized controlled trial, *JAMA* 292:2221–2236, 2004.

30. Brixius K, Middeke M, Lichtenthal A, et al: Nitric oxide, erectile dysfunction and beta-blocker treatment (MR NOED study): benefit of nebivolol versus metoprolol in hypertensive men, *Clin Exp Pharmacol Physiol* 34:327–331, 2007.

31. Bell DS, Lukas MA, Holdbrook FK, Fowler MB: The effect of carvedilol on mortality risk in heart failure patients with diabetes: results of a meta-analysis, *Curr Med Res Opin* 22:287–296, 2006.

32. MacMahon S, Neal B, Tzourio C, et al: Randomised trial of a perindopril-based blood-pressure-lowering regimen among 6105 individuals with previous stroke or transient ischaemic attack, *Lancet* 358:1033–1041, 2001.

33. Turner R, Holman R, Stratton I, et al: Tight blood pressure control and risk of macrovascular and microvascular complications in type 2 diabetes: UKPDS 38, *BMJ* 317:703–713, 1998.

34. Cushman WC, Evans GW, Byington RP, et al: Effects of intensive blood-pressure control in type 2 diabetes mellitus, *N Engl J Med* 362:1575–1585, 2010.

35. Gerstein HC, Miller ME, Byington RP, et al: Effects of intensive glucose lowering in type 2 diabetes, *N Engl J Med* 358:2545–2559, 2008.

36. Ginsberg HN, Elam MB, Lovato LC, et al: Effects of combination lipid therapy in type 2 diabetes mellitus, *N Engl J Med* 362:1563–1574, 2010.

37. Holman RR, Paul SK, Bethel MA, et al: Long-term follow-up after tight control of blood pressure in type 2 diabetes, *N Engl J Med* 359:1565–1576, 2008.

38. Holman RR, Paul SK, Bethel MA, et al: 10-year follow-up of intensive glucose control in type 2 diabetes, *N Engl J Med* 359:1577–1589, 2008.

39. Paulis L, Steckelings UM, Unger T: Key advances in antihypertensive treatment, *Nat Rev Cardiol* 9:276–285, 2012.

40. Schlaich MP, Sobotka PA, Krum H, et al: Renal sympathetic-nerve ablation for uncontrolled hypertension, *N Engl J Med* 361:932–934, 2009.

41. Esler MD, Krum H, Sobotka PA, et al: Renal sympathetic denervation in patients with treatment-resistant hypertension (the Symplicity HTN-2 Trial): a randomised controlled trial, *Lancet* 376:1903–1909, 2010.

42. Anderson KM, Odell PM, Wilson PW, Kannel WB: Cardiovascular disease risk profiles, *Am Heart J* 121:293–298, 1991.

43. Anderson KM, Wilson PW, Odell PM, Kannel WB: An updated coronary risk profile. A statement for health professionals, *Circulation* 83:356–362, 1998.

44. Stevens RJ, Kothari V, Adler AI, Stratton IM: The UKPDS risk engine: a model for the risk of coronary heart disease in type II diabetes (UKPDS 56), *Clin Sci* 101:671–679, 2001.

45. Kengne AP, Patel A, Marre M, et al: Contemporary model for cardiovascular risk prediction in people with type 2 diabetes, *Eur J Cardiovasc Prev Rehabil* 18:393–398, 2011.

46. van der Heijden AA, Ortegon MM, Niessen LW, et al: Prediction of coronary heart disease risk in a general, pre-diabetic, and diabetic population during 10 years of follow-up: accuracy of the Framingham, SCORE, and UKPDS risk functions: the Hoorn Study, *Diabetes Care* 32:2094–2098, 2009.

47. Kengne AP, Patel A, Colagiuri S, et al: The Framingham and UK Prospective Diabetes Study (UKPDS) risk equations do not reliably estimate the probability of cardiovascular events in a large ethnically diverse sample of patients with diabetes: the Action in Diabetes and Vascular Disease: Preterax and Diamicron-MR Controlled Evaluation (ADVANCE) Study, *Diabetologia* 53:821–831, 2010.

48. Nilsson PM, Cederholm J, Zethelius BJ, et al: Trends in blood pressure control in patients with type 2 diabetes: data from the Swedish National Diabetes Register (NDR), *Blood Press* 20:348–354, 2011.

49. Braga M, Casanova A, Teoh H, et al: Treatment gaps in the management of cardiovascular risk factors in patients with type 2 diabetes in Canada, *Can J Cardiol* 26:297–302, 2010.

50. Suh DC, Kim C-M, Choi I-S, et al: Trends in blood pressure control and treatment among type 2 diabetes with comorbid hypertension in the United States: 1988–2004, *J Hypertens* 27:1908–1916, 2009.

51. Vijayaraghavan M, He G, Stoddard P, Schillinger D: Blood pressure control, hypertension, awareness, and treatment in adults with diabetes in the United States-Mexico border region, *Pan Am J Public Health* 28:164–173, 2010.

52. McLean DL, Simpson SH, McAlister FA, Tsuyuki RT: Treatment and blood pressure control in 47,964 people with diabetes and hypertension: a systematic review of observational studies, *Can J Cardiol* 22:855–860, 2006.

53. Al-Shehri AM: Blood pressure control among type 2 diabetics, *Saudi Med J* 29:718–722, 2008.

54. Bunnag P, Plengvidhya N, Deerochanawong C, et al: Thailand diabetes registry project: prevalence of hypertension, treatment and control of blood pressure in hypertensive adults with type 2 diabetes, *J Med Assoc Thai* 89(Suppl 1):S72–S77, 2006.

15 Effect of Lipid Management on Coronary Heart Disease Risk in Patients with Diabetes

Michel P. Hermans, Sylvie A. Ahn, and Michel F. Rousseau

OVERVIEW

This chapter describes strategies for and effects of therapeutic lifestyle changes and/or pharmacologic interventions with lipid-lowering medications on coronary heart disease (CHD) risk in patients with diabetes mellitus (DM), focusing on the most recent data from randomized clinical trials in the context of contemporary clinical care.

Planning a strategy to manage dyslipidemia for CHD risk reduction for patients with DM can be partitioned into five steps: (1) identifying lipid-related risk factors for CHD, including those related to unhealthy lifestyle behaviors; (2) assessing and then stratifying CHD risk; (3) determining which among these risk factors are modifiable through interventions affecting lifestyle combined with timely and appropriate medications; (4) confirming effectiveness of various lipid interventions on CHD outcome reduction in clinical trials; and (5) translating the expected gains to common, unselected DM patients most likely to benefit from these interventions.

Coronary Heart Disease Risk Among Patients with Diabetes and Dyslipidemia

To better understand CHD risk for patients with versus without DM in the context of lipid management, it is informative to analyze baseline characteristics of DM patients participating in landmark lipid-lowering clinical trials such as trials focused exclusively on patients with DM, or those that report data on a sufficient number of patients making up DM subgroups. For the present summary, data were considered from trials with a high proportion of patients with DM at baseline (>15%) and/or trials that enrolled at least 100 patients with

prevalent DM. Data from 47 lipid trials comprising 198,930 patients, of whom 65,558 had prevalent DM, are summarized in **Tables 15-1** (alphabetically by trial name acronym) and **15-2** (ordered by descending numbers of participants with DM), with abbreviations used to describe respective trial outcomes defined in **Table 15-3**.[1–82] Except for the Acute Coronary Syndrome Israeli Survey (ACSIS),[9] all studies were randomized controlled trials, most of which evaluated monotherapy with a statin or a fibrate versus placebo. A few randomized controlled trials studied a combined lipid-lowering intervention (statin plus fibrate; statin plus ezetimibe); Steno-2 was a randomized comparison of a multifactorial intervention versus usual care, with statins and/or fibrates used as part of a comprehensive global cardiovascular disease (CVD) risk intervention strategy in patients with DM and albuminuria.[73]

The baseline characteristics of patients participating in clinical trials and substudies that included only patients with DM (n = 46,326 patients) are described in **Table 15-4**, and ranked by baseline low-density lipoprotein (LDL) cholesterol (LDL-C). Mean age at entry was 60.3 years and, similar to lipid intervention trials not focusing specifically on DM, men accounted for more than two thirds of the patients. Most DM patients in these studies are assumed to have had type 2 diabetes mellitus (T2DM) given the relative prevalence of T2DM versus type 1 diabetes mellitus (T1DM) in the age groups studied (see **Chapter 1**), with a few trials specifically allowing inclusion of patients with T1DM, and most trials not differentiating DM type for eligibility.

Average baseline lipid levels in the trials surveyed did not meet contemporary targets for lipid management in DM patients (see later), with mean LDL-C 129 mg/dL (3.3 mmol/L); non–high-density lipoprotein (HDL) cholesterol (non–HDL-C)

MANAGEMENT OF CORONARY HEART DISEASE RISK AND DISEASE IN PATIENTS WITH DIABETES

TABLE 15-1 Trials on Lipid Management of Coronary Heart Disease (CHD) Risk

ACRONYM	REFERENCES	STUDY NAME	IDENTIFIER	PHARMACEUTICAL SPONSOR (SJ/LLD(S) SUPPLIERS
4D	1	Die Deutsche Diabetes Dialyse studie		Pfizer
4S	2-4	Scandinavian Simvastatin Survival Study		Merck
4S (substudy)	4	Scandinavian Simvastatin Survival Study (diabetes substudy)		Merck
A to Z	5	Aggrastat to Zocor		Merck
ACCORD-Lipid	6-8	Action to Control Cardiovascular Risk in Diabetes - Lipid arm	NCT00000620	Abbott; Amylin Ph.; AstraZeneca; Bayer; GSK; King Ph.; Merck; Novartis; NovoNordisk; SanofiAventis; Takeda
ACCORD-Lipid (AD subgroup)	7	Action to Control Cardiovascular Risk in Diabetes - Lipid arm (AD subgroup)	NCT00000620	same as above
ACSIS	9	Acute Coronary Syndrome Israeli Surveys Data		
AFCAPS/TexCAPS	10,11	Air Force/Texas Coronary Atherosclerosis Prevention Study		Merck
AIM-HIGH	12,13	Atherothrombosis Intervention in Metabolic Syndrome with Low HDL/High Triglycerides: Impact on Global Health Outcomes	NCT00120289	Abbott; Merck
ALERT	14	Assessment of Lescol in Renal Transplantation		Novartis
ALLHAT-LLT	15	Antihypertensive and Lipid-Lowering treatment to prevent Heart Attack Trial	NCT00000542	AstraZeneca; Bristol-Myers Squibb; Pfizer
ASCOT-LLA	16, 17	Anglo-Scandinavian Cardiac Outcomes Trial - Lipid Lowering Arm		Pfizer; Servier; Leo; Solvay
ASCOT-LLA (substudy)	17	Anglo-Scandinavian Cardiac Outcomes Trial - Lipid Lowering Arm (diabetes substudy)		Pfizer; Servier; Leo; Solvay
ASPEN	18	Atorvastatin as Prevention of CHD Endpoints in patients with Non-insulin dependent diabetes mellitus		Pfizer
AURORA	19, 20	A Study to Evaluate the Use of Rosuvastatin in Subjects or Regular Hemodialysis: an Assessment of Survival and Cardiovascular Events	NCT00240331	AstraZeneca
AURORA (substudy)	20	A Study to Evaluate the Use of Rosuvastatin in Subjects on Regular Hemodialysis: an Assessment of Survival and Cardiovascular Events (diabetes substudy)	NCT00240331	AstraZeneca
AVERT	21	Atorvastatin Versus Revascularization Treatment		Parke-Davis
BIP	22, 23	Bezafibrate Infarction Prevention		Boehringer Mannheim
CARDS	24	Collaborative Atorvastatin Diabetes Study	NCT0327418	Pfizer
CARE	25-27	Cholesterol and Recurrent Events		Bristol-Myers Squibb
CARE (substudy)	27	Cholesterol and Recurrent Events (diabetes substudy)		Bristol-Myers Squibb
DAIS	28, 29	Diabetes Atherosclerosis Intervention Study		Fournier
DIS	30	Diabetes Intervention Study		VEB Berlin
Extended-ESTABLISH	31	Demonstration of the Beneficial Effect on Atherosclerotic Lesions by Serial Volumetric Intravascular Ultrasound Analysis during Half a Year After Coronary Event		
FIELD	32-34	Fenofibrate Intervention and Event Lowering in Diabetes	ISRCTN64783481	Fournier
FIELD (AD subgroup)	32, 33	Fenofibrate Intervention and Event Lowering in Diabetes (AD subgroup)	ISRCTN64783481	Fournier
FIELD (MetS subgroup)	34	Fenofibrate Intervention and Event Lowering in Diabetes (MetS subgroup)	ISRCTN64783481	Fournier
GISSI-Prevenzione	35	Gruppo Italiano per lo Studio della Sopravvivenza nell'Infarto miocardico - Prevenzione		
GREACE	36, 37	Greek Atorvastatin and Coronary-heart-disease Evaluation		
GREACE (substudy)	37	Greek Atorvastatin and Coronary-heart-disease Evaluation - subgroup with diabetes		
HHS	38, 39	Helsinki Heart Study		Warner-Lambert

HHS (substudy)	39	Helsinki Heart Study (diabetes substudy)		Warner-Lambert
HPS—MRC/BHF	40, 41	Medical Research Council and British Heart Foundation Heart Protection Study		Merck
HPS—MRC/BHF (substudy)	41	Medical Research Council and British Heart Foundation Heart Protection Study (diabetes substudy)		Merck
HPS2-THRIVE	42	Heart Protection Study 2—Treatment of HDL to Reduce the Incidence of Vascular Events	NCT00461630	Merck
IDEAL	43, 44	Incremental Decrease in End Points Through Aggressive Lipid Lowering	NCT00159835	Pfizer
IMPROVE-IT	45	Improved Reduction of Outcomes: Vytorin Efficacy International Trial: Comparison of ezetimibe/simvastatin versus simvastatin monotherapy on cardiovascular outcomes in patients with acute coronary syndromes	NCT00202878	Merck; Shering Plough
JAPAN-ACS	46	Japan Assessment of Pitavastatin and Atorvastatin in Acute Coronary Syndrome	NCT00242944	Kowa
LDS	47	Lipids in Diabetes Study		Bayer
LEADER	48, 49	Lower Extremity Arterial Disease Event Reduction	ISRCTN41194621	Boehringer Mannheim
LIPID	50-52	Long-term Intervention with Pravastatin in Ischaemic Disease		Bristol-Myers Squibb
LIPS	53	Lescol Intervention Prevention Study		Novartis
MEGA	54	Management of Elevated Cholesterol in the Primary Prevention Group of Adult Japanese	NCT00211705	Sankyo
MIRACL	55-57	Myocardial Ischaemia Reduction with Aggressive Cholesterol Lowering		Parke-Davis
PACT	58	Pravastatin in Acute Coronary Treatment		Bristol-Myers Squibb
Post-CABG (FU)	59, 60	Post Coronary Artery Bypass Graft		Merck; Bristol-Myers Squibb
PROACTIVE	61, 62	Prospective Pioglitazone Clinical Trial in Macrovascular Events		Takeda; Eli Lilly
PROSPER	63	Prospective Study of Pravastatin in the Elderly at Risk		Bristol-Myers Squibb
PROVE IT-TIMI 22	64-66	Pravastatin or Atorvastatin Evaluation and Infection Therapy—Thrombolysis in Myocardial Infarction 22		Bristol-Myers Squibb; Sankyo
PROVE IT-TIMI 22 (substudy)	65	Pravastatin or Atorvastatin Evaluation and Infection Therapy—Thrombolysis in Myocardial Infarction 22 (diabetes substudy)		Bristol-Myers Squibb; Sankyo
REVEAL	67	Randomized Evaluation of the Effects of Anacetrapib Through Lipid Modification	NCT01252953	Merck
REVERSAL	68	Reversal of Atherosclerosis with Aggressive Lipid Lowering	NCT00380939	Pfizer
SENDCAP	69	St. Mary's, Ealing, Northwick Park Diabetes Cardiovascular Disease Prevention study		Boehringer Mannheim
SHARP	70	Study of Heart and Renal Protection	NCT00125593	Merck; Shering Plough
SPARCL	71, 72	Stroke Prevention by Aggressive Reduction of Cholesterol Levels	NCT00147602	Pfizer
SPARCL (substudy)	72	Stroke Prevention by Aggressive Reduction of Cholesterol Levels (diabetes substudy)	NCT00147602	Pfizer
Steno-2	73	Steno-2 Study	NCT00320008	Novo-Nordisk
TNT	74-78	Treating to New Targets study	NCT00327691	Pfizer
TNT (substudy)	78	Treating to New Targets study (diabetes study)		Pfizer
VA-HIT	79-81	Veterans Affairs High-Density Lipoprotein Intervention Trial	NCT00283335	Parke-Davis
VA-HIT (substudy)	81	Veterans Affairs High-Density Lipoprotein Intervention Trial (diabetes substudy)	NCT00283335	Parke-Davis
VA Cooperative Study	82	Veteran Administration Cooperative Study of Atherosclerosis, Neurology Section		

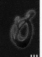

MANAGEMENT OF CORONARY HEART DISEASE RISK AND DISEASE IN PATIENTS WITH DIABETES

TABLE 15-2 Trials of Lipid-Lowering Therapy by Numbers of Diabetic Patients at Inclusion

ACRONYM	PUBLICATION YEAR	CHD RISK	PATIENTS (n)	DIABETES (n)	DIABETES (%)	THERAPY	CHD-RELATED OUTCOMES*
FIELD	2005	PP and SP	9795	9795	100	Fibrate	C; B+D+I+M
FIELD (MetS SS)	2009	PP and SP	8183	8183	100	Fibrate	C; B+D+I+M
HPS—MRC/BHF	2002	PP and SP	20,536	5963	29	Statin	C; A+G
HPS—MRC/BHF (DSS)	2003	PP and SP	5963	5963	100	Statin	E+B
ACCORD—Lipid	2010	PP and SP	5518	5518	100	Fibrate	C; J+D
PROACTIVE	2005	SP	5238	5238	100	Glitazone	C; A+J+H+M
LDS	ET	PP	4026	4026	100	Statin and/or fibrate	C; K+P+J+M
ALLHAT-LLT	2002	PP and SP	10,355	3638	35	Statin	A
ACSIS	2012	ACS	8982	3063	34	Fibrate	C; A+I+L+M
CARDS	2004	PP	2838	2838	100	Statin	C; H+M+T
ASCOT-LLA	2003	PP	10,305	2532	25	Statin	J+G
ASCOT-LLA (DSS)	2005	PP	2532	2532	100	Statin	B
ASPEN	2006	PP	2410	2410	100	Statin	C; D+J+M+O+L
SHARP	2011	PP and SP	9270	2094	23	Statin and ezetimibe	C; J+G+M
FIELD (AD subgroup)	2009	PP and SP	2014	2014	100	Fibrate	C; B+D+I+M
MEGA	2006	PP	7832	1632	21	Statin	C; I+L+M+P
TNT	2005	SP	10,001	1501	15	Statin	C; G+J+O+T
TNT (DSS)	2006	SP	1501	1501	100	Statin	C; G+J+O+T
4D	2005	PP and SP	1255	1255	100	Statin	C; D+J
AIM-HIGH	2011	SP	3414	1158	34	Niacin	C; G+J+H+M
A to Z	2004	ACS	4497	1059	24	Statin	C; D+J+H
IDEAL	2005	SP	8888	1057	12	Statin	C; G+J+O
PROVE IT–TIMI 22 (DSS)	2006	ACS	978	978	100	Statin	C; A+I+L+M
ACCORD-Lipid (AD SS)	2010	PP and SP	941	941	100	Fibrate	C; J+D
SPARCL	2006	SP	4731	794	17	Statin	
SPARCL (DSS)	2011	SP	794	794	100	Statin	
LIPID	1998	SP	9014	782	9	Statin	G
VA-HIT	1999	SP	2531	769	30	Fibrate	C; J+G
VA-HIT (DSS)	2002	SP	769	769	100	Fibrate	C; J+G
DIS	1991	PP	761	761	100	Fibrate	E
PROVE IT–TIMI 22	2004	ACS	4162	734	18	Statin	C; A+I+L+M
AURORA	2009	PP and SP	2776	731	26	Statin	C; J+D
AURORA (DSS)	2011	PP and SP	731	731	100	Statin	C; G+J
MIRACL	2001	ACS	3086	715	23	Statin	C; A+J+O+L
PROSPER	2002	PP and SP	5804	623	11	Statin	C; G+J
CARE	1998	SP	4159	586	14	Statin	G+J
CARE (DSS)	1998	SP	586	586	100	Statin	G+J+M
GISSI-Prevenzione	2000	SP	4271	582	14	Statin	C; A+I
PACT	2004	ACS	3408	478	14	Statin	C; A+I+L
DAIS	2001	PP and SP	418	418	100	Fibrate	R
ALERT	2003	PP and SP	2102	396	19	Statin	C; G+J+M
GREACE	2002	SP	1600	313	20	Statin	C; A+J+L+Q+M
GREACE (DSS)	2003	SP	313	313	100	Statin	C; A+J+L+Q+M
BIP	2000	SP	3090	309	10	Fibrate	C; K+J+P
LEADER	2002	PP and SP	1568	268	17	Fibrate	E
4S	1994	SP	4444	202	5	Statin	A
4S (DSS)	1997	SP	202	202	100	Statin	A

TABLE 15-2 Trials of Lipid-Lowering Therapy by Numbers of Diabetic Patients at Inclusion—cont'd

ACRONYM	PUBLICATION YEAR	CHD RISK	PATIENTS (n)	DIABETES (n)	DIABETES (%)	THERAPY	CHD-RELATED OUTCOMES*
LIPS	2002	SP	1677	202	12	Statin	C; G+J+M
SENDCAP	1998	PP	164	164	100	Fibrate	
Steno-2	2008	PP and SP	160	160	100	Statin and/or fibrate	A
AFCAPS/TexCAPS	1998	PP	6605	155	2	Statin	C; E
HHS (DSS)	1992	PP	135	135	100	Fibrate	C; K+J+G
VA Cooperative Study	1973	SP	532	128	24	Fibrate	A+B
Post-CABG (FU)	2000	SP	1351	116	9	Statin	C; D+J+M
HHS	1987	PP	4081	108	3	Fibrate	C; K+J+G
REVERSAL	2004	SP	502	95	19	Statin	R
JAPAN-ACS	2009	SP	252	74	29	Statin	R
Extended-ESTABLISH	2010	ACS	180	66	37	Statin	C; A+H
AVERT	1999	SP	341	52	15	Statin	E
Total (n)			198,930	65,558			

ACS = Acute coronary syndrome; AD = atherogenic dyslipidemia; DSS = diabetes substudy; ET = early termination; FU = follow-up; LLA = lipid-lowering arm; LLT = lipid-lowering therapy; MetS = metabolic syndrome; PP = primary prevention; SP = secondary prevention; SS = substudy.
*See **Table 15-1** for acronym definition and **Table 15-3** for outcome categories.

TABLE 15-3 Outcomes Classification

CATEGORIES	DESCRIPTION	CODE
Total mortality	All-cause death	A
CV composite	All CV events (including procedures)	B
	MACE	C
	CV death	D
Cardiac	Total CHD and major coronary events	E
	Nonfatal CHD	F
	Cardiac death or fatal CHD	G
	ACS or ACE	H
	All MI	I
	Nonfatal MI	J
	Fatal MI	K
	Unstable or hospitalization-requiring AP	L
	Coronary revascularization (PCI or CABG)	M
	Life-threatening arrhythmias	N
	Resuscitation for cardiac arrest	O
	Sudden death	P
	CHF	Q
Coronary imaging	Angiographic CAD progression, change in coronary atheroma volume	R
Cerebrovascular	All major cerebrovascular events	S
	All stroke and TIA	T
	Nonfatal stroke	U
	Fatal stroke	V
	Carotid revascularization	W
CV composite	Non-CHD MACE	X
Other mortality	Non-CHD CV death	Y
Peripheral	Any PAD event (including revascularization and leg amputation)	Z

ACE = acute coronary event; AP = angina pectoris; CABG = coronary artery bypass graft; CAD = coronary artery disease; CHF = congestive heart failure; CV = cardiovascular; MACE = major adverse cardiovascular event; MI = myocardial infarction; PAD = peripheral arterial disease; PCI = percutaneous coronary intervention; TIA = transient ischemic attack.

166 mg/dL (4.3 mmol/L); HDL-C 42 mg/dL (1.1 mmol/L); and triglycerides (TGs; triacylglycerols) 180 mg/dL (2.0 mmol/L). In most diabetes trials and DM subgroup analyses, LDL-C was calculated, with routine direct measurement in only three studies: 4D; HPS—MRC/BHF (DM subgroup); and PROACTIVE.[1,41,61,62] Mean baseline apolipoprotein B100 (apo B) concentration was 115 mg/dL, a value also beyond generally accepted targets, as inferred from studies in which baseline apo B level was available in the reports.*

In addition to elevated and/or unsatisfactory LDL-C levels at study entry, the frequent findings of low HDL-C together with elevated fasting TGs are consistent with the assumption of a high prevalence of atherogenic dyslipidemia in these DM patients at enrollment (see **Table 15-4** and **Chapter 10**). Similarly, data from studies in which baseline apo B was measured concomitantly with LDL-C reveal a high prevalence of increased small, dense LDL particles—a pattern commonly observed in T2DM (see **Chapter 10**).[83–93]

Given the high cardiovascular (CV) risk associated with DM (see **Chapters 7, 9,** and **10**), observed event rates in reported lipid trials are influenced by the proportion of patients with DM enrolled. The rates of primary CV outcome events among patients with DM across lipid intervention trials in primary prevention, secondary prevention, and post–acute coronary syndrome (ACS) patient populations are summarized in **Table 15-5**, arranged by decreasing hazard, with significantly higher rates among those with versus without DM across the spectrum of clinical indication.

To estimate CHD risk or to better characterize it for specific patients groups, there are other complementary determinations in addition to total cholesterol and LDL-C levels measurements. Non–HDL-C, apo B, and LDL particle (LDL-P) concentration are closely associated with obesity, DM, insulin resistance or hyperinsulinemia, and other markers of dysmetabolism in conditions of increased cardiometabolic risk, such as T2DM. Their determination, in addition to

*References 24, 28, 29, 32-34, 41, 65, 69, 72, 78.

MANAGEMENT OF CORONARY HEART DISEASE RISK AND DISEASE IN PATIENTS WITH DIABETES

TABLE 15-4 Baseline Characteristics of Diabetes Trials and Substudies Ranked by Low-Density Lipoprotein (LDL) Cholesterol (LDL-C) at Inclusion

ACRONYM	PATIENTS (n)	MALES (%)	WHITE CAUCASIANS (%)	MEAN AGE (YR)	INCLUSION CRITERIA	DM TYPE	DM DURATION (years)	HBA1C (%)	TC	NON-HDL-C	apo B	LDL-C	HDL-C	TG
HHS (DSS)	135	100	Most	49	Non-HDL-C ≥200 mg/dL	T2DM	4.5		292	246		200	46	214
GREACE (DSS)	313	56	Most	55	Prior MI or >70% stenosis in one or more vessels; TC >100; TGs <400 mg/dL	T2DM (92%)	10.5	7.5	271	236		189	35	221
4S (DSS)	202	78	Most	60	MI or angina; TC 213-309 mg/dL; TGs <221 mg/dL	DM			259	216		186	43	150
SENDCAP	164	71	56	51	T2DM; no CV history	T2DM	5	9.5	223	184	131	142	39	198
CARE (DSS)	586	80	85	61	MI history; TC <240 mg/dL; LDL-C 115-174 mg/dL; TG <350 mg/dL	DM			206	168		136	38	164
Steno-2	160	74	Most	55	T2DM with microalbuminuria	T2DM	5.8	8.6	210	170		133	40	159
DAIS	418	73	96	57	T2DM with CAD	T2DM	8.6	7.5	215	176	116	131	39	229
SPARCL (DSS)	794	61		64	Diabetes and stroke or TIA	T2DM			208	162	134	131	46	155
ASCOT-LLA (DSS)	2532	76	90	64	T2DM with HBP; no CHD; ≥3 CV RF's	T2DM			205	159		128	46	168
4D	1255	54	Most	66	T2DM; ESRD on hemodialysis	T2DM	18	6.7	218	182		125	36	261
HPS-MRC/BHF (DSS)	5963	70	Most	62	Diabetes	T2DM (90%)	27	7	220	179	110	124	41	204
LDS	4026	75	91	61	LDL-C 58-155 mg/dL; TG <400 mg/dL	T2DM	6	8	174	128		120	46	133
FIELD	9795	63	Most	62	T2DM; TC 116-251 mg/dL and TC/HDL-C ≥4 or TG 89-443 mg/dL	T2DM	5	6.9	195	152	97	119	43	173
CARDS	2838	68	95	62	T2DM; low or normal LDL-C; at least one of: DRP; albumin; smoking; HBP	T2DM	8	7.9	207	153	117	117	54	173
PROACTIVE	5238	66	99	62	T2DM with macrovascular disease	T2DM	9.5	8.1	199	154		114	45	198
ASPEN	2410	66	84	61	T2DM; LDL-C above contemporary guidelines	T2DM	8	7.8	194	147		113	47	147
VA-HIT (DSS)	769	72	14	65	Diabetes plus CHD; HDL-C ≤40 mg/dL; LDL-C ≤140 mg/dL	DM			172	141		108	31	166
PROVE IT-TIMI 22 (DSS)	978	72	85	60	Post-ACS status	DM			178	140	100	101	38	171
ACCORD-Lipid	5518	69	69	62	T2DM; high CV risk	T2DM	10	8.3	175	137		100	38	164
AURORA (DSS)	731	66	76	65	DM patients with ESRD on chronic hemodialysis	DM			174	131		97	43	168
TNT (DSS)	1501	73	89	63	DM and stable CHD; LDL-C <130 mg/dL	DM	8.5	7.4	175	130	113	96	45	171
Total	46326													
Mean		70.6		60.3			9.6	7.8	208	166	115	129	42	180

All lipid values in mg/dL.

See **Table 15-1** for acronym definitions and **Table 15-2** for primary outcome descriptions.

apo B = Apolipoprotein B100; DRP = diabetic retinopathy; ESRD = end-stage renal disease; HbA1c = glycated hemoglobin A1c; HBP = high blood pressure; HDL-C = high-density lipoprotein cholesterol; RF = risk factor; T2DM = type 2 diabetes mellitus; TC = total cholesterol; TG = triglycerides (triacylglycerols).

TABLE 15-5 Primary Outcome Rates (Comparator Arm), Baseline Atherogenic Lipids, and apo B from Lipid-Lowering Trials

	TRIALS WITH DIABETIC SUBPOPULATIONS AT ENTRY							DIABETES TRIALS AND DIABETES SUBSTUDIES					
	Age (yr)	Diabetes (%)	Non-HDL-C	LDL-C	apo B	Primary Outcome (% per yr)		Age (yr)	Diabetes (%)	Non-HDL-C	LDL-C	apo B	Primary Outcome (% per yr)
Acute Coronary Syndrome													
ACSIS	63	34	168	96		75.0	PROVE IT–TIMI 22 (DSS)	60	100	140	101	100	15.9
MIRACL	65	23	159	124	132	56.1							
PACT	61	14				15.5							
PROVE IT-TIMI 22	58	18	143	106	102	13.1							
A to Z	61	24	146	112		7.7							
ESTABLISH (FU)	62	37	137	115	86	7.1							
Secondary Prevention													
AVERT	59	15	179	143		13.9	GREACE (DSS)	55	100	236	189		10.1
GREACE	60	20	225	193		8.3	PROACTIVE	62	100	154	114		7.5
LIPS	60	12	162	131		6.8	CARE (DSS)	61	100	168	136		7.4
VA Cooperative Study	55	24				6.3	VA-HIT (DSS)	65	100	141	108		7.1
AIM-HIGH	64	34	111	74	83	5.4	4S (DSS)	60	100	216	186		4.6
Post-CABG (FU)	62	9	187	156		5.4	TNT (DSS)	63	100	130	96	113	3.7
VA-HIT	64	30	143	111	96	4.3							
GISSI-Prevenzione	60	14	183	152		3.1							
CARE	59	14	170	139		2.6							
BIP	60	10	177.4	148		2.4							
TNT	61	15	128	97	111	2.2							
IDEAL	62	12	151	122	119	2.2							
4S	59	5	214	188	133	2.1							
LIPID	62	9	182	150		1.4							
Primary and Secondary Prevention													
AURORA	64	26	131	100	82	7.8	AURORA (DSS)	65	100	131	97		10.8
LEADER	68	17	172	131		5.2	4D	66	100	182	125		9.6
PROSPER	75	11	170	147		5.1	HPS—MRC/BHF (DSS)	62	100	179	124	110	5.2
HPS—MRC/BHF	62	29	187	131	114	2.9	Steno-2	55	100	170	133		3.8
SHARP	62	23	146	107	92	2.7	ACCORD-Lipid (AD)		100				3.7
ALLHAT-LLT	66	35	176	146		2.6	ACCORD-Lipid	62	100	137	100		2.4
ALERT	50	19	197	158		2.5	FIELD	62	100	152	119	97	1.2
Primary Prevention													
AFCAPS/TexCAPS	58	2	184	150		1.1	ASPEN	61	100	147	113		3.8
ASCOT-LLA	63	25	162	131		0.9	ASCOT-LLA (DSS)	64	100	159	128		3.6
HHS	47	3	223	189		0.8	CARDS	62	100	153	117	110	2.3
MEGA	58	21	184	157		0.5	HHS (DSS)	49	100	246	200	117	2.1
							DIS	46	100				1.6

All lipid measurements represent baseline values (in mg/dL).
See **Table 15-1** for acronyms definition and **Table 15-2** for primary outcomes description.

LDL-C measurement, may provide information before and after introduction of lipid-lowering therapies, to assess CV risk at baseline and residual vascular risk after intervention. Compared with on-treatment LDL-C, these may help to clarify some aspects of risk and response to therapy, but their combined measurement is not routinely recommended in DM.

In addition to non–HDL-C, apo B, and LDL-P determination, screening for atherogenic dyslipidemia, before any lipid-lowering intervention, is an easy and inexpensive means to determine residual vascular risk associated with low HDL-C, high TGs, and their determinants. As a result of lack of agreement on cutoffs for HDL-C and TGs, this is rarely performed in routine practice. An alternative approach to defining atherogenic dyslipidemia as the combined occurrence of high TG levels plus low HDL-C uses the ratio of TG to HDL-C. Because both TG and HDL-C levels are continuous risk variables with mutually additive associations with residual vascular risk, computing a ratio of fasting TGs to HDL-C provides a summary metric for the severity of atherogenic dyslipidemia, calibrated as a continuous rather than a dichotomous variable. Given the extreme right skewness of TG values, assessing atherogenic dyslipidemia using log(TGs)/HDL-C may be more clinically informative than an untransformed ratio.[91,92]

LIPID MANAGEMENT STRATEGIES TO REDUCE CARDIOVASCULAR RISK

Therapeutic Lifestyle Changes

The cardiometabolic abnormalities underlying CHD risk in T2DM and their potentially reversible components under the influence of various therapeutic lifestyle changes make the population with these abnormalities particularly suitable to respond positively to such interventions, provided they are applied early (i.e., in primary prevention) and maintained long term (see Chapters 5 and 12). Long-term compliance with therapeutic lifestyle changes must be optimized and regularly assessed and reinforced, because it is often difficult for patients with DM to comply long term with dietary and lifestyle advice. This is all the more relevant because the hallmark of atherogenic dyslipidemia (low HDL-C and high TGs) and all three other defining components of the metabolic syndrome are responsive to therapeutic lifestyle changes (see Chapters 4, 5, and 12).

Lifestyle approaches and dietary strategies to lower LDL-C and TGs and raise HDL-C as well as the effects of dietary carbohydrate restriction on atherogenic dyslipidemia, fatty acid partitioning, and metabolic syndrome have been previously reviewed.[94,95] The American Diabetes Association (ADA) recommends that DM patients on low-carbohydrate diets undergo lipid profile monitoring and that the ratios of dietary intake of carbohydrates, proteins, and fat be individually adjusted to the metabolic requirements and preferences of patients. With regard to dietary intake of saturated and *trans*-saturated fatty acids, both modulators of LDL-C levels, there are no specific data available for patients with DM, and recommended dietary goals for DM patients are currently those, by default, of individuals with established CHD. Thus, saturated fat intake should not exceed 7% of total calories, and intake of *trans*-saturated fatty acids should be reduced.[96]

Unfortunately, for most T2DM patients in real-life conditions it is very hard to follow the current recommendations regarding dietary and physical activity for DM for the long

term and/or with the required intensity. This underscores the importance of systems-based lifestyle interventions (see Chapter 12). Even for those who are able to implement lifestyle changes, many will not achieve sufficiently low LDL-C, non–HDL-C, and apo B and/or improve atherogenic dyslipidemia components through therapeutic lifestyle changes alone and will require lifelong therapy with one or more lipid-lowering drugs. For example, in the Action for Health in Diabetes (Look AHEAD) trial, 5145 overweight or obese adults with T2DM were randomized to intensive lifestyle intervention focusing on weight loss and increased leisure-time physical activity versus standard care diabetes support and education.[97] Despite greater and sustained weight loss, greater reductions in glycated hemoglobin, and improvements in fitness in the intensive lifestyle arm, there was no difference achieved between the groups in LDL-C. The overall trial failed to demonstrate mortality improvement, as discussed in Chapter 12.

Drugs Targeting Low-Density Lipoprotein Cholesterol

Given the predominant role of LDL-C as the major lipid-related modifiable risk factor for CHD in nondiabetic and diabetic patients, most of the pivotal studies have investigated the benefit on CHD outcomes of pharmacologic agents whose main effect is to reduce LDL-C levels (Fig. 15-1). Most of the clinical evidence of a beneficial effect on CHD of a decrease in total cholesterol and/or LDL-C was derived from landmark clinical trials with statins in nondiabetic and diabetic cohorts. In contrast, it is currently not established whether other nonstatin drugs specifically targeting LDL-C (ezetimibe; bile acid binders; proprotein convertase subtilisin/kexin type 9 [PCSK9] inhibitors) (Fig. 15-2), or with an LDL-C– lowering component among other lipid- and lipoprotein-modulating

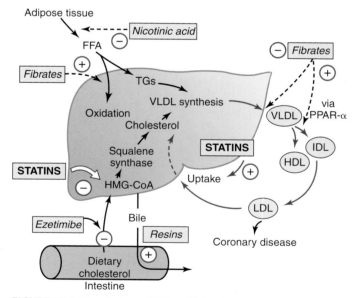

WHERE LIPID-LOWERING DRUGS ACT

FIGURE 15-1 Sites of action of lipid-modifying drugs. Hepatic import and export of lipids is crucial to the sites of action of lipid-lowering drugs. Proposed mechanism of action of statins, fibrates, and nicotinic acid. FFA = Free fatty acid; HMG-CoA = 3-hydroxy-3-methylglutaryl-coenzyme A; IDL = intermediate-density lipoprotein; PPAR-α = peroxisome proliferator–activated receptor alpha; VLDL = very low-density lipoprotein. *(Figure copyright L.H. Opie, 2012. From Gotto AM, Opie LH: Drugs for the Heart. Philadelphia, Saunders, 2013, pp 398-435.)*

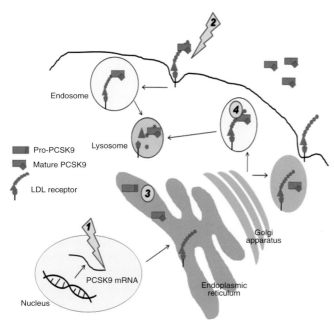

FIGURE 15-2 PCSK9 inhibition. Proprotein convertase subtilisin/kexin type 9 (PCSK9): from structure–function relation to therapeutic inhibition. *(From Tibolla G, Norata GD, Artali R, et al. Proprotein convertase subtilisin/kexin type 9 (PCSK9): from structure-function relation to therapeutic inhibition. Nutr Metab Cardiovasc Dis 21:835-843, 2011.)*

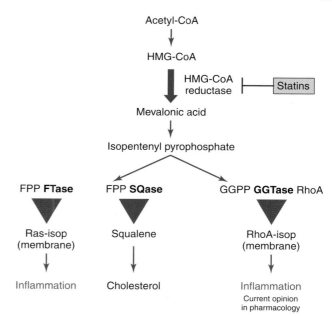

FIGURE 15-3 Mechanism of action of statins. The mechanism by which statins could be used for the treatment of COPD patients seems to be the same as that observed for cholesterol lowering. HMG-CoA, 3-hydroxy-3-methylglutaryl coenzyme A; FPP = farnesyl pyrophosphate; FTase = farnesyl protein transferase; SQase = squalene synthase; GGPP = geranylgeranyl diphosphate; GGTase = geranylgeranyl protein transferase. *(From Matera MG, Calzetta L, Rinaldi B, et al. Treatment of COPD: moving beyond the lungs. Curr Opin Pharmacol 12:315-22, 2012.)*

effects (niacin, fibrates) have a beneficial influence on cardiovascular events in nondiabetic or diabetic patients.

3-Hydroxy-3-Methylglutaryl-Coenzyme a (HMG-CoA) Reductase Inhibitors: the Statins

Statins inhibit the 3-hydroxy-3-methylglutaryl-coenzyme A (HMG-CoA) reductase, upregulating hepatic expression of LDL receptors and increasing uptake of circulating LDL (**Fig. 15-3**), and thereby decreasing circulating cholesterol (total cholesterol, LDL-C, and non–HDL-C) as a result of lowered LDL-P numbers. As a direct consequence, statins also reduce levels of apo B, the major atherogenic apolipoprotein, of which a single structural molecule is present on each LDL-P, as well as on each of their TG-rich lipoprotein precursors (very low-density lipoproteins [VLDLs]; intermediate-density lipoproteins [IDL]; and VLDL remnants).

In general, patients with and without diabetes respond similarly to statins with regard to LDL-C reduction, with response similarly dependent on drug choice, dose choice, and individual response. Proportional reductions in LDL-C levels on statin treatment range from 20% to 40% for less potent statins (fluvastatin, lovastatin, and pravastatin), 30% to 45% for simvastatin, and 40% to more than 50% for the most potent statins (atorvastatin, rosuvastatin, and pitavastatin). In the vast majority of diabetic and nondiabetic patients, long-term statin use is safe and effective.[98–108]

Patients with Diabetes in Key Statin Trials

Numerous studies have demonstrated the effectiveness of statins to reduce primary CHD outcomes in primary and secondary prevention settings and post-ACS events; the risk reduction after LDL-C lowering parallels the magnitude of the achieved LDL-C decrease in populations with and without diabetes. The studies having established the beneficial effect of statins on CHD risk in patients with DM selected for the present review comprised a total of 20,103 DM

patients, followed for a mean duration of 4.0 years. Average (1 standard deviation) on-treatment LDL-C decreased to a mean 81 (standard deviation [SD] 18) mg/dL (2.1 [SD 0.5] mmol/L). This corresponds to absolute and relative reductions of 48 mg/dL (1.2 mmol/L) and 36%, respectively. With respect to non–LDL lipids, mean on-statin HDL-C was 46 (4) mg/dL (1.2 [0.1] mmol/L); non–HDL-C was 114 (19) mg/dL (3.0 [0.5] mmol/L); and TG was 144 (12) mg/dL (1.6 [0.1] mmol/L) (**Table 15-6**).

In the active arms of statin trials (n = 10,077), a total of 1638 primary outcome events (5.3%/year) were observed, versus 2022 outcomes (7.0 %/year) in the comparator arms (n = 10,026), with a weighted and adjusted hazard ratio (HR) of 0.76 (95% confidence interval [CI] 0.65 to 0.84) favoring statin treatment. As a class, for each 1 mg/dL (0.03 mmol/L) reduction in LDL-C achieved on statin, the HR of incident CHD was reduced on average by 0.5%. This translated into a 19.5% primary outcome reduction for every 1 mmol/L (40 mg/dL) decrease of LDL-C. The mean absolute risk reduction for composite major adverse CV events in statin trials was 6.0%; the mean relative risk reduction (RRR) was 25%. The average number needed to treat for 5 years to prevent one major adverse CV event was 16 patients. Qualitatively similar effects are evident when analyzing the component endpoints of all-cause mortality (HR 0.88; 95% CI 0.65-1.01) and fatal CHD events (HR 0.59; 95% CI 0.48-0.97), although pooled analysis of death alone failed to achieve statistical significance (see **Table 15-6**).

Meta-analyses of Statin Efficacy Among Diabetes Mellitus Patients

In the Cholesterol Treatment Trialists' Collaboration (CTT) prospective meta-analysis of data from 90,056 participants in 14 statin randomized controlled trials (among whom 21% had DM), statin therapy safely reduced 5-year incidence of major adverse coronary events (MACEs) and coronary

TABLE 15-6 Statins Effects on Lipids and apo B and Primary Outcome (Ranked by Low-Density Lipoprotein Cholesterol [LDL-C] Reduction) in Diabetes Trials and Substudies

ACRONYMS	ACTIVE ARM (n)	CONTROL ARM (n)	FOLLOW-UP (yr)	THERAPY	DOSAGE (mg)	CONTROL	LDL-C	HDL-C	NON-HDL-C	TG	apo B	DELTA LDL-C (mg)	DELTA LDL-C (%)	EVENTS ACTIVE ARM (n)	ANNUAL RATE (%)	EVENTS CONTROL (n)	ANNUAL RATE (%)	HR	95% CI	P	ARR (%)	RRR (%)	5-YEAR NNT
GREACE (DSS)	161	152	3	atorva	23.7	Usual care	97	43	123	142		−92	−49	20	4.1	46	10.1	0.41		<.0001	17.8	59	3
4S (DSS)	105	97	5.4	simva	20-40	Placebo	119	46	143	134		−67	−36	15	2.6	24	4.6	0.58		.087	10.5	42.3	
4D	619	636	4	atorva	20	Placebo	72					−53	−42	226	9.1	243	9.6	0.96	0.77-1.1	.37	1.7	4.4	
SPARCL (DSS)	395	399	4.9	atorva	80	Placebo	81	48	106	137		−50	−38										
ASCOT-LLA (DDS)	1258	1274	3.3	atorva	10	Placebo	81	47	108	136		−47	−37	116	2.8	151	3.6	0.78	0.61-0.98	.036	2.6	22.2	25
CARDS	1428	1410	3.9	atorva	10	Placebo	70	55	99	140	90	−47	−40	83	1.5	127	2.3	0.65	0.48-0.83	.001	3.2	35.5	24
PROVE IT-TIMI 22 (DSS)	499	479	2	atorva	80	prava 40	57					−44	−44	142	14.2	152	15.9	0.88		.28	3.3	10.3	
AURORA (DSS)	388	343	2.8	rosuva	10	Placebo	54	45	83	146		−43	−39	85	7.8	104	10.8	0.72	0.51-0.90	.008	8.4	27.7	7
CARE (DSS)	282	304	5	prava	40	Placebo	96	40	130	143		−40	−27	81	5.7	112	7.4	0.78		<.0001	8.1	22	12
HPS—MRC/BHF (DSS)	2978	2985	4.8	simva	40	Placebo	89	41	136	177	84	−35	−28	601	4.2	748	5.2	0.81	0.19-0.30	<.0001	4.9	19.5	20
ASPEN	1211	1199	4	atorva	10	Placebo	79	48	108	141		−34	−30	166	3.4	180	3.8	0.91	0.73-1.12	.341	1.3	8.7	
TNT (DSS)	753	748	4.9	atorva	80	atorva 10	77	45	106	145		−19	−20	103	2.8	135	3.7	0.76	0.58-0.97	.026	4.4	24.2	22
Total (n = 20,103)	10,077	10,026												1638		2022							
Mean			4.0				81	46	114	144		−48	−36		5.3		7.0	0.76			6.0	25	16

All lipids measurements correspond to on-treatment values (in mg/dL).
See **Table 15-1** for acronyms definition and **Table 15-2** for primary outcomes description.
ARR = Absolute risk reduction; atorva = atorvastatin; CI = confidence interval; NNT = number needed to treat; prava = pravastatin; rosuva = rosuvastatin; RRR = relative risk reduction; simva = simvastatin.

revascularization by approximately 20% per 40 mg/dL (1.0 mmol/L) LDL-C reduction, and largely independent of baseline LDL-C.[109] Other meta-analyses have confirmed these observations that statins effectively reduce CHD outcomes with or without DM in both primary and secondary prevention populations,[110–112] including meta-analyses focused only on statin efficacy among DM participants.[111]

Patients with DM could possibly benefit even more from the cardioprotective effects of statins than those without DM,[110] and the authors of the CTT meta-analysis of 18,686 diabetic patients from 14 randomized controlled trials went as far as to recommend considering statin therapy for all patients with DM and elevated risk for incident CV events, based on the 21% proportional reduction in MACE for every 40 mg/dL (1.0 mmol/L) LDL-C reduction.[111] However, this may overestimate statin efficacy to some degree because of the exclusion from the analyses of data from the ASPEN trial, which was a DM-specific trial of atorvastatin that failed to demonstrate statistically significant differences in CV outcomes.[18]

Statin Use, Glucose Homeostasis, and New-Onset Diabetes

Much has been discussed with regard to cholesterol metabolism, use of statins, and drug-induced pancreatic beta cell dysfunction,[113–121] with a modest diabetogenic action of statins increasingly considered an infrequent, likely dose-dependent side effect affecting most of the drugs within the class. Incident diabetes cases observed in randomized controlled statin trials have been reported and included in meta-analysis of data from eight landmark trials (A to Z; ASCOT-LLA; GREACE; HPS—MRC/BHF; IDEAL; JUPITER; SPARCL; TNT).* On a population basis, statins may cause marginal increases in blood glucose—both fasting and postprandial—in predisposed individuals. This translates into a slight increase in glycated hemoglobin A1c (HbA1c) and for patients with baseline values just below diagnostic thresholds leads to a small excess in incident DM cases for statin versus control patients. In most patients with small increases in HbA1c, this observation is of uncertain clinical relevance. For patients already diagnosed with DM, subtle deterioration of glycemic control and/or a rise in HbA1c, if it occurs, appear equally modest, even verging on the trivial when put into perspective with the cumulative rise in blood glucose over years associated with the relentless loss of residual beta cell function.

Because major randomized controlled trials investigate very large numbers of patients, such an effect, however small, may produce highly significant statistics, despite limited clinical relevance. Indeed, the ratio between number needed to treat (to avoid occurrence of one major CHD event) versus number needed to harm (i.e., new-onset diabetes or glucose control worsening in patients with already known T2DM) remains unquestionably in favor of using statins to lower LDL-C, whatever a patient's glucose homeostasis at the time of statin initiation,[120] an opinion underpinned by the recent American College of Cardiology (ACC), American Heart Association (AHA), and the European Society of Cardiology (ESC) cholesterol treatment guidelines.[122,150]

Ezetimibe

Ezetimibe is a selective blocker of intestinal cholesterol absorption, which binds to Niemann-Pick C1-like 1 (NPC1L1) receptors in the gut (**Fig. 15-4**). Whereas ezetimibe monotherapy moderately lowers LDL-C (<20%), it markedly reduces it when coadministered with a statin. Ezetimibe counteracts, in a complementary manner, the intestinal absorption of cholesterol that is often upregulated by statins; this upregulation reduces the LDL-C–lowering effectiveness of statins in patients with high intestinal ability to reabsorb cholesterol from the intestinal lumen whenever hepatic synthesis is constrained by statin inhibition of HMG-CoA reductase. Combination therapy with statin plus ezetimibe may represent an alternative approach to further reduce LDL-C when statin monotherapy is insufficient to lower LDL-C to target levels, as confirmed in a lipid-lowering efficacy meta-analysis.[123]

With regard to CHD outcomes data, the clinical evidence for benefit of ezetimibe is currently limited. In the SHARP trial, 9270 patients with advanced renal disease (among whom 23% had diabetes at inclusion) were randomly assigned to treatment with simvastatin 20 mg plus ezetimibe 10 mg daily versus matching placebo with mean trial follow-up of 4.9 years. There was a significant reduction in major atherosclerotic events (coronary death, MI, ischemic stroke, or any revascularization procedure) in the simvastatin-ezetimibe group versus placebo, with an HR of 0.84 (CI 0.74-0.94; $P=0.0021$) with a number needed to treat for 5 years of 47 patients. In SHARP, the treatment response in the subgroup of patients with DM did not differ from the findings of the overall trial.[70] However, it remains unclear as to what extent each of the lipid-lowering drugs that were combined contributed to the results.

IMPROVE-IT is ongoing and is comparing the effects of a combination of simvastatin (40 mg)+ezetimibe (10 mg) daily versus simvastatin (40 mg) alone in 18,000 very high-risk patients with ACS, among whom a large subgroup (22%) had DM at enrollment.[45]

The ARBITER 6-HALTS Trial (Arterial Biology for the Investigation of the Treatment Effects of Reducing Cholesterol 6-HDL and LDL Treatment Strategies in Atherosclerosis) investigated, in an open-label design, the effect of ezetimibe (10 mg) versus extended-release (ER) niacin (2000 mg) daily in 315 patients with CHD or CHD equivalent (among whom 40% had DM at inclusion), given on top of background statin therapy. The trial was terminated early on the basis of a prespecified interim analysis showing superiority of ER niacin over ezetimibe on carotid artery intima-media thickness regression ($P<.001$).[124] It should be noted that the study design, by isolating niacin's additional actions on HDL-C and TGs from its LDL-C–lowering effects, could have disadvantaged detection of a beneficial effect of long-term ezetimibe therapy. Thus, part of atherosclerosis regression in the ER niacin arm could theoretically be ascribed to changes in components of atherogenic dyslipidemia. Given the high proportion of patients with DM in ARBITER 6-HALTS trial, a specific analysis of the respective benefits of these two lipid-lowering approaches in these patients would be of great interest. At the time of writing this chapter, no definitive data either support or call into question the effectiveness of ezetimibe, alone or in combination with statins, to reduce CHD events in patients with DM.

Drugs Targeting High-Density Lipoprotein Cholesterol

Given the epidemiologic evidence of a link between a low HDL-C level (or a decreased number of HDL) and increased CHD risk in nondiabetic and diabetic populations, it was

---

*References 5, 16, 17, 36, 40, 44, 71, 75, 119-121.

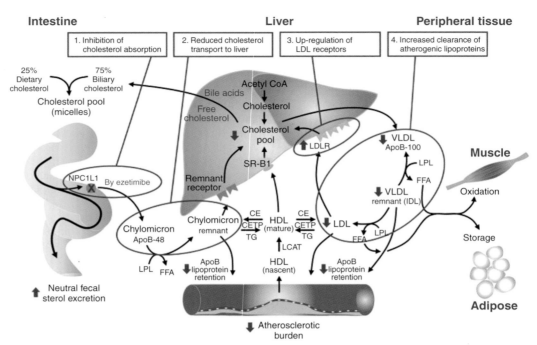

FIGURE 15-4 Ezetimibe mechanism of action. Mechanism of action for reduction of atherogenic ApoB-containing lipoproteins by ezetimibe, and potential effects on atherosclerotic burden. ApoB=Apolipoprotein B; CE=cholesteryl ester; CETP=cholesteryl ester transfer protein; FFA=free fatty acid; HDL=high-density lipoprotein; IDL=intermediate-density lipoprotein; LCAT=lecithin-cholesterol acyltransferase; LDL=low-density lipoprotein; LPL=lipoprotein lipase; NPC1L1=Niemann-Pick C1 Like 1 sterol transporter; SR-B1=scavenger receptor type B1; TG=triglyceride; VLDL=very low-density lipoprotein. *(From Davis HR, Lowe RS, Neff DR. Atherosclerosis 215: 266-278, 2011.)*

logical to target HDL-C levels and/or the number of HDL particles as lipid-related modifiable CV risk factors in DM patients. However, several classes of drugs that alter HDL-C levels and/or function have failed to yield significant improvements in CV risk, as described in the following section. And although treatment with fibric acid derivatives (fibrates) does have a modest effect on raising HDL-C, their principal mechanism of action modulates circulating TG levels, and therefore this class of medications will be reviewed in the following section on TGs.

Niacin

Niacin (nicotinic acid) is a broad-spectrum lipid-altering drug with multiple effects on lipids and lipoproteins. In hepatocytes, niacin inhibits microsomal diacylglycerol acyltransferase 2 (DGAT2), resulting in decreased TG synthesis, lowered VLDL assembly, and increased intrahepatic apo B degradation (**Fig. 15-5**). Niacin impairs apo B and VLDL secretion; decreases TG, apo B, non–HDL-C, LDL-C, and lipoprotein(a) levels; and also reduces the number of VLDL (especially TG-rich VLDL) and small dense LDL-Ps. Niacin

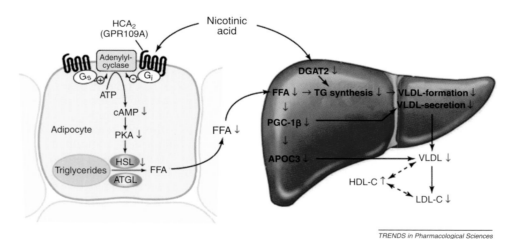

TRENDS in Pharmacological Sciences

FIGURE 15-5 Niacin (nicotinic acid) mechanisms of action. Potential mechanisms underlying the antidyslipidemic effects of nicotinic acid. Activation of the nicotinic acid receptor HCA$_2$ on adipocytes via the heterotrimeric G protein, Gi, leads to inhibition of adenylyl cyclase. Decreased cAMP levels via reduced activation of protein kinase A (PKA) results in an inhibition of lipolysis. Owing to this antilipolytic effect, free fatty acid (FFA) plasma levels drop, and triglyceride (TG) synthesis in the liver is reduced resulting in decreased very-low-density lipoprotein (VLDL) formation. A reduced supply of FFAs to the liver also suppresses hepatic expression of PPARγ coactivator-1β (PGC-1β) and of apolipoprotein C3 (APOC3). Decreased PGC-1β expression reduces VLDL formation and secretion. Under in vitro conditions, nicotinic acid has also been shown to inhibit triglyceride synthesis by a direct inhibitory effect on diacylglycerol acyltransferase 2 (DGAT2). The reduced expression of APOC3 may contribute to the decrease in VLDL levels by increasing VLDL turnover. Reduced VLDL levels result in reduced LDL cholesterol levels. How HDL cholesterol levels increase in unclear. This effect may be due to decreased expression of the cholesterol ester transfer protein (CETP) or the decreased exchange of triglycerides from VLDL and LDL particles against cholesterol esters of HDL particles. ATGL=adipocyte triglyceride lipase; HSL=hormone sensitive lipase. For details, see text. *(From Lukasova M, Hanson J, Tunaru S, et al. Nicotonic acid (niacin): new lipid-independent mechanisms of action and therapeutic potentials. Trends Pharmacol Sci 32:700-707, 2011.)*

also decreases liver fractional catabolism of apo A-I–HDL, increasing the levels of apo A-I and HDL-C, and raising type 2 HDL number. In adipose tissue, niacin modulates TG lipolysis and fatty acid mobilization. The range of niacin's lipid effects theoretically means that it could be a choice drug to treat LDL-C and/or atherogenic dyslipidemia in DM patients with low HDL-C, elevated small dense LDL particles, and/or hypertriglyceridemia.

Niacin use, especially at the beginning of treatment, often causes vasocutaneous flushing, whereas chronic niacin intake may impair insulin sensitivity, causing DM in some patients and, in those with DM, adversely influencing glucose control.[125] To mitigate flushing, ER formulations of niacin or a fixed-dose combination of niacin with laropiprant, an antiflush pharmacologic agent, have been introduced. However, recent large clinical trials of these formulations have failed to demonstrate reduction in CV risk, with the clinical benefit suggested in earlier studies challenged by small sample sizes and high dropout rates as a result of flushing.

Niacin Clinical Trial Results

In the Coronary Drug Project (CDP), a trial comprising 3908 men with a history of MI with mean study follow-up of 6.2 years, there was a significant reduction in the primary outcome (all-cause mortality) with niacin (3000 mg) daily versus placebo. Of note, the beneficial effect became evident only years after the end of the study. Whereas the prevalence of diabetes at enrollment was not reported, the benefits of niacin were observed irrespective of the presence of impaired fasting glucose, DM, and/or a metabolic syndrome at inclusion.[126] In the Stockholm Ischaemic Heart Disease study, conducted in 555 patients with a history of MI over a mean follow-up of 5 years, there was a significant reduction in total mortality (HR 0.74; $P=0.05$) and CHD mortality (HR 0.64; $P<.01$) with niacin (3000 mg) plus clofibrate (2000 mg) daily versus placebo.[127] In the HDL-Atherosclerosis Treatment Study (HATS), conducted in 160 patients with CHD, low HDL-C, and normal LDL-C (among whom 16% had DM at inclusion) over a mean follow-up of 3 years, the risk of the composite primary endpoint (CHD death, MI, stroke, revascularization for ischemic symptoms) was 90% lower ($P=0.03$) with a combination of niacin (2000 to 4000 mg) plus simvastatin (10 to 20 mg) daily versus placebo.[128]

As summarized earlier, the ARBITER 6-HALTS trial compared the addition of ezetimibe (10 mg) versus ER niacin (2000 mg) daily in 315 patients (of whom 40% had diabetes) with CHD or CHD equivalent, given on top of background statin therapy. The trial was terminated early based on a prespecified interim analysis showing superiority of ER niacin over ezetimibe on carotid artery intima-media thickness regression ($P<.001$).[124]

The Atherothrombosis Intervention in Metabolic Syndrome with Low HDL/High Triglycerides: Impact on Global Health Outcomes (AIM-HIGH) trial was conducted in 3414 patients with prior CVD (among whom 34% had DM and 80% a metabolic syndrome at inclusion). The trial was interrupted early because of futility after a mean follow-up of 3 years at the time of termination; there was no benefit of ER niacin (1500 to 2000 mg) daily versus placebo, given in addition to standardized background LDL-C–lowering therapy with simvastatin 40 to 80 mg plus or minus ezetimibe 10 mg daily to maintain LDL-C levels at 40 to 80 mg/dL (1.03 to 2.07 mmol/L). Whereas the primary composite outcome of CHD death, MI, ACS, ischemic

stroke, and/or symptom-driven revascularization was not reduced (HR 1.02; CI 0.87-1.21; $P=0.80$), broad-spectrum improvements in lipids and lipoproteins—increased HDL-C, decreased TG, and lowered LDL-C—were recorded after addition of ER niacin. Of interest, there were no significant interactions with respect to primary endpoint occurrence according to presence or absence of DM at inclusion. However, a post hoc analysis found a 36% relative reduction of the primary outcome ($P=0.032$) in a subgroup of 439 patients with marked atherogenic dyslipidemia (defined as TGs ≥ 200 mg/dL [≥ 2.3 mmol/L] and HDL-C <32 mg/dL [<0.83 mmol/L]).[129,130]

In HPS2-THRIVE, the risk of the composite primary endpoint (nonfatal MI or CHD death; stroke or [non]coronary revascularization) was not significantly different among 25,673 patients with either MI or cerebrovascular disease or peripheral arterial disease, or with DM plus CHD (the latter amounting to 32% of enrolled patients) randomized to ER niacin + laropiprant (2000 mg + 40 mg) or placebo over a median follow-up of 3.9 years, given in addition to standardized background LDL-C–lowering therapy (simvastatin 40 mg $\pm$ ezetimibe 10 mg daily) to maintain a total cholesterol target of 135 mg/dL (3.5 mmol/L).[42,131] There were, on the other hand, significant increases with ER niacin + laropiprant in diabetic complications (HR 1.55; CI 1.34-1.78; $P<0.0001$); new-onset DM (HR 1.27; CI 1.14-1.41; $P<0.0001$); and other side effects (infection; gastrointestinal effects; musculoskeletal, bleeding, and skin adverse events).

In a systematic meta-regression review of 9959 patients treated with niacin to reduce CVD, a significant reduction in incidence of the composite endpoints of any CV events was reported (HR 0.75; CI 0.59-0.96; $P=0.02$), irrespective of on-treatment HDL-C changes.[132] In the setting of subpopulations with DM, as for ezetimibe, a formal demonstration of the effectiveness of niacin, ER niacin, or niacin/laropiprant, alone or in combination with statins, to reduce CHD events is not currently available. Based on the negative results of these most recent large-scale clinical outcomes trials of niacin preparations, in 2013 the European Medicines Agency (EMA) recommended that the marketing, supply, and authorizations of three identical niacin + laropiprant products for the treatment of adults with dyslipidemia be suspended across the European Union; none of the formulations had been approved for use in the United States.

Cholesteryl Ester Transfer Protein Inhibition

Cholesteryl ester transfer protein (CETP) mediates intravascular transfer and exchange of cholesteryl ester and TG between TG-rich lipoproteins (and their remnants) and HDL. An antiatherogenic potential has been suggested on the basis of a considerable rise in HDL-C, combined with a substantial decrease in LDL-C, lipoprotein(a), and apo B levels after pharmacologic inhibition of CETP. Clinical results for the first two CETP inhibitors were, however, problematic. Torcetrapib development was stopped because of higher rates of CV events and mortality in the ILLUMINATE (Investigation of Lipid Level Management to Understand Its Impact in Atherosclerotic Events) trial comprising 15,067 patients, of whom 44% had DM at inclusion. Development of the CETP inhibitor dalcetrapib was also discontinued because of ineffectiveness, based on data from the dal-OUTCOMES trial in 15,871 ACS patients, 25% of whom had DM at baseline.

Regarding other CETP inhibitors under study, there has not been any general safety issue reported in ongoing prospective outcomes studies so far. REVEAL and ACCELERATE (A Study of Evacetrapib in High-Risk Vascular Disease) are currently evaluating whether the broad range of lipid modifications induced by CETP inhibition translate into CV risk reduction in patients with a past MI, cerebrovascular atherosclerotic disease, peripheral arterial disease, and/or DM with evidence of symptomatic CHD (REVEAL), and in patients with high-risk vascular disease (past ACS, cerebrovascular atherosclerotic disease, peripheral arterial disease, and/or DM with coronary artery disease [ACCELERATE]).[67,133–138]

Drugs Targeting Triglycerides

Because pharmacologic lowering of LDL-C by statins (alone or combined with ezetimibe) has minimal effects on HDL-C and TG levels, atherogenic dyslipidemia remains frequent among patients treated for elevated LDL-C, even when LDL-C targets are achieved. Among the currently available medications targeting TG and atherogenic dyslipidemia (see **Chapter 10**), fibrates, niacin, and omega-3 fatty acids are known to improve one or more lipid abnormalities characteristic of DM, including atherogenic dyslipidemia components.

Fibric Acid Derivatives (Fibrates)

Fibrates are pharmacologic agonists of PPAR-α, which are nuclear receptors that coordinately regulate gene transcription. Activated PPAR-α regulates genes involved in lipoprotein metabolism, including apo A-I and apo A-II (HDL particle formation); lipoprotein lipase (TG-rich particles lipolysis); apo C-III (decreasing TG-rich particle numbers and small dense LDL particles); apo A-V (decreasing TG levels); adenosine triphosphate (ATP)–binding cassette transporter A1 (ABCA1) (promoting cholesterol efflux and reverse cholesterol transport); scavenger receptor B1 (HDL capture and catabolism); and transrepression of nuclear factor κB and activator protein 1 transcription factors (anti-inflammatory and parietal vascular protection) (**Fig. 15-6**). Reported effects of fibrates on lipids and lipoproteins among DM patients participating in clinical outcomes trials include mean on-treatment TG levels of 147 (SD 29) mg/dL (1.7 [SD 0.3] mmol/L), with absolute and relative mean reductions of 39 mg/dL (0.4 mmol/L) and 19%, respectively. Average on-treatment LDL-C was 120 (37) mg/dL (3.1 [1.0] mmol/L); HDL-C 41 (5) mg/dL (1.1 [0.1] mmol/L); non–HDL-C 152 (43) mg/dL (3.9 [1.1] mmol/L; and apo B 108 (28) mg/dL.*

Most clinical trials of fibrates have included patients without and with DM; the DM subsets were most often too small for meaningful conclusions to be drawn about efficacy specifically in patients with DM.† Two trials have evaluated the effects of fenofibrate specifically in high-risk DM populations. The FIELD trial investigated the effects of fenofibrate (200 mg/day) versus placebo in 9795 patients with T2DM with or at risk for CVD, with a primary composite outcome of CHD death or nonfatal MI. Eligibility criteria also included total cholesterol (TC) 116 to 251 mg/dL (3.0 to 6.5 mmol/L) and either TC/HDL-C ≥4 or TGs 89 to 443 mg/dL (1.0 to

5.0 mmol/L). Over a mean follow-up of 5 years with 544 primary endpoint events occurring, differences in the primary outcome were not statistically different (HR 0.89; CI 0.75-1.05).[32–34] The ACCORD-Lipid trial investigated the effects of fenofibrate (160 mg/day) versus placebo, each added to background simvastatin therapy, in 5518 patients with DM and high CV risk with a primary composite outcome of CV death, MI, or stroke. Over a mean follow-up of 4.7 years with 601 primary outcome events for analysis, there was no significant difference between the groups (HR 0.92; 95% CI 0.79-1.08).[6–8]

Although fenofibrate therapy was ineffective to reduce risk for the primary composite outcome in the overall cohort, analyses of the prespecified subgroup (17%) of patients with atherogenic dyslipidemia at inclusion (defined as fasting TGs >204 mg/dL [2.3 mmol/L] and HDL-C <34 mg/dL [<0.9 mmol/L]) yielded a statistically significant 31% reduction ($P < .05$). The implications of ACCORD-Lipid are threefold: (1) T2DM patients with atherogenic dyslipidemia have a 70% increase in relative risk for CHD compared with those without atherogenic dyslipidemia, even when LDL-C is controlled with simvastatin; (2) addition of fenofibrate to simvastatin appears to reduce CV events, although with noted limitations of subset analyses in an overall neutral trial; and (3) such dual therapy was well tolerated.

General Limitations of the Available Fibrate Data

The most significant limitation of the totality of the fibrate data is the failure to limit the evaluation to patients with atherogenic dyslipidemia, with trials evaluating broad CV risk cohorts or cohorts with DM with or without atherogenic dyslipidemia. This limitation is highlighted by the biologic plausibility of the atherogenic influence of high TGs combined with low HDL-C; the known mechanism of action of the fibrates; and subanalyses across multiple trials consistently demonstrating efficacy of fibrates in patients with the combination of high TGs and low HDL-C. Thus, the fragmented amount of direct clinical evidence results from a lack of randomized clinical trials, on a large scale, comparing fibrates and statins head to head, or investigating the additional effect of fibrates (versus placebo) in combination therapy with statins in long-term studies that would have included only patients with high TGs, or atherogenic dyslipidemia, with and without DM. For these reasons, until further data come available, it is most appropriate to interpret the evidence to date regarding fibrate effects on CHD outcomes in light of the following: lipid characteristics at entry, including hypercholesterolemia versus non-LDL dyslipidemia and average TG levels; concomitant treatment with statins at entry, or statin admission during follow-up; and CV risk of enrollees at baseline, including that related to the proportion of patients with DM, the latter usually with T2DM at presentation, comorbid with atherogenic dyslipidemia and/or hypertriglyceridemia.

Omega-3 Fatty Acids

Oral supplementation with omega-3 (n-3) fatty acids (marine-derived eicosapentaenoic acid [EPA] and docosahexaenoic acid [DHA] and plant-derived alpha-linolenic acid [ALA]) decreases hypertriglyceridemia, inhibits platelet aggregation, improves plaque stability and endothelial function, and prevents certain arrhythmias. It is on the basis of these observations that large clinical outcomes trials have

---

*References 6-8, 28-30, 32-34, 39, 69, 81.
†References 22, 23, 38, 39, 48, 49, 79-82.

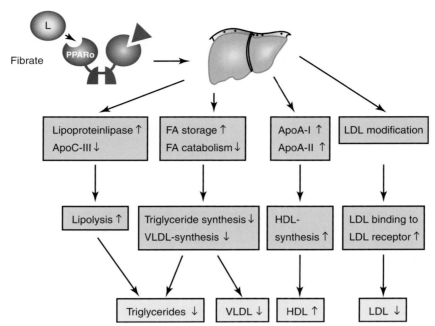

FIGURE 15-6 Fibrates mechanisms of action.

been conducted to evaluate the potential benefits of these supplements on CV events and death.

In the Japan Eicosapentaenoic Acid Lipid Intervention Study (JELIS), 18,645 patients with hypercholesterolemia (among whom 16% had DM at inclusion) were given EPA (1.8 g/day) plus statin versus statin alone during a mean follow-up of 4.6 years. There was a significant reduction in the primary outcome of developing any MACE (HR 0.81; CI 0.69-0.95; $P=0.011$). In the small subgroup of patients with atherogenic dyslipidemia at enrollment (TGs $\geq$150 mg/dL ($\geq$1.7 mmol/L) and HDL-C below 40 mg/dL (<1.0 mmol/L; 5% of the total study population), n-3 supplementation was associated with a significant 53% RRR.[143,144] Similarly, in a subanalysis stratified by glucose status within the first 6 months of the trial, 4565 patients with DM or impaired fasting glucose had a 22% ($P=0.048$) reduction in the primary composite event with EPA treatment.[145]

In the Outcome Reduction with an Initial Glargine Intervention (ORIGIN) trial, 12,536 patients with dysglycemia (impaired fasting glucose or glucose intolerance [18%] or diabetes [82%]), among whom 59% had a history of MI, stroke, or revascularization were randomized to EPA (465 mg) and DHA (375 mg) daily versus placebo, with the primary outcome of CV death. Over a median 6.2 years, EPA or DHA had no significant effect on the primary outcome that occurred in 1155 patients (HR 1.01; 0.87-1.17; $P=0.93$).[146]

A meta-analysis of 20 trials in 68,680 patients who received supplementation of, on average, 1.51 g of omega fatty acids per day failed to demonstrate a decrease in total mortality, cardiac death, sudden death, MI, or stroke.[147] All in all, the benefits of supplementation with omega-3 fatty acids are discordant according to studies, and generally disappointing in recent clinical trials and meta-analyses. Although large numbers of patients have been included in completed trials of n-3 supplementation, meta-analysis of efficacy has not been reported.

Other Trials with Lipid Intervention in Diabetes Mellitus Patients

In the PROACTIVE randomized placebo-controlled CV outcomes trial, addition of pioglitazone, a glucose-lowering PPAR-γ agonist that has some degree of PPAR-α agonism, versus placebo resulted in complementary improvement in lipids and lipoproteins as a result of pioglitazone's pleiotropic effects on lipid metabolism and fatty acid oxidation. In PROACTIVE, patients with T2DM patients and prevalent CVD were randomized to receive pioglitazone (target dose 45 mg daily) versus placebo. The incidence of the primary composite outcome (death, MI, stroke, unstable angina, coronary or peripheral revascularization, amputation) was not statistically different between the groups (HR 0.90; CI 0.80-1.02), but the prioritized secondary outcome of death, MI, or stroke did demonstrate superiority of pioglitazone (HR 0.84; CI 0.72-0.98) with an absolute risk reduction of 3.4%, a RRR of 16%, and a 3-year number needed to treat of 29 patients.[61,62] It remains unclear to what extend the lipid-modifying properties of pioglitazone have influenced these results.

In the intensified multifactorial Steno-2 intervention study, which combined lipid-lowering agents (statin and/or fibrate), renin-angiotensin system blockers, aspirin, and tight glucose regulation in patients with T2DM and microalbuminuria, a significant and pronounced reduction in all-cause mortality was observed (HR 0.60; CI 0.32-0.89; $P=0.02$), amounting to an absolute risk reduction of 20%; a RRR of 40%; and a number needed to treat for 5 years of 13 patients.[73] One must nevertheless acknowledge the limited statistical precision of these estimates, as the overall trial randomized only 160 participants, who experienced a limited total number of incident events. Furthermore, it is not possible, because of the multifactorial design, to quantify the beneficial component related to lowering of LDL-C or other lipids from those related to improvement in nonlipid risk factors.

The Anglo-Danish-Dutch Study of Intensive Treatment In People with Screen Detected Diabetes in Primary Care

(ADDITION-Europe) investigated 3057 newly diagnosed patients with T2DM randomized to either routine care or intensive treatment of CV multiple risk factors. Despite improvement in cholesterol levels, blood pressure, and HbA1c, there was no significant reduction in CV events (HR 0.83; CI 0.65-1.05) or total mortality (HR 0.91; 0.69-1.21).[148]

CLINICAL PRACTICE GUIDELINES FOR LIPID-LOWERING THERAPIES

Most published guidelines for lipid management advocate intensive lowering of elevated LDL-C in adult patients with hypercholesterolemia, based on therapeutic lifestyle interventions and with statin therapy as the primary pharmacologic intervention. Because of their heightened CV risk, patients with DM are a choice group to benefit from widespread statin use in primary or secondary CV prevention, irrespective of baseline LDL-C levels. Thus, DM patients without overt CVD are often considered as having CHD risk equivalency, and on that basis the LDL-C levels to trigger statin initiation and commensurate LDL-C targets are often lower than those for nondiabetic patients.[99,149,151–155] All in all, most guidelines and consensus statements from diabetes or cardiology scientific societies regarding management of dyslipidemia for patients with DM advocate aggressive lowering of LDL-C. In addition to therapeutic lifestyle changes, statin therapy is considered the mainstay of dyslipidemia management (ADA; European Association for the Study of Diabetes [EASD]; European Society of Cardiology [ESC]; European Atherosclerosis Society [EAS]; National Cholesterol Education Program; Canadian Cardiovascular Society; ACC).[98–108,150]

2011 European Society of Cardiology and European Atherosclerosis Society Guidelines for the Management of Dyslipidemias

The 2011 ESC/EAS guidelines for the management of dyslipidemias endorse the use of the SCORE risk estimating equation to categorize patients into risk categories, on which recommendations for lipid management are based. Four categories based on total CV risk are listed; patients with DM are, in general, at very high or high risk, especially those with T2DM.[98]

- *Very high risk:* patients with documented CV disease, previous MI, ACS, coronary revascularization and other arterial revascularization procedures, ischemic stroke, or peripheral arterial disease; patients with DM plus target organ damage (e.g., microalbuminuria); patients with moderate to severe chronic kidney disease; and patients whose calculated 10-year SCORE risk for fatal CV disease is 10% or higher
- *High risk:* patients with markedly elevated single risk factors (e.g., familial dyslipidemias) and patients with 10-year SCORE risk of 5% to 10%
- *Moderate risk:* patients with 10-year SCORE risk of 1% to 5%, with risk modulated according to family history of premature CAD, abdominal obesity, physical activity, HDL-C, TGs, C-reactive protein, lipoprotein(a), fibrinogen, homocysteine, apo B, and social class
- *Low risk:* individuals with 10-year SCORE risk below 1%

In this context, all patients at very high or high risk should be treated with medical therapy in addition to professional advice on lifestyle changes, whereas those at moderate risk

should receive lifestyle advice with or without lipid-modifying medication(s), and low-risk patients should be treated with lifestyle advice alone.[98] The guidelines recommend pretreatment lipid profile assessment with LDL-C as the primary focus; TGs and HDL-C may be considered to complement risk assessment and to refine therapeutic choice; and apo B measurement is recommended for better risk characterization of patients with DM and/or the metabolic syndrome. LDL-C is the paramount treatment target, whereas total cholesterol is an alternative treatment target if other analyses are unavailable. TGs should be monitored during treatment of patients with hypertriglyceridemia, but measurement of on-treatment HDL-C is not recommended as a therapeutic target, nor are calculations of on-treatment apo B/apo A-I and non–HDL-C/HDL-C ratios. Non–HDL-C is a secondary target for patients with DM and/or the metabolic syndrome; apo B is also a secondary treatment target.[98] In all T2DM patients, bringing LDL-C below 100 mg/dL (<2.6 mmol/L) is the primary target. Non–HDL-C below 130 mg/dL (<3.4 mmol/L) and overall apo B below 100 mg/dL are secondary targets (class I recommendation; level of evidence B). In patients with T2DM and CHD or CKD, and in those without CHD older than 40 years with one or more other CHD risk factors or markers of target organ damage, the primary goal is to lower LDL-C to below 70 mg/dL (<1.8 mmol/L), and the secondary goals are to bring non–HDL-C to below 100 mg/dL (<2.6 mmol/L) and apo B to below 80 mg/dL (class I recommendation; level of evidence B). In all patients with T1DM and in the presence of microalbuminuria and renal disease, LDL-C lowering by at least 30%, with statins as first choice and eventually with a drug combination, is recommended irrespective of baseline LDL-C (class I recommendation; level of evidence C).[98]

2013 European Society of Cardiology and European Association for the Study of Diabetes Guidelines on Diabetes, Prediabetes, and Cardiovascular Diseases

The 2013 ESC guidelines on diabetes, prediabetes, and CVD developed in collaboration with the EASD recommend classification of patients with DM as being at very high risk or high risk for CVD depending on the presence of concomitant risk factor and target organ damage. They do not recommend assessment of CVD risk in DM patients based on scores developed for the general population. Estimation of urinary albumin excretion rate is indicated when risk stratification of DM patients is performed, whereas screening for silent myocardial ischemia may be considered in selected high-risk DM patients.[150]

Statin therapy is recommended for patients with T1DM and T2DM at very high risk (diabetes with at least an additional cardiovascular risk factor or target organ damage), with an LDL-C target of below 70 mg/dL (<1.8 mmol/L), or at least a 50% reduction of LDL-C when this target cannot be attained. Treatment with a statin is also recommended for patients with T2DM at high risk, with an LDL-C target of below 100 mg/dL (<2.6 mmol/L). For T1DM patients at high risk, statin use may also be considered irrespective of baseline LDL-C. A secondary goal of on-treatment non–HDL-C below 100 mg/dL (<2.6 mmol/L) may be considered in patients with DM at very high risk, and of below 130 mg/dL (<3.4 mmol/L) in patients at high risk. In addition, intensification of statin therapy should be considered before combination therapy with ezetimibe. Finally, the use of drugs that increase HDL-C levels to prevent CVD in T2DM is not recommended.[150] Recommendations from other major scientific associations are often consensual with respect to primary and secondary lipid and lipoprotein targets to be achieved through therapeutic lifestyle changes and lipid-lowering drugs, alone or in combination in patients with DM, in primary prevention or secondary prevention.[98–108]

2013 American College of Cardiology and American Heart Association Guidelines for the Treatment of Blood Cholesterol to Reduce Atherosclerotic Cardiovascular Risk in Adults: Global Risk Assessment for Primary Prevention

The 2013 ACC/AHA Guideline on the Treatment of Blood Cholesterol to Reduce Atherosclerotic Cardiovascular Risk in Adults: Global Risk Assessment for Primary Prevention recommends the use of the Pooled Cohort Equations to estimate 10-year atherosclerotic CVD risk in both white and black men and women and to more accurately identify higher-risk individuals for statin therapy, focusing this treatment on those most likely to benefit.[122] This guideline proposes a paradigmatic revision of the management of hypercholesterolemia, which is the subject of ongoing debate. Thus, for secondary CV prevention (with or without DM), high-intensity statin therapy (atorvastatin 40 to 80 mg or rosuvastatin 20 to 40 mg/day) is recommended to lower LDL-C by 50% or more on average, with combination therapy to be considered if a 50% reduction is not achieved. For patients 40 to 75 years old with T1DM or T2DM in primary prevention whose LDL-C is 70 to 189 mg/dL (1.8 to 4.9 mmol/L), absolute 10-year risk of atherosclerotic CVD should be computed using the Pooled Cohort Equations. If the calculated risk is below 7.5%, moderate-intensity statin therapy is advocated (atorvastatin 10 to 20 mg; rosuvastatin 5 to 10 mg; simvastatin 20 to 40 mg; pravastatin 40 to 80 mg; lovastatin 40 mg; ER fluvastatin 80 mg; fluvastatin 2×40 mg; pitavastatin 2 to 4 mg—all daily doses); if calculated absolute risk is 7.5% or higher, high-intensity statin therapy (as defined earlier) is recommended.[122]

Reconciling Discordance in the Guidelines

Simultaneous achievement of several therapeutic targets inevitably leads to consider the pros and cons of two escalation approaches: one that involves using several lipid-lowering medications with complementary mechanisms of action, and another that advocates dose-titration of monotherapy. With regard to multiple lipid target achievements in DM patients, the frequent joint presence of atherogenic dyslipidemia is associated with lower success in achieving recommended targets for managing hypercholesterolemia—namely, achieving targets for three modifiable risk factors: LDL-C, non–HDL-C, and apo B. Such low achievement was found in a large proportion (one third) of very high-risk T2DM patients despite very low on-statin LDL-C levels.[93] Given currently available medications, combined attainment of LDL-C, non–HDL-C, and apo B targets will require titration or permutation of statins, reinforcement of therapeutic lifestyle changes, and/or combination lipid-lowering therapy.

Thus, a lipid-lowering therapy policy solely guided by an LDL-C target may not systematically deliver synchronous attainment of all atherogenic cholesterol targets, because lipid-lowering drugs do not produce strictly proportional decreases in LDL-C, LDL-P, non–HDL-C, and apo B.[93,156–158] More than 90% of circulating apo B belongs to LDL-Ps, which account for the bulk of non–HDL-C, meaning that discordant rates of achievement of targets for LDL-C versus apo B and/or non–HDL-C hints at potential unaddressed modifiable residual CV risk. Many recommendations include evaluation of and targeting therapy toward other non-LDL components of dyslipidemia, especially raised TGs and/or low HDL-C in subgroups with high CHD risk once LDL-C is at target. Along these lines, the lower the on-treatment LDL-C level achieved, the more likely that all four critical variables used to assess hypercholesterolemia (LDL-C, LDL-P, non–HDL-C, and apo B) will attain their respective targets.

With regard to baseline and on-treatment non–HDL-C and apo B levels and LDL-C, a joint consensus statement issued by the ADA and the ACC Foundation recommends two sets of triple targets for patients at high or very high cardiometabolic risk, respectively. LDL-C, non–HDL-C, and apo B levels below 100 mg/dL (<2.6 mmol/L), below 130 mg/dL (<3.4 mmol/L), and below 90 mg/dL, respectively, are recommended for patients with DM but without major CHD risk factors. LDL-C, non–HDL-C, and apo B levels below 70 mg/dL (<1.8 mmol/L), below 100 mg/dL (<2.6 mmol/L), and below 80 mg/dL, respectively, are recommended for patients with the highest CHD risk—that is, known CHD or DM plus one or more additional major CHD risk factors.[105]

Regarding individual components of atherogenic dyslipidemia, or the presence of atherogenic dyslipidemia in high-risk patients reaching recommended levels of LDL-C, a recent EAS consensus statement recommends for male and female patients with TGs of 150 mg/dL (≥1.7 mmol/L) or higher and/or HDL-C below 40 mg/dL (<1.0 mmol/L) the consideration of intensified LDL-C lowering (the largest decrease being reached by maximizing statin therapy and/or the addition of ezetimibe) or combination of lipid-lowering therapy with niacin (although currently not marketed in Europe and the United States) or a fibrate—after intensifying therapeutic lifestyle changes, addressing secondary dyslipidemias, and checking patient compliance. Based on clinical outcome and safety data for combined statin plus fibrate therapies, fenofibrate is the preferred fibrate among the class to be added to a statin.[83–85,88,89,108,159]

Titration of the statin dose or use of more potent statins are options most often used when further reduction in LDL-particle concentration is contemplated. Other combination therapies can also be used in selected patients, associating a statin (in addition to therapeutic lifestyle changes) with ezetimibe, niacin, or fibrates to reach all LDL-related targets. In addition, such combinatory strategies can contribute to improvement in other non-LDL features of diabetic dyslipidemia. Determining whether this will reduce CHD outcomes will require dedicated outcome studies with DM patients for each association.

Unmet Clinical Needs and Future Directions

At present, results from trials evaluating the effects of lipid-lowering medications other than (or added to) statins on CHD outcomes have been either disappointing or inconclusive, especially when baseline LDL-C was normal or controlled with statins (with or without ezetimibe) and/or whenever the annual CV event rate during follow-up was relatively low compared with older landmark trials. Regarding statins, evidence of the effectiveness of the entire class, in terms of reduction of occurrence of composite primary outcomes, is undeniable in DM patients.

The presently unmet need for definitive proof of efficacy of current lipid-lowering drugs on all components of lipid-related CHD in patients with DM is attributable to a variety of causes. There have been few DM-specific trials; most of the available evidence has been derived from post hoc analyses of DM subgroups. Within the aggregate DM dataset, the relatively few cumulative events available for analyses challenge statistical power for efficacy assessments, especially for assessment of effects on individual components of the endpoints analyzed (**Table 15-7**). This is confounded by the inclusion in several trials of patients at lower risk than planned, resulting in low event rates and marginal statistical

TABLE 15-7 Statin Efficacy on Coronary Heart Disease Outcomes in Patients with Diabetes Mellitus (DM)*

DRUG(s)	DOSE (mg)	ACRONYM	OUTCOME	HR	P	5-YEAR NNT
Simvastatin	20-40	4S (DM subgroup)	All MI	0.27		
Atorvastatin	23.7	GREACE (DM subgroup)	Fatal CHD	0.38	= 0.042	15
Atorvastatin	10	CARDS	Fatal MI	0.39		
Atorvastatin	23.7	GREACE (DM subgroup)	Primary	0.41	< 0.0001	3
Atorvastatin	80	PROVE IT–TIMI 22 (DM subgroup)	UAP	0.42	= 0.003	9
Atorvastatin	23.7	GREACE (DM subgroup)	All CV events	0.43	= 0.0001	4
Atorvastatin	23.7	GREACE (DM subgroup)	All-cause mortality	0.48	= 0.049	14
Atorvastatin	80	SPARCL (DM subgroup)	Total CHD	0.49	= 0.01	23
Pravastatin	40	CARE (DM subgroup)	Fatal MI	0.54		
Simvastatin	20-40	4S (DM subgroup)	All-cause mortality	0.58		
Simvastatin	20-40	4S (DM subgroup)	Primary	0.58	= 0.087	
Atorvastatin	10	CARDS	Nonfatal MI	0.60		
Simvastatin	40	HPS—MRC/BHF (DM subgroup)	Nonfatal MI	0.64	= 0.0002	49
Atorvastatin	10	CARDS	Primary	0.65	= 0.001	24
Simvastatin	20-40	4S (DM subgroup)	Fatal CHD	0.65	= 0.242	
Simvastatin	20-40	4S (DM subgroup)	Total CHD	0.65	= 0.015	5
Atorvastatin	10	CARDS	ACS	0.65		
Atorvastatin	80	SPARCL (DM subgroup)	All CV events	0.67	= 0.01	11
Simvastatin	20-40	4S (DM subgroup)	PCI, CABG	0.69	= 0.265	
Atorvastatin	10	CARDS	PCI, CABG	0.70		
Pravastatin	40	CARE (DM subgroup)	PCI, CABG	0.71	= 0.04	9
Atorvastatin	10	CARDS	All CV events	0.71	= 0.001	20
Atorvastatin	20	4D	Fatal MI	0.72		
Rosuvastatin	10	AURORA (DM subgroup)	Primary	0.72	= 0.008	7
Atorvastatin	10	CARDS	All-cause mortality	0.73	= 0.059	
Atorvastatin	10	ASPEN	All MI	0.74	= 0.1	
Rosuvastatin	10	AURORA (DM subgroup)	Fatal CHD	0.74		
Atorvastatin	80	TNT (DM subgroup)	Fatal CHD	0.74	= 0.203	
Simvastatin	40	HPS—MRC/BHF (DM subgroup)	Total CHD	0.74	< 0.0001	29
Atorvastatin	80	PROVE IT–TIMI 22 (DM subgroup)	All MI	0.75	= 0.11	
Atorvastatin	80	TNT (DM subgroup)	Primary	0.76	= 0.026	22
Atorvastatin	10	CARDS	UAP	0.77		
Atorvastatin	10	ASCOT-LLA (DM subgroup)	All CV events	0.77	= 0.036	24
Pravastatin	40	CARE (DM subgroup)	All MI	0.77		
Pravastatin	40	CARE (DM subgroup)	Total CHD	0.77	= .05	
Atorvastatin	10	ASCOT-LLA (DM subgroup)	Primary	0.78	= .036	25
Pravastatin	40	CARE (DM subgroup)	Primary	0.78	< .0001	12
Atorvastatin	80	TNT (DM subgroup)	Nonfatal MI	0.79	= .202	
Atorvastatin	80	TNT (DM subgroup)	All CV death	0.79	> .05	
Atorvastatin	20	4D	PCI, CABG	0.79		
Simvastatin	40	HPS—MRC/BHF (DM subgroup)	Primary	0.81	< .0001	20
Atorvastatin	80	TNT (DM subgroup)	Total CHD	0.81		
Simvastatin	40	HPS—MRC/BHF (DM subgroup)	Fatal CHD	0.81	= .02	63

TABLE 15-7 Statin Efficacy on Coronary Heart Disease Outcomes in Patients with Diabetes Mellitus (DM)—cont'd

DRUG(s)	DOSE (mg)	ACRONYM	OUTCOME	HR	P	5-YEAR NNT
Atorvastatin	10	ASPEN	Sudden death	0.81		
Pravastatin	40	CARE (DM subgroup)	Nonfatal MI	0.82		
Atorvastatin	20	4D	Fatal CHD	0.83	= .08	
Atorvastatin	80	TNT (DM subgroup)	All CV events	0.85	= .044	22
Atorvastatin	80	PROVE IT–TIMI 22 (DM subgroup)	Primary	0.88	= .28	
Pravastatin	40	CARE (DM subgroup)	UAP	0.89		
Atorvastatin	20	4D	Nonfatal MI	0.91	= .42	
Atorvastatin	10	ASPEN	Primary	0.9	= .341	
Atorvastatin	20	4D	Sudden death	0.95		
Atorvastatin	20	4D	All-cause mortality	0.95	= .33	
Atorvastatin	80	PROVE IT–TIMI 22 (DM subgroup)	All-cause mortality	0.95	= .75	
Atorvastatin	20	4D	Primary	0.96	= .37	
Atorvastatin	10	ASPEN	PCI, CABG	0.97		
Pravastatin	40	CARE (DM subgroup)	Fatal CHD	0.97		
Atorvastatin	10	ASPEN	All CV death	1.02		NA
Atorvastatin	10	ASPEN	UAP	1.02		NA
Atorvastatin	80	SPARCL (DM subgroup)	All-cause mortality	1.03	= .82	NA
Atorvastatin	80	TNT (DM subgroup)	All-cause mortality	1.09		NA
Atorvastatin	10	CARDS	Sudden death	2.47		NA

See **Table 15-1** for acronym definition and references.
NA = not applicable (HR >1.00); UAP = unstable angina pectoris.
*Trials listed by descending order of HR reduction;

power, and use of suboptimal eligibility criteria in the context of the study medication being evaluated. For example, the inclusion of patients in the FIELD or ACCORD-Lipid trials without requiring hypertriglyceridemia and/or atherogenic dyslipidemia remains difficult to defend, given the prevalence of atherogenic dyslipidemia in DM patients and the mechanism of action of the PPAR-α agonist tested.

SUMMARY

Patients with DM, especially T2DM, are at very high risk of CHD, particularly because of the high prevalence of LDL-C and non–LDL-C dyslipidemias and other comorbidities. Large clinical trials have unambiguously demonstrated the elevated risk for CHD in DM, and the significant CHD risk reduction that can be achieved by statins in both primary and secondary prevention populations. With regard to other lipid-lowering medications, instead of or added to statin therapy, there are currently insufficient data to guide clinical recommendations and use, overall and in DM populations specifically. Therefore, support for pharmacologic treatment of diabetic dyslipidemia remains grounded on pathophysiological considerations, epidemiologic associations, and signals based on post hoc analyses from selected clinical trials. All guidelines recognize a higher risk of CHD in patients with DM, even in situations of primary prevention, compared with nondiabetic patients. This recognition underlies the current recommendations, generally converging, which advocate targeting of LDL-C as the major modifiable lipid risk factor for CHD in DM patients, although there is ongoing debate regarding the clinical relevance of the concept of therapeutic target values for LDL-C versus matching intensity of drug with estimated CVD risk. In addition, there remains debate about

whether other therapeutic targets should be pursued, such as non–HDL-C, apo B, TGs, and HDL-C in patients treated with lipid-lowering agents.[160]

The lipid-lowering effects of drugs under development make them potentially attractive to improve both standard care and other aspects of dyslipidemia management in patients with DM. This includes screening for and targeting the high residual vascular risk that persists in DM patients whose LDL-C is controlled on statins and that is present in patients with inadequate LDL-C levels and the risk of persistently high LDL-C in patients with severe statin intolerance. The future challenge will be to identify and to bring a greater majority of patients with DM to meet their personalized optimal levels of LDL-C and non–LDL-C, to further reduce the occurrence of CHD.

References

1. Wanner C, Krane V, März W, et al: the German Diabetes and Dialysis Study Investigators: Atorvastatin in patients with type 2 diabetes mellitus undergoing hemodialysis, *N Engl J Med* 353:238–248, 2005.
2. Randomised trial of cholesterol lowering in 4444 patients with coronary heart disease: the Scandinavian Simvastatin Survival Study (4S), *Lancet* 344:1383–1389, 1994.
3. Kjekshus J, Pedersen TR, for the Scandinavian Simvastatin Survival Study Group: Reducing the risk of coronary events: evidence from the Scandinavian Simvastatin Survival Study (4S), *Am J Cardiol* 76:64C–68C, 1995.
4. Pyorala K, Pedersen TR, Kjekshus J, et al: the 4S Study Group: Cholesterol lowering with simvastatin improves prognosis of diabetic patients with coronary heart disease. A subgroup analysis of the Scandinavian Simvastatin Survival Study (4S), *Diabetes Care* 20:614–620, 1997.
5. de Lemos JA, Blazing MA, Wiviott SD, et al: the A to Z Investigators: Early intensive vs a delayed conservative simvastatin strategy in patients with acute coronary syndromes, *JAMA* 292:1307–1316, 2004.
6. ACCORD Study Group, Buse JB, Bigger JT, et al: Action to control cardiovascular risk in diabetes (ACCORD) trial: design and methods, *Am J Cardiol* 99:21j–33j, 2007.
7. ACCORD Study Group, Ginsberg HN, et al: Effects of combination lipid therapy in type 2 diabetes mellitus, *N Engl J Med* 362:1563–1574, 2010.
8. Elam M, Lovato L, Ginsberg H: The ACCORD-Lipid study: implications for treatment of dyslipidemia in type 2 diabetes mellitus, *Clin Lipidol* 6:9–20, 2011.
9. Tenenbaum A, Medvedofsky D, Fisman EZ, et al: Cardiovascular events in patients received combined fibrate/statin treatment versus statin monotherapy: acute coronary syndrome Israeli Surveys Data, *PLoS One* 7:e35298, 2012.
10. Downs JR, Beere PA, Whitney E, et al: Design and rationale of the Air Force/Texas coronary atherosclerosis prevention study (AFCAPS/TexCAPS), *Am J Cardiol* 80:287–293, 1997.
11. Downs JR, Clearfield M, Weis S, et al: the AFCAPS/TexCAPS Research Group: Primary prevention of acute coronary events with lovastatin in men and women with average cholesterol levels. Results from AFCAPS/TexCAPS, *JAMA* 279:1615–1622, 1998.

12. The AIM-HIGH Investigators: The role of niacin in raising high-density lipoprotein cholesterol to reduce cardiovascular events in patients with atherosclerotic cardiovascular disease and optimally treated low-density lipoprotein cholesterol: baseline characteristics of study participants. The atherothrombosis intervention in metabolic syndrome with low HDL/high triglycerides: impact on global health outcomes (AIM-HIGH) trial, *Am Heart J* 161:538–543, 2011.
13. The AIM-HIGH Investigators: Niacin in patients with low HDL cholesterol levels receiving intensive statin therapy, *N Engl J Med* 365:2255–2267, 2011.
14. Holdaas H, Fellström B, Jardine AG, et al: the ALERT Study Investigators: Effect of fluvastatin on cardiac outcomes in renal transplant recipients: a multicentre, randomised, placebo-controlled trial, *Lancet* 361:2024–2031, 2003.
15. The ALLHAT Officers and Coordinators for the ALLHAT Collaborative Research Group: Major outcomes in moderately hypercholesterolemic, hypertensive patients randomized to pravastatin vs usual care: the antihypertensive and lipid-lowering treatment to prevent heart attack trial (ALLHAT-LLT), *JAMA* 288:2998–3007, 2002.
16. Sever PS, Dahlöf B, Poulter NR, et al: the ASCOTT Investigators: Prevention of coronary and stroke events with atorvastatin in hypertensive patients who have average or lower-than-average cholesterol concentrations, in the Anglo-Scandinavian Cardiac Outcomes Trial-Lipid Lowering Arm (ASCOTT-LLA): a multicentre randomised controlled trial, *Lancet* 361:1149–1158, 2003.
17. Sever PS, Poulter NR, Dahlöf B, et al: the ASCOTT Investigators: Reduction in cardiovascular events with atorvastatin in 2532 patients with type 2 diabetes. Anglo-Scandinavian Cardiac Outcomes Trial-Lipid Lowering Arm (ASCOTT-LLA), *Diabetes Care* 28:1151–1157, 2005.
18. Knopp RH, D'Emden M, Smilde JG, et al: the ASPEN Study Group: Efficacy and safety of atorvastatin in the prevention of cardiovascular end points in subjects with type 2 diabetes. The atorvastatin study for prevention of coronary heart disease endpoints in non–insulin-dependent diabetes mellitus (ASPEN), *Diabetes Care* 29:1478–1485, 2006.
19. Felström BC, Jardine AG, Schmeider RE, et al: the AURORA Study Group: Rosuvastatin and cardiovascular events in patients undergoing hemodialysis, *N Engl J Med* 360:1395–1407, 2009.
20. Holdaas H, Holme I, Schmeider RE, et al: the AURORA Study Group: Rosuvastatin in diabetic hemodialysis patients, *J Am Soc Nephrol* 22:1335–1341, 2011.
21. Pitt B, Waters D, Brown WV, et al: the AVERT Investigators: Aggressive lipid-lowering therapy compared with angioplasty in stable coronary artery disease, *N Engl J Med* 341:70–76, 1999.
22. The BIP Study Group: Secondary prevention by raising HDL cholesterol and reducing triglycerides in patients with coronary artery disease. The Bezafibrate Infarction Prevention (BIP) Study, *Circulation* 102:21–27, 2000.
23. Goldenberg I, Boyko V, Tennenbaum A, et al: Long-term benefit of high-density lipoprotein cholesterol-raising therapy with bezafibrate. 16-year mortality follow-up of the Bezafibrate Infarction Prevention Trial, *Arch Intern Med* 169:508–514, 2009.
24. Colhoun HM, Betteridge DJ, Durrington PN, et al: the CARDS Investigators: Primary prevention of cardiovascular disease with atorvastatin in type 2 diabetes in the Collaborative Atorvastatin Diabetes Study (CARDS): multicentre randomised placebo-controlled trial, *Lancet* 364:685–696, 2004.
25. Sacks FM, Pfeffer MA, Moye LA, et al: the CARE Investigators: The effect of pravastatin on coronary events after myocardial infarction in patients with average cholesterol levels, *N Engl J Med* 335:1001–1009, 1996.
26. Lewis SJ, Sacks FM, Mitchell JS, et al: the CARE Investigators: Effect of pravastatin on cardiovascular events in women after myocardial infarction: the Cholesterol and Recurrent Events (CARE) Trial, *J Am Coll Cardiol* 32:140–146, 1998.
27. Goldberg RB, Mellies MJ, Sacks FM, et al: the CARE Investigators: Cardiovascular events and their reduction with pravastatin in diabetic and glucose-intolerant myocardial infarction survivors with average cholesterol levels. Subgroup analyses in the Cholesterol And Recurrent Events (CARE) Trial, *Circulation* 98:2513–2519, 1998.
28. Diabetes Atherosclerosis Intervention Study Investigators: Effect of fenofibrate on progression of coronary artery disease in type 2 diabetes: the Diabetes Atherosclerosis Intervention Study, a randomised study, *Lancet* 357:905–910, 2001.
29. Vakkilainen J, Steiner G, Ansquer JC, et al: the DAIS Group: Relationships between low-density lipoprotein particle size, plasma lipoproteins, and progression of coronary artery disease. The Diabetes Atherosclerosis Intervention Study (DAIS), *Circulation* 107:1733–1737, 2003.
30. Hanefeld M, Fischer S, Schmechel H, et al: Diabetes Intervention Study. Multi-intervention trial in newly diagnosed NIDDM, *Diabetes Care* 14:308–317, 1991.
31. Dohi T, Miyauchi K, Okazaki S, et al: Early intensive statin treatment for six months improves long-term clinical outcomes in patients with acute coronary syndrome (Extended-ESTABLISH trial): a follow-up study, *Atherosclerosis* 210:497–502, 2010.
32. The FIELD Study Investigators: Fenofibrate intervention and event lowering in diabetes (FIELD) study: baseline characteristics and short-term effects of fenofibrate [ISRCTN64783481], *Cardiovasc Diabetol* 4:13, 2005.
33. The FIELD Study Investigators: Effects of long-term fenofibrate therapy on cardiovascular events in 9795 people with type 2 diabetes mellitus (the FIELD study): randomised controlled trial, *Lancet* 366:1849–1861, 2005.
34. Scott R, O'Brien R, Fulcher G, et al: the FIELD Study Investigators: Effects of fenofibrate treatment on cardiovascular disease risk in 9795 individuals with type 2 diabetes and various components of the metabolic syndrome. The Fenofibrate Intervention and Event Lowering in Diabetes (FIELD) study, *Diabetes Care* 32:493–498, 2009.
35. GISSI Prevenzione Investigators (Gruppo Italiano per lo Studio della Soprovvivenza nell'Infarto Miocardico): Results of the low-dose (20 mg) pravastatin GISSI Prevenzione trial in 4271 patients with recent myocardial infarction: do stopped trials contribute to overall knowledge? *Ital Heart J* 1:810–820, 2000.
36. Athyros VG, Papageorgiou AA, Mercouris BR, et al: Treatment with atorvastatin to the national cholesterol educational program goal versus "usual" care in secondary coronary heart disease prevention. The Greek Atorvastatin and Coronary-heart-disease Evaluation (GREACE) study, *Curr Med Res Opin* 18:220–228, 2002.
37. Athyros VG, Papageorgiou AA, Symeonidis AN, et al: the GREACE Study Collaborative Group: Early benefit from structured care with atorvastatin in patients with coronary heart disease and diabetes mellitus. A subgroup analysis of the GREACE Study, *Angiology* 54:679–690, 2003.
38. Heikki Frick M, Elo O, Haapa K, et al: Helsinki Heart Study: primary-prevention trial with gemfibrozil in middle-aged men with dyslipidemia: safety of treatment, changes in risk factors, and incidence of coronary heart disease, *N Engl J Med* 317:1237–1245, 1987.
39. Koskinen P, Mänttäri M, Manninen V, et al: Coronary heart disease incidence in NIDDM patients in the Helsinki Heart Study, *Diabetes Care* 15:820–825, 1992.
40. Heart Protection Study Collaborative Group: MRC/BHF Heart Protection Study of cholesterol lowering with simvastatin in 20536 high-risk individuals: a randomised placebo-controlled trial, *Lancet* 360:7–22, 2002.
41. Heart Protection Study Collaborative Group: MRC/BHF Heart Protection Study of cholesterol lowering with simvastatin in 5963 people with diabetes: a randomised placebo-controlled trial, *Lancet* 361:2005–2016, 2003.
42. HPS2-THRIVE. Treatment of HDL to Reduce the Incidence of Vascular Events. ClinicalTrials.gov identifier: NCT00461630. Study design and status available at: www.clinicaltrials.gov.
43. Pedersen TR, Faergeman O, Kastelein JJP, et al: the IDEAL Study Group: Design and baseline characteristics of the incremental decrease in end points through aggressive lipid lowering study, *Am J Cardiol* 94:720–724, 2004.
44. Pedersen TR, Faergeman O, Kastelein JJP, et al: the IDEAL Study Group: High-dose atorvastatin vs usual-dose simvastatin for secondary prevention after myocardial infarction. The IDEAL Study: a randomised controlled trial, *JAMA* 294:2437–2445, 2005.
45. Cannon CP, Giugliano RP, Blazing MA, et al: the IMPROVE-IT Investigators: Rationale and design of IMPROVE-IT (IMProved Reduction of Outcomes: Vytorin Efficacy International Trial): comparison of ezetimibe/simvastatin versus simvastatin monotherapy on cardiovascular outcomes in patients with acute coronary syndromes, *Am Heart J* 156:826–832, 2008.
46. Hiro T, Kimura T, Morimoto T, et al: the Japan-ACS Investigators: Effect of intensive statin therapy on regression of coronary atherosclerosis in patients with acute coronary syndrome. A multicenter randomized trial evaluated by volumetric intravascular ultrasound using pitavastatin versus atorvastatin (JAPAN-ACS [Japan Assessment of Pitavastatin and Atorvastatin in Acute Coronary Syndrome] Study), *J Am Coll Cardiol* 54:293–302, 2009.
47. Price HC, Clarke PM, Gray AM, Holman RR: Life expectancy in individuals with type 2 diabetes: implications for annuities, *Med Decis Making* 30:409–414, 2010.
48. Meade TW: the MRC General Practice Research Framework and Participating Vascular Clinics: Design and intermediate results of the Lower Extremity Arterial Disease Event Reduction (LEAD) trial of bezafibrate in men with lower extremity arterial disease, *Curr Control Trials Cardiovasc Med* 2:195–204, 2001.
49. Meade T, Zuhrie R, Cook C: Cooper J on behalf of MRC General Practice Research Framework: Bezafibrate in men with lower extremity arterial disease: randomised controlled trial, *BMJ* 325:1139, 2002.
50. The Lipid Study Group: Design features and baseline characteristics of the LIPID (Long-Term Intervention With Pravastatin in Ischemic Disease) Study: a randomized trial in patients with previous acute myocardial infarction and/or unstable angina pectoris, *Am J Cardiol* 76:474–479, 1995.
51. The Lipid Study Group: Prevention of cardiovascular events and death with pravastatin in patients with coronary heart disease and a broad range of initial cholesterol levels, *N Engl J Med* 339:1349–1357, 1998.
52. The Lipid Study Group: Long-term effectiveness and safety of pravastatin in 9014 patients with coronary heart disease and average cholesterol concentrations: the LIPID trial follow-up, *Lancet* 359:1379–1387, 2002.
53. Serruys PW, de Feyter P, Macaya C, et al: the Lescol Intervention Prevention Study (LIPS) Investigators: Fluvastatin for prevention of cardiac events following successful first percutaneous coronary intervention. A randomized controlled trial, *JAMA* 287:3215–3222, 2002.
54. Nakamura H, Arakawa K, Itakura H, et al: for the MEGA Study Group: Primary prevention of cardiovascular disease with pravastatin in Japan (MEGA Study): a prospective randomised controlled trial, *Lancet* 368:1155–1163, 2006.
55. Schwartz GG, Oliver MF, Ezekowitz MD, et al: Rationale and design of the Myocardial Ischemia Reduction with Aggressive Cholesterol Lowering (MIRACL) Study that evaluates atorvastatin in unstable angina pectoris and in non–Q-wave acute myocardial infarction, *Am J Cardiol* 81:578–581, 1998.
56. Schwartz GG, Olsson AG, Ezekowitz MD, et al: The MIRACL Study Investigators: Effects of atorvastatin on early recurrent ischemic events in acute coronary syndromes. The MIRACL Study: a randomized controlled trial, *JAMA* 285:1711–1718, 2001.
57. Olsson AG, Schwartz GG, Szarek M, et al: High-density lipoprotein, but not low-density lipoprotein cholesterol levels influence short-term prognosis after acute coronary syndrome: results from the MIRACL trial, *Eur Heart J* 26:890–896, 2005.
58. Thompson PL, Meredith I, Amerena J, et al: the PACT Investigators: Effect of pravastatin compared with placebo initiated within 24 hours of onset of acute myocardial infarction or unstable angina: the Pravastatin in Acute Coronary Treatment (PACT) trial, *Am Heart J* 48: e1–e8, 2004.
59. The Post Coronary Artery Bypass Graft Trial Investigators: The effect of aggressive lowering of low-density lipoprotein cholesterol levels and low-dose anticoagulation on obstructive changes in saphenous-vein coronary-artery bypass grafts, *N Engl J Med* 336:153–162, 1997.
60. Knatterud GL, Rosenberg Y, Campeau L, et al: the Post CABG Investigators: Long-term effects on clinical outcomes of aggressive lowering of low-density lipoprotein cholesterol levels and low-dose anticoagulation in the Post Coronary Artery Bypass Graft Trial, *Circulation* 102:157–165, 2000.
61. Charbonnel B, Dormandy J, Erdmann E, et al: the PROActive Study Group: The prospective pioglitazone clinical trial in macrovascular events (PROactive), *Diabetes Care* 27: 1647–1653, 2004.
62. Dormandy JA, Charbonnel B, Eckland DJA, et al: the PROActive Investigators: Secondary prevention of macrovascular events in patients with type 2 diabetes in the PROactice Study (PROspective pioglitAzone Clinical Trial In macro Vascular Events): a randomised controlled trial, *Lancet* 366:1279–1289, 2005.
63. Shepherd J, Blauw GJ, Murphy MB, et al: the PROSPER Study Group: Pravastatin in elderly individuals at risk of vascular disease (PROSPER): a randomised controlled trial, *Lancet* 360:1623–1630, 2002.
64. Cannon CP, Braunwald E, McCabe CH, et al: the PROVE-IT-TIMI22 Investigators: Intensive versus moderate lipid lowering with statins after acute coronary syndromes, *N Engl J Med* 350:1495–1504, 2004.
65. Ahmed S, Cannon CP, Murphy SA, Braunwald E: Acute coronary syndromes and diabetes: is intensive lipid lowering beneficial? Results of the PROVE-IT-TIMI22 trial, *Eur Heart J* 27:2323–2329, 2006.
66. Miller M, Cannon CP, Murphy SA, et al: the PROVE-IT-TIMI22 Investigators: Impact of triglyceride levels beyond low-density lipoprotein cholesterol after acute coronary syndrome in the PROVE-IT-TIMI22 trial, *J Am Coll Cardiol* 51:724–730, 2008.
67. REVEAL - Randomized Evaluation of the Effects of Anacetrapib Through Lipid-modification ClinicalTrials.gov. identifier: NCT01252953. Study design and status available at: www.clinicaltrials.gov.
68. Nissen SE, Tuzcu EM, Schoenhagen P, et al: the REVERSAL Investigators: Effect of intensive compared with moderate lipid-lowering therapy on progression of coronary atherosclerosis. A randomized controlled trial, *JAMA* 291:1071–1080, 2004.
69. Elkeles RS, Diamond JR, Poulter C, et al: the SENDCAP Study Group: Cardiovascular outcomes in type 2 diabetes. A double-blind placebo-controlled study of bezafibrate: the St. Mary's Ealing, Northwick Park Diabetes Cardiovascular Disease Prevention (SENDCAP) study, *Diabetes Care* 21:641–648, 1998.
70. Baigent C, Landray MJ, Reith C, et al: the SHARP Investigators: The effects of lowering LDL cholesterol with simvastatin plus ezetimibe in patients with chronic kidney disease (Study of Heart and Renal Protection):a randomised placebo-controlled trial, *Lancet* 377:2181–2192, 2011.
71. The SPARCL Investigators: High-dose atorvastatin after stroke or transient ischemic attack, *N Engl J Med* 355:549–559, 2006.
72. Callahan A, Amarenco P, Goldstein LB, et al: the SPARCL Investigators: Risk of stroke and cardiovascular events after ischemic stroke or transient ischemic attack in patients with type 2 diabetes or metabolic syndrome. Secondary analysis of the Stroke Prevention by Aggressive Reduction in Cholesterol Levels (SPARCL) trial, *Arch Neurol* 68:1245–1251, 2011.
73. Gaede P, Lund-Andersen H, Parving HH, Pedersen O: Effects of a multifactorial intervention on mortality in type 2 diabetes, *N Engl J Med* 358:580–591, 2008.
74. Waters DD, Guyton JR, Herrington DM, et al: the TNT Steering Committee Members and Investigators: Treating to new targets (TNT) study: does lowering low-density lipotrotein cholesterol

levels below currently recommended guidelines yield incremental clinical benefit? *Am J Cardiol* 93:145–148, 2004.

75. LaRosa JC, Grundy SM, Waters DD, et al: the TNT Investigators: Intensive lipid lowering with atorvastatin in patients with stable coronary disease, *N Engl J Med* 352:1425–1435, 2005.

76. Shepherd J, Kastelein JJP, Bittner V, et al: the TNT Investigators: Effect on intensive lipid lowering with atorvastatin on renal function in patients with coronary heart disease: the Treating to New Targets (TNT) Study, *Clin J Am Soc Nephrol* 2:1131–1139, 2007.

77. Barter P, Gotto AM, LaRosa JC, et al: the TNT Investigators: HDL cholesterol, very low levels of LDL cholesterol, and cardiovascular events, *N Engl J Med* 357:1301–1310, 2007.

78. Shepherd J, Barter P, Carmena R, et al: the TNT Investigators: Effect of lowering LDL cholesterol substantially below currently recommended levels in patients with coronary heart disease and diabetes. The Treating to New Targets (TNT) study, *Diabetes Care* 29:1220–1226, 2006.

79. Bloomfield Rubins H, Robins SJ, Collins D, et al: the VA-HIT Study Group: Gemfibrozil for the secondary prevention of coronary heart disease in men with low levels of high-density lipotrotein cholesterol, *N Engl J Med* 341:410–418, 1999.

80. Robins SJ, Collins D, Wittes JT, et al: the VA-HIT Study Group: Relation of gemfibrozil treatment and lipid levels with major coronary events. VA-HIT: a randomized controlled trial, *JAMA* 285:1585–1591, 2001.

81. Bloomfield Rubins H, Robins SJ, Collins D, et al: the VA-HIT Study Group: Diabetes, plasma insulin, and cardiovascular disease. Subgroup analysis from the Department of Veterans Affairs High-Density Lipoprotein Intervention Trial (VA-HIT), *Arch Intern Med* 162:2597–2604, 2002.

82. The Veterans Administration Cooperative Study Group: The treatment of cerebrovascular disease with clofibrate. Final report of the Veterans Administration Cooperative Study of Atherosclerosis, Neurology Section, *Stroke* 4:684–693, 1973.

83. Hermans MP, Fruchart JC: Reducing residual vascular risk in patients with atherogenic dyslipidaemia: where do we go from here? *Clin Lipidol* 5:811–826, 2010.

84. Hermans MP, Fruchart JC: Reducing vascular events risk in patients with dyslipidaemia: an update for clinicians, *Ther Adv Chronic Dis* 2:307–323, 2011.

85. Hermans MP, Ahn SA, Rousseau MF: Residual vascular risk in T2DM: the next frontier. In Zimering MB, editor: *Recent advances in the pathogenesis, prevention and management of type 2 diabetes and its complications*, Rijeka (Croatia), 2011, Intech, pp 45–66.

86. Fruchart J-C, Sacks F, Hermans MP, et al: Executive statement: the Residual Risk Reduction Initiative: a call to action to reduce residual vascular risk in dyslipidemic patients. A condensed position paper by the Residual Risk Reduction Initiative (R3i), *Diab Vasc Dis Res* 5:319–335, 2008.

87. Fruchart J-C, Sacks F, Hermans MP, et al: for the Residual Risk Reduction Initiative: The Residual Risk Reduction Initiative: a call to action to reduce residual vascular risk in patients with dyslipidemia, *Am J Cardiol* 102(Suppl):1–34, 2008.

88. Hermans MP: Impact of fenofibrate on type 2 diabetes patients with features of the metabolic syndrome: subgroup analysis from FIELD, *Curr Cardiol Rev* 6:112–118, 2010.

89. Fruchart J-C, Sacks FM, Hermans MP: Implications of the ACCORD lipid study : perspective from the Residual Risk Reduction Initiative (R3i), *Curr Med Res Opin* 26:1793–1797, 2010.

90. Hermans MP, Sacks F, Ahn SA, Rousseau MF: Non–HDL-cholesterol as valid surrogate to apolipoprotein B100 measurement in diabetes: Discriminant Ratio and unbiased equivalence, *Cardiovasc Diabetol* 10:20, 2011.

91. Hermans MP, Ahn SA, Rousseau MF: Log(TG)/HDL-C is related to both residual cardiometabolic risk and beta-cell function loss in type 2 diabetes males, *Cardiovasc Diabetol* 9:88, 2010.

92. Hermans MP, Ahn SA, Rousseau MF: The atherogenic dyslipidemia ratio [log(TG)/HDL-C] is associated with residual vascular risk, beta-cell function loss and microangiopathy in type 2 diabetes females, *Lipids Health Dis* 11:132, 2012.

93. Querton L, Buysschaert M, Hermans MP: Hypertriglyceridemia and residual dyslipidemia in statin-treated, high-risk diabetic patients achieving very-low plasma LDL-cholesterol levels, *J Clin Lipidol* 6:434–442, 2012.

94. Volek JS, Fernandez ML, Feinman RD, Phinney SD: Dietary carbohydrate restriction induces a unique metabolic state positively affecting AD, fatty acid partitioning, and metabolic syndrome, *Prog Lipid Res* 47:307–318, 2008.

95. Katcher HI, Hill AM, Lanford JL, et al: Lifestyle approaches and dietary strategies to lower LDL-cholesterol and triglycerides and raise HDL-cholesterol, *Endocrinol Metab Clin North Am* 38:45–78, 2009.

96. Bantle JP, Wylie-Rosett J, Albright AL, et al: American Diabetes Association Nutrition recommendations and interventions for diabetes: a position statement of the American Diabetes Association, *Diabetes Care* 31(Suppl 1):S61–S78, 2008.

97. Look AHEAD Research Group, Wing RR, Bolin P, et al: Cardiovascular effects of intensive lifestyle intervention in type 2 diabetes, *N Engl J Med* 369:145–154, 2013.

98. European Association for Cardiovascular Prevention and Rehabilitation, Reiner Z, Catapano AL, et al: ESC Committee for Practice Guidelines (CPG) 2008–2010 and 2010–2012 Committees: ESC/EAS Guidelines for the management of dyslipidaemias: the Task Force for the management of dyslipidaemias of the European Society of Cardiology (ESC) and the European Atherosclerosis Society (EAS), *Eur Heart J* 32:1769–1818, 2011.

99. American Diabetes Association: Standards of medical care in diabetes - 2012, *Diabetes Care* 35(Suppl 1):S11–S63, 2012.

100. National Cholesterol Education Program (NCEP) Expert Panel on Detection, Evaluation, and Treatment of High Blood Cholesterol in Adults (Adult Treatment Panel III): Third report of the National Cholesterol Education Program (NCEP) Expert Panel on Detection, Evaluation, and Treatment of High Blood Cholesterol in Adults (Adult Treatment Panel III) final report, *Circulation* 106:3143–3421, 2002.

101. Grundy SM, Cleeman JI, Merz CN, et al: Implications of recent clinical trials for the National Cholesterol Education Program Adult Treatment Panel III guidelines, *Circulation* 110:227–239, 2004.

102. Grundy SM, Cleeman JI, Daniels SR, et al: American Heart Association, National Heart, Lung, and Blood Institute: Diagnosis and management of the metabolic syndrome: an American Heart Association/National Heart, Lung, and Blood Institute Scientific Statement, *Circulation* 112:2735–2752, 2005.

103. Graham I, Atar D, Borch-Johnsen K, et al: European guidelines on cardiovascular disease prevention in clinical practice. Fourth Joint Task Force of the European Society of Cardiology and other Societies on Cardiovascular Disease Prevention in Clinical Practice. Executive summary, *Eur Heart J* 28:2375–2414, 2007.

104. Buse JB, Ginsberg HN, Bakris GL, et al: American Heart Association, American Diabetes Association: Primary prevention of cardiovascular diseases in people with diabetes mellitus: a scientific statement from the American Heart Association and the American Diabetes Association., *Circulation* 115:114–126, 2007.

105. Brunzell JD, Davidson M, Furberg CD, et al: Lipoprotein management in patients with cardiometabolic risk: consensus conference report from the American Diabetes Association and the American College of Cardiology Foundation, *J Am Coll Cardiol* 51:1512–1524, 2008.

106. Genest J, McPherson R, Frohlich J, et al: 2009 Canadian Cardiovascular Society/Canadian guidelines for the diagnosis and treatment of dyslipidemia and prevention of cardiovascular disease in the adult - 2009 recommendations, *Can J Cardiol* 25:567–579, 2009.

107. Greenland P, Alpert JS, Beller GA, et al: American College of Cardiology Foundation, American Heart Association: 2010 ACCF/AHA guideline for assessment of cardiovascular risk in asymptomatic adults: a report of the American College of Cardiology Foundation/American Heart Association Task Force on Practice Guidelines, *J Am Coll Cardiol* 56:e50–e103, 2010.

108. Chapman MJ, Ginsberg HN, Amarenco P, et al: European Atherosclerosis Society Consensus Panel: Triglyceride-rich lipoproteins and high-density lipoprotein cholesterol in patients at high risk of cardiovascular disease: evidence and guidance for management, *Eur Heart J* 32:1345–1361, 2011.

109. CTT-Cholesterol treatment trialists' (CTT) Collaborators: Efficacy and safety of cholesterol-lowering treatment: prospective meta-analysis of data from 90056 participants in 14 randomised trials of statins, *Lancet* 366:1267–1278, 2005.

110. Costa J, Borges M, David C, Vaz Carneiro A: Efficacy of lipid lowering drug treatment for diabetic and non-diabetic patients: meta-analysis of randomised controlled trials, *BMJ* 332:1115–1118, 2006.

111. CTT-Cholesterol treatment trialists' (CTT) Collaborators: Efficacy of cholesterol-lowering therapy in 18,686 people with diabetes in 14 randomised trials of statins: a meta-analysis, *Lancet* 371:117–125, 2008.

112. Brugts JJ, Yetgin T, Hoeks SE, et al: The benefits of statins in people without established cardiovascular disease but with cardiovascular risk factors: meta-analysis of randomised controlled trials, *BMJ* 338:B2376, 2009.

113. Brunham LR, Kruit JK, Pape TD, et al: Cell ABCA1 influences insulin secretion, glucose homeostasis and response to thiazolidinedione treatment, *Nat Med* 13:340–347, 2007.

114. Brunham LR, Kruit JK, Verchere CB, Hayden MR: Cholesterol in islet dysfunction and type 2 diabetes, *J Clin Invest* 118:403–408, 2008.

115. Fryirs M, Barter PJ, Rye KA: Cholesterol metabolism and pancreatic beta-cell function, *Curr Opin Lipidol* 20:159–164, 2009.

116. Kruit JK, Brunham LR, Verchere CB, Hayden MR: HDL and LDL cholesterol significantly influence beta-cell function in type 2 diabetes mellitus, *Curr Opin Lipidol* 21:178–185, 2010.

117. Kruit JK, Kremer PHC, Kai L, et al: Cholesterol efflux via ATP-binding cassette transporter A1 (ABCA1) and cholesterol uptake via the LDL receptor influences cholesterol-induced impairment of beta cell function in mice, *Diabetologia* 53:1110–1119, 2010.

118. von Eckardstein A, Sibler RA: Possible contributions of lipoproteins and cholesterol to the pathogenesis of diabetes mellitus type 2, *Curr Opin Lipidol* 22:26–32, 2011.

119. Preiss D, Seshasai SRK, Welsh P, et al: Risk of incident diabetes with intensive-dose compared with moderate-dose statin therapy. A meta-analysis, *JAMA* 305:2556–2564, 2011.

120. Jukema JW, Cannon CP, de Craen AJM, et al: The controversies of statin therapy. Weighing the evidence, *J Am Coll Cardiol* 60:875–881, 2012.

121. Ridker PM, Pradhan A, MacFadyen JG, et al: Cardiovascular benefits and diabetes risks of statin therapy in primary prevention: an analysis from the JUPITER trial, *Lancet* 380:565–571, 2012.

122. Stone NJ, Robinson J, Lichtenstein AH, et al: 2013 ACC/AHA guideline on the treatment of blood cholesterol to reduce atherosclerotic cardiovascular risk in adults: a report of the American College of Cardiology/American Heart Association Task Force on Practice Guidelines, *J Am Coll Cardiol*, 2013, Nov 12.

123. Morrone D, Weintraub WS, Toth PP, et al: Lipid-altering efficacy of ezetimibe plus statin and statin monotherapy and identification of factors associated with treatment response: a pooled analysis of over 21,000 subjects from 27 clinical trials, *Atherosclerosis* 223:251–261, 2012.

124. Villines TC, Stanek EJ, Devine PJ, et al: The ARBITER 6-HALTS Trial (Arterial Biology for the Investigation of the Treatment Effects of Reducing Cholesterol 6-HDL and LDL Treatment Strategies in Atherosclerosis): final results and the impact of medication adherence, dose, and treatment duration, *J Am Coll Cardiol* 55:2721–2726, 2010.

125. Kamanna VS, Kashyap ML: Mechanism of action of niacin, *Am J Cardiol* 101(Suppl):20B–26B, 2008.

126. Coronary Drug Project Research Group: Clofibrate and niacin in coronary heart disease, *JAMA* 231:360–381, 1975.

127. Carlson LA, Rosenhamer G: Reduction of mortality in the Stockholm Ischaemic Heart Disease Secondary Prevention Study by combined treatment with clofibrate and nicotinic acid, *Acta Med Scand* 223:405–418, 1988.

128. Brown BG, Zhao XQ, Chait A, et al: Simvastatin and niacin, antioxidant vitamins, or the combination for the prevention of coronary disease, *N Engl J Med* 345:1583–1592, 2001.

129. AIM-HIGH Investigators, Boden WE, Probstfield JL, Anderson T, et al: Niacin in patients with low HDL cholesterol levels receiving intensive statin therapy, *N Engl J Med* 365:2255–2267, 2011.

130. Guyton JR, Slee AE, Anderson T, et al: Relationship of lipoproteins to cardiovascular events: the AIM-HIGH Trial (Atherothrombosis Intervention in Metabolic Syndrome With Low HDL/High Triglycerides and Impact on Global Health Outcomes), *J Am Coll Cardiol* 62:1580–1584, 2013.

131. HPS2-THRIVE Collaborative Group: HPS2-THRIVE randomized placebo-controlled trial in 25 673 high-risk patients of ER niacin/laropiprant: trial design, pre-specified muscle and liver outcomes, and reasons for stopping study treatment, *Eur Heart J* 34:1279–1291, 2013.

132. Lavigne PM, Karas RH: The current state of niacin in cardiovascular disease prevention: a systematic review and meta-regression, *J Am Coll Cardiol* 61:440–446, 2013.

133. Barter PJ, Caulfield M, Eriksson M, et al: ILLUMINATE Investigators: Effects of torcetrapib in patients at high risk for coronary events, *N Engl J Med* 357:2109–2122, 2007.

134. Schwartz GG, Olsson AG, Abt M, et al: Effects of dalcetrapib in patients with a recent acute coronary syndrome, *N Engl J Med* 367:2089–2099, 2012.

135. Fruchart JC, Davignon J, Hermans MP, et al: Residual macrovascular risk in 2013: what have we learned? *Cardiovasc Diabetol*, 2013, in press.

136. A Study of Evacetrapib in High-Risk Vascular Disease (ACCELERATE) [http://clinicaltrials.gov/show/NCT01687998].

137. Forrest MJ, Bloomfield D, Briscoe RJ, et al: Torcetrapib-induced blood pressure elevation is independent of CETP inhibition and is accompanied by increased circulating levels of aldosterone, *Br J Pharmacol* 154:1465–1473, 2008.

138. Li C, Zhang W, Zhou F, et al: Cholesteryl ester transfer protein inhibitors in the treatment of dyslipidemia: a systematic review and meta-analysis, *PLoS One* 8:e77049, 2013.

139. Birjmohun RS, Hutten BA, Kastelein JJP, Stroes ESG: Efficacy and safety of high-density lipoprotein cholesterol-increasing compounds. A meta-analysis of randomized controlled trials, *J Am Coll Cardiol* 45:185–197, 2005.

140. Jun M, Foote C, Lv J, et al: Effects of fibrates on cardiovascular outcomes: a systematic review and meta-analysis, *Lancet* 375:1875–1884, 2010.

141. Lee M, Saver JL, Towfighi A, et al: Efficacy of fibrates for cardiovascular risk reduction in persons with AD: a meta-analysis, *Atherosclerosis* 217:492–498, 2011.

142. Jun M, Zhu B, Tonelli M, et al: Effects of fibrates in kidney disease. A systematic review and meta-analysis, *J Am Coll Cardiol* 60:2061–2071, 2012.

143. Yokoyama M, Origasa H, Matsuzaki M, et al: Effects of eicosapentaenoic acid on major coronary events in hypercholesterolaemic patients (JELIS): a randomized open-label, blinded endpoint analysis, *Lancet* 369:1090–1098, 2007.

144. Saito Y, Yokoyama M, Origasa H, et al: Effects of EPA on coronary artery disease in hypercholesterolemic patients with multiple risk factors: sub-analysis of primary prevention cases from the Japan EPA Lipid Intervention Study (JELIS), *Atherosclerosis* 200:135–140, 2008.

145. Oikawa S, Yokoyama M, Origasa H, et al: Suppressive effect of EPA on the incidence of coronary events in hypercholesterolemia with impaired glucose metabolism: subanalysis of the Japan EPA Lipid Intervention Study (JELIS), *Atherosclerosis* 206:535–539, 2009.

146. Bosch J, Gerstein HC, Dagenais GR, et al: for the ORIGIN Trial Investigators: n-3 fatty acids and cardiovascular outcomes in patients with dysglycemia, *N Engl J Med* 367:309–318, 2012.

147. Rizos EC, Ntzani EE, Bika E, et al: Association between omega-3 fatty acid supplementation and risk of major cardiovascular disease events: a systematic review and meta-analysis, *JAMA* 308:1024–1033, 2012.

148. Griffin SJ, Borch-Johnsen K, Davies MJ, et al: Effect of early intensive multifactorial therapy on 5-year cardiovascular outcomes in individuals with type 2 diabetes detected by screening (ADDITION-Europe): a cluster-randomised trial, *Lancet* 378:156–167, 2011.

149. Hermans MP: Diabetic macro- and microvascular disease in type 2 diabetes, *Diabetes Vasc Dis Res* 4(Suppl 2):7–11, 2007.

150. Task Force Members, Rydén L, Grant PJ, et al: ESC Guidelines on diabetes, pre-diabetes, and cardiovascular diseases developed in collaboration with the EASD: the Task Force on diabetes, pre-diabetes, and cardiovascular diseases of the European Society of Cardiology (ESC) and developed in collaboration with the European Association for the Study of Diabetes (EASD), *Eur Heart J* 34:3035–3087, 2013.

151. Haffner SM, Lehto S, Rönnemaa T, et al: Mortality from coronary heart disease in subjects with type 2 diabetes and in non-diabetic subjects with and without prior myocardial infarction, *N Engl J Med* 339:229–234, 1998.

152. Juutilainen A, Lehto S, Rönnemaa T, et al: Type 2 diabetes as a 'coronary heart disease equivalent'. An 18-year prospective population-based study in Finnish subjects, *Diabetes Care* 28:2901–2907, 2005.

153. Buyken AE, von Eckardstein A, Schulte H, et al: Type 2 diabetes mellitus and risk of coronary heart disease: results of the 10-year follow-up of the PROCAM study, *Eur J Cardiovasc Prev Rehabil* 14:230–236, 2007.

154. Mazzone T, Chait A, Plutzky J: Cardiovascular disease risk in type 2 diabetes mellitus: insights from mechanistic studies, *Lancet* 371:1800–1809, 2008.

155. Schramm TK, Gislason GH, Køber L, et al: Diabetes patients requiring glucose-lowering therapy and non-diabetics with a prior myocardial infarction carry the same cardiovascular risk: a population study of 3.3 million people, *Circulation* 117:1945–1954, 2008.

156. Ballantyne CM, Raichlen JS, Cain VA: Statin therapy alters the relationship between apolipoprotein B and low-density lipoprotein cholesterol and non–high-density lipoprotein cholesterol targets in high-risk patients: the MERCURY II (Measuring Effective Reductions in Cholesterol Using Rosuvastatin) trial, *J Am Coll Cardiol* 52:626–632, 2008.

157. Sulkes D, Brown BG, Krauss RM, et al: The editor's roundtable: expanded versus standard lipid panels in assessing and managing cardiovascular risk, *Am J Cardiol* 101: 828–842, 2008.

158. Sniderman A, Williams K, Cobbaert C: ApoB versus non–HDL-C: what to do when they disagree, *Curr Atheroscler Rep* 11:358–363, 2009.

159. Hermans MP: Prevention of microvascular diabetic complications by fenofibrate: lessons from FIELD and ACCORD, *Diab Vasc Dis Res* 8:180–189, 2011.

160. EAS Guidelines Committee: *New guidelines in USA: how do they compare with the EAS/ESC guidelines for the management of dyslipidaemia?* EAS website updates, November 22th, 2013. www.eas-society.org/News.aspx?newsId=316.

16 Effect of Antiplatelet Therapy on Coronary Heart Disease Risk in Patients with Diabetes Mellitus

Michelle L. O'Donoghue and Deepak L. Bhatt

Platelets play a central role in the pathobiology of atherogenesis and atherothrombosis. Therefore therapies that are directed toward platelet inhibition are widely used in patients with established coronary heart disease (CHD) or in moderate- to high-risk individuals for primary prevention of cardiovascular (CV) events.[1] As our armamentarium of potent antiplatelet therapies continues to expand, there is growing interest in identifying the appropriate groups of patients who will derive the greatest benefit from more potent therapies. To that end, several studies over the past few decades have highlighted that individuals with diabetes mellitus (DM) exhibit abnormalities in platelet function that place them at increased risk of adverse outcomes, as compared with their nondiabetic counterparts (see also **Chapter 10**).[2] Although the mechanisms that contribute to platelet hyperreactivity in diabetic patients continue to be elucidated, it appears that diabetic platelets are characterized by the dysregulation of several signaling pathways that occur both at the level of the platelet receptor and with subsequent downstream signaling.[3,4] In addition, glycosylation may impair endothelial function and promote oxidative stress, thereby further promoting platelet reactivity and procoagulant activity.[1] There is therefore a priori biologic plausibility to support the concept that diabetic patients may derive enhanced benefit from particular therapies directed toward blocking the platelet. However, differences in platelet biology in diabetic patients may also contribute to diminished antiplatelet drug responsiveness. This chapter reviews the use of established and novel oral antiplatelet therapies in diabetic patients for use in primary or secondary prevention of CV events.

ASPIRIN

To date, aspirin remains the cornerstone of antiplatelet therapy in the primary and secondary prevention of CV events. Aspirin selectively acetylates the hydroxyl group of a serine residue leading to irreversible inhibition of the cyclooxygenase-1 (COX-1) enzyme.[5] In turn, inhibition of the COX-1 enzyme blocks downstream production of thromboxane A_2 (TXA$_2$; **Fig. 16-1**), thereby preventing thromboxane-mediated platelet aggregation and vasoconstriction. Because the platelet is enucleate, it is unable to

resynthesize COX-1 and the effects of aspirin persist throughout the lifetime of the platelet.[5]

Aspirin in Primary Prevention

Although its role in secondary prevention is well established, the clinical efficacy of aspirin in primary prevention remains an ongoing area of investigation. Several large primary prevention trials of aspirin have been conducted in the general population, and investigators have subsequently evaluated the benefit of aspirin within their diabetic subgroups.[6-8] Although limited by small numbers of diabetic patients and by post hoc design, many trials were able to demonstrate a consistent benefit of aspirin in the primary prevention of CV events for both their diabetic and nondiabetic patients.[6,7] These results were supported by the Early Treatment Diabetic Retinopathy Study (ETDRS), which included a mixed population of 3711 patients with DM with or without a history of CHD who were randomized to aspirin 650 mg daily or placebo.[9] Although aspirin did not reduce the primary endpoint of all-cause death (hazard ratio [HR] 0.91, 95% confidence interval [CI] 0.75-1.11), a favorable trend was observed toward a reduction in fatal or nonfatal myocardial infarction (MI) at 5 years that did not achieve statistical significance (HR 0.83, 95% CI 0.66-1.04).[9]

In contrast, a benefit for aspirin could not be definitively demonstrated in diabetic patients enrolled in the Primary Prevention Project (PPP), a randomized trial of low-dose aspirin (100 mg daily) versus placebo in 4495 patients with one or more CV risk factors.[8] Although underpowered to detect a significant benefit within the diabetic subgroup (n = 1031), the investigators were unable to demonstrate a significant reduction in CV death, MI, or stroke in diabetic patients (HR 0.90, 95% CI 0.50-1.62) or in total CV events (HR 0.89, 95% CI 0.62-1.26). Moreover, an unfavorable trend was observed toward an increased risk of CV death (HR 1.23, 95% CI 0.69-2.19) in aspirin-treated diabetic patients. In contrast, a more consistent benefit was seen with aspirin in nondiabetic patients with regard to reduction in the risk of CV death, MI, or stroke (HR 0.59, 95% CI 0.37-0.94), total CV events (HR 0.69, 95% CI 0.53-0.90), and CV death (HR 0.32, 95% CI 0.14-0.72).[8]

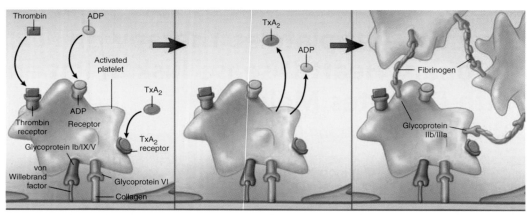

FIGURE 16-1 The platelet has multiple ligands that contribute to pathways leading to platelet activation including thrombin, adenosine diphosphate (ADP), von Willebrand factor, and thromboxane A_2 (TXA$_2$). The activated platelet then releases prothrombotic factors including ADP and TXA$_2$, thereby further amplifying platelet activation. A platelet latticework is formed when fibrinogen cross-links activated platelets via the glycoprotein IIb/IIIa receptor. The P2Y12 subtype of the ADP receptor is the site of action for established and novel compounds, including ticlopidine, clopidogrel, prasugrel, ticagrelor, and elinogrel. *(Modified from Bhatt DL: Intensifying platelet inhibition—navigating between Scylla and Charybdis, N Engl J Med 357:2078-2081, 2007.)*

Because individual trials of aspirin therapy in primary prevention enrolled relatively few diabetic patients, De Berardis and colleagues combined data from six trials and 10,117 patients to examine the clinical efficacy of aspirin to reduce major CV events in primary prevention.[10] The meta-analysis demonstrated a benefit of aspirin in the overall study population, yet the authors were unable to identify a statistically significant benefit in the diabetic subgroup. Although a directional trend was observed, aspirin did not significantly reduce the risk of major CV events in diabetic patients as compared with placebo (HR 0.90, 95% CI 0.81-1.00). Furthermore, aspirin did not reduce either CV mortality (HR 0.94, 95% CI 0.72-1.23) or all-cause mortality (HR 0.93, 95% CI 0.82-1.05) in diabetic patients. However, limitations of the meta-analysis included evidence of significant heterogeneity across trials for key endpoints including MI. To that end, aspirin significantly reduced the risk of MI in men (HR 0.57, 95% CI 0.34-0.94), but did not reduce the risk of MI in women (HR 1.08, 95% CI 0.71-1.65; P for interaction $=0.056$). Because women had a higher prevalence of DM, sex-restricted enrollment in some of the trials may have contributed to the observed heterogeneity.[6,11] Consistent findings were observed in an updated meta-analysis that included individuals with DM across nine trials of aspirin in primary prevention. Aspirin reduced the risk of CHD events by 9%, but the results were not statistically significant (relative risk 0.91, 95% CI 0.79-1.05). Similarly, the use of aspirin was associated with a nonsignificant 10% reduction in the risk of stroke (relative risk 0.90, 95% CI 0.71-1.13; **Fig. 16-2**).[12] These findings therefore raised concerns that the antiplatelet effects of aspirin were insufficient to attenuate risk of CV events in diabetic patients with baseline abnormalities in platelet function.

Because subgroup analyses from randomized trials may yield spurious results, dedicated trials of aspirin for primary prevention in diabetic patients have since been completed or are still ongoing. The Japanese Primary Prevention of Atherosclerosis with Aspirin for Diabetes (JPAD) study was the first prospectively designed trial to evaluate the use of low-dose aspirin (81 or 100 mg daily) versus placebo in 2539 type 2 diabetic patients in Japan aged 30 to 85 years and without a known history of atherosclerotic disease.[13] After a median of 4.37 years, only 154 atherosclerotic events (including fatal or

nonfatal ischemic heart disease, fatal or nonfatal stroke, and peripheral arterial disease [PAD]) occurred during follow-up and the trial was therefore unable to demonstrate clinical efficacy with aspirin in diabetic patients despite a directional trend (HR 0.80, 95% CI 0.58-1.10, $P=0.16$).[13] In addition to being underpowered, other limitations of the trial included its open label design, which introduced the possibility of bias. However, among the subgroup of patients older than 65 years, aspirin reduced the risk of atherosclerotic events by 32% ($P=0.047$). The incidence of hemorrhagic stroke or gastrointestinal (GI) bleeding was low and did not differ significantly between groups.[13]

Subsequently, the Prevention of Progression of Arterial Disease and Diabetes (POPADAD) trial evaluated the efficacy of low-dose aspirin (100 mg daily) versus placebo in 1276 adults in Scotland older than 40 years with type 1 or type 2 DM and an ankle brachial pressure index below 0.99 in the absence of symptomatic CV disease.[14] Although the trial was relatively small, the incidence of CV events (death from congestive heart failure [CHF] or stroke, nonfatal MI or stroke, or amputation because of critical limb ischemia) was almost identical between treatment arms during a median of 6.7 years follow-up (116 versus 117 events; HR 0.98, 95% CI 0.76-1.26). Aspirin did not reduce the risk of death from CHD or stroke (HR 1.23, 95% CI 0.79-1.93). GI bleeding was infrequent, and its incidence did not differ between groups.[14]

In light of these conflicting data, the use of aspirin in primary prevention continues to be a topic of debate. In particular, any signal suggesting efficacy must be weighed against the potential risks of treatment. In a large population-based cohort of individuals in Italy, the use of aspirin was associated with a relative 55% increased incidence of major bleeding over a median of 5.7 years in the overall cohort, as compared with patients not taking aspirin.[15] The risk of bleeding was increased in individuals over the age of 70, those with a higher risk of GI disease, and by concomitant use of NSAIDs. Irrespective of aspirin use, patients with DM were observed to have a 36% higher incidence of major bleeding episodes, including an increased risk of GI and intracranial bleeding, as compared with nondiabetic patients.[15] Of interest, the use of aspirin did not appear to

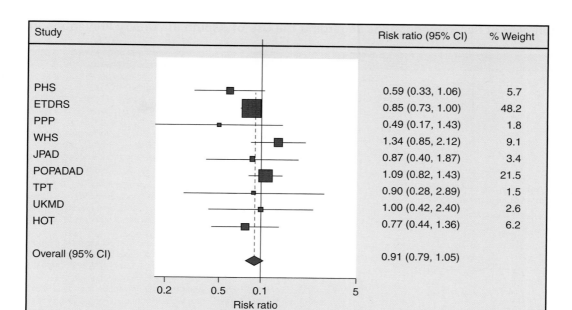

A

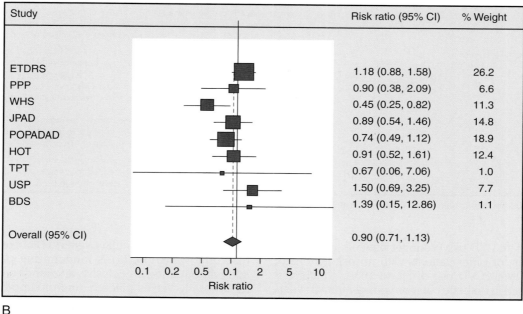

B

FIGURE 16-2 A meta-analysis of randomized trials that examined the effects of aspirin on the risk on CHD events **(A)** and stroke **(B)** in diabetic patients without an overt history of CV disease. Although there was a directional trend toward a reduction in the risk of CHD events and stroke with aspirin in diabetic patients, this benefit was not statistically significant. *(From Pignone M, Alberts MJ, Colwell JA, et al: Aspirin for primary prevention of cardiovascular events in people with diabetes: a position statement of the American Diabetes Association, a scientific statement of the American Heart Association, and an expert consensus document of the American College of Cardiology Foundation, Circulation 121:2694-2701, 2010.)*

be associated with an increased risk of bleeding for diabetic patients. However, it remains unknown whether the absence of a bleeding signal with aspirin in diabetic patients might be explained by a diminished pharmacodynamic response to aspirin in diabetic patients with abnormal platelet biology, or attributable to other factors.

Based on the weight of the evidence to date, the American Diabetes Association (ADA) updated its recommendations in 2010 to consider low-dose aspirin therapy (75 to 162 mg/day) in primary prevention in diabetic individuals (men older than 50 years, women older than 60 years) at increased CV risk (10-year risk greater than 10%) with at least one or more major CV risk factor including family history of CV disease, hypertension, albuminuria, dyslipidemia, or current tobacco use (**Table 16-1**).[16] In 2010, an expert panel that included representatives from the ADA, the American College of Cardiology Foundation (ACCF), and the American Heart Association (AHA) issued similar recommendations that included the use of aspirin (75 to 162 mg/day) in individuals (men older than 50 years, women older than 60 years) at increased CV risk (10-year risk >10%) and with established CV risk factors, who were not believed to be at increased risk of bleeding.[12] They also noted that low-dose (75-162 mg/day) aspirin could be considered for those with

TABLE 16-1 Summary of Recommendations Regarding the Use of Aspirin in Primary Prevention in Diabetic Individuals

ORGANIZATION	YEAR	RECOMMENDATION
American Diabetes Association[16]	2014	Consider aspirin therapy (75-162 mg/day) as a primary prevention strategy in those with type 1 or type 2 DM at increased CV risk (10-year risk >10%). This includes most men older than 50 years or women older than 60 years who have at least one additional major risk factor (family history of CVD, hypertension, smoking, dyslipidemia, or albuminuria). (Level of evidence: C) There is not sufficient evidence to recommend aspirin for primary prevention in lower-risk individuals, such as men younger than 50 years or women younger than 60 years without other major risk factors. In patients in these age groups with multiple other risk factors, clinical judgment is required. (C)
ADA, American Heart Association (AHA), American College of Cardiology Foundation (ACCF)[12]	2010	Low-dose (75-162 mg/day) aspirin use for prevention is reasonable for adults with DM and no previous history of vascular disease who are at increased CVD risk (10-year risk of CVD events >10%) and who are not at increased risk for bleeding (based on a history of previous GI bleeding or peptic ulcer disease or concurrent use of other medications that increase bleeding risk, such as NSAIDS or warfarin). Adults with diabetes who are at increased CVD risk include most men over age 50 years and women over age 60 years who have one or more of the following additional major risk factors: smoking, hypertension, dyslipidemia, family history of premature CVD, and albuminuria. (ACCF/AHA Class IIa, level of evidence B; ADA level of evidence C) Aspirin should not be recommended for CVD prevention for adults with DM at low CVD risk (men younger than 50 years and women younger than 60 years with no major additional CVD risk factors; 10-year CVD risk under 5%) because the potential adverse effects from bleeding offset the potential benefits. (ACCF/AHA Class III, level of evidence C; ADA level of evidence C) Low-dose (75-162 mg/day) aspirin use for prevention might be considered for those with DM at intermediate CVD risk (younger patients with one or more risk factors, or older patients with no risk factors, or patients with 10-year CVD risk of 5%-10%) until further research is available. (ACCF/AHA Class IIb, level of evidence C; ADA level of evidence E)
U.S. Preventive Services Task Force[17,18]	2009	In men aged 45-79 years, encourage aspirin use when potential CVD benefit (MIs prevented) outweighs the potential harm of GI hemorrhage (irrespective of whether the individual has DM). In women aged 55-79 years, encourage aspirin use when potential CVD benefit (ischemic strokes prevented) outweighs the potential harm of gastrointestinal hemorrhage (irrespective of whether the individual has DM). Do not encourage aspirin use for MI prevention in men younger than 45 years or for stroke prevention in women younger than 55 years (irrespective of whether the individual has DM). There is insufficient evidence to recommend the use of aspirin for primary prevention in individuals aged 80 years or older.
European Society of Cardiology[19]	2012	Antiplatelet therapy with aspirin is not recommended for people with DM who do not have clinical evidence of atherosclerotic disease. (Level of evidence A)

CVD = Cardiovascular disease; NSAIDs = nonsteroidal anti-inflammatory drugs.

DM at intermediate CVD risk (younger patients with one or more risk factors, or older patients with no risk factors, or patients with 10-year CVD risk of 5% to 10%).[12] Aspirin is not recommended in diabetic patients younger than 21 years because of the risk of Reye syndrome, and the role of aspirin in diabetic patients younger than 30 years remains largely untested. The U.S. Preventive Services Task Force has recommended aspirin use in men aged 45 to 79 years and women 55 to 79 years but has not differentiated their recommendations on the presence or absence of DM.[17,18] In contrast, the European Society of Cardiology guidelines for CV prevention do not recommend aspirin for primary prevention regardless of baseline risk, including in patients with DM (see **Table 16-1**).[19]

Because trials to date have yielded inconclusive results, the net clinical benefit of aspirin in the primary prevention of CV events in diabetic patients remains an ongoing area of investigation (**Table 16-2**). The Aspirin and Simvastatin Combination for Cardiovascular Events Prevention Trial in Diabetes (ACCEPT-D, ISRCTN48110081) study is an open-label trial that is randomizing individuals with type 1 or type 2 DM and without clinical evidence of vascular disease to aspirin with statin or statin alone to evaluate whether aspirin will reduce a first CV event. Similarly, the ongoing ASCEND

(A Study of Cardiovascular Events in Diabetes) trial (clinical-trials.gov NCT00135226) is randomizing patients with DM and without known occlusive arterial disease to 100 mg of aspirin daily versus placebo and/or supplementation with 1 g of omega-3 fatty acids daily or placebo.

Aspirin in Secondary Prevention

Although the role of aspirin in primary prevention continues to be investigated, the use of aspirin in stable and unstable secondary prevention is well established. Whereas smaller studies had been suggestive, the first randomized trial that definitively demonstrated aspirin's efficacy in patients with acute MI was the Second International Study of Infarct Survival (ISIS-2), which demonstrated a 23% reduction in the odds of vascular death with aspirin at 5 weeks when compared with placebo.[20] Subsequent trials have since demonstrated a consistent benefit for aspirin across the spectrum of acute coronary syndrome (ACS) (see also **Chapter 21**).[1]

The Antithrombotic Trialists' Collaboration (ATC) combined data from 287 secondary prevention studies of oral antiplatelet agents, mostly aspirin, and included a total of 212,000 individuals with acute vascular disease, established vascular disease, or risk factors for vascular disease.[21]

TABLE 16-2 Ongoing Trials of Aspirin for Primary Prevention in Individuals with Type 1 or Type 2 DM

TRIAL NAME	DESIGN	POPULATION	INTERVENTION	OUTCOME
Aspirin and Simvastatin Combination for Cardiovascular Events Prevention Trial in Diabetes (ACCEPT-D; ISRCTN48110081)	Open label, randomized, parallel group	Approximately 5170 patients; type 1 or type 2 DM without clinical evidence of vascular disease and with an indication for statin therapy	Aspirin (100 mg/day) plus simvastatin versus simvastatin alone	CV death, MI, stroke, or CV hospitalization
A Study of Cardiovascular Events in Diabetes trial (ASCEND; clinicaltrials.gov NCT00135226)	Double-blind, 2 × 2 factorial randomized design	Approximately 15,480 patients; type 1 or type 2 DM, older than 40 years, and without known history of vascular disease	Aspirin (100 mg/day) versus placebo (2 × 2: 1 g/day omega-3 ethyl esters versus placebo)	Vascular death, MI, or stroke (excluding cerebral hemorrhage)

Overall, in patients with established CV disease, antiplatelet therapy reduced the odds of recurrent CV events by 22% and of nonfatal stroke by 25%. Although individuals with DM had a higher absolute event rate than nondiabetic patients, the relative benefit of antiplatelet therapy toward reducing vascular events was consistent across patient groups. For every 1000 diabetic patients treated with aspirin, it was estimated that 42 vascular events could be prevented with use of antiplatelet therapy.[21]

Of note, it was observed in the ATC analysis that lower doses of aspirin (75 to 150 mg/day) appeared to be as efficacious as high doses of aspirin (>150 mg/day). Furthermore, the use of lower doses of aspirin was associated with a reduced risk of bleeding complications as compared with higher doses. The evidence to support the use of lower doses of aspirin was also supported by an observational analysis from the Clopidogrel for High Atherothrombotic Risk and Ischemic Stabilization, Management, and Avoidance (CHARISMA) trial that demonstrated that aspirin doses exceeding 100 mg daily were not associated with increased efficacy as compared with lower doses in patients with stable CV disease or CV risk factors.[22] Moreover, there was an unfavorable trend toward a higher risk of CV death, MI, or stroke (adjusted HR 1.16, 95% CI 0.93-1.14) and increased risk of severe or life-threatening bleeding (adjusted HR 1.30, 95% CI 0.83-2.04) when aspirin doses above 100 mg daily were combined with clopidogrel. More recently, the question of optimal aspirin dosage was directly addressed in a randomized clinical trial of low-dose (325 mg loading dose, 75 to 100 mg daily) versus higher-dose aspirin (325 mg loading dose, 300 to 325 mg daily) in patients with ACS.[23] The use of higher-dose aspirin did not reduce the risk of CV death, MI, or stroke (HR 0.97, 95% CI 0.86-1.09) as compared with low-dose aspirin after 30 days, but increased the risk of minor bleeding by 13% (HR 1.13, 95% CI 1.00-1.27, $P=0.04$).[23]

The ADA currently recommends the use of low-dose aspirin (75 to 162 mg/day) for secondary prevention of CV events (including stroke) in all diabetic patients without contraindication. Based on the strength of the data, the use of low-dose aspirin is now supported by the ACC/AHA guidelines in patients after non–ST-elevation ACS or percutaneous coronary intervention (PCI) (see also **Chapter 21**).[24,25]

P2Y12 RECEPTOR ANTAGONISTS

Although CV events are not always platelet mediated, platelet activation and aggregation may occur in the presence of aspirin through pathways unrelated to TXA_2 (see **Fig. 16-1**). Therefore this unmet need has prompted the development of alternate oral antiplatelet drugs to use in combination with or as a substitute for aspirin. The P2Y1 and P2Y12 receptors on the platelet cell surface play a tandem role in contributing to platelet activation and aggregation via adenosine diphosphate (ADP)–dependent pathways. The P2Y1 receptor is responsible for an initial weak and transient phase of platelet aggregation, whereas ADP signaling pathways mediated by G_i-coupled P2Y12 receptor activation lead to sustained platelet aggregation and stabilization of the platelet aggregate.[26] The P2Y12 receptor is the target for many established and novel antiplatelet agents, including ticlopidine, clopidogrel, prasugrel, ticagrelor, elinogrel, and cangrelor.

Ticlopidine

Ticlopidine was the first thienopyridine to be approved for clinical use, in 1991. It is a first-generation thienopyridine that irreversibly blocks the ADP P2Y12 receptor and thereby prevents platelet activation and aggregation mediated by ADP signaling pathways.[27] When combined with aspirin, ticlopidine has been shown to reduce the risk of CV events in patients undergoing coronary stenting as compared with aspirin monotherapy or aspirin with warfarin.[27] However, an unfavorable safety profile (including risk of neutropenia) and slow onset of action led the way for clopidogrel to emerge shortly thereafter as the preferred thienopyridine in appropriate settings.

Clopidogrel

When compared with ticlopidine, clopidogrel has been shown to have similar efficacy in addition to improved safety and tolerability[27] and faster pharmacodynamic effects after a loading dose.[28] In a meta-analysis that combined data from 13,995 patients in randomized trials and registries of ticlopidine versus clopidogrel, the use of clopidogrel was associated with a significant reduction in mortality and recurrent ischemic events when compared with ticlopidine and had fewer side effects.[29] The efficacy of clopidogrel monotherapy (75 mg/day) versus aspirin (325 mg/day) in secondary prevention was evaluated in the Clopidogrel versus Aspirin in Patients at Risk of Ischaemic Events (CAPRIE) trial.[30] The CAPRIE trial compared clopidogrel (75 mg/day) versus aspirin (325 mg/day) in 19,185 patients with established atherosclerotic disease, including recent MI, recent stroke, or symptomatic PAD. Overall, clopidogrel monotherapy significantly reduced the risk of vascular death, MI, or ischemic stroke by 8.7% compared with aspirin alone ($P=0.043$) and reduced the risk of GI bleeding ($P=0.05$).[30] Patients with DM in the trial (n=3866) were observed to have approximately a threefold higher event rate compared with their nondiabetic counterparts.[31] Overall, the relative risk reduction (RRR) of clopidogrel versus aspirin for reducing vascular events was statistically similar in diabetic and nondiabetic patients (12.5% versus 6.1%, respectively, P for interaction $= 0.36$).[31] However, because of the higher absolute event rate in diabetic patients and the trend toward a greater RRR, clopidogrel conferred a greater absolute benefit in diabetic patients. To that end, the number of events (vascular death, MI, stroke, rehospitalization with ischemia, bleeding) prevented per 1000 patients per year was 21 in diabetic patients versus 9 in nondiabetic patients treated with clopidogrel as compared with aspirin. The absolute benefit of clopidogrel further improved to 38 events prevented per 1000 patients per year in insulin-treated patients with diabetes treated with clopidogrel as compared with aspirin (**Fig. 16-3**).[31] Following the publication of the CAPRIE findings, the ADA issued recommendations that clopidogrel be used as monotherapy in very high-risk diabetic patients and as an alternative to aspirin in intolerant patients.[32]

Although individuals with DM have higher platelet reactivity, randomized trials have been unable to demonstrate a greater relative benefit for clopidogrel in diabetic versus nondiabetic patients. The Clopidogrel in Unstable Angina to Prevent Recurrent Events (CURE) trial enrolled 12,562 patients with non–ST-elevation ACS and randomized them to clopidogrel versus placebo on a background of aspirin for up to 1 year.[33] After a mean of 9 months, clopidogrel reduced the risk of vascular death, MI, or stroke by 20% compared with placebo (HR 0.80, 95% CI 0.72-0.90). This clinical benefit was associated with a 38% increase in the risk of major bleeding (3.7% versus 2.7%, $P < 0.001$) but no increase in the risk of fatal bleeding.[33] The benefit of clopidogrel appeared early but was maintained beyond 30 days (HR 0.82; 95% CI 0.70-0.95). Consistent with prior studies, diabetic patients in the trial ($n = 2840$) were observed to have almost a two-fold higher rate of CV events (14.2% versus 7.9%) as compared with their nondiabetic counterparts, thereby translating into a greater absolute benefit from clopidogrel. However, the relative benefit of clopidogrel was grossly similar in diabetic and nondiabetic patients with an approximate 17% RRR in the primary endpoint in diabetic patients, as compared with 20% in the overall population.[33]

More recently, the clinical efficacy of clopidogrel was evaluated in a nonrandomized analysis of a large nationwide Danish registry of patients who had survived 30 days after an MI.[34] After multivariable adjustment and propensity-score matching, clopidogrel was associated with a smaller reduction in all-cause mortality (adjusted HR 0.89, 95% CI 0.79-1.00 versus 0.75, 95% CI 0.70-0.80, P interaction $= 0.001$) and CV mortality (adjusted HR 0.93, 0.81-1.06 versus 0.77, 95% CI 0.72-0.83, P interaction $= 0.01$) in patients with DM, as compared with those who did not have diabetes. Clopidogrel was associated with only a marginal difference in the risk of death or reinfarction in either patient group (0.91, 0.87-0.96 versus 1.00, 0.91-1.10, P interaction $= 0.08$).[34] However, this differential association for clopidogrel between diabetic and nondiabetic patients was not observed in patients undergoing PCI, and no differential association was observed between patient groups with regard to the efficacy of aspirin.[35] Limitations of this analysis included the fact that use of clopidogrel was not randomized and therefore there is the risk of confounding despite adjustments having been made for known confounders. Supporting this hypothesis, clopidogrel appeared to have a greater magnitude of association toward reduced risk of death as compared with the risk of reinfarction, a finding not supported by existing trials.[35]

Notwithstanding the limitations of a nonrandomized analysis, there are mechanistic data to support the hypothesis that clopidogrel may have diminished efficacy in diabetic patients. Pharmacodynamic studies have demonstrated that almost two thirds of diabetic patients have an inadequate response to clopidogrel.[36] Moreover, platelet aggregation on dual antiplatelet therapy is even further heightened in insulin-treated diabetic patients, as compared with those who do not require insulin therapy (**Fig. 16-4**).[37] The latter finding is perhaps explained by the fact that insulin inhibits platelet aggregation by suppressing the P2Y12 pathway. Because diabetic patients have a loss of responsiveness to insulin, there is subsequent upregulation of the P2Y12 pathway, leading to heightened platelet reactivity and diminished response to antiplatelet agents.

Multiple trials have examined the benefit of clopidogrel and the optimal timing of loading dose administration in patients undergoing PCI. Because clopidogrel is a prodrug, approximately 6 hours are required to attain steady state

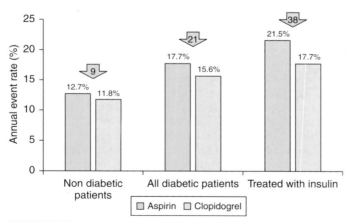

FIGURE 16-3 The number of events (vascular death, MI, stroke, or rehospitalization for ischemia or bleeding) prevented per 1000 patients per year treated with clopidogrel instead of aspirin in nondiabetic patients, all diabetic patients, and diabetic patients treated with insulin in the CAPRIE trial. *(Modified from Bhatt DL, Marso SP, Hirsch AT, et al: Amplified benefit of clopidogrel versus aspirin in patients with diabetes mellitus, Am J Cardiol 90:625-628, 2002.)*

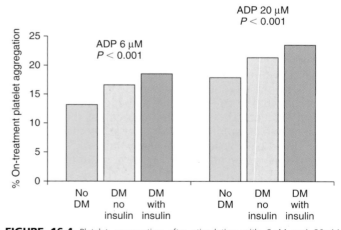

FIGURE 16-4 Platelet aggregation after stimulation with 6 μM and 20 μM adenosine diphosphate (ADP) in nondiabetic patients, non–insulin-treated diabetic patients, and insulin-dependent diabetic patients. on stable doses of dual antiplatelet therapy. *(Modified from Angiolillo DJ, Bernardo E, Ramirez C, et al. Insulin therapy is associated with platelet dysfunction in patients with type 2 diabetes mellitus on dual oral antiplatelet treatment, J Am Coll Cardiol 48:298-304, 2006.)*

concentrations after a 300-mg loading dose. The PCI-CURE substudy examined outcomes for those patients enrolled in the CURE trial who underwent PCI (see also **Chapter 21**).[38] The CURE trial enrolled 12,562 patients with non–ST-elevation acute coronary syndromes (NSTE-ACS) and randomized them to clopidogrel (300-mg loading dose, 75 mg daily) versus placebo on a background of aspirin. Those patients who were pretreated with clopidogrel before PCI and who continued clopidogrel for up to 1 year had a 31% lower risk of CV death or MI compared with patients who were not pretreated and who were treated for only 4 weeks after PCI. Although numerically smaller in magnitude, this benefit was comparable in diabetic patients in whom clopidogrel reduced the risk of CV death or MI by 23% compared with placebo after PCI.[38]

Similar early and long-term benefits with clopidogrel were demonstrated in the Clopidogrel for the Reduction of Events during Observation (CREDO) trial, in which patients were randomized to a loading dose of clopidogrel 3 to 24 hours before PCI and then to continued maintenance therapy with clopidogrel beyond the first month after the procedure, compared with patients who were not administered a loading dose and were treated with clopidogrel for only 28 days after PCI.[39] Overall, patients randomized to early and sustained clopidogrel treatment had a 26.9% reduction in the risk of death, MI, or stroke. It is important to note that there appeared to be continued benefit for long-term treatment with clopidogrel throughout the treatment period of 1 year.[39] As was seen in the diabetic subgroup of the PCI-CURE substudy, the relative benefit of clopidogrel in diabetic patients was comparable, but numerically smaller, than that seen in nondiabetic patients (11.2% RRR, 95% CI 46.2% to −46.8 versus 32.8% RRR, 95% CI 51.6%-6.8%).[39]

Higher loading (600 mg) and maintenance doses (150 mg daily for 6 days) of clopidogrel were compared with standard doses of clopidogrel in patients after ACS in the Clopidogrel and Aspirin Optimal Dose Usage to Reduce Recurrent Events—Seventh Organization to Assess Strategies in Ischemic Syndromes (CURRENT-OASIS 7) trial (see also **Chapter 21**).[23] Although double-dosing did not reduce the risk of 30-day CV events in the overall study population (HR 0.94, 95% CI 0.83-1.06), the higher-dose regimen was associated with a reduced risk of CV death, MI, or stroke (HR 0.86, 95% CI 0.74-0.99) in the cohort of patients who underwent PCI. However, the higher dose of clopidogrel also increased the risk of major bleeding by 42% (HR 1.42, 95% CI 1.09-1.83). There was no evidence of heterogeneity by DM status for the primary efficacy endpoint (*P* for interaction = 0.32).[23]

The use of dual antiplatelet therapy in stable secondary prevention and high-risk primary prevention was evaluated in the CHARISMA trial.[40] Overall, clopidogrel did not reduce the risk of CV events when compared with placebo, and there was no evidence of interaction by DM status. In a post hoc analysis, the subgroup of patients with prior MI, ischemic stroke, or symptomatic PAD showed a 17% RRR with dual antiplatelet therapy.[41] In contrast, there was no clear benefit and an increased risk of bleeding in high-risk patients in the absence of established vascular disease (**Fig. 16-5**). Of note, the primary prevention cohort was enriched with diabetic patients based on the entry criteria. Therefore the results of the CHARISMA trial do not support the use of dual antiplatelet therapy in diabetic patients for primary prevention, but ongoing trials may demonstrate a benefit for more

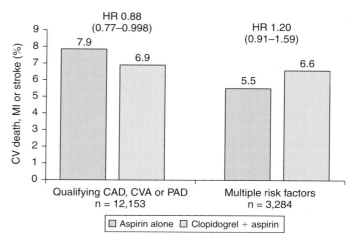

FIGURE 16-5 The relative effect (HR, 95% CI) of clopidogrel versus placebo in patients with symptomatic atherosclerotic disease or multiple risk factors in the CHARISMA trial. In subgroup analyses, clopidogrel reduced the risk of CV death, MI, or stroke in patients with symptomatic atherosclerotic disease, but not in patients who only had multiple risk factors in the absence of symptoms. The diabetic population was enriched in the latter group.[40] *(Modified from Bhatt DL, Fox KA, Hacke W, et al: Clopidogrel and aspirin versus aspirin alone for the prevention of atherothrombotic events,* N Engl J Med 354:1706-1717, 2006.)

prolonged dual antiplatelet therapy in patients with established vascular disease.

Another area of ongoing investigation is the optimal duration of dual antiplatelet therapy after PCI (see also **Chapter 17**). Several studies have demonstrated that there is an increased risk of adverse outcomes after discontinuation of clopidogrel.[42] In a study of 749 patients with DM who underwent stenting, the use of more prolonged dual antiplatelet therapy was associated with a reduced risk of death or MI in patients after bare metal stent placement (*P* = 0.01) and a reduced risk of death in patients with a drug-eluting stent (DES) (*P* = 0.03).[43] However, many of the analyses to date have been observational in design, and therefore it is plausible that the results might be explained by confounding. In particular, clopidogrel is often discontinued in the setting of bleeding or surgery, which may independently place a patient at increased risk of CV events.

To date, only a small number of studies have addressed the optimal duration of dual antiplatelet therapy with a randomized design. The Prolonging Dual Antiplatelet Treatment after Grading Stent-Induced Intimal Hyperplasia Study (PRODIGY) trial randomized 2013 patients who had undergone PCI to dual antiplatelet therapy for a period of 6 versus 24 months.[44] The incidence of CV death, MI, or stroke was observed to be similar in both treatment arms (10.1% versus 10.0%, *P* = 0.92), whereas the incidence of bleeding (Bleeding Academic Research Consortium [BARC] type 2, 3, and 5) was higher for patients who continued dual antiplatelet therapy for 24 months (7.4% versus 3.5%, *P* < 0.001). Similar findings were seen in two trial populations that were composed of 2701 patients in Korea who were randomized to aspirin alone versus continued dual antiplatelet therapy 12 months after PCI.[45] Although the study was underpowered because of a low event rate, more prolonged dual antiplatelet therapy failed to demonstrate any signal toward clinical efficacy.[45] In a second study underpowered to assess noninferiority, a similar lack of efficacy was demonstrated for dual-antiplatelet therapy beyond

6 months in patients undergoing placement of a DES.[46] The efficacy and safety of prolonged dual antiplatelet therapy beyond 12 months are currently undergoing evaluation in the larger Dual Antiplatelet Therapy (DAPT) Study (clinical-trials.gov NCT00977938). The DAPT trial is enrolling patients after PCI and then randomizing those patients who are event free after 12 months to an additional 18 months of treatment with a thienopyridine versus placebo.

Clopidogrel Response Variability

There exists significant interindividual variability in pharmacodynamic response to clopidogrel.[47] In turn, diabetic patients with an inadequate response to clopidogrel are at increased risk of CV events.[48] The estimated prevalence of individuals with an inadequate response to clopidogrel varies considerably depending on the applied definitions, type of assay, dose of clopidogrel, and patient population. In patients undergoing elective PCI, it has been described that approximately 31% of individuals will have less than 10% inhibition of platelet aggregation (IPA) at 24 hours as measured by light transmission aggregometry after a 300-mg loading dose of clopidogrel.[49] It is important to note there is evidence that the prevalence of clopidogrel hyporesponders is higher in patients with DM and is highest in patients requiring insulin therapy (see **Fig. 16-4**).[37] In the Optimizing Antiplatelet Therapy in Diabetes Mellitus (OPTIMUS) trial, individuals with DM had higher baseline platelet reactivity, and almost two thirds of diabetic patients were demonstrated to have an inadequate response to clopidogrel.[36] Higher baseline platelet reactivity and diminished response to clopidogrel may therefore in part explain the persistent risk of CV events that is observed in diabetic patients.

It remains unknown whether specific genetic, cellular, and clinical causes may contribute to the higher prevalence of clopidogrel hyporesponders in diabetic patients. Regardless of DM status, several studies have demonstrated that clopidogrel-treated patients with at least one copy of a reduced-function *CYP2C19* allele have an increased risk of CV events after undergoing PCI[50]; however, genotype appears to explain only a small fraction of observed interpatient variability.[51] In diabetic patients, in the setting of excess insulin, there is evidence to suggest that platelets develop insulin resistance leading to upregulation of the P2Y12 receptor[52] and heightened platelet reactivity.[53] Additional cellular factors that may contribute to the observed attenuation in response in diabetic patients include alterations in calcium metabolism,[54] increased ADP exposure, and accelerated platelet turnover.[55]

Because patients with DM may have upregulation of the P2Y12 receptor, there has been interest in using a higher dose of clopidogrel to help overcome pharmacodynamic resistance. In the OPTIMUS trial, the use of 150 mg of clopidogrel daily resulted in greater IPA than the 75-mg dose in diabetic patients with poor pharmacodynamic response to clopidogrel. However, despite the use of the 150-mg maintenance dose, a substantial fraction of diabetic patients continued to have high post-treatment platelet reactivity. Similar findings were observed in Gauging Responsiveness with a VerifyNow P2Y12 Assay—Impact on Thrombosis and Safety (GRAVITAS) (see also **Chapter 17**),[56] a trial of 2214 patients with high on-treatment platelet reactivity with clopidogrel after placement of a DES; the patients were randomized to high-dose (600-mg loading dose then 150 mg daily) or standard-dose (75 mg daily) clopidogrel. The prevalence

of high on-treatment platelet reactivity was observed to be higher among diabetic patients, and as a consequence almost half the patients who were determined to have high on-treatment platelet reactivity had diabetes. Although higher doses of clopidogrel reduced the in vitro prevalence of pharmacodynamic clopidogrel hyporesponders, clopidogrel 150 mg daily failed to reduce the risk of CV events as compared with standard dosing in these high-risk patients. Therefore there are no prospective data that support routine platelet function testing at the present time.

Prasugrel

Prasugrel is a third-generation thienopyridine that irreversibly binds to the P2Y12 receptor to inhibit platelet activation and aggregation. Although the active metabolites of both clopidogrel and prasugrel have similar affinity for the P2Y12 receptor in vitro, prasugrel achieves more rapid and more potent IPA than clopidogrel. It is hypothesized that this is because of its more efficient pathway of drug metabolism and activation.[57] Clopidogrel requires two separate CYP-dependent oxidative steps to form its active metabolite, and most of the prodrug is metabolized by esterases that shunt the drug toward a dead-end inactive pathway. In contrast, esterases assist with activation of the prasugrel prodrug, and prasugrel is oxidized to its active metabolite in a single CYP-dependent step.[58] After a 60-mg loading dose, prasugrel has been shown to significantly inhibit platelets within 30 minutes of ingestion.[57] In contrast, a 300-mg loading dose of clopidogrel requires approximately 6 hours to achieve steady-state, and a 600-mg loading dose takes approximately 2 hours to demonstrate clinically relevant antiplatelet effects. In addition to its enhanced potency, prasugrel demonstrates diminished interpatient variability as compared with clopidogrel.[47]

The Trial to Assess Improvement in Therapeutic Outcomes by Optimizing Platelet Inhibition with Prasugrel—Thrombolysis in Myocardial Infarction (TRITON-TIMI) 38 enrolled 13,608 patients with ACS and undergoing PCI to prasugrel (60-mg loading dose, 10 mg daily) or clopidogrel (300-mg loading dose, 75 mg daily) on a background of aspirin (see also **Chapter 21**).[59] After a median of 14.5 months, prasugrel significantly reduced the risk of CV death, MI, or stroke by 19% as compared with clopidogrel (HR 0.81, 95% CI 0.73-0.90). Furthermore, prasugrel significantly reduced the risk of MI (9.7% versus 7.4%, $P < 0.001$), urgent target-vessel revascularization (3.7% versus 2.5%, $P < 0.001$), and stent thrombosis (2.4% versus 1.1%, $P < 0.001$).[59] The benefit of prasugrel appeared early, and landmark analyses demonstrated that the benefit appeared to persist over time. Although the incidence of bleeding was low, prasugrel significantly increased the risk of non–coronary artery bypass graft (CABG) surgery–related TIMI major bleeding by 32%, including a significant increase in the risk of life-threatening and fatal bleeding.[60] Subsequent post hoc analyses demonstrated the patients with a history of stroke or TIA do not appear to benefit from prasugrel and may incur harm from more potent antiplatelet therapy. In addition, a net clinical benefit was not observed in patients aged older than 75 years or weighing less than 60 kilograms.

Of interest, the balance between efficacy and safety for prasugrel compared with clopidogrel appeared most favorable in diabetic patients enrolled in the TRITON-TIMI 38 trial with DM.[61] Of the 3146 patients with DM, prasugrel

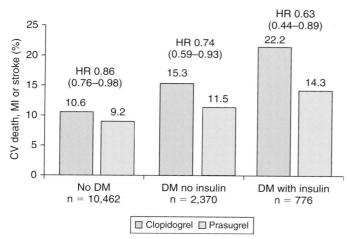

FIGURE 16-6 Clinical events and relative benefit (HR, 95% CI) of prasugrel versus clopidogrel for patients without DM, diabetic patients not treated with insulin, and insulin-treated diabetic patients in the TRITON-TIMI 38 trial. The relative benefit of prasugrel versus clopidogrel appeared to be enhanced in diabetic patients, and further benefit was observed in those patients requiring insulin therapy.[61] *(Modified from Wiviott SD, Braunwald E, Angiolillo DJ, et al: Greater clinical benefit of more intensive oral antiplatelet therapy with prasugrel in patients with diabetes mellitus in the trial to assess improvement in therapeutic outcomes by optimizing platelet inhibition with prasugrel—Thrombolysis in Myocardial Infarction 38,* Circulation 118:1626-1636, 2008.)

significantly reduced the risk of CV death, MI, or stroke by 30% (HR 0.70, 95% CI 0.58-0.85, $P < 0.001$, P interaction = 0.09) and this benefit was further increased to 37% in insulin-treated patients (HR 0.63, 95% CI 0.44–0.89, **Fig. 16-6**).[61] Prasugrel reduced the risk of MI by 40% in diabetic patients (HR 0.60, 95% CI 0.48-0.76), as opposed to by 18% in nondiabetic patients (HR 0.82, 95% CI 0.72-0.95, P interaction = 0.02). Also, prasugrel reduced the risk of stent thrombosis in the overall diabetic cohort (3.6% versus 2.0%, HR 0.52, 95% CI 0.33-0.84), and this benefit was further enhanced in diabetic patients requiring insulin (5.7% versus 1.8%, HR 0.31, 95% CI 0.12-0.77). Although diabetic patients had a higher absolute rate of bleeding, prasugrel did not appear to substantially increase the risk of major bleeding as compared with clopidogrel in this high-risk patient group (2.6% versus 2.5%, HR 1.06, 95% CI 0.66-1.69). Because of the higher event rate and greater benefit of prasugrel in insulin-treated patients, the absolute risk reduction in CV events with prasugrel was 8% indicating that only 13 insulin-treated diabetic patients would need to be treated to prevent one ischemic event, contrasted with a number-needed-to-treat of 26 for DM patients not on insulin. The observations from the diabetic subgroup of the TRITON-TIMI 38 trial therefore support the hypothesis that the achieved degree of platelet reactivity is an important predictor of outcome. Because individuals with DM have higher baseline platelet reactivity and diminished pharmacodynamic response to clopidogrel, it is plausible that diabetic patients derive enhanced benefit from this more potent antiplatelet therapy that is able to attain lower levels of on-treatment platelet reactivity.

The Prasugrel in Comparison to Clopidogrel for Inhibition of Platelet Activation and Aggregation—Thrombolysis in Myocardial Infarction 44 (PRINCIPLE-TIMI 44) trial was a two-phase study of 201 patients undergoing PCI that compared the pharmacodynamic response to prasugrel (60-mg loading dose, 10 mg daily) with higher-dose clopidogrel (600-mg loading dose, 150 mg daily).[57] Prasugrel achieved greater IPA as compared with higher-dose clopidogrel in

both the loading dose and maintenance dose phases. The rate of patients who were hyporesponsive to clopidogrel (IPA ≤20% in response to 20 μM ADP) was higher in diabetic patients than nondiabetic patients at all timepoints. In contrast, no hyporesponders were observed for patients on prasugrel at 6 hours regardless of diabetes status.[57] Consistent findings were observed in the OPTIMUS-3 trial, which exclusively enrolled patients with DM.[62] In OPTIMUS-3, individuals with DM and coronary artery disease (CAD) were randomized to prasugrel (60-mg loading dose, 10 mg daily) or clopidogrel (600-mg loading dose, 150 mg daily) over two 1-week treatment periods separated by a 2-week washout. Prasugrel achieved greater platelet inhibition than high-dose clopidogrel at 4 hours after a loading dose. This difference was maintained throughout the loading dose and maintenance phase (from 1 hour through 7 days, $P < 0.001$). Prasugrel reduced the number of diabetic patients with an inadequate response to thienopyridine therapy as compared with high-dose clopidogrel.[62]

After the publication of the TRITON-TIMI 38 trial findings, the Targeted Platelet Inhibition to Clarify the Optimal Strategy to Medically Manage Acute Coronary Syndromes (TRILOGY ACS) trial compared the long-term efficacy of prasugrel (10 mg daily) versus clopidogrel (75 mg daily) in 7243 patients with ACS who were managed medically without coronary revascularization (see also **Chapter 21**).[63] A lower dose of prasugrel (5 mg daily) was used in patients who weighed less than 60 kg or were older than 75 years. The primary analysis was restricted to patients younger than 75 years. In this patient group, prasugrel did not significantly reduce the risk of CV death, MI, or stroke as compared with clopidogrel (HR 0.91, 95% CI 0.79-1.05). The findings were consistent in the subset of 2811 patients with DM (HR 0.90, 95% CI 0.73-1.09, P interaction = 0.71). The prespecified analysis of first or recurrent ischemic events (all components of the primary endpoint) suggested a lower risk for prasugrel among patients under the age of 75 years (HR 0.85; 95% CI 0.72 to 1.00; $P = 0.04$). Rates of severe and intracranial bleeding were similar in the two groups in all age groups.[63] Therefore the findings of the TRILOGY ACS trial do not support the use of prasugrel in patients who are managed without coronary revascularization.

The 2012 Focused Update to the ACCF/AHA Guidelines for the Management of Patients with non–ST-elevation ACS offers a class I recommendation for the use of clopidogrel, prasugrel, or ticagrelor (see later) on a background of aspirin in patients with unstable angina (UA) or non–ST-segment myocardial infarction (NSTEMI) who are undergoing PCI, with no distinction in the recommendations with regard to drug of choice based on DM status (see also **Chapter 21**).[24] If prasugrel is used, it should be given promptly and no later than 1 hour after PCI once the coronary anatomy is defined and the decision is made to proceed with PCI (see also **Chapters 17** and **22**). Based on the findings from TRITON-TIMI 38, prasugrel should not be administered to patients with a history of stroke or transient ischemic attack (TIA). In patients over the age of 75 years, the use of prasugrel is generally not recommended but may be considered in high-risk patients such as those with DM. A lower dose of 5 mg daily can be considered in patients over the age of 75 or who weigh less than 60 kg. Prasugrel should be continued for at least 12 months in ACS patients who undergo PCI. Earlier discontinuation of a P2Y12 receptor inhibitor can be considered in patients in whom the anticipated morbidity from bleeding exceeds its benefits.

Ticagrelor

Ticagrelor is the first reversibly binding oral P2Y12 receptor antagonist.[64] It is a nonthienopyridine and does not require metabolism to form its active metabolite. It has been shown to bind the P2Y12 receptor with a noncompetitive binding mechanism toward ADP. Similar to prasugrel, ticagrelor demonstrates rapid onset of action and decreased interpatient variability as compared with clopidogrel. Because of an elimination half-life of 7 hours and its reversible binding characteristics, it is administered twice daily. However, its antiplatelet effects have been shown to extend to approximately 120 hours.[64] Although it is more potent than clopidogrel, its ability to inhibit platelet aggregation is roughly equivalent to that of clopidogrel at 24 hours after drug discontinuation because of its faster offset kinetics. Ticagrelor may therefore be less likely than clopidogrel to increase the risk of bleeding in patients who require surgery 48 to 120 hours after the last dose.[64]

The Study of Platelet Inhibition and Patient Outcomes (PLATO) trial evaluated the safety and efficacy of ticagrelor in 18,624 patients across the spectrum of ACS (see also **Chapter 21**).[65] Patients were randomized to clopidogrel (300- to 600-mg loading dose, 75 mg daily) or ticagrelor (180-mg loading dose, 90 mg daily). At 12 months, ticagrelor reduced the risk of vascular death, MI, or stroke by 16% (HR 0.84, 95% CI 0.77-0.92), as compared with clopidogrel. In addition, ticagrelor reduced the risk of death from vascular causes (4.0% versus 5.1%, $P=0.001$) and all-cause mortality (4.5%, versus 5.9% with clopidogrel, $P<0.001$), but increased the risk of non–CABG-related Thrombolysis in Myocardial Infarction (TIMI) major bleeding by 25% ($P=0.03$). Of the P2Y12 inhibitors that have been evaluated to date, ticagrelor is the only drug to have demonstrated a mortality benefit across the spectrum of ACS. However, ticagrelor did not increase the risk of fatal bleeding ($P=0.66$) or CABG-related major bleeding ($P=0.32$).

The relative benefit of ticagrelor appeared to be comparable in diabetic and nondiabetic patients in PLATO, although the absolute benefits were greater in insulin-treated diabetic patients.[66] Ticagrelor reduced the risk of vascular death, MI, or stroke by 12% in diabetic patients (HR 0.88, 95% CI 0.76-1.03) versus 17% in nondiabetic patients (HR 0.83, 95% CI 0.74-0.92, P interaction $=0.49$; **Fig. 16-7**). Similarly, in diabetic patients, ticagrelor reduced the risk of all-cause mortality (HR 0.82, 95% CI 0.66-1.01) and stent thrombosis (HR 0.65, 95% CI 0.36-1.17) to an extent that was consistent with the overall cohort. Ticagrelor tended to increase non–CABG-related PLATO major bleeding in both diabetic and nondiabetic patients (HR 1.13, 95% CI 0.86-1.49; HR 1.22, 95% CI 1.01-1.46, respectively, P interaction $= .69$). There was no heterogeneity in the efficacy or safety of ticagrelor with regard to patients who were or were not treated with insulin.[66]

If diabetic patients indeed derive enhanced benefit from more potent antiplatelet therapy after ACS, it is unclear why these findings were not observed in the PLATO trial. In patients who are hyporesponsive to clopidogrel, switching to ticagrelor has been shown to inhibit platelet aggregation to the same extent as it does when clopidogrel-responsive patients are treated with ticagrelor.[67] In this same study,

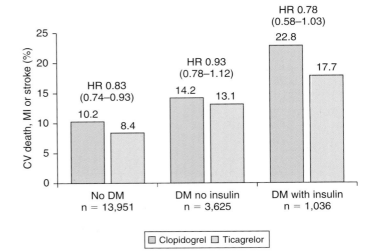

FIGURE 16-7 Clinical events and comparative efficacy (HR, 95% CI) of ticagrelor versus clopidogrel for patients without DM, diabetic patients not treated with insulin, and patients with diabetes treated with insulin in the PLATO trial. The absolute benefit of ticagrelor appeared largest in diabetic patients treated with insulin, although the relative benefits were similar in all three groups.[66] (Modified from James S, Angiolillo DJ, Cornel JH, et al: Ticagrelor vs. clopidogrel in patients with acute coronary syndromes and diabetes: a substudy from the PLATelet inhibition and patient Outcomes (PLATO) trial, Eur Heart J 31:3006-3016, 2010.)

almost all patients treated with ticagrelor (25% of whom had diabetes) achieved platelet reactivity levels below the threshold that has been shown to be associated with an increased risk of ischemic events regardless of their clopidogrel response status.[67]

There are limited head-to-head data to compare the pharmacodynamic or clinical efficacy of prasugrel with that of ticagrelor. In a study of 44 patients with ACS (23% of whom had DM) and high on-treatment platelet reactivity on clopidogrel, patients were randomized in a double-blind crossover design to either ticagrelor 90 mg twice daily or prasugrel 10 mg daily without a loading dose for 15 days before crossing over to the alternate therapy.[68] At the end of the two treatment periods, ticagrelor achieved a greater degree of platelet inhibition than prasugrel ($P<0.001$). Both drugs were effective at reducing platelet reactivity below the predefined threshold for poor response.[68] It remains unknown whether the two drugs would demonstrate similar clinical efficacy if compared in a large-scale head-to-head clinical trial or if similar pharmacodynamic effects would have been observed if a loading dose of the drugs had been administered.

Unlike with prasugrel, the benefit of ticagrelor has not been directly assessed in a dedicated trial population of patients managed without PCI. However, in the PLATO trial, ticagrelor reduced the risk of vascular death, MI, or stroke in patients who were intended to be managed noninvasively (HR 0.85, 95% CI 0.73-1.00, $P=0.04$), of whom 29% eventually underwent PCI.[69] Ticagrelor is the first of the two novel P2Y12 antagonists to be evaluated in a population of patients with stable CAD. The ongoing Prevention with Ticagrelor of Secondary Thrombotic Events in High-Risk Patients with Prior Acute Coronary Syndrome—Thrombolysis in Myocardial Infarction (PEGASUS-TIMI) 54 trial (clinicaltrials.gov NCT01225562) has enrolled intermediate- to high-risk individuals with a history of MI in the past 1 to 3 years to one of two doses of ticagrelor (60 mg or 90 mg twice daily) or placebo on a background of low-dose aspirin.[69a] The trial will directly address the clinical efficacy of ticagrelor in patients with stable CAD and will also help to assess the optimal duration of dual antiplatelet therapy in patients after MI. As well, The Effect of Ticagrelor on Health Outcomes in Diabetes Mellitus Patients Intervention Study (THEMIS) trial is evaluating the efficacy and safety of ticagrelor (90 mg twice daily) in patients with type 2 diabetes mellitus and either a documented history of obstructive coronary artery disease or prior coronary revascularization (clinicaltrials.gov NCT01991795).

OTHER ANTIPLATELET MEDICATIONS

Cilostazol

Cilostazol is a phosphodiesterase III inhibitor that raises cyclic adenosine monophosphate (cAMP) levels in platelets and vascular smooth muscle cells, leading to inhibition of platelet activation and arteriolar vasodilation.[70] When cilostazol was added to a background of dual antiplatelet therapy, nonrandomized studies demonstrated that this agent appeared to reduce the risk of stent thrombosis[71,72] and ischemic events,[72,73] without a significant increase in bleeding. Thus far, randomized trials of triple antiplatelet therapy in patients after PCI have yielded conflicting results, although most trials have been underpowered for clinical outcomes (see also **Chapter 17**).[74] In the Efficacy of Cilostazol on Ischemic Complications after Drug-Eluting Stent Implantation (CILON-T) trial, the addition of cilostazol failed to reduce the risk of cardiac death, nonfatal MI, ischemic stroke, or target lesion revascularization in patients after DES implantation (8.5% versus 9.2%, $P=0.74$), despite achieving a reduction in platelet reactivity.[74] In contrast, in a second trial of patients after ACS undergoing PCI, cilostazol reduced the risk of cardiac death, nonfatal MI, stroke, or target vessel revascularization (10.3% versus 15.1%, $P=0.011$) when added to aspirin and clopidogrel.[75] In the latter study, the benefit of cilostazol appeared to be enhanced in patients with high-risk clinical or angiographic features, including DM (n=263, 9.9% versus 18.9%, HR 0.47, 95% CI 0.23-0.96).[75]

These findings are supported by pharmacodynamic data that have shown that cilostazol enhances inhibition of P2Y12 signaling in diabetic patients.[76] Cilostazol combined with standard-dose clopidogrel reduces platelet reactivity to a greater extent than clopidogrel 150 mg daily in patients with type 2 DM.[77] The greater pharmacodynamic effect of cilostazol in diabetic patients was observed regardless of whether or not patients carried genetic polymorphisms that have been shown to influence response to clopidogrel.[77] These findings may in part explain the ability of cilostazol to reduce the risk of ischemic events in high-risk patients. To that end, the antiplatelet effects of cilostazol appear to be enhanced in diabetic patients[78] and patients with high on-treatment platelet reactivity.[79,80]

In addition to its antiplatelet effects, cilostazol is hypothesized to exert pleiotropic effects including inhibition of neointimal hyperplasia. Supporting this concept, a systematic review that combined data from 23 randomized trials of cilostazol suggested that it may reduce the risk of in-stent restenosis (RR 0.60, 95% CI 0.49-0.73) and need for repeat revascularization (RR 0.69, 95% CI 0.55-0.86) without a significant increase in bleeding (RR 0.71, 95% CI 0.43-1.16) in patients after PCI.[81] In a dedicated trial of diabetic patients receiving a DES, the addition of cilostazol to aspirin and clopidogrel reduced angiographic restenosis and extent of late

luminal loss, thereby leading to a lower rate of target lesion revascularization at 9 months as compared with dual antiplatelet therapy alone.[82] Although the study was underpowered for clinical events, major adverse cardiac events tended to be lower in the triple than in the dual antiplatelet therapy group (3.0% versus 7.0%, $P=0.066$).[82] However, the use of cilostazol is limited by a high frequency of side effects including headache, GI disturbance, and palpitations. Larger, more definitive studies of cilostazol are therefore needed before it can be routinely used as an adjunct to dual antiplatelet therapy after coronary stenting.

Dipyridamole

Dipyridamole exhibits a number of properties that contribute to platelet inhibition and vasodilation. Dipyridamole inhibits thromboxane synthase leading to reduced TXA_2 production and thereby reduced platelet activation.[83] It inhibits adenosine deaminase and cellular reuptake of adenosine into platelets, erythrocytes, and endothelial cells causing extracellular adenosine levels to rise.[83] Dipyridamole is also a phosphodiesterase inhibitor leading to higher cAMP and cyclic guanosine monophosphate (cGMP) levels within platelets and endothelial cells and thereby blocking response to ADP via the P2Y12 receptor and enhancing nitric oxide signaling.[83,84]

Although there are limited data to support the use of dipyridamole in patients with CHD, its use has been extensively studied in patients with cerebrovascular disease in combination with aspirin. In the European Stroke Prevention Study (ESPS), the combination of aspirin (330 mg) and dipyridamole (75 mg) three times daily reduced the risk of all-cause mortality or stroke by 33.5% compared with placebo in patients with a recent stroke or TIA.[85] Moreover, the benefit appeared to be further enhanced in diabetic versus nondiabetic patients (48% versus 32%, respectively).[86] Furthermore, it appears that the effects of dipyridamole and aspirin are additive.[87] In patients with recent stroke or TIA, the combination of dipyridamole (400 mg daily) and aspirin (50 mg daily) reduced the risk of stroke by 37% compared with placebo, whereas dipyridamole alone reduced the risk of stroke by 16% and aspirin alone by 18%.[87] In the open-label European/Australasian Stroke Prevention in Reversible Ischaemia Trial (ESPRIT), the combination of aspirin plus dipyridamole (200 mg twice daily) reduced the risk of CV death, MI, stroke, or major bleeding by 20% (HR 0.80, 95% CI 0.66-0.98), as compared with aspirin alone (30 to 325 mg daily) in patients with a history of an acute cerebrovascular event.[88] An increased frequency of headache contributed to a higher rate of discontinutation in the dipyridamole group.[88] Currently there is no role for dipyridamole for the purpose of reduction of coronary risk.

PROTEASE-ACTIVATED RECEPTOR 1 ANTAGONISTS

Vorapaxar

Thrombin stimulates platelet activation via protease-activated receptor 1 (PAR-1), the major thrombin receptor on the platelet cell surface. Although extensive research has been directed toward the ADP-dependent P2Y12 receptor, thrombin is the most potent platelet agonist.[89] Because aspirin and clopidogrel do not interfere with

PAR-1–dependent platelet activation, patients on standard dual antiplatelet therapy remain at risk of recurrent CV events via alternate pathways of platelet activation.

Vorapaxar is a competitive and selective antagonist of PAR-1 that acts by binding at or near the tethered ligand binding site.[89] Because PAR-1 receptor antagonists selectively interfere with thrombin-mediated platelet activation without disrupting the coagulation cascade or ADP-dependent platelet activation, it was hypothesized that PAR-1 receptor antagonists might reduce the risk of ischemic events without significantly increasing the risk of bleeding. This hypothesis was supported by phase II studies that suggested trends toward efficacy with increasing doses of vorapaxar and without a significant increase in major bleeding.[90]

Vorapaxar was subsequently evaluated in two large-scale clinical trials of patients with stable atherosclerotic disease or ACS, the Trial to Assess the Effects of SCH 530348 in Preventing Heart Attack and Stroke in Patients with Atherosclerosis (TRA2°P-TIMI 50) and the Trial to Assess the Effects of SCH 530348 in Preventing Heart Attack and Stroke in Patients with Acute Coronary Syndrome (TRA-CER), respectively. In January 2011, the joint Data and Safety Monitoring Board for the two trials reported an excess in intracranial hemorrhage in patients with a history of stroke. As a consequence, the study drug was discontinued in the TRA2°P-TIMI 50 trial for patients with a history of stroke, but the trial continued to completion in patients with a history of MI or PAD. The TRA-CER trial was stopped prematurely after reaching its prespecified number of primary endpoints.

In the 26,449 patients with stable atherosclerotic disease enrolled in the TRA2°P-TIMI 50 trial, vorapaxar (2.5 mg daily) significantly reduced the risk of CV death, M, or stroke by 13% and the risk of CV death, MI, stroke, or urgent coronary revascularization by 12% (HR 0.88, 95% CI 0.82-0.95) as compared with placebo during a median follow-up of 2.5 years.[91] Although vorapaxar reduced the risk of recurrent CV events, vorapaxar increased the risk of moderate or severe bleeding by 66% (HR 1.66, 95% CI 1.43-1.93), including a significant increase in the risk of intracranial hemorrhage. The rate of fatal bleeding was not significantly increased in the vorapaxar group. The efficacy and safety of vorapaxar were consistent in patients with or without DM (P interaction = 0.61 for CV death, MI, or stroke; P interaction = 0.79 for GUSTO moderate or severe bleeding). No heterogeneity was observed on the basis of background thienopyridine use.

The balance between efficacy and safety appeared to be most favorable for vorapaxar in patients with a history of MI more than 1 month before randomization in the TRA°2P-TIMI 50 trial.[92] Of the 17,779 patients within this prespecified subgroup, vorapaxar significantly reduced the risk of CV death, MI, or stroke by 20% (HR 0.80, 95% CI 0.72-0.89), including a 21% reduction in the risk of MI (HR 0.79, 95% CI 0.70-0.89) and a 34% reduction in the risk of ischemic stroke (HR 0.66, 95% CI 0.48-0.89). Moderate or severe bleeding remained more common in patients treated with vorapaxar as compared with patients on placebo (HR 1.61, 95% CI 1.31-1.97). Within this subgroup of patients, intracranial hemorrhage was infrequent and not statistically increased for patients on vorapaxar (0.6% versus 0.4%, P = 0.076).[92]

Despite an observed trend toward efficacy, vorapaxar was not superior to placebo for the management of patients with ACS in the TRA-CER trial.[93] Vorapaxar (40-mg loading dose, 2.5 mg daily) did not significantly reduce the risk of the primary endpoint of CV death, MI, recurrent ischemia with hospitalization, or urgent coronary revascularization (HR 0.92, 95% CI 0.85-1.017) in patients after ACS. Vorapaxar did reduce the key secondary endpoint of CV death, MI, or stroke by 11% compared with placebo (HR 0.89, 95% CI 0.81-0.98), including a 12% reduction in MI (HR 0.88, 95% CI 0.79-0.98). Consistent with the findings from the TRA°2P-TIMI 50 trial, vorapaxar increased the risk of GUSTO moderate or severe bleeding (HR 1.35, 95% CI 1.16-1.58) and intracranial hemorrhage (HR 3.39, 95% CI 1.78-6.45) in patients after ACS.

Atopaxar

Atopaxar (E5555) is a second orally active, reversible, small molecule inhibitor that selectively inhibits PAR-1 activation by binding at or near the tethered ligand binding site. Although vorapaxar and atopaxar share similarities, vorapaxar exhibits a much longer half-life (165 to 311 hours) and achieves 50% recovery of platelet function at 4 weeks after treatment discontinuation. In contrast, atopaxar has an approximate plasma half-life of 22 to 26 hours.[89]

The phase II Lessons from Antagonizing the Cellular Effects of Thrombin (LANCELOT) program evaluated the safety tolerability of atopaxar in patients after ACS or with stable CAD.[89,94,95] In patients after ACS, atopaxar significantly reduced Holter-detected ischemia without a clear increase in major bleeding compared with placebo.[89] Similar findings were observed in patients with CAD, including a nonsignificant trend toward reduced ischemic events.[94] In a focused platelet function substudy, atopaxar achieved rapid and sustained platelet inhibition via the PAR-1 receptor.[89,94] Although the drug was generally well tolerated, liver transaminase elevation and relative QTc prolongation were observed with the highest doses of atopaxar. To date, atopaxar has not been evaluated in phase III testing.

FUTURE DIRECTIONS

As the prevalence of DM continues to grow, there will be an urgent need to develop therapies that may help to attenuate CV risk in this high-risk population. In addition to the antiplatelet drugs reviewed in this chapter, several novel antiplatelet drugs remain in development. Cangrelor is a direct-acting and reversible intravenous P2Y12 receptor inhibitor whose use has been studied in the setting of PCI[96,97] and as a bridge to surgery for patients off oral P2Y12 inhibition.[98] Picotamide inhibits TXA$_2$ synthase and TXA$_2$ receptors and has been proposed as an alternative to aspirin.[99] Because the drug blocks TXA$_2$ through pathways independent of COX-1, it may offer enhanced benefit to diabetic patients who respond inadequately to aspirin.[99] As more potent or alternate antiplatelet therapies undergo clinical evaluation, continued emphasis will need to be placed on achieving the optimal balance between efficacy and safety.

References

1. Ferreiro JL, Angiolillo DJ: Diabetes and antiplatelet therapy in acute coronary syndrome, *Circulation* 123:798–813, 2011.
2. Bhatt DL: What makes platelets angry: diabetes, fibrinogen, obesity, and impaired response to antiplatelet therapy? *J Am Coll Cardiol* 52:1060–1061, 2008.
3. Vinik AI, Erbas T, Park TS, Davi G: Platelet dysfunction in type 2 diabetes, *Diabetes Care* 24:1476–1485, 2001.
4. Ferroni P, Basili S, Falco A, et al: Platelet activation in type 2 diabetes mellitus, *J Thromb Haemost* 2:1282–1291, 2004.
5. Patrono C, Garcia Rodriguez LA, Landolfi R, Baigent C: Low-dose aspirin for the prevention of atherothrombosis, *N Engl J Med* 353:2373–2383, 2005.

6. Final report on the aspirin component of the ongoing Physicians' Health Study. Steering Committee of the Physicians' Health Study Research Group, *N Engl J Med* 321:129–135, 1989.

7. Hansson L, Zanchetti A, Carruthers SG, et al: Effects of intensive blood-pressure lowering and low-dose aspirin in patients with hypertension: principal results of the Hypertension Optimal Treatment (HOT) randomised trial. HOT Study Group, *Lancet* 351:1755–1762, 1998.

8. de Gaetano G: Low-dose aspirin and vitamin E in people at cardiovascular risk: a randomised trial in general practice. Collaborative Group of the Primary Prevention Project, *Lancet* 357:89–95, 2001.

9. Aspirin effects on mortality and morbidity in patients with diabetes mellitus. Early Treatment Diabetic Retinopathy Study report 14. ETDRS Investigators, *JAMA* 268:1292–1300, 1992.

10. De Berardis G, Sacco M, Strippoli GF, et al: Aspirin for primary prevention of cardiovascular events in people with diabetes: meta-analysis of randomised controlled trials, *BMJ* 339:b4531, 2009.

11. Ridker PM, Cook NR, Lee IM, et al: A randomized trial of low-dose aspirin in the primary prevention of cardiovascular disease in women, *N Engl J Med* 352:1293–1304, 2005.

12. Pignone M, Alberts MJ, Colwell JA, et al: Aspirin for primary prevention of cardiovascular events in people with diabetes: a position statement of the American Diabetes Association, a scientific statement of the American Heart Association, and an expert consensus document of the American College of Cardiology Foundation, *Circulation* 121:2694–2701, 2010.

13. Ogawa H, Nakayama M, Morimoto T, et al: Low-dose aspirin for primary prevention of atherosclerotic events in patients with type 2 diabetes: a randomized controlled trial, *JAMA* 300:2134–2141, 2008.

14. Belch J, MacCuish A, Campbell I, et al: The prevention of progression of arterial disease and diabetes (POPADAD) trial: factorial randomised placebo controlled trial of aspirin and antioxidants in patients with diabetes and asymptomatic peripheral arterial disease, *BMJ* 337:a1840, 2008.

15. De Berardis G, Lucisano G, D'Ettorre A, et al: Association of aspirin use with major bleeding in patients with and without diabetes, *JAMA* 307:2286–2294, 2012.

16. American Diabetes Association. Standards of medical care in diabetes, *Diabetes Care* 37(Suppl 1):S14–S80, 2014.

17. Wolff T, Miller T, Ko S: Aspirin for the primary prevention of cardiovascular events: an update of the evidence for the U.S. Preventive Services Task Force, *Ann Intern Med* 150:405–410, 2009.

18. Aspirin for the prevention of cardiovascular disease: U.S. Preventive Services Task Force recommendation statement, *Ann Intern Med* 150:396–404, 2009.

19. Perk J, De Backer G, Gohlke H, et al: European guidelines on cardiovascular disease prevention in clinical practice (version 2012). The Fifth Joint Task Force of the European Society of Cardiology and Other Societies on Cardiovascular Disease Prevention in Clinical Practice (constituted by representatives of nine societies and by invited experts). Developed with the special contribution of the European Association for Cardiovascular Prevention & Rehabilitation (EACPR), *Eur Heart J* 33:1635–1701, 2012.

20. Randomised trial of intravenous streptokinase, oral aspirin, both, or neither among 17,187 cases of suspected acute myocardial infarction: ISIS-2. ISIS-2 (Second International Study of Infarct Survival) Collaborative Group, *Lancet* 2:349–360, 1988.

21. Collaborative meta-analysis of randomised trials of antiplatelet therapy for prevention of death, myocardial infarction, and stroke in high risk patients, *BMJ* 324:71–86, 2002.

22. Steinhubl SR, Bhatt DL, Brennan DM, et al: Aspirin to prevent cardiovascular disease: the association of aspirin dose and clopidogrel with thrombosis and bleeding, *Ann Intern Med* 150:379–386, 2009.

23. CURRENT-OASIS 7 Investigators, Mehta SR, Bassand JP, Chrolavicius S, et al: Dose comparisons of clopidogrel and aspirin in acute coronary syndromes, *N Engl J Med* 363:930–942, 2010.

24. 2012 Writing Committee Members, Jneid H, Anderson JL, Wright RS, et al: 2012 ACCF/AHA focused update of the guideline for the management of patients with unstable angina/Non-ST-elevation myocardial infarction (updating the 2007 guideline and replacing the 2011 focused update): a report of the American College of Cardiology Foundation/American Heart Association Task Force on practice guidelines, *Circulation* 126:875–910, 2012.

25. Levine GN, Bates ER, Blankenship JC, et al: 2011 ACCF/AHA/SCAI guideline for percutaneous coronary intervention: a report of the American College of Cardiology Foundation/American Heart Association Task Force on Practice Guidelines and the Society for Cardiovascular Angiography and Interventions, *Circulation* 124:e574–e651, 2011.

26. Gachet C: ADP receptors of platelets and their inhibition, *Thromb Haemost* 86:222–232, 2001.

27. Bertrand ME, Rupprecht HJ, Urban P, Gershlick AH, for the CLASSICS Investigators: Double-blind study of the safety of clopidogrel with and without a loading dose in combination with aspirin compared with ticlopidine in combination with aspirin after coronary stenting: the clopidogrel aspirin stent international cooperative study (CLASSICS), *Circulation* 102:624–629, 2000.

28. Cadroy Y, Bossavy JP, Thalamas C, et al: Early potent antithrombotic effect with combined aspirin and a loading dose of clopidogrel on experimental arterial thrombogenesis in humans, *Circulation* 101:2823–2828, 2000.

29. Bhatt DL, Bertrand ME, Berger PB, et al: Meta-analysis of randomized and registry comparisons of ticlopidine with clopidogrel after stenting, *J Am Coll Cardiol* 39:9–14, 2002.

30. A randomised, blinded, trial of clopidogrel versus aspirin in patients at risk of ischaemic events (CAPRIE). CAPRIE Steering Committee, *Lancet* 348:1329–1339, 1996.

31. Bhatt DL, Marso SP, Hirsch AT, et al: Amplified benefit of clopidogrel versus aspirin in patients with diabetes mellitus, *Am J Cardiol* 90:625–628, 2002.

32. Colwell JA: Aspirin therapy in diabetes, *Diabetes Care* 27(Suppl 1):S72–S73, 2004.

33. Yusuf S, Zhao F, Mehta SR, et al: Effects of clopidogrel in addition to aspirin in patients with acute coronary syndromes without ST-segment elevation, *N Engl J Med* 345:494–502, 2001.

34. Andersson C, Lyngbæk S, Nguyen CD, et al: Association of clopidogrel treatment with risk of mortality and cardiovascular events following myocardial infarction in patients with and without diabetes, *JAMA* 308:882–889, 2012.

35. Bhatt DL: Antiplatelet therapy following myocardial infarction in patients with diabetes, *JAMA* 308:921–922, 2012.

36. Angiolillo DJ, Shoemaker SB, Desai B, et al: Randomized comparison of a high clopidogrel maintenance dose in patients with diabetes mellitus and coronary artery disease: results of the Optimizing Antiplatelet Therapy in Diabetes Mellitus (OPTIMUS) study, *Circulation* 115:708–716, 2007.

37. Angiolillo DJ, Bernardo E, Ramírez C, et al: Insulin therapy is associated with platelet dysfunction in patients with type 2 diabetes mellitus on dual oral antiplatelet treatment, *J Am Coll Cardiol* 48:298–304, 2006.

38. Mehta SR, Yusuf S, Peters RJ, et al: Effects of pretreatment with clopidogrel and aspirin followed by long-term therapy in patients undergoing percutaneous coronary intervention: the PCI-CURE study, *Lancet* 358:527–533, 2001.

39. Steinhubl SR, Berger PB, Mann JT 3rd, , et al: Early and sustained dual oral antiplatelet therapy following percutaneous coronary intervention: a randomized controlled trial, *JAMA* 288:2411–2420, 2002.

40. Bhatt DL, Fox KA, Hacke W, et al: Clopidogrel and aspirin versus aspirin alone for the prevention of atherothrombotic events, *N Engl J Med* 354:1706–1717, 2006.

41. Bhatt DL, Flather MD, Hacke W, et al: Patients with prior myocardial infarction, stroke, or symptomatic peripheral arterial disease in the CHARISMA trial, *J Am Coll Cardiol* 49:1982–1988, 2007.

42. Ho PM, Peterson ED, Wang L, et al: Incidence of death and acute myocardial infarction associated with stopping clopidogrel after acute coronary syndrome, *JAMA* 299:532–539, 2008.

43. Brar SS, Kim J, Brar SK, et al: Long-term outcomes by clopidogrel duration and stent type in a diabetic population with de novo coronary artery lesions, *J Am Coll Cardiol* 51:2220–2227, 2008.

44. Valgimigli M, Campo G, Monti M, et al: Short- versus long-term duration of dual-antiplatelet therapy after coronary stenting: a randomized multicenter trial, *Circulation* 125:2015–2026, 2012.

45. Park SJ, Park DW, Kim YH, et al: Duration of dual antiplatelet therapy after implantation of drug-eluting stents, *N Engl J Med* 362:1374–1382, 2010.

46. Gwon HC, Hahn JY, Park KW, et al: Six-month versus 12-month dual antiplatelet therapy after implantation of drug-eluting stents: the Efficacy of Xience/Promus Versus Cypher to Reduce Late Loss After Stenting (EXCELLENT) randomized, multicenter study, *Circulation* 125:505–513, 2012.

47. O'Donoghue M, Wiviott SD: Clopidogrel response variability and future therapies: clopidogrel: does one size fit all? *Circulation* 114:e600–e606, 2006.

48. Angiolillo DJ, Bernardo E, Sabate M, et al: Impact of platelet reactivity on cardiovascular outcomes in patients with type 2 diabetes mellitus and coronary artery disease, *J Am Coll Cardiol* 50:1541–1547, 2007.

49. Gurbel PA, Bliden KP, Hiatt BL, O'Connor CM: Clopidogrel for coronary stenting: response variability, drug resistance, and the effect of pretreatment platelet reactivity, *Circulation* 107:2908–2913, 2003.

50. Mega JL, Simon T, Collet JP, et al: Reduced-function CYP2C19 genotype and risk of adverse clinical outcomes among patients treated with clopidogrel predominantly for PCI: a meta-analysis, *JAMA* 304:1821–1830, 2010.

51. Shuldiner AR, O'Connell JR, Bliden KP, et al: Association of cytochrome P450 2C19 genotype with the antiplatelet effect and clinical efficacy of clopidogrel therapy, *JAMA* 302:849–857, 2009.

52. Michno A, Bielarczyk H, Pawelczyk T, et al: Alterations of adenine nucleotide metabolism and function of blood platelets in patients with diabetes, *Diabetes* 56:462–467, 2007.

53. Ferreira IA, Mocking AI, Feijge MA, et al: Platelet inhibition by insulin is absent in type 2 diabetes mellitus, *Arterioscler Thromb Vasc Biol* 26:417–422, 2006.

54. Li Y, Woo V, Bose R: Platelet hyperactivity and abnormal Ca(2⁺) homeostasis in diabetes mellitus, *Am J Physiol Heart Circ Physiol* 280:H1480–H1489, 2001.

55. Guthikonda S, Alviar CL, Vaduganathan M, et al: Role of reticulated platelets and platelet size heterogeneity on platelet activity after dual antiplatelet therapy with aspirin and clopidogrel in patients with stable coronary artery disease, *J Am Coll Cardiol* 52:743–749, 2008.

56. Price MJ, Berger PB, Teirstein PS, et al: Standard- versus high-dose clopidogrel based on platelet function testing after percutaneous coronary intervention: the GRAVITAS randomized trial, *JAMA* 305:1097–1105, 2011.

57. Wiviott SD, Trenk D, Frelinger AL, et al: Prasugrel compared with high loading- and maintenance-dose clopidogrel in patients with planned percutaneous coronary intervention: the Prasugrel in Comparison to Clopidogrel for Inhibition of Platelet Activation and Aggregation-Thrombolysis in Myocardial Infarction 44 trial, *Circulation* 116:2923–2932, 2007.

58. Jakubowski JA, Winters KJ, Naganuma H, Wallentin L: Prasugrel: a novel thienopyridine antiplatelet agent. A review of preclinical and clinical studies and the mechanistic basis for its distinct antiplatelet profile, *Cardiovasc Drug Rev* 25:357–374, 2007.

59. Wiviott SD, Braunwald E, McCabe CH, et al: Prasugrel versus clopidogrel in patients with acute coronary syndromes, *N Engl J Med* 357:2001–2015, 2007.

60. Bhatt DL: Intensifying platelet inhibition—navigating between Scylla and Charybdis, *N Engl J Med* 357:2078–2081, 2007.

61. Wiviott SD, Braunwald E, Angiolillo DJ, et al: Greater clinical benefit of more intensive oral antiplatelet therapy with prasugrel in patients with diabetes mellitus in the trial to assess improvement in therapeutic outcomes by optimizing platelet inhibition with prasugrel-Thrombolysis in Myocardial Infarction 38, *Circulation* 118:1626–1636, 2008.

62. Angiolillo DJ, Badimon JJ, Saucedo JF, et al: A pharmacodynamic comparison of prasugrel vs. high-dose clopidogrel in patients with type 2 diabetes mellitus and coronary artery disease: results of the Optimizing anti-Platelet Therapy In diabetes MellitUS (OPTIMUS)-3 Trial, *Eur Heart J* 32:838–846, 2011.

63. Roe MT, Armstrong PW, Fox KA, et al: Prasugrel versus clopidogrel for acute coronary syndromes without revascularization, *N Engl J Med* 2012.

64. Gurbel PA, Bliden KP, Butler K, et al: Randomized double-blind assessment of the ONSET and OFFSET of the antiplatelet effects of ticagrelor versus clopidogrel in patients with stable coronary artery disease: the ONSET/OFFSET study, *Circulation* 120:2577–2585, 2009.

65. Wallentin L, Becker RC, Budaj A, et al: Ticagrelor versus clopidogrel in patients with acute coronary syndromes, *N Engl J Med* 361:1045–1057, 2009.

66. James S, Angiolillo DJ, Cornel JH, et al: Ticagrelor vs. clopidogrel in patients with acute coronary syndromes and diabetes: a substudy from the PLATelet inhibition and patient Outcomes (PLATO) trial, *Eur Heart J* 31:3006–3016, 2010.

67. Gurbel PA, Bliden KP, Butler K, et al: Response to ticagrelor in clopidogrel nonresponders and responders and effect of switching therapies: the RESPOND study, *Circulation* 121:1188–1199, 2010.

68. Alexopoulos D, Galati A, Xanthopoulou I, et al: Ticagrelor versus prasugrel in acute coronary syndrome patients with high on-clopidogrel platelet reactivity following percutaneous coronary intervention: a pharmacodynamic study, *J Am Coll Cardiol* 60:193–199, 2012.

69. James SK, Roe MT, Cannon CP, et al: Ticagrelor versus clopidogrel in patients with acute coronary syndromes intended for non-invasive management: substudy from prospective randomised PLATelet inhibition and patient Outcomes (PLATO) trial, *BMJ* 342:d3527, 2011.

69a. Bonaca MP, Bhatt DL, Braunwald E, et al: Design and rationale for the Prevention of Cardiovascular Events in Patients With Prior Heart Attack Using Ticagrelor Compared to Placebo on a Background of Aspirin–Thrombolysis in Myocardial Infarction 54 (PEGASUS-TIMI 54) trial, *Am Heart J* 167:437–444, 2014a.

70. Schrör K: The pharmacology of cilostazol, *Diabetes Obes Metab* 4(Suppl 2):S14–S19, 2002.

71. Lee SW, Park SW, Hong MK, et al: Triple versus dual antiplatelet therapy after coronary stenting: impact on stent thrombosis, *J Am Coll Cardiol* 46:1833–1837, 2005.

72. Lee SW, Park SW, Yun SC, et al: Triple antiplatelet therapy reduces ischemic events after drug-eluting stent implantation: Drug-Eluting stenting followed by Cilostazol treatment REduces Adverse Serious cardiac Events (DECREASE registry), *Am Heart J* 159:284–291 e1, 2010.

73. Chen KY, Rha SW, Li YJ, et al: Triple versus dual antiplatelet therapy in patients with acute ST-segment elevation myocardial infarction undergoing primary percutaneous coronary intervention, *Circulation* 119:3207–3214, 2009.

74. Suh JW, Lee SP, Park KW, et al: Multicenter randomized trial evaluating the efficacy of cilostazol on ischemic vascular complications after drug-eluting stent implantation for coronary heart disease: results of the CILON-T (influence of CILostazol-based triple antiplatelet therapy ON ischemic complication after drug-eluting stenT implantation) trial, *J Am Coll Cardiol* 57:280–289, 2011.

75. Han Y, Li Y, Wang S, et al: Cilostazol in addition to aspirin and clopidogrel improves long-term outcomes after percutaneous coronary intervention in patients with acute coronary syndromes: a randomized, controlled study, *Am Heart J* 157:733–739, 2009.

76. Angiolillo DJ, Capranzano P, Goto S, et al: A randomized study assessing the impact of cilostazol on platelet function profiles in patients with diabetes mellitus and coronary artery disease on dual antiplatelet therapy: results of the OPTIMUS-2 study, *Eur Heart J* 29:2202–2211, 2008.

77. Jeong YH, Tantry US, Park Y, et al: Pharmacodynamic effect of cilostazol plus standard clopidogrel versus double-dose clopidogrel in patients with type 2 diabetes undergoing percutaneous coronary intervention, *Diabetes Care* 2012.

78. Angiolillo DJ, Capranzano P, Ferreiro JL, et al: Impact of adjunctive cilostazol therapy on platelet function profiles in patients with and without diabetes mellitus on aspirin and clopidogrel therapy, *Thromb Haemost* 106:253–262, 2011.

79. Capranzano P, Ferreiro JL, Ueno M, et al: Pharmacodynamic effects of adjunctive cilostazol therapy in patients with coronary artery disease on dual antiplatelet therapy: impact of high on-treatment platelet reactivity and diabetes mellitus status, *Catheter Cardiovasc Interv* 2012.

80. Jeong YH, Lee SW, Choi BR, et al: Randomized comparison of adjunctive cilostazol versus high maintenance dose clopidogrel in patients with high post-treatment platelet reactivity: results of the ACCEL-RESISTANCE (Adjunctive Cilostazol Versus High Maintenance Dose Clopidogrel in Patients With Clopidogrel Resistance) randomized study, *J Am Coll Cardiol* 53:1101–1109, 2009.

81. Biondi-Zoccai GG, Lotrionte M, Anselmino M, et al: Systematic review and meta-analysis of randomized clinical trials appraising the impact of cilostazol after percutaneous coronary intervention, *Am Heart J* 155:1081–1089, 2008.

82. Lee SW, Park SW, Kim YH, et al: Drug-eluting stenting followed by cilostazol treatment reduces late restenosis in patients with diabetes mellitus the DECLARE-DIABETES Trial (A Randomized Comparison of Triple Antiplatelet Therapy with Dual Antiplatelet Therapy After Drug-Eluting Stent Implantation in Diabetic Patients), *J Am Coll Cardiol* 51:1181–1187, 2008.

83. Kim HH, Liao JK: Translational therapeutics of dipyridamole, *Arterioscler Thromb Vasc Biol* 28: s39–s42, 2008.

84. Aktas B, Utz A, Hoenig-Liedl P, et al: Dipyridamole enhances NO/cGMP-mediated vasodilator-stimulated phosphoprotein phosphorylation and signaling in human platelets: in vitro and in vivo/ex vivo studies, *Stroke* 34:764–769, 2003.

85. European stroke prevention study. ESPS Group, *Stroke* 21:1122–1130, 1990.

86. Sivenius J, Laakso M, Riekkinen P Sr., et al: European stroke prevention study: effectiveness of antiplatelet therapy in diabetic patients in secondary prevention of stroke, *Stroke* 23:851–854, 1992.

87. Diener HC, Cunha L, Forbes C, et al: European stroke prevention study. 2. Dipyridamole and acetylsalicylic acid in the secondary prevention of stroke, *J Neurol Sci* 143:1–13, 1996.

88. Halkes PH, van Gijn J, Kappelle LJ, et al: Aspirin plus dipyridamole versus aspirin alone after cerebral ischaemia of arterial origin (ESPRIT): randomised controlled trial, *Lancet* 367:1665–1673, 2006.

89. O'Donoghue ML, Bhatt DL, Wiviott SD, et al: Safety and tolerability of atopaxar in the treatment of patients with acute coronary syndromes: the lessons from antagonizing the cellular effects of Thrombin-Acute Coronary Syndromes Trial, *Circulation* 123:1843–1853, 2011.

90. Becker RC, Moliterno DJ, Jennings LK, et al: Safety and tolerability of SCH 530348 in patients undergoing non-urgent percutaneous coronary intervention: a randomised, double-blind, placebo-controlled phase II study, *Lancet* 373:919–928, 2009.

91. Morrow DA, Braunwald E, Bonaca MP, et al: Vorapaxar in the secondary prevention of atherothrombotic events, *N Engl J Med* 366:1404–1413, 2012.

92. Scirica BM, Bonaca MP, Braunwald E, et al: Vorapaxar for secondary prevention of thrombotic events for patients with previous myocardial infarction: a prespecified subgroup analysis of the TRA 2° P-TIMI 50 trial, *Lancet* 2012.

93. Tricoci P, Huang Z, Held C, et al: Thrombin-receptor antagonist vorapaxar in acute coronary syndromes, *N Engl J Med* 366:20–33, 2012.

94. Wiviott SD, Flather MD, O'Donoghue ML, et al: Randomized trial of atopaxar in the treatment of patients with coronary artery disease: the lessons from antagonizing the cellular effect of thrombin-coronary artery disease trial, *Circulation* 123:1854–1863, 2011.

95. Goto S, Ogawa H, Takeuchi M, et al: Double-blind, placebo-controlled Phase II studies of the protease-activated receptor 1 antagonist E5555 (atopaxar) in Japanese patients with acute coronary syndrome or high-risk coronary artery disease, *Eur Heart J* 31:2601–2613, 2010.

96. Bhatt DL, Lincoff AM, Gibson CM, et al: Intravenous platelet blockade with cangrelor during PCI, *N Engl J Med* 361:2330–2341, 2009.

97. Harrington RA, Stone GW, McNulty S, et al: Platelet inhibition with cangrelor in patients undergoing PCI, *N Engl J Med* 361:2318–2329, 2009.

98. Angiolillo DJ, Firstenberg MS, Price MJ, et al: Bridging antiplatelet therapy with cangrelor in patients undergoing cardiac surgery: a randomized controlled trial, *JAMA* 307:265–274, 2012.

99. Neri Serneri GG, Coccheri S, Marubini E, Violi F: Picotamide, a combined inhibitor of thromboxane A2 synthase and receptor, reduces 2-year mortality in diabetics with peripheral arterial disease: the DAVID study, *Eur Heart J* 25:1845–1852, 2004.

was significantly better in nondiabetic patients (60.1% versus 82.6%; $P=0.02$). After 8 years, repeat revascularization was necessary in 65.3% of PTCA patients but in only 26.5% of CABG patients ($P<0.001$). The Coronary Angioplasty versus Bypass Revascularization Investigation (CABRI) trial randomized 1054 patients with multivessel disease to either CABG or PTCA.[43] The overall 1-year mortality was no different between CABG (2.7%) and PTCA (3.9%). However, in the 122 randomized patients who had diabetes, there was a nonsignificant trend toward better survival in the CABG group at 2 years (96% versus 85%), a significantly lower incidence of re-revascularization procedures (2.0% versus 11.8%; $P<0.001$), and significantly better relief of angina ($P<0.001$). The overall composite rate of major adverse coronary and cerebral events (MACCEs), which included strokes and the need for repeat revascularization, was significantly lower in CABG patients (11.3% versus 19.1%; $P=0.016$).

Coronary Artery Bypass Graft Surgery versus Percutaneous Coronary Intervention with Bare Metal Stents

The high incidence of restenosis with PTCA led to the emergence of coronary stents. Several trials compared the results of revascularization with CABG versus bare metal stents (BMS). In the Arterial Revascularization Therapies Study (ARTS), a total of 1205 patients were randomly assigned to treatment with PCI or CABG. The event-free survival at 1 year in patients with diabetes was significantly lower in the BMS group (63.4% versus 84.4%; $P<0.001$) because of the higher incidence of repeat revascularization (21.6% versus 12.4%).[44] The difference was largely the result of a lower rate of complete revascularization in patients undergoing PCI with BMS versus CABG (70.5% versus 84.1%; $P<0.001$). Overall, 5-year mortality in patients with diabetes was higher in the BMS group (13.4% versus 8.3%), but this did not reach statistical significance. However, in patients undergoing PCI with BMS, 5-year mortality was higher in patients with versus without diabetes (13.4% versus 6.8%; $P=0.03$) whereas there was no statistical difference in mortality of patients with versus without diabetes in the CABG group (8.3% versus 7.5%; $P=0.8$). In BMS patients, the need for repeat revascularization was significantly higher in patients with versus without diabetes (42.9% versus 27.5%; $P=0.002$). In the Stent Or Surgery (SOS) trial, diabetic patients undergoing CABG had significantly decreased mortality after 6 years compared with patients treated with BMS (10.9% versus 6.8%; $P=0.02$).[45] Hlatky and colleagues analyzed data from 10 randomized trials comparing CABG with PTCA and BMS in 7812 patients.[46] Over a median follow-up of 5.9 years, mortality in patients with diabetes was 30% lower in the CABG group compared with the PCTA and BMS group. In contrast, mortality was increased in diabetic patients undergoing PTCA or BMS (20.0% versus 12.3%; $P=0.014$).

Coronary Artery Bypass Graft Surgery versus Percutaneous Coronary Intervention with Drug-Eluting Stents

In earlier studies comparing CABG versus PCI with PTCA or BMS, the difference in MACCE was driven by the need for repeat revascularization procedures in the PTCA-BMS diabetic patients. It was hoped that the introduction of drug-eluting stents (DESs) with concomitant more aggressive

antiplatelet therapy would reduce post-PCI restenosis, stent thrombosis and clinical events and make it a more attractive revascularization option for patients with diabetes mellitus.

The Coronary Artery Revascularization in Diabetes (CARDIA) trial was the first randomized trial of CABG versus coronary stenting using DES in diabetic patients with multivessel disease.[47] In this multicenter study, 510 diabetic patients were randomized to CABG or BMS in earlier phases of the trial, and subsequently in the later phases to DESs. DESs were used in 69% of the PCI group. The primary outcome was the composite of all-cause mortality, MI, or stroke. The secondary outcomes included the need for repeat revascularization. After 1 year, there was no difference in the primary composite outcome (10.5% CABG versus 13.0% PCI; $P=0.39$). However, there was a significant reduction in the combination of the primary endpoint and the need for repeat revascularization in favor of CABG patients (11.3% CABG versus 19.3% PCI; $P=0.02$). The rate of MIs was also significantly higher in the PCI group ($P=0.016$). After 1 year, symptoms had improved in both groups; however, patients randomized to CABG had significantly less angina ($P<0.001$).

BARI 2D

The BARI 2D trial compared aggressive medical management with immediate revascularization using either CABG or PCI versus aggressive medical management alone in patients with diabetes and multivessel CHD.[41] Patients were randomized by the treating physician to either prompt revascularization or medical therapy and then randomized to glucose-lowering treatment with either insulin-sensitizing agents (metformin and/or thiazolidinediones) or insulin providers (sulfonylureas and/or insulin). The primary outcome of the study was survival at 5 years. Secondary endpoints included the composite score of death, MI, or stroke.

Before randomization, the mode of revascularization was determined collaboratively by an interventional cardiologist and a cardiac surgeon. Patients prospectively selected for CABG versus PCI (with BMS and/or DES) had more three-vessel and proximal left anterior descending artery (LAD) disease. By the end of the trial, 42% of patients initially randomized to medical therapy had undergone some type of revascularization procedure. In the primary analysis, there was no statistical difference between the randomized comparator groups of medical therapy versus immediate revascularization for 5-year survival (87.8% versus 88.3%). In a subanalysis of those patients randomized to immediate revascularization, there was no statistical difference in 5-year survival between patients selected for the PCI stratum and those selected for the CABG stratum (88.3% versus 87.8%; $P=0.97$). There was also no difference in secondary endpoints. When compared with medical therapy for all patients, there was no difference in primary or secondary endpoints in patients undergoing PCI. However, a significantly larger number of CABG patients were free from the secondary endpoints of death, MI, or stroke than in the medical treated group (77.6% versus 69.5%; $P=0.01$).

The Synergy between Percutaneous Coronary Intervention with Taxus and Cardiac Surgery (SYNTAX) study compared CABG versus the Taxus Express DES in patients with and without diabetes mellitus and three-vessel disease.[48] After 1 year, the risk of repeat revascularization was higher with DES than CABG in patients with diabetes (6.4% versus 20.3%) or without diabetes (5.7% versus 11.1%). Mortality was higher with

DES, with more complex lesions than in CABG patients (4.1% versus 13.5%). Mack and coworkers compared three-year outcomes of DES with CABG in patients with and without diabetes as part of the SYNTAX trial.[49] MACCE (major adverse coronary and cerebral events) rates were higher in those with versus without diabetes receiving DESs, largely because of an increased need for repeat revascularization. Although diabetes increased MACCE rates among patients receiving DES, the presence of diabetes had little impact on outcomes after CABG. The presence of diabetes significantly increased 3-year MACCE rate, mortality, and need for repeat revascularization in DES patients, but not in patients undergoing CABG. The SYNTAX score is a measure of complexity of the coronary lesion—presence of occlusion, length of the lesion, degree of calcification, and presence of ulceration–with higher scores representing more complex disease. There was no difference in MACCE rate in DES versus CABG in other diabetic or non-diabetic patients with a SYNTAX score below 22. However, in patients with SYNTAX scores higher than 33, the MACCE rate was significantly higher in both diabetic and nondiabetic patients undergoing DES versus CABG. Banning and coworkers further analyzed the MACCE outcomes (death, stroke, MIs, and need for repeat revascularization) in diabetic patients with a SYNTAX score above 33.[48] Overall mortality was significantly increased in patients with DES versus CABG. The need for repeat revascularization was three times higher in DES patients. There was no difference in the incidence of strokes between DES and CABG groups.

Certain subgroups of diabetic patients may also benefit more from particular revascularization strategies. Ohno and colleagues found that in patients with diabetic retinopathy there is a survival benefit of CABG over PCI.[50] Patients with diabetic retinopathy have an increased incidence of CHF and cardiomyopathy, and the results of CABG in this group are especially poor.[51] In a retrospective study of 223 diabetic patients undergoing CABG, Ohno and colleagues found that the 12-year survival was 82% for patients without retinopathy, 56% for patient with mild to moderate, non-proliferative retinopathy, 36% for patients with severe nonproliferative retinopathy, and only 12% for patients with proliferative retinopathy.[52]

Previous trials comparing CABG versus PCI have been criticized because state of the art techniques for PCI or CABG were not used. In an attempt to overcome these limitations, the Future Revascularization Evaluation in Patients with Diabetes Mellitus: Optimal Management of Multivessel Disease (FREEDOM) trial used contemporary PCI and CABG techniques and the latest medical therapies, including dual anti-platelet agents, to determine whether CABG or PCI with DES is the optimal method to revascularize patients with diabetes mellitus who have multivessel coronary disease.[53] The study prospectively randomized 1900 patients with diabetes mellitus and multivessel disease to either CABG or PCI with DES at 140 centers throughout the world from 2005 to 2010. The primary outcome was a composite of all-cause mortality, non-fatal MI, and nonfatal stroke. After 5 years, the incidence of the primary outcome was 26.6% in the PCI group—significantly higher than in patients undergoing CABG (18.7%; $P = 0.005$). PCI patients also had a significantly higher rate of MIs (13.9% versus 6%; $P < 0.0001$) and experienced a higher overall mortality (16.3% versus 10.9%; $P < 0.001$). The incidence of stroke was higher in the CABG group (5.2% versus 2.4%; $P = 0.03$), mainly because of an increased rate of events in the first 30 days after surgery. These results were independent of the SYNTAX score. At 12 months, PCI patients required significantly more repeat revascularization procedures (13% versus 5%; $P < 0.0001$). The FREEDOM trial adds further support to the premise that in diabetic patients with multivessel disease, CABG is the preferred method for coronary revascularization.

The Optimal Strategy for Coronary Revascularization in Patients with Diabetes and Multivessel Coronary Artery Disease (Fig. 18-1 and also see Chapter 17)

The BARI 2D trial demonstrated that for patients with diabetes mellitus and stable multivessel coronary artery disease, optimal medical therapy rather than immediate revascularization with PCI or CABG is an appropriate and effective first-line strategy.[39] In patients in whom medical therapy has failed and who have left main and severe multivessel disease, CABG appears to offer the best therapy. It results in better long-term survival, freedom from recurrent MIs, and need for repeat revascularization.[54–56] CABG offers more complete revascularization, especially in patients with more

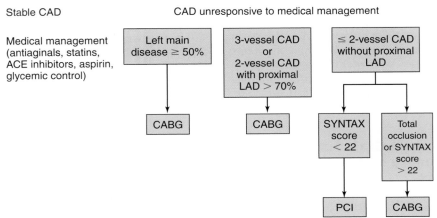

MANAGEMENT OF CORONARY DISEASE IN PATIENTS WITH DIABETES MELLITUS

FIGURE 18-1 Management of coronary disease in patients with diabetes mellitus. ACE = Angiotensin-converting enzyme; CABG = coronary artery bypass graft surgery; CAD = coronary artery disease; LAD = left anterior descending artery; PCI = percutaneous coronary intervention; SYNTAX = Synergy between Percutaneous Coronary Intervention with Taxus and Cardiac Surgery trial.

BOX 18-4 Perioperative Glucose Management after the Intensive Care Unit

Target Goals
Blood glucose <180 mg/dL in postprandial state
Blood glucose 100-140 mg/dL in fasting and premeal states
Goals are best achieved with subcutaneous insulin combining intermediate- and rapid-acting insulin agents.
Oral agents are resumed when target glucose levels are maintained and the patient is tolerating a normal diet.
Metformin should *not* be restarted until the patient is documented to have normal renal function.

scheduled basal insulin regimen when they meet the following criteria:

- A stable IV insulin infusion rate is maintained for at least 4 hours in the fasting state.
- The patient is extubated and off pressor agents.
- The patient is ready to receive oral, enteral, or parenteral nutrition.[107]

Our goals during the non-ICU phase of the patient's hospital stay are as follows (**Box 18-4**):

- Target a blood glucose level below 180 mg/dL in the postprandial state.
- Achieve a blood glucose level of 100 to 140 mg/dL in the fasting and premeal states after transfer to the floor.

The best method to achieve consistent glycemic control in clinically stable patients with diabetes is with scheduled basal or bolus insulin therapy. This is accomplished best with subcutaneous insulin that combines long- or intermediate-acting insulin with rapid-acting insulin administered simultaneously with nutritional intake.

References

1. Flaherty JD, Davidson CJ: Diabetes and coronary revascularization, *JAMA* 293:1501, 2005.
2. Kip KE, Faxon DP, Detre KM, et al: The National Heart, Lung and Blood Institute percutaneous transluminal coronary angioplasty registry, *Circulation* 94:1818, 1996.
3. Kapur A, Malik IS, Bagger JP, et al: The Coronary Artery Revascularization in Diabetes (CARDia) trial: background aims and design, *Am Heart J* 149:13, 2005.
4. Clough RA, Leavitt BJ, Morton JR, et al: The effect of comorbid illness on mortality outcomes in cardiac surgery, *Arch Surg* 137:428, 2002.
5. Thourani VH, Weintraub WS, Stein B, et al: Influence of diabetes mellitus on early and late outcomes after coronary artery bypass grafting, *Ann Thorac Surg* 67:1045, 1999.
6. Braxton JH, Marrin CA, McGrath PD, et al: Mediastinitis and long-term survival after coronary artery bypass graft surgery. Northern New England Cardiovascular Disease Study Group, *Ann Thorac Surg* 70:2004, 2000.
7. Herlitz J, Wognsen GB, Karlson BW, et al: Mortality, mode of death and risk indicators for death during 5 years after coronary artery bypass grafting amongst patients with and without a history of diabetes mellitus, *Coron Artery Dis* 11:339, 2000.
8. Liv JY, Birkmeyer NJ, Sanders JH, et al: Risks of morbidity and mortality in dialysis patients undergoing coronary artery bypass surgery, *Circulation* 102:2973, 2000.
9. Birkmeyer JD, O'Connor GT, Quinton HB, et al: The effect of peripheral vascular disease on in-hospital mortality rates with coronary artery bypass surgery, *J Vasc Surg* 21:445, 1995.
10. Stein B, Weintraub WS, Gebhart S, et al: Influence of diabetes mellitus on early and late outcomes after percutaneous transluminal coronary angioplasty, *Circulation* 91:979, 1995.
11. Mehta RH, Honeycutt E, Patel VD, et al: Relationship of the time interval between cardiac catheterization and elective coronary artery bypass surgery with postprocedural acute kidney injury, *Circulation* 124(1):5149, 2011.
12. Smith LR, Harrell FE, Rankin JS, et al: Determinants of early versus late cardiac death in patients undergoing coronary artery bypass graft surgery, *Circulation* 84 II:245, 1991.
13. Carson JL, Scholz PM, Chen AY, et al: Diabetes mellitus increases short-term mortality and morbidity in patients undergoing coronary artery bypass graft surgery, *J Am Coll Cardiol* 40:418, 2002.
14. Morricone L, Ranucci M, Dentis, et al: Diabetes and complications after cardiac surgery: comparison with a non-diabetic population, *Acta Diabetol* 36:77, 1999.
15. Bucerius J, Gummert JF, Borger MA, et al: Stroke after cardiac surgery: a risk factor analysis of 16,184 consecutive adult patients, *Ann Thorac Surg* 75:472, 2003.
16. Rao V, Ivanou J, Weisel RD, et al: Predictors of low cardiac output syndrome after coronary artery bypass, *J Thorac Cardiovasc Surg* 112:38, 1996.
17. Woods SE, Smith JM, Sohail S, et al: The influence of type 2 diabetes mellitus in patients undergoing coronary artery bypass graft surgery. An 8-year prospective cohort study, *Chest* 126:1789, 2004.
18. Calafiore AM, Di Mauro M, Di Giammarco G, et al: Effect of diabetes on early and late survival after isolated first coronary bypass surgery in multi-vessel disease, *J Thorac Cardiovasc Surg* 125:144, 2003.
19. van Straten AH, Soliman Hamad MA, van Zundert, et al: Diabetes and survival after coronary artery bypass grafting: comparison with an age and sex-matched population, *Eur J Cardiothorac Surg* 37:1068, 2010.
20. Mohammadi S, Dagenais F, Mathieu P, et al: Long-term impact of diabetes and its comorbidities in patients undergoing isolated primary coronary artery bypass graft surgery, *Circulation* 116:220, 2007.
21. O'Keefe JH, Blackstone EH, Sergeant P, et al: The optimal mode of coronary revascularization for diabetics. A risk-adjusted long-term study comparing coronary angioplasty and coronary bypass surgery, *Eur Heart J* 19:1696, 1998.
22. Weintraub WS, Stein B, Kosinski A, et al: Outcome of coronary bypass surgery versus coronary angioplasty in diabetic patients with multi-vessel coronary artery disease, *J Am Coll Cardiol* 31:10, 1998.
23. Morris JJ, Smith LR, Jones RH, et al: Influence of diabetes and mammary artery grafting on survival after coronary bypass, *Circulation* 81:275, 1991.
24. Szabo Z, Hakanson E, Svedjeholm R: Early postoperative outcome and medium-term survival in 540 diabetic and 2,239 non-diabetic patients undergoing coronary artery bypass grafting, *Ann Thorac Surg* 74:712, 2002.
25. Leavitt BJ, Sheppard L, Maloney C, et al: Effect of diabetes and associated conditions on long-term survival after coronary artery bypass graft surgery, *Circulation* 110:41, 2004.
26. Trachiotis GD, Weintraub WS, Johnston TS, et al: Coronary artery bypass grafting in patients with advanced left ventricular dysfunction, *Ann Thorac Surg* 66:1632, 1998.
27. Whang W, Bigger JT Jr., Diabetes and outcomes of coronary artery bypass graft surgery in patients with severe left ventricular dysfunction: results from The CABG Patch Trial database. The CABG Patch Trial Investigators and Coordinators, *J Am Coll Cardiol* 36:1166, 2000.
28. Kaul TK, Agnihorn AK, Fields BL, et al: Coronary artery bypass grafting in patients with an ejection fraction of twenty percent or less, *J Thorac Cardiovasc Surg* 111:1001, 1996.
29. Milano CA, White WD, Smith R, et al: Coronary artery bypass in patients with severely depressed ventricular function, *Ann Thorac Surg* 56:487, 1993.
30. Bell DS: Diabetic cardiomyopathy: a unique entity or a complication of coronary artery disease? *Diabetes Care* 18:708, 1995.
31. van der Meer, Hillege HL, van Gilst WH, et al: A comparison of internal mammary artery and saphenous vein grafts after coronary artery bypass surgery: no difference in 1-year occlusion rates and clinical outcomes, *Circulation* 90:2367, 1994.
32. Alderman EL, Carley SD, Fisher LD, et al: Five-year angiographic follow-up of factors associated with progression of coronary artery disease in the Coronary Artery Surgery Study (CASS), *J Am Coll Cardiol* 22:1141, 1993.
33. Singh SK, Desai ND, Petroff SD, et al: The impact of diabetic status on coronary artery bypass graft patency. Insights from the radial artery patency study, *Circulation* 118:222, 2008.
34. Choudhary BP, Antoniades C, Brading AF, et al: Diabetes mellitus as a predictor for radial artery vaso-reactivity in patients undergoing coronary after bypass grafting, *J Am Coll Cardiol* 50:1047, 2007.
35. Hirotani T, Kameda T, Kumamoto T, et al: Effects of coronary artery bypass grafting using internal mammary arteries for diabetic patients, *J Am Coll Cardiol* 34:532, 1999.
36. Endo M, Tomizawa Y, Nishida H: Bilateral versus unilateral internal mammary revascularization in patients with diabetes, *Circulation* 108:1343, 2003.
37. Matsa M, Paz Y, Gurevitch J, et al: Bilateral skeletonized internal thoracic artery grafts in patients with diabetes mellitus, *J Thorac Cardiovasc Surg* 121:668, 2001.
38. The BARI Investigators: Influence of diabetes on 5-year mortality and morbidity in a randomized trial comparing CABG and PTCA in patients with multi-vessel disease: the Bypass Angioplasty Revascularization Investigation (BARI), *N Engl J Med* 335:217, 1996.
39. The BARI Investigators: Seven-year outcome in the Bypass Angioplasty Revascularization Investigation by treatment and diabetic status, *J Am Coll Cardiol* 35:1122, 2000.
40. Rogers WJ, Alderman EL, Chaitman BR, et al: The BARI Study Group: Bypass Angioplasty Revascularization Investigation (BARI): baseline clinical and angiographic data, *Am J Cardiol* 75:9C, 1995.
41. The BARI Investigators: A randomized trial of therapies for type 2 diabetes and coronary artery disease, *N Engl J Med* 360(24):2503, 2009.
42. King SB, Kosinski AS, Guyton RA, et al: Eight-year mortality in the Emory Angioplasty versus Surgery Trial (EAST). J Am Coll Cardiol 35: 1116–21, 2000.
43. Kurbaan AS, Bowkaer TJ, Ilsley CD, et al: Difference in the mortality of the CABRI diabetic and non-diabetic populations and its relation to coronary artery disease and the revascularization mode, *Am J Cardiol* 87:947, 2001.
44. Abizaid A, Costa MA, Centemero M, et al: Clinical and economic impact of diabetes mellitus on percutaneous and surgical treatment of multi-vessel coronary disease patients: insights from the Arterial Revascularization Therapy Study (ARTS) trial, *Circulation* 104:533, 2001.
45. Booth J, Clayton T, Pepper J, et al: Randomized, controlled trial of coronary artery bypass surgery versus percutaneous coronary intervention in patients with multi-vessel coronary artery disease. Six-year follow-up for the Stent or Surgery (SOS) trial, *Circulation* 118:381, 2008.
46. Hlatky MA, Boothroyd DB, Bravata DM, et al: Coronary artery bypass surgery compared with percutaneous coronary interventions for multi-vessel disease: a collaborative analysis of individual patient data from ten randomized trials, *Lancet* 373:1190, 2009.
47. Kapur A, Hall RJ, Malik IS, et al: Randomized comparison of percutaneous coronary intervention with coronary artery bypass grafting in diabetic patients. 1-year results of the CARDia (Coronary Artery Revascularization in Diabetes) trial, *J Am Coll Cardiol* 55:432, 2010.
48. Banning AP, Westaby S, Morice MC, et al: Diabetic and non-diabetic patients with left main and/or 3-vessel coronary artery disease: comparison of outcomes with cardiac surgery and paclitxel-eluting stents, *J Am Coll Cardiol* 55:1067, 2010.
49. Mack MJ, Banning AP, Serruys PW, et al: Bypass versus drug-eluting stents at 3 years in SYNTAX patients with diabetes or metabolic syndrome, *Ann Thorac Surg* 92:240, 2011.
50. Ohno T, Ohashi T, Asakura T, et al: Impact of diabetic retinopathy on cardiac outcome after coronary artery bypass graft surgery: prospective observational study, *Ann Thorac Surg* 81:608, 2006.
51. Wong TY, Rosamond W, Chang PP, et al: Retinopathy and risk of congestive heart failure, *JAMA* 293:63, 2005.
52. Ohno T, Ando J, Ono M, et al: The beneficial effect of coronary-artery-bypass surgery on survival in patients with diabetic retinopathy, *Eur J Cardiothorac Surg* 30:881, 2006.
53. Farkouth ME, Domanski M, Sleeper LA, et al: Strategies for multi-vessel revascularization in patients with diabetes, *N Engl J Med* 367:2375, 2012.
54. Boden NE, Taggart DP: Diabetes with coronary disease – a moving target amid evolving therapies? *N Engl J Med* 360:2570, 2009.
55. Chaitman BR, Hardison RM, Adler D, et al: The bypass angioplasty revascularization investigation 2 diabetes randomized trial of different treatment strategies in type 2 diabetes mellitus with stable ischemic heart disease: impact of treatment strategy on cardiac mortality and myocardial infarction, *Circulation* 120:2529, 2009.
56. Hollis LD, Smith PK, Anderson R, et al: ACCF/AHA guideline for coronary artery bypass graft surgery. A report of the American College of Cardiology Foundation/American Heart Association Task Force on Practice Guidelines, *J Am Coll Cardiol* 58:123, 2011.
57. Roffi M, Chew DP, Mukherjee D, et al: Platelet glycoprotein IIb/IIIa inhibitors reduce mortality in diabetic patients with non-ST segment elevation acute coronary syndromes, *Circulation* 104:2767, 2001.
58. Laskey WK, Selzer F, Vlachos HA, et al: Comparison of in-hospital and one-year outcomes in patients with and without diabetes mellitus undergoing percutaneous catheter intervention (from the National Heart, Lung, and Blood Institute Dynamic Registry), *Am J Cardiol* 90:1062, 2002.
59. Choi D, Kim SK, Choi SH, et al: Preventative effects of rosiglitazone on restenosis after coronary stent implantation in patients with type 2 diabetes, *Diabetes Care* 27:2654, 2004.

60. Luciani N, Nasso G, Guadino M, et al: Coronary artery bypass grafting in type II diabetic patients: a comparison between insulin-dependent and non-insulin dependent patients at short and mid-term follow-up, *Ann Thorac Surg* 76:1149, 2003.

61. Kubal C, Srinivasan AK, Grayson AD, et al: Effect of risk-adjusted diabetes on mortality and morbidity after coronary artery bypass graft surgery, *Ann Thorac Surg* 79:1570, 2005.

62. Estrada CA, Young JA, Nifong LW, et al: Outcomes and perioperative hyperglycemia in patients with or without diabetes mellitus undergoing coronary artery bypass grafting, *Ann Thorac Surg* 75:1392, 2003.

63. Opie LH: Effects of regional ischemia on metabolism of glucose and fatty acids. Relative rates of aerobic and anaerobic energy production during myocardial infarction and comparison with effects of anoxia, *Circulation* 38:152, 1976.

64. Sowers JR, Epstein M: Diabetes mellitus and associated hypertension, vascular disease, and nephropathy, *Hypertension* 26:869, 1995.

65. Schmidt AM, Yan SD, Wautier JL, et al: Activation of receptor for advanced glycation end-points: a mechanism for chronic vascular dysfunction in diabetic vasculopathy and atherosclerosis, *Circ Res* 84:489, 1999.

66. Viassara H: Recent progress in advanced glycation end-products and diabetic complications, *Diabetes* 46:519, 1997.

67. Dandena P, Algada A, Mohauty P, et al: Insulin inhibits intranuclear nuclear factor kappa B and simulates 1 kappa B in mononuclear cells in obese subjects: evidence for anti-inflammatory effect, *J Clin Endocrinol Metab* 86:3257, 2001.

68. Guerci B, Bohme P, Kearney-Schwartz A, et al: Endothelial dysfunction and type-2 diabetes, *Diabetes Metab* 27:436, 2001.

69. Park JT, Takahara N, Gabriele A, et al: Induction of endothelin-1 expression by glucose. An effect on protein kinase-c activation, *Diabetes* 49:1239, 2001.

70. Lazar HL, Joseph L, San Mateo C, et al: Expression of inducible nitric oxide synthase in conduits used in patients with diabetes mellitus undergoing coronary revascularization, *J Card Surg* 25:120, 2010.

71. Guzik TS, Mussa S, Gastaldi D, et al: Mechanisms of increased vascular superoxide production in human diabetes mellitus: role of NAD(1)H Oxidase and endothelial nitric oxide synthase, *Circulation* 105:1656, 2001.

72. Davi G, Catalan I, Averna M: Thromboxane biosynthesis and platelet function in type II diabetes mellitus, *N Engl J Med* 322:1769, 1990.

73. Marfella R, Esposito K, Gionata R, et al: Circulating adhesion molecules in humans: role of hyperglycemia and hyperinsulinemia, *Circulation* 201:2247, 2000.

74. Suzuka K, Kono T: Evidence that insulin causes translocation of glucose transport activity to the plasma membrane from intracellular storage site, *Proc Natl Acad Sci U S A* 77:2542, 1980.

75. Langovche L, Vanhorebeek I, Vlaselaers D, et al: Intensive insulin therapy protects the endothelium of critically ill patients, *J Clin Invest* 115:1177, 2005.

76. Johassen AK, Jack MN, Ejos OD, et al: Myocardial protection by insulin at reperfusion requires early administration and is medicated via AKT and p70s6 kinase cell-survival signaling, *Circ Res* 89:1191, 2001.

77. Gao F, Gao E, Yur, et al: Nitric oxide mediates the antiapoptotic effect of insulin in myocardial ischemia-reperfusion: the roles of p13-kinase, AKT, and endothelial nitric oxide synthase phosphorylation, *Circulation* 105:1497, 2002.

78. Svensson S, Svedjeholm R, Ekroth R: Trauma metabolism of the heart: uptake of substrates and effects of insulin early after cardiac operations, *J Thorac Cardiovasc Surg* 99:1063, 1990.

79. Rao V, Merante F, Weisel RD, et al: Insulin stimulates pyruvate dehydrogenase and protects human ventricular cardiomyocytes from simulated ischemia, *J Thorac Cardiovasc Surg* 116:485, 1998.

80. Dandona P, Aljada A, Mohanty P, et al: Insulin inhibits intranuclear factor KB and stimulates KB in mononuclear cells in obese subjects: evidence for an anti-inflammatory effect, *J Clin Endocrinol Metab* 86:7357, 2001.

81. Doenst T, Wiseysundera D, Karkouti K, et al: Hyperglycemia during cardiopulmonary bypass is an independent risk factor for mortality in patients undergoing cardiac surgery, *J Thorac Cardiovasc Surg* 130:1140, 2005.

82. Fish LH, Weaver TW, Moore AL, et al: Value of postoperative blood glucose in predicting complications and length of stay after coronary artery bypass grafting, *Am J Cardiol* 92:74, 2003.

83. McAlister FA, Man J, Bistritz L, et al: Diabetes and coronary artery bypass surgery: an examination of perioperative glycemic control and outcomes, *Diabetes Care* 26:1518, 2003.

84. Imran SA, Random TB, Buth KR, et al: Impact of admission serum glucose level on in-hospital outcomes following coronary artery bypass grafting surgery, *Can J Cardiol* 26:151, 2010.

85. Székely A, Levin J, Miao Y, et al: Impact of hyperglycemia on perioperative mortality after coronary artery bypass graft surgery, *J Thorac Cardiovasc Surg* 142:430, 2001.

86. Duncan AE, Abd-Elsayed A, Maheshwari A, et al: Risk of intraoperative and postoperative blood glucose concentrations in predicting outcomes after cardiac surgery, *Anesthesiology* 112:860, 2010.

87. Golden SH, Peart-Vigilance C, Kao WH, et al: Perioperative glycemic control and the risk of infectious complications in a cohort of adults with diabetes, *Diabetes Care* 22:1408, 1999.

88. Kerr K, Furnary A, Grunkemeier G, et al: Glucose control lowers the risk of wound infections in diabetics after open heart operations, *Ann Thorac Surg* 63:365, 1997.

89. Anderson RE, Klerdal K, Ivert T: Fasting blood glucose and mortality after coronary artery bypass graft surgery, *Eur Heart J* 26:1513, 2005.

90. Malmberg K, Ryden L, Efendic S, et al: Randomized trial of insulin-glucose infusion followed by subcutaneous insulin treatment in diabetic patients with acute myocardial infarction (DIGAMI Study): effects on mortality at 1 year, *J Am Coll Cardiol* 26:57, 1995.

91. DIGAMI Study Group: Prospective, randomized study of intensive insulin treatment on long-term survival after acute myocardial infarction in patients with diabetes mellitus, *Br Med J* 314:1512, 1997.

92. Lazar HL, Chipkin SR, Fitzgerald CA, et al: Tight glycemic control in diabetic coronary artery bypass graft patients improves perioperative outcomes and decreases recurrent ischemic events, *Circulation* 109:1497, 2004.

93. Furnary AP, Gao G, Grunkemeier GL, et al: Continuous insulin infusion reduces mortality in patients with diabetes undergoing coronary artery bypass grafting, *J Thorac Cardiovasc Surg* 125:1007, 2003.

94. Furnary A, Wu Y, Bookin S: Effect of hyperglycemia and continuous intravenous insulin infusions on outcomes of cardiac surgical procedures: the Portland Diabetic Project, *Endocr Pract* 10(Suppl 2):21, 2004.

95. Hruska LA, Smith JM, Hendy MP, et al: Continuous insulin infusion reduces infectious complications in diabetes following coronary surgery, *J Card Surg* 20:402, 2005.

96. Rassias AJ, Marrin CA, Arruda, et al: Insulin infusion improves neutrophil function in diabetic cardiac surgery patients, *Anesth Analg* 88:1011, 1996.

97. van den Berghe G, Wouters P, Weekers F, et al: Intensive insulin therapy in critically ill patients, *N Engl J Med* 345:1359, 2001.

98. D'Alessandro C, Leprince P, Golmard JL, et al: Strict glycemic control reduces EuroScore expected mortality in diabetic patients undergoing myocardial revascularization, *J Thorac Cardiovasc Surg* 134:29, 2007.

99. NICE-SUGAR Study Investigators, Finfer S, Chittock DR, Su SY, et al: Intensive versus conventional glucose control in critically ill patients, *N Engl J Med* 360:1283, 2009.

100. Acton to control Cardiovascular Risk in Diabetes Study Group, Gerstein HC, Miller ME, Byinton RP, et al: Effects of intensive glucose lowering in type 2 diabetes, *N Engl J Med* 358:2545, 2008.

101. The UK Prospective Diabetes Study (UKPDS) Group: Effect of intensive blood-glucose control with metformin on complications in overweight patients with type 2 diabetes. (UKPDS 34), *Lancet* 352:854, 1993.

102. ADVANCE Collaborative Group, Patel A, MacMahond A, Chalmer J, et al: Intensive blood glucose control and vascular outcomes in patients with type 2 diabetes, *N Engl J Med* 358:2560, 2008.

103. Lazar HL, McDonnell MM, Chipkin S, et al: Effects of aggressive vs moderate glycemic control on clinical outcomes in diabetic coronary artery bypass graft patients, *Ann Surg* 254(3):458, 2011.

104. Bhamidipati CM, LaPar DJ, Stukenborg GJ, et al: Superiority of moderate control of hyperglycemia to tight control in patients undergoing coronary artery bypass grafting, *J Thorac Cardiovasc Surg* 141:1, 2010.

105. Qaseem A, Humphrey LL, Chou R, et al: For the Clinical Guidelines Committee of the American College of Physicians: Use of intensive insulin therapy for the management of glycemic control in hospitalized patients. A clinical practice guideline from the American College of Physicians, *Ann Intern Med* 154:260, 2011.

106. Alexanian SM, McDonnell ME, Akhtar S: Creating a perioperative glycemic control program, *Anesthesiol Res Pract* 46:59, 2011.

107. McDonnell ME, Alexanian SM, White L, Lazar HL: A primer for achieving glycemic control in the cardiac surgical patient, *J Card Surg* 27:470, 2012.

108. Friedberg SJ, Lan YW, Blum JJ, Gregerman RI: Insulin absorption: a major factor in apparent insulin resistance and the control of type 2 diabetes mellitus, *Metabolism* 55:614, 2006.

109. Varghese P, Gleason V, Sorokin R, et al: Hypoglycemia in hospitalized patients treated with antihyperglycemia agents, *J Hosp Med* 2:234, 2007.

110. London MJ, Grunwald GK, Shroyer AL, et al: Association of fast-track cardiac management and low-dose to moderate-dose glucocorticoid administration with perioperative hyperglycemia, *J Cardiothorac Vasc Anesth* 14:631, 2000.

111. Chaney MA, Nikolov MP, Blakeman BP, et al: Attempting to maintain normoglycemia during cardiopulmonary bypass with insulin may initiate postoperative hypoglycemia, *Anesth Analg* 89:1091, 1999.

112. Goldberg PA, Siegel MD, Sherwin RS, et al: Implementation of a safe and effective insulin infusion protocol in a medical intensive care unit, *Diabetes Care* 27:461, 2004.

113. Krikorian A, Ismail-Beigi F, Moghissi ES: Comparisons of different insulin infusion protocols: a review of recent literature, *Curr Opin Clin Nutr Metab Care* 13:198, 2009.

114. Donihi A, Rea R, Haas L, et al: Safety and effectiveness of a standardized 80-150 gm/dL IV insulin infusion protocol in the Medical Intensive Care Unit: > 11,000 hours of experience, *Diabetes* 55:459, 2006.

115. Davidson PC, Steed RD, Bode BW: Glucommander: a computer-directed intravenous insulin system shown to be safe, simple, and effective in 120,618 hours of operation, *Diabetes Care* 28:2418, 2005.

116. Juneja R, Roudebush C, Kumar N, et al: Utilization of a computerized intravenous insulin infusion program to control blood glucose in the intensive care unit, *Diabetes Technol Ther* 9:232, 2007.

117. Newton CA, Smiley D, Bode BW, et al: A comparison study of continuous insulin infusion protocols in the medical intensive care unit: computer-guided vs. standard column-based algorithms, *J Hosp Med* 5:432, 2010.

118. DeStantis AJ, Schmeltz LR, Schmidt K, et al: Inpatient management of hyperglycemia: the Northwestern experience, *Endocr Pract* 12:491, 2006.

119. Rea RS, Donihi AC, Bobeck M, et al: Implementing an intravenous insulin infusion protocol in the intensive care unit, *Am J Health Syst Pharm* 64:385, 2007.

120. Lazar HL, McDonnell M, Chipkin SR, et al: The Society of Thoracic Surgeons Practice guideline series: blood glucose management during adult cardiac surgery, *Ann Thorac Surg* 87:663, 2009.

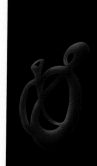

PART IV

EPIDEMIOLOGY AND MANAGEMENT OF ACUTE CORONARY SYNDROMES IN PATIENTS WITH DIABETES

19 Epidemiology of Acute Coronary Syndromes in Patients with Diabetes

Anselm K. Gitt

GLOBAL BURDEN OF CARDIOVASCULAR DISEASE AND DIABETES

Cardiovascular diseases are the number one cause of death worldwide.[1] In 2008, approximately 17.3 million people died from cardiovascular disease, accounting for approximately one third of all deaths; an estimated 7.3 million were caused by coronary heart disease and another 6.2 million by stroke.[2] Until recently, cardiovascular diseases were more frequent in the developed countries, but during the past years low- and middle-income countries have been disproportionally affected. According to the 2010 Global Status Report of the World Health Organization on noncommunicable diseases, over 80% of cardiovascular disease deaths take place in low- and middle-income countries, with no differences between men and women,[1] predominantly as a result of ischemic heart disease (**Fig. 19-1**).[2] Furthermore, the number of people who die from cardiovascular diseases will increase to reach 23.3 million by 2030; ischemic heart disease will remain the single leading cause of death in 2030 (**Fig. 19-2**).[3]

The most important behavioral risk factors of cardiovascular diseases are unhealthy diet, physical inactivity, and tobacco use. These may contribute to raised blood pressure, abnormal blood lipids, raised blood glucose, and overweight and obesity. The increasing frequencies of obesity and sedentary lifestyles—major risk factors for the development of type 2 diabetes, in both developed and developing countries—will further contribute to diabetes being a growing clinical and public health problem worldwide.

The International Diabetes Federation (IDF) reports that 371 million people had diabetes in 2012 (see also **Chapter 1**). The worldwide prevalence of diabetes was 8.4% in the population aged 20 to 79 years, including an estimated 50% (29.2% to 81.2%) of whom had undiagnosed diabetes; there were large differences in prevalence and proportions diagnosed among different regions and countries worldwide (**Fig. 19-3**).[4]

In 2012, 4.8 million people died from complications of diabetes mellitus.[4] In the ranking of causes of death, diabetes will move from rank 11 in the year 2002 to rank 7 in 2030 (**Table 19-1**).[3]

INTERHEART,[5] a large-scale standardized, case-control study involving 15,152 patients with acute myocardial infarction and 14,820 controls, examined the relationship between important cardiovascular risk factors, such as hypertension, diabetes mellitus, and lifestyle, and myocardial infarction in 52 countries worldwide. The study identified diabetes mellitus to be associated with a more than doubled adjusted odds for the development of myocardial infarction (odds ratio [OR] 2.37, 95% confidence interval [CI] 2.07-2.71) for the overall population after adjustment for all other risk factors.[5]

In a population-based study in Denmark, all 3.3 million inhabitants at least 30 years of age and older were identified through the Danish Civil Registration System and followed for 5 years from 1997 to 2002 by individual-level linkage of nationwide registers to estimate cardiovascular risk associated with diabetes mellitus.[6] Diabetes patients receiving glucose-lowering medications and individuals without diabetes, both with and without prior myocardial infarction,

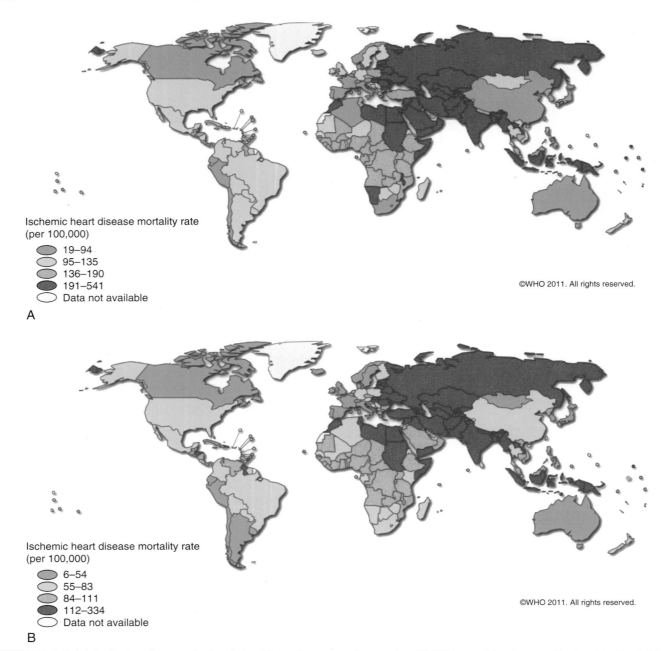

Ischemic heart disease mortality rate
(per 100,000)

- 19–94
- 95–135
- 136–190
- 191–541
- Data not available

A

Ischemic heart disease mortality rate
(per 100,000)

- 6–54
- 55–83
- 84–111
- 112–334
- Data not available

B

FIGURE 19-1 Global distribution of age standardized ischemic heart disease mortality rates (per 100,000) in men (A) and women (B). *(Data from Mendis S, Puska P, Norrving B, eds: Global atlas on cardiovascular disease prevention and control. Geneva, Switzerland, 2011, World Health Organization (WHO). Available at http://whqlibdoc.who.int/publications/2011/9789241564373_eng.pdf.)*

were compared. Regardless of age and sex the hazard ratios (HRs) for cardiovascular death were as high in patients with diabetes mellitus without prior myocardial infarction as in nondiabetic patients with prior myocardial infarction (HR in men 2.42 and 2.44, respectively, and $P=0.60$; HR in women 2.45 and 2.62, respectively, and $P<0.001$; **Fig. 19-4**).[6] Based on these data, diabetes mellitus might be seen as a coronary artery disease risk equivalent. The incidence rates of myocardial infarction during the 5 years of follow-up in this study in men and women with diabetes and without prior myocardial infarction were 7.3% and 6.9%, respectively; for those with diabetes and prior myocardial infarction, the incidence rates were 23.7% and 25.0%, respectively (**Table 19-2**, **Fig. 19-5**).[6]

Further population-based studies with long-term follow-up describing the prevalence of acute coronary syndromes (ACSs) in patients with diabetes are lacking. Available data on patients with diabetes are heterogeneous, because diabetic patients with a long duration of the disease have a different cardiovascular risk than patients with shorter disease duration. The type of diabetes treatment—that is, insulin versus noninsulin—also correlates with risk for ACS, most likely reflecting differences in underlying disease severity. In the ideal setting, information regarding the long-term risk of a patient with newly diagnosed diabetes mellitus for coronary artery disease and its complications would be desirable, but data on the long-term risk of cardiovascular events for patients with new onset of diabetes are scarce. This

TABLE 19-4 Mortality at 30 Days and 1 Year of Patients With Versus Without Diabetes Presenting With Unstable Angina, Non-ST-segment Elevation MI, or ST-segment Elevation MI in 11 Independent Randomized Controlled Trials Evaluating Acute Coronary Syndrome Therapy from 1997 to 2006

| | MORTALITY AT 30 DAYS | | | MORTALITY AT 1 YEAR* | | |
| | INCIDENCE, % | | | INCIDENCE, % | | |
	With Diabetes	Without Diabetes	Adjusted OR (95% CI)†	With Diabetes	Without Diabetes	Adjusted OR (95% CI)‡
UA or NSTEMI	2.1	1.1	1.78 (1.24-2.56)	7.2	3.1	1.65 (1.30-2.10)
STEMI	8.5	5.4	1.40 (1.24-1.57)	13.2	8.1	1.22 (1.08-1.38)
All ACS	6.4	4.4	1.40 (1.26-1.56)	11.2	6.8	1.33 (1.20-1.48)

*Reported as Kaplan-Meier event rates at 12 months (360 days).
†Adjusted for age; sex; region of enrollment; smoking status; history of hypertension; prior myocardial infarction; congestive heart failure; coronary artery bypass graft surgery; systolic blood pressure; heart rate; creatinine clearance at enrollment; use of aspirin, beta blockers, angiotensin-converting enzyme (ACE) inhibitors, or angiotensin II receptor blockers (ARBs); and hypolipidemic therapy during hospitalization for ACS. Infarct location and administration of thrombolytics were also included in the STEMI model.
‡Aspirin, beta blockers, ACE inhibitors or ARBs, thienopyridines, and lipid lowering therapy at time of discharge were included in the model.
Data from Donahoe SM, Stewart GC, McCabe CH, et al: Diabetes and mortality following acute coronary syndromes, *JAMA* 298:765-775, 2007.

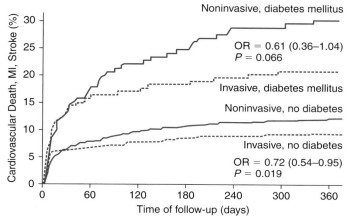

FIGURE 19-6 Outcome of patients with non-ST-segment elevation acute coronary syndromes with and without diabetes mellitus stratified by randomized treatment strategy (invasive versus noninvasive) in the FRISC II trial. *(Modified from Norhammar A, Malmberg K, Diderholm E, et al: Diabetes mellitus: the major risk factor in unstable coronary artery disease even after consideration of the extent of coronary artery disease and benefits of revascularization, J Am Coll Cardiol 43:585-591, 2004.)*

(TRITON-TIMI 38) trial (23.1% with diabetes)[28] and the Study of Platelet Inhibition and Patient Outcomes (PLATO)[29] (25.0% with diabetes) comparing prasugrel and ticagrelor, respectively, with clopidogrel for the treatment of ACS. In both studies comparing different strategies of platelet inhibition in ACS, patients with versus without diabetes had significantly higher 1-year mortality (**Table 19-5**) independent of the treatment strategies (**Figs. 19-7** and **19-8**). (See also **Chapter 15**.)

Despite advances in the treatment of ACS on data from numerous RCTs, the magnitude of excess mortality associated with diabetes among patients with ACSs remains considerable, independent of the chosen treatment strata.

Diabetes in Registry Studies of Acute Coronary Syndromes

A range of prospective registries of patients with ACS are currently providing a wealth of standardized data regarding patient characteristics, clinical practices, and outcomes worldwide.

As part of the Euro Heart Survey Program of the European Society of Cardiology (ESC), several surveys and registries on treatment and outcome of ACS were undertaken from 2000 to 2008. The ACS I survey prospectively enrolled 10,484 patients across Europe in 2000 and 2001,[30] of whom 2352 (23.0%) had diabetes mellitus, 562 were treated with diet alone, 1112 received oral glucose lowering therapy alone, 561 were on insulin alone, and 117 received both oral and insulin treatment. The in-hospital mortality was significantly higher for patients with diabetes than for those without diabetes for STEMI (9.8% versus 5.7%), with an adjusted risk of in-hospital mortality of 1.6 (95% CI 1.2-2.1)[31]; insulin-treated patients had the worst mortality.

In the ACS II survey, conducted in 2004, 6385 patients with ACS were enrolled, of whom 1587 (25.0%) had prevalent diabetes.[32] In-hospital mortality was significantly higher in patients with diabetes for both STEMI (7.3% versus 4.6%) and NSTE-ACS (3.6% versus 1.9%).[33] Patients with diabetes had a significantly increased 1-year mortality after both STEMI and NSTE-ACS, with an even more pronounced difference in the latter patient group (**Fig. 19-9**). In a multivariable analysis adjusting for differences in baseline characteristics and in acute and long-term treatment, diabetes had an independent 37% increased odds for 1-year mortality (OR 1.37, 95% CI 1.09-.71).[33]

GRACE was a prospective observational study of patients hospitalized with ACS at 94 hospitals in 14 countries. In a subset of 16,116 patients hospitalized from April 1999 to September 2001, 25.0% had prevalent diabetes. Franklin and colleagues[10] reported that patients with diabetes were less likely to be treated according to guidelines and had an increased risk for heart failure, renal failure, cardiogenic shock, and death (**Table 19-6**).[10]

The CRUSADE quality improvement initiative compared adherence to treatment recommendations from the American College of Cardiology Foundation (ACCF)/American Heart Association (AHA) guidelines for NSTE-ACS among 46,410 patients from 413 U.S. hospitals. In this NSTE-ACS population, 33.1% of patients had prevalent diabetes.[34] Similar to the results from the GRACE registry,[10] patients with diabetes were less likely to receive guideline-recommended treatments. Hospital mortality was 5.4% in non–insulin-treated diabetes, 6.8% in patients with insulin-treated diabetes, and 4.4% in nondiabetic patients. The adjusted odds for death was 1.14 (95% CI 1.02-1.29) for non–insulin-treated diabetes and 1.29 (1.12-1.49) for insulin-treated diabetes as compared with patients without diabetes.[34] The odds for reinfarction as well as for congestive heart failure and red blood cell transfusion was similarly increased in the subset of patients with diabetes (**Table 19-7**).[34]

TABLE 19-5 Comparison of Patient Characteristics and Outcomes of Patients With and Without Diabetes in the TRITON and PLATO Trials

	TRITON TRIAL[29]			PLATO TRIAL[28]		
	Diabetes N = 3146 (23.1%)	No Diabetes N = 10,462 (76.9%)	*P*-Value	Diabetes N = 4662 (25.0%)	No Diabetes N= 13,951 (75.0%)	*P*-Value
Baseline Characteristics						
STEMI (%)	28.7	40.8	< 0.001	21.0	27.0	< 0.001
NSTE-ACS (%)	68.5	56.4	< 0.001	79	73	< 0.001
Age (yr)	63	60	< 0.001	64	61	< 0.001
Age older than 75 yr (%)	15.0	13.0	< 0.001	17.4	14.8	< 0.001
Women (%)	33.0	24.0	< 0.001	34.8	26.2	< 0.001
BMI (kg/m^2)	29.0	27.0	< 0.001	28.7	27.0	< 0.001
Hypertension (%)	80.0	59.0	< 0.001	81.6	60.1	< 0.001
Smoker (%)	27.0	41.0	< 0.001	24.8	39.6	< 0.001
Prior MI (%)	23.0	16.0	< 0.001	27.0	18.4	< 0.001
Prior CABG (%)	12.0	6.0	< 0.001	10.0	4.6	< 0.001
MI (%)	10.7	8.0	< 0.001	8.7	5.6	< 0.001
Composite Outcome Observed in the Trials						
CV death, MI, stroke (%)	14.6	9.9	< 0.001	15.2	9.3	< 0.001

CV = Cardiovascular.
Modified from Wiviott SD, Braunwald E, Angiolillo DJ, et al. Greater clinical benefit of more intensive oral antiplatelet therapy with prasugrel in patients with diabetes mellitus in the Trial to AssessImprovement in Therapeutic Outcomes by Optimizing Platelet Inhibition with Prasugrel—Thrombolysis in Myocardial Infarction 38, Circulation 2008;118:1626-36 and James S, Angiolillo DJ, Cornel JH, et al. Ticagrelor vs. clopidogrel in patients with acute coronary syndromes and diabetes: a substudy from the PLATelet inhibition and patient Outcomes (PLATO) trial, Euro Heart J 2010; 31:3006-3016.

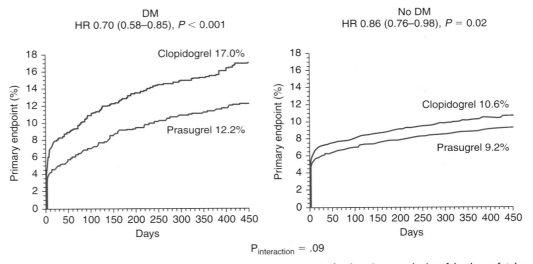

FIGURE 19-7 Kaplan-Meier curves for prasugrel versus clopidogrel stratified by diabetes status for the primary endpoint of death, nonfatal myocardial infarction, nonfatal stroke. *(Modified from Wiviott SD, Braunwald E, Angiolillo DJ, et al: Greater clinical benefit of more intensive oral antiplatelet therapy with prasugrel in patients with diabetes mellitus in the Trial to Assess Improvement in Therapeutic Outcomes by Optimizing Platelet Inhibition with Prasugrel—Thrombolysis in Myocardial Infarction 38, Circulation 118:1626-1636, 2008.)*

All reported ACS registries come to the common conclusion that ACS patients with diabetes are less likely to receive guideline-recommended treatment and are more likely to experience short- and long-term adverse events. The Euro Heart Survey on Diabetes and the Heart[35] recruited 3488 patients to study the prevalence of abnormal glucose regulation in adult patients with coronary artery disease, of whom two thirds presented with unstable coronary artery disease. Anselmino and colleagues[36] examined the impact of adherence to guidelines for medical treatment (evidence-based medication [EBM]) and for revascularization

in patients with and without diabetes on long-term cardiovascular events (death, myocardial infarction, and stroke). Increased use of both EBM and revascularization was associated with lower event rates in patients with diabetes (11.6% versus 14.7% for EBM; 9.9% versus 16.9% for revascularization; **Fig. 19-10**). Although no separate analysis was provided to discriminate between patients with stable and unstable coronary artery disease, these data encourage the improved implementation of evidence-based guidelines to decrease adverse cardiovascular events, especially in patients with diabetes.

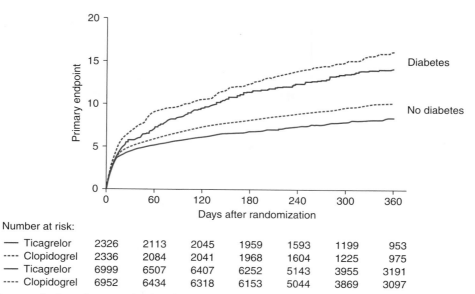

Number at risk:							
— Ticagrelor	2326	2113	2045	1959	1593	1199	953
---- Clopidogrel	2336	2084	2041	1968	1604	1225	975
— Ticagrelor	6999	6507	6407	6252	5143	3955	3191
---- Clopidogrel	6952	6434	6318	6153	5044	3869	3097

FIGURE 19-8 Kaplan-Meier curves for ticagrelor versus clopidogrel stratified by diabetes status for the primary endpoint of death, nonfatal myocardial infarction, nonfatal stroke. *(Modified from James S, Angiolillo DJ, Cornel JH, et al: Ticagrelor vs. clopidogrel in patients with acute coronary syndromes and diabetes: a substudy from the PLATelet inhibition and patient Outcomes (PLATO) trial,* Eur Heart J *31:3006-3016, 2010.)*

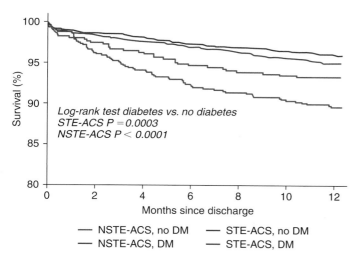

FIGURE 19-9 Kaplan–Meier curves for ST-segment elevation MI and non-ST-segment elevation acute coronary syndromes stratified by diabetes status for all-cause mortality during 1 year after hospitalization. The increase in mortality among patients with diabetes was even more pronounced in patients with non-ST-segment elevation acute coronary syndromes. *(Modified from Hasin T, Hochadel M, Gitt AK, et al: Comparison of treatment and outcome of acute coronary syndrome in patients with versus patients without diabetes mellitus,* Am J Cardiol *103:772-778, 2009.)*

UNDIAGNOSED DIABETES IN PATIENTS WITH CARDIOVASCULAR DISEASE AND ACUTE CORONARY SYNDROME EVENTS

Glucose intolerance and the associated traditional risk factors for cardiovascular disease, such as dyslipidemia and hypertension, might be present for many years before the diagnosis of diabetes mellitus is made.[37]

The Euro Heart Survey on Diabetes and the Heart[35] was undertaken to study the prevalence of abnormal glucose regulation in adult patients with coronary artery disease in Europe. A total of 4196 patients referred to a cardiologist because of CAD were enrolled, of whom 2107 were admitted on an acute basis (91% with ACS) and 2854 for elective consultation. Within the ACS population, 31.5% of patients had known diabetes mellitus. An oral glucose tolerance test (OGTT) was performed to characterize glucose metabolism in patients without previously known diabetes. In the 923 patients with ACS and without known diabetes, OGTT identified an additional 22% with newly diagnosed diabetes and a further 36% with either impaired fasting glucose (IFG) or impaired glucose tolerance (IGT) (**Fig. 19-11**). In addition to the patients with known diabetes in this population, most patients with ACS seen by cardiologists had pathologic

TABLE 19-6 The Association Between Diabetes Mellitus and Outcomes in Consecutive Patients With Acute Coronary Syndromes Participating in the GRACE-Registry

OUTCOME	STEMI*	NSTEMI*	UA*
Death	1.48 (1.03-2.13)	1.14 (0.85-1.52)	1.41 (1.02-1.95)
Cardiogenic shock	1.08 (0.76-1.53)	1.09 (0.79-1.50)	1.33 (0.88-2.02)
Heart failure	1.74 (1.43-2.11)	1.88 (1.60-2.21)	1.80 (1.50-2.18)
Renal failure	1.50 (1.00-2.23)	1.72 (1.32-2.25)	2.12 (1.45-3.08)

Comparison of patients with versus without diabetes for each endpoint.
NSTEMI = Non-ST-segment elevation myocardial infarction; STEMI = ST-segment elevation myocardial infarction; UA = unstable angina.
*Data are adjusted odds ratio (95% confidence interval).
Data from Franklin K, Goldberg RJ, Spencer F, et al: Implications of diabetes in patients with acute coronary syndromes. The Global Registry of Acute Coronary Events, *Arch Intern Med* 164:1457-1463; 2004.

TABLE 19-7 Clinical Outcomes in Patients With versus Without Diabetes Presenting With Non-ST-segment Elevation Acute Coronary Syndromes in the CRUSADE Registry

Clinical Outcome	No Diabetes	All Type 2 Diabetes	Insulin-Treated Diabetes	ADJUSTED ODDS RATIO (95% CI)	
				All Type 2 Diabetes*	Insulin-Treated Diabetes†
n	31,049	9,773	5,588		
Death (%)	4.4	5.4	6.8	1.14 (1.02-1.29)	1.29 (1.12-1.49)
Reinfarction (%)	3.2	3.5	3.8	1.07 (0.96-1.19)	1.07 (0.93-1.24)
Congestive heart failure (%)	8.0	12.4	13.7	1.25 (1.16-1.34)	1.19 (1.09-1.31)
Shock (%)	2.5	3.2	3.5	1.22 (1.05-1.41)	1.18 (0.97-1.44)
Red blood cell transfusion (%)	12.9	17.4	20.8	1.31 (1.23-1.40)	1.51 (1.40-1.63)

*No diabetes versus type 2 diabetes.
†No diabetes versus insulin-treated diabetes.
Data from Brogan GX Jr, Peterson ED, Mulgund J, et al: Treatment disparities in the care of patients with and without diabetes presenting with non-ST-segment elevation acute coronary syndromes, *Diabetes Care* 29:9-14, 2006.

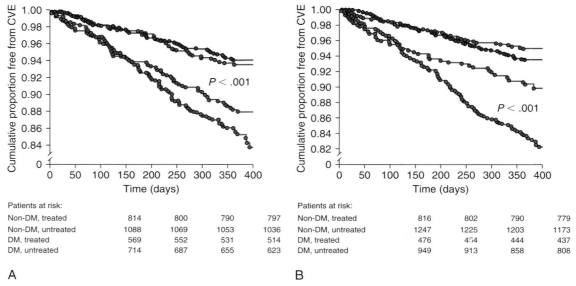

Patients at risk:

Non-DM, treated	814	800	790	797
Non-DM, untreated	1088	1069	1053	1036
DM, treated	569	552	531	514
DM, untreated	714	687	655	623

Non-DM, treated	816	802	790	779
Non-DM, untreated	1247	1225	1203	1173
DM, treated	476	454	444	437
DM, untreated	949	913	858	808

A   B

FIGURE 19-10 Kaplan-Meier curves cardiovascular events (CVE) comparing patients with and without DM who received evidence-based medicine (EBM, left panel) and who were revascularized or not (right panel). Non-DM without EBM / revascularization (blue circles), with EBM / revascularization (purple circles) and DM without EBM/ revascularization (green circles) with EBM / revascularization (red circles). CVE = Cardiovascular events. *(Modified from Anselmino M, Malmberg K, Ohrvik J, Rydén L; Euro Heart Survey Investigators: Evidence-based medication and revascularization: powerful tools in the management of patients with diabetes and coronary artery disease: a report from the Euro Heart Survey on diabetes and the heart,* Eur J Cardiovasc Prev Rehabil 15:216-23, 2008.)

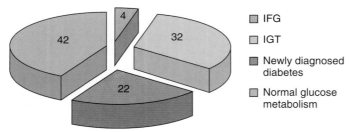

IFG
IGT
Newly diagnosed diabetes
Normal glucose metabolism

FIGURE 19-11 Glucose metabolism according to oral glucose tolerance tests in 923 patients admitted to the hospital for acute coronary syndromes without previously known diabetes. *(Modified from Bartnik M, Rydén L, Ferrari R, et al: The prevalence of abnormal glucose regulation in patients with coronary artery disease across Europe. The Euro Heart Survey on diabetes and the heart,* Eur Heart J 25:1880-1890, 2004.)

glucose metabolism. The 1-year follow-up of this survey demonstrated that patients with newly diagnosed diabetes had a significantly higher mortality than patients with normal glucose metabolism (HR 2.0, 95% CI 1.1-3.6) (**Fig. 19-12**).[38]

The ESC and the European Association for the Study of Diabetes (EASD) published joint guidelines on the management

of diabetes, prediabetes, and cardiovascular diseases.[39] Based on the findings of the Euro Heart Survey on Diabetes and the Heart,[35] it is recommended that screening for potential type 2 diabetes mellitus in patients with cardiovascular disease be initiated with hemoglobin A1c (HbA1c) and fasting plasma glucose (FPG) testing and that an OGTT be added if HbA1c and FPG are inconclusive.

The appropriateness of the routine performance of an OGTT to screen for diabetes during hospitalization for ACS has been controversial. Ye and colleagues[40] performed a meta-analysis of 15 prospective cohort studies assessing the accuracy and reproducibility of an OGTT in ACS (10 studies) and non-ACS (5 studies) patient populations. They reported that the OGTT in patients with ACS was as accurate as in non-ACS patients, and concluded that it was reasonable to screen patients hospitalized for ACS for otherwise undiagnosed diabetes mellitus using an OGTT.

A recently published subanalysis of the randomized Early Glycoprotein IIb/IIIa Inhibition in Non–ST-Segment Elevation Acute Coronary Syndrome (EARLY-ACS) trial examined the prevalence of previously undiagnosed diabetes or

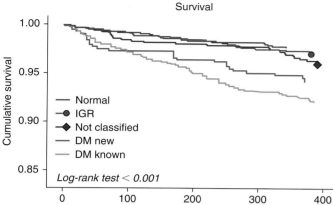

FIGURE 19-12 One-year outcome in relation to glycometabolic state in the Euro Heart Survey on Diabetes and the Heart of the European Society of Cardiology. Normal = normal glucose metabolism; DM known = previously known diabetes; DM new = newly diagnosed diabetes; IGR = impaired glucose regulation (impaired fasting glucose and/or impaired glucose tolerance); not classified = patients not classified, because no oral glucose tolerance test (OGTT) or fasting plasma glucose was performed. *(Modified from Lenzen M, Ryden L, Ohrvik J, et al: Diabetes known or newly detected, but not impaired glucose regulation, has a negative influence on 1-year outcome in patients with coronary artery disease: a report from the Euro Heart Survey on Diabetes and the Heart,* Eur Heart J *27:2969-2974, 2006.)*

prediabetes and associations with ischemic outcomes among NSTE-ACS patients.[41] Patients were classified as having previously undiagnosed diabetes or prediabetes based on available data of FPG or HbA1c; no OGTT was performed in the trial. Of 8795 patients with available data of known diabetes or at least one of the reported glucose values, 2860 (32.5%) had known diabetes, 1069 (12.2%) were classified as having previously undiagnosed diabetes, and 947 (10.8%) were classified as having prediabetes. Both, patients with known diabetes and patients with previously undiagnosed diabetes had higher 30-day mortality (adjusted OR 1.40, 95% CI 1.01-1.93; and adjusted OR 1.65, 95% CI 1.09-2.48, respectively). Patients with prediabetes had similar

30-day death or MI outcomes as compared with patients with normal glucose metabolism. One-year mortality was higher for patients with known diabetes (adjusted HR 1.38, 95% CI 1.13-1.67) but not for patients with previously undiagnosed diabetes or prediabetes (**Fig. 19-13**).[41]

SUMMARY

Diabetes mellitus is a well-known risk factor for the development of cardiovascular diseases. The prevalence of diabetes will continue to grow worldwide, with about one-half of coronary artery disease patients with diabetes presently undiagnosed. Based on observational data, current guidelines therefore recommend screening for abnormal glucose metabolism in patients with coronary artery disease including those with ACS. This will be of clinical importance because both patients with known diabetes and those with newly diagnosed diabetes are less likely to receive evidence-based treatments and are more likely to develop cardiovascular adverse events. Reflecting the currently available epidemiologic data, diabetes will continue to have a strong impact on the incidence and outcomes of ACS in the future.

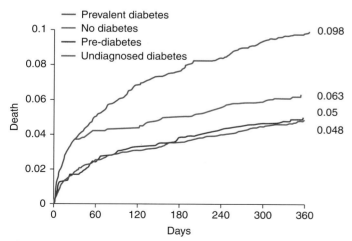

FIGURE 19-13 Unadjusted 1-year Kaplan-Meier mortality curves according to diabetes diagnosis group in patients with NSTE-ACS. Results of a subanalysis of the EARLY-ACS trial. Diagnosed = patients with known diabetes; no diabetes = patients with normal glucose metabolism; prediabetes = patients with fasting glucose greater than or equal to 110 and less than 126 mg/dL; undiagnosed = patients with previously undiagnosed diabetes, but fasting glucose greater than or equal to 126 mg/dL or HbA1c greater than or equal to 6.5% with no previous diabetes history. *(Modified from Giraldez RR, Clare RM, Lopes RD, et al: Prevalence and clinical outcomes of undiagnosed diabetes mellitus and prediabetes among patients with high-risk non-ST-segment elevation acute coronary syndrome,* Am Heart J *165:918-925.e2, 2013.)*

References

1. *Global status report on noncommunicable diseases 2010,* 2011. at http://whqlibdoc.who.int/publications/2011/9789240686458_eng.pdf.
2. *Global Atlas on cardiovascular disease prevention and control,* 2011. at http://whqlibdoc.who.int/publications/2011/9789241564373_eng.pdf.
3. Mathers CD, Loncar D: Projections of global mortality and burden of disease from 2002 to 2030, *PLoS Med* 3:e442, 2006.
4. *IDF diabetes update 2012,* 2012. at www.idf.org/diabetesatlas.
5. Yusuf S, Hawken S, Ounpuu S, et al: Effect of potentially modifiable risk factors associated with myocardial infarction in 52 countries (the INTERHEART study): case-control study, *Lancet* 364:937–952, 2004.
6. Schramm TK, Gislason GH, Kober L, et al: Diabetes patients requiring glucose-lowering therapy and nondiabetics with a prior myocardial infarction carry the same cardiovascular risk: a population study of 3.3 million people, *Circulation* 117:1945–1954, 2008.
7. Steg PG, Lopez-Sendon J, Lopez de Sa E, et al: External validity of clinical trials in acute myocardial infarction, *Arch Intern Med* 167:68–73, 2007.
8. Brown ML, Gersh BJ, Holmes DR, et al: From randomized trials to registry studies: translating data into clinical information, *Nat Clin Pract Cardiovasc Med* 5:613–620, 2008.
9. Donahoe SM, Stewart GC, McCabe CH, et al: Diabetes and mortality following acute coronary syndromes, *JAMA* 298:765–775, 2007.
10. Franklin K, Goldberg RJ, Spencer F, et al: Implications of diabetes in patients with acute coronary syndromes. The Global Registry of Acute Coronary Events, *Arch Intern Med* 164:1457–1463, 2004.
11. Gitt AK, Bueno H, Danchin N, et al: The role of cardiac registries in evidence-based medicine, *Eur Heart J* 31:525–529, 2010.
12. Granger CB, Gersh BJ: Clinical trials and registries in cardiovascular disease: competitive or complementary? *Eur Heart J* 31:520–521, 2010.
13. Fox KA, Steg PG, Eagle KA, et al: Decline in rates of death and heart failure in acute coronary syndromes, 1999-2006, *JAMA* 297:1892–1900, 2007.
14. Mehta RH, Roe MT, Chen AY, et al: Recent trends in the care of patients with non-ST-segment elevation acute coronary syndromes: insights from the CRUSADE initiative, *Arch Intern Med* 166:2027–2034, 2006.
15. Schiele F, Hochadel M, Tubaro M, et al: Reperfusion strategy in Europe: temporal trends in performance measures for reperfusion therapy in ST-elevation myocardial infarction, *Eur Heart J* 31:2614–2624, 2010.
16. Cannon CP, Braunwald E, McCabe CH, et al: Intensive versus moderate lipid lowering with statins after acute coronary syndromes, *N Engl J Med* 350:1495–1504, 2004.
17. Cannon CP, McCabe CH, Wilcox RG, et al: Oral glycoprotein IIb/IIIa inhibition with orbofiban in patients with unstable coronary syndromes (OPUS-TIMI 16) trial, *Circulation* 102:149–156, 2000.
18. Cannon CP, Weintraub WS, Demopoulos LA, et al: Comparison of early invasive and conservative strategies in patients with unstable coronary syndromes treated with the glycoprotein IIb/IIIa inhibitor tirofiban, *N Engl J Med* 344:1879–1887, 2001.
19. Wiviott SD, Antman EM, Winters KJ, et al: Randomized comparison of prasugrel (CS-747, LY640315), a novel thienopyridine P2Y12 antagonist, with clopidogrel in percutaneous coronary intervention: results of the Joint Utilization of Medications to Block Platelets Optimally (JUMBO)-TIMI 26 trial, *Circulation* 111:3366–3373, 2005.
20. Wiviott SD, Morrow DA, Frederick PD, et al: Performance of the thrombolysis in myocardial infarction risk index in the National Registry of Myocardial Infarction-3 and -4: a simple index that predicts mortality in ST-segment elevation myocardial infarction, *J Am Coll Cardiol* 44:783–789, 2004.
21. Antman EM, Louwerenborg HW, Baars HF, et al: Enoxaparin as adjunctive antithrombin therapy for ST-elevation myocardial infarction: results of the ENTIRE-Thrombolysis in Myocardial Infarction (TIMI) 23 Trial, *Circulation* 105:1642–1649, 2002.
22. Antman EM, Morrow DA, McCabe CH, et al: Enoxaparin versus unfractionated heparin with fibrinolysis for ST-elevation myocardial infarction, *N Engl J Med* 354:1477–1488, 2006.
23. Ohman EM, Van de Werf F, Antman EM, et al: Tenecteplase and tirofiban in ST-segment elevation acute myocardial infarction: results of a randomized trial, *Am Heart J* 150:79–88, 2005.
24. Giugliano RP, Roe MT, Harrington RA, et al: Combination reperfusion therapy with eptifibatide and reduced-dose tenecteplase for ST-elevation myocardial infarction: results of the integrilin and tenecteplase in acute myocardial infarction (INTEGRITI) Phase II Angiographic Trial, *J Am Coll Cardiol* 41:1251–1260, 2003.

25. Intravenous NPA for the treatment of infarcting myocardium early; InTIME-II, a double-blind comparison of single-bolus lanoteplase vs accelerated alteplase for the treatment of patients with acute myocardial infarction, *Eur Heart J* 21:2005–2013, 2000.

26. de Lemos JA, Blazing MA, Wiviott SD, et al: Early intensive vs a delayed conservative simvastatin strategy in patients with acute coronary syndromes: phase Z of the A to Z trial, *JAMA* 292:1307–1316, 2004.

27. Norhammar A, Malmberg K, Diderholm E, et al: Diabetes mellitus: the major risk factor in unstable coronary artery disease even after consideration of the extent of coronary artery disease and benefits of revascularization, *J Am Coll Cardiol* 43:585–591, 2004.

28. Wiviott SD, Braunwald E, Angiolillo DJ, et al: Greater clinical benefit of more intensive oral antiplatelet therapy with prasugrel in patients with diabetes mellitus in the trial to assess improvement in therapeutic outcomes by optimizing platelet inhibition with prasugrel-Thrombolysis in Myocardial Infarction 38, *Circulation* 118:1626–1636, 2008.

29. James S, Angiolillo DJ, Cornel JH, et al: Ticagrelor vs. clopidogrel in patients with acute coronary syndromes and diabetes: a substudy from the PLATelet inhibition and patient Outcomes (PLATO) trial, *Eur Heart J* 31:3006–3016, 2010.

30. Hasdai D, Behar S, Wallentin L, et al: A prospective survey of the characteristics, treatments and outcomes of patients with acute coronary syndromes in Europe and the Mediterranean basin; the Euro Heart Survey of Acute Coronary Syndromes (Euro Heart Survey ACS), *Eur Heart J* 23:1190–1201, 2002.

31. Hasdai D, Behar S, Boyko V, et al: Treatment modalities of diabetes mellitus and outcomes of acute coronary syndromes, *Coron Artery Dis* 15:129–135, 2004.

32. Mandelzweig L, Battler A, Boyko V, et al: The second Euro Heart Survey on acute coronary syndromes: characteristics, treatment, and outcome of patients with ACS in Europe and the Mediterranean Basin in 2004, *Eur Heart J* 27:2285–2293, 2006.

33. Hasin T, Hochadel M, Gitt AK, et al: Comparison of treatment and outcome of acute coronary syndrome in patients with versus patients without diabetes mellitus, *Am J Cardiol* 103:772–778, 2009.

34. Brogan GX Jr., Peterson ED, Mulgund J, et al: Treatment disparities in the care of patients with and without diabetes presenting with non-ST-segment elevation acute coronary syndromes, *Diabetes Care* 29:9–14, 2006.

35. Bartnik M, Ryden L, Ferrari R, et al: The prevalence of abnormal glucose regulation in patients with coronary artery disease across Europe. The Euro Heart Survey on diabetes and the heart., *Eur Heart J* 25:1880–1890, 2004.

36. Anselmino M, Malmberg K, Ohrvik J, et al: Evidence-based medication and revascularization: powerful tools in the management of patients with diabetes and coronary artery disease: a report from the Euro Heart Survey on diabetes and the heart, *Eur J Cardiovasc Prev Rehabil* 15:216–223, 2008.

37. Volpe M, Camm J, Coca A, et al: The cardiovascular continuum refined: a hypothesis, *Blood Press* 19:273–277, 2010.

38. Lenzen M, Ryden L, Ohrvik J, et al: Diabetes known or newly detected, but not impaired glucose regulation, has a negative influence on 1-year outcome in patients with coronary artery disease: a report from the Euro Heart Survey on diabetes and the heart, *Eur Heart J* 27:2969–2974, 2006.

39. Ryden L, Grant PJ, Anker SD, et al: ESC Guidelines on diabetes, pre-diabetes, and cardiovascular diseases developed in collaboration with the EASD: the Task Force on diabetes, pre-diabetes, and cardiovascular diseases of the European Society of Cardiology (ESC) and developed in collaboration with the European Association for the Study of Diabetes (EASD), *Eur Heart J* 34:3035–3087, 2013.

40. Ye Y, Xie H, Zhao X, et al: The oral glucose tolerance test for the diagnosis of diabetes mellitus in patients during acute coronary syndrome hospitalization: a meta-analysis of diagnostic test accuracy, *Cardiovasc Diabetol* 11:155, 2012.

41. Giraldez RR, Clare RM, Lopes RD, et al: Prevalence and clinical outcomes of undiagnosed diabetes mellitus and prediabetes among patients with high-risk non-ST-segment elevation acute coronary syndrome, *Am Heart J* 165:918–925 e2, 2013.

20 Hyperglycemia and Acute Coronary Syndromes

Association with Outcomes and Management

Mikhail Kosiborod

The observation that elevated glucose can occur in patients hospitalized with acute coronary syndromes (ACS; unstable angina, non–ST-segment elevation myocardial infarction [NSTEMI], and ST-segment elevation myocardial infarction [STEMI]) was made many decades ago.[1] Since then, numerous studies have documented that hyperglycemia is common, affects patients with and without established diabetes, and is associated with adverse outcomes, with a graded, incremental increase in the risk of mortality and complications observed across the spectrum of glucose elevations.[2-26] However, many gaps in knowledge remain. These include first and foremost the need for a better understanding of whether the glucose level is simply a risk marker of greater illness severity or a risk factor with a direct causal relationship to the adverse outcomes in patients with ACS. Furthermore, it remains unclear whether interventions to lower glucose in patients with ACS can improve patient outcomes, and if so, what the optimal targets, therapeutic strategies, and timing for such interventions should be during ACS events.

This chapter reviews what is presently known about the association between glucose levels and outcomes of patients hospitalized with ACS; describes the available data with regard to inpatient glucose management in this patient population, as well as comparative data across the spectrum of critically ill hospitalized patients; addresses the controversies in this field; and offers practical recommendations for patient management based on the existing data.

DEFINITION OF HYPERGLYCEMIA DURING ACUTE CORONARY SYNDROME

There is presently no uniform definition of what constitutes hyperglycemia in the setting of ACS. Prior studies used various blood glucose cut points ranging from 110 mg/dL or higher to 200 mg/dL or higher.[2] This uncertainty is compounded by variation in timing of glucose level assessments in this context. Most prior studies defined hyperglycemia based on the first available (admission or "on-arrival") glucose value,[2-11] whereas others used fasting glucose[12-17] as well as glucose values averaged over a period of time, such as the first 24 hours,[18-20] the first 48 hours, or the entire duration of hospitalization.[21] The American Heart Association (AHA) scientific statement on hyperglycemia and acute coronary syndrome suggests use of a random glucose level of above 140 mg/dL observed at any point over the course of hospitalization for ACS as the definition of hyperglycemia.[22] This recommendation is based in part on epidemiologic studies demonstrating that admission, mean 24-hour, 48-hour, and hospitalization glucose levels above approximately 120-140 mg/dL are associated with increased mortality risk,[7,18,19,21] and that decline in glucose levels below approximately 140 mg/dL during ACS hospitalization is associated with better survival,[23] although no cause-and-effect conclusions can be drawn from these data because of their observational nature.

It is important to note that the nature of the relationship between higher glucose levels and greater risk of mortality differs in patients with and without diabetes, with a paradoxically greater magnitude of association in those without versus those with prevalent diabetes.* The risk of mortality gradually rises when glucose levels exceed approximately 110-120 mg/dL in patients without diabetes, whereas in patients with established diabetes this risk does not increase significantly until glucose levels exceed approximately 200 mg/dL.[7,21] Thus, different thresholds may be appropriate to define hyperglycemia depending on the presence or absence of known diabetes.

PREVALENCE OF ELEVATED GLUCOSE LEVELS IN ACUTE CORONARY SYNDROME

Numerous studies have documented that elevated glucose levels occur commonly in patients hospitalized with ACS.[2-26] Although the definition of hyperglycemia varies across studies, the largest investigations show that the overall

---

*References 7, 9, 10, 12, 21, 23.

prevalence of elevated glucose levels (>140 mg/dL) at the time of hospital admission varies from 51% to 58%.[7,21] It is important to note that more than 50% of patients with ACS who have hyperglycemia on hospital arrival do not have known diabetes.[7]

Although glucose levels normalize in some ACS patients after admission (either spontaneously or as a result of targeted pharmacologic interventions),[24] persistent hyperglycemia remains present in more than 40% of patients throughout the course of hospitalization, and the prevalence of severe, sustained hyperglycemia (average hospitalization glucose >200 mg/dL) is approximately 14%.[21,25] Although persistent hyperglycemia occurs more commonly in patients with versus without established diabetes (78% versus 26%, respectively),[26] more than 40% of patients with persistent hyperglycemia do not have previously diagnosed diabetes.[21]

THE RELATIONSHIP BETWEEN GLUCOSE LEVELS AND MORTALITY IN ACUTE CORONARY SYNDROME

Multiple studies have now proven a powerful, independent relationship between elevated glucose and increased risk of mortality and other adverse clinical outcomes in patients hospitalized with ACS.[2-26] Plausible pathophysiologic underpinnings potentially contributing to these observed associations derive from a plethora of ex vivo, animal, and human studies that show that hyperglycemia may mediate adverse effects on inflammation, cell injury, apoptosis, ischemic myocardial metabolism, endothelial function, the coagulation cascade, and platelet aggregation in the setting of acute ischemia.[22,27] The association between higher glucose and greater mortality risk has been established across various glucose metrics[2-26,28] and across the spectrum of ACS[3] and applies to both short- and longer-term outcomes.[7,21]

The relationship between hyperglycemia and adverse outcomes among patients with ACS has been quantitatively summarized based on data from a large series of relatively small human studies collected over a period of three decades by Capes and colleagues.[2] This systematic overview demonstrated that among ACS patients without known diabetes, the relative risk of in-hospital mortality was 3.9 times higher in those with initial glucose 110 mg/dL or higher compared

with normoglycemic patients (95% confidence interval [CI] 2.9-5.4). Among ACS patients with established diabetes, those with initial glucose of 180 mg/dL or higher had a 70% increase in the relative risk of in-hospital mortality, as compared with normoglycemic patients. More recent studies confirmed these findings and extended them across the broader range of ACS to include STEMI, NSTEMI, and unstable angina, demonstrating a significant increase in the risk of short- and long-term mortality, as well as incident heart failure in hyperglycemic ACS patients both with and without diabetes.[3,9,10] The largest observational study to date to address this issue used the data from Cooperative Cardiovascular Project and showed a near-linear relationship between higher admission glucose and greater risk of mortality at 30 days and at 1 year in more than 140,000 patients hospitalized with AMI.[7] A similar relationship between elevated glucose and increased risk of death was also shown with other glucose metrics, such as postadmission fasting glucose,[12,15-17] and with outcomes other than mortality, including such intermediates associated with adverse clinical outcomes as the "no-reflow phenomenon" following percutaneous coronary intervention (PCI)[29]; greater infarct size[7,21]; worse left ventricular systolic function[5]; and contrast-mediated acute kidney injury.[30,31]

The association between hyperglycemia and increased risk of death is not limited to the initial stages of ACS hospitalization. To the contrary, in a study of almost 17,000 patients hospitalized with acute myocardial infarction (AMI) in 40 U.S. hospitals, persistently elevated glucose during hospitalization was a better discriminator of adverse events than hyperglycemia on admission (C statistic 0.70 versus 0.62, $P < 0.0001$).[21] There was a significant, gradual increase in the risk of in-hospital mortality with rising mean hospitalization glucose levels (**Fig. 20-1**). Observational analyses from randomized clinical trials of glucose-insulin-potassium (GIK) therapy and of targeted glucose control in ACS also confirm the relationship between persistent hyperglycemia and increased mortality risk.[18,20]

Another important observation is that the nature of the relationship between higher glucose levels and increased mortality is different in patients with and without established diabetes.[7,21] Regardless of the glucose metrics used, the mortality risk starts rising at considerably lower glucose levels, and increases at a much steeper slope, in patients without previously diagnosed diabetes than in those with

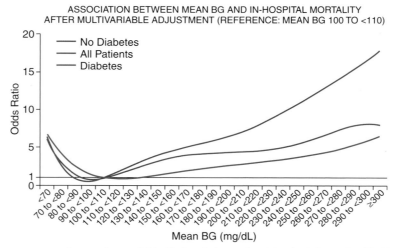

FIGURE 20-1 The association between average glucose values and risk of in-hospital mortality. BG = Blood glucose. (*Modified from Kosiborod M, Inzucchi SE, Krumholz HM, et al:* Circulation *117:1018-1027, 2008.*)

established diabetes (see **Fig. 20-1**). This phenomenon has been recently confirmed in other critically ill patient populations[32] and is not well understood. Several possible explanations have been proposed. Many patients with hyperglycemia in the absence of known diabetes actually have diabetes that simply was not recognized or treated before hospitalization,[33] representing a higher-risk cohort because other undiagnosed and untreated cardiovascular risk factors may be more prevalent in this group. Moreover, whereas the effect of targeted glucose control and insulin therapy in this clinical setting remains uncertain, nondiabetic ACS patients with hyperglycemia are less likely to be treated with insulin than those with established diabetes, even when glucose levels are markedly elevated.[7,28] Further contributing to this consistent observation is the fact that patients with established diabetes tend to have clustering of numerous risk factors that contribute to clinical risk, which may attenuate the magnitude of risk independently associated with any single factor, such as hyperglycemia. Finally, it is possible that higher degrees of stress and illness severity are required to produce similar degrees of hyperglycemia in patients without known diabetes compared with those with established diabetes.

DYNAMIC CHANGES IN GLUCOSE LEVELS DURING ACUTE CORONARY SYNDROME AND MORTALITY

Adding to the growing body of data on the relationship between hyperglycemia and adverse events in hospitalized ACS patients, several studies have shown that dynamic changes in glucose values are also strongly associated with patient survival. In post hoc analyses of data from the Complement and Reduction of Infarct Size after Angioplasty or Lytics (CARDINAL) trial, a randomized clinical trial that investigated the effect of a complement inhibitor, pexelizumab, in 1903 patients with STEMI, a decline in glucose of 30 mg/dL or more during the first 24 hours of hospitalization was associated with lower risk of 30-day mortality compared with the groups who had either no change or an increase in glucose values.[23] Similarly, in a study of approximately 8000 patients hospitalized with ACS in the United States who had

hyperglycemia (glucose >140 mg/dL) on arrival, glucose normalization after admission was associated with better patient survival, even after adjustment for confounders (**Fig. 20-2**).[24] Whereas glucose normalization took place after insulin administration in some patients, many patients experienced normalization of their glucose values spontaneously (without any glucose-lowering interventions). It is interesting to note that improved survival was observed regardless of whether glucose normalization occurred as the result of insulin therapy or happened spontaneously. In fact, it was glucose normalization, and not insulin therapy per se, that was associated with better outcomes. These observational analyses highlight the uncertainty with regard to whether normalization of glucose levels during hospitalization simply identifies a lower-risk group of patients, reflects differences in patient care, or has a direct beneficial impact on survival.

CLINICAL TRIALS OF GLUCOSE CONTROL IN PATIENTS WITH ACUTE CORONARY SYNDROME

Although the strong relationship between elevated glucose levels and greater risk of death in patients with ACS is incontrovertible, one critical question remains unanswered: Is hyperglycemia a direct mediator of increased mortality and complications in patients with ACS, or is it simply a marker of greater disease severity and comorbidity? To definitively answer this question, large randomized clinical trials of target-driven intensive glucose control in hospitalized ACS patients are required. Because no such clinical outcomes trial has been performed to date, this issue continues to be highly controversial and cannot presently be addressed with certainty. Nevertheless, some insights may be gained from critical appraisal of the findings from small clinical trials of targeted glucose control in the ACS setting and trials of GIK therapy that used a hyperinsulinemic, hyperglycemic infusion strategy, as well as data from studies of targeted glucose control conducted in non-ACS clinical settings.

Because of marked variability in the insulin-infusion strategies used and the hypotheses tested across the clinical trials to date, one must first establish several key parameters to appropriately identify those randomized studies that

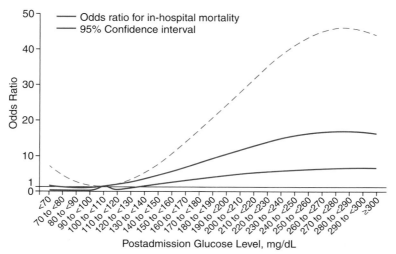

FIGURE 20-2 Glucose normalization and survival during hospitalization for acute myocardial infarction. *(Modified from Kosiborod M, Inzucchi SE, Krumholz HM, et al: Glucose normalization and outcomes in patients with acute myocardial infarction, Arch Intern Med 169:438-446, 2009.)*

provide useful information with regard to the effect of targeted glucose control in the ACS setting. These parameters include the following:

- The presence of hyperglycemia at the time of patient randomization, with or without an antecedent diabetes diagnosis, because targeted glucose management is unlikely to yield benefit in the absence of hyperglycemia.
- Target-driven glucose control as the primary tested intervention, with substantially lower glucose targets in the intervention versus control arm.
- The achievement of a clinically and statistically significant difference in glucose values between intervention and control groups postrandomization.
- The assessment of treatment effects on meaningful patient outcomes, as opposed to intermediate endpoints.

To date, no ACS trial has fulfilled all of these criteria with any degree of rigor. A few studies fulfilling some but not all of these criteria are summarized in **Table 20-1**. The trial most closely satisfying the listed parameters is the Diabetes Insulin-Glucose in Acute Myocardial Infarction (DIGAMI) trial, with a number of key caveats with regard to its interpretation.[34] In DIGAMI, patients presenting within 24 hours of acute MI symptoms with diabetes or initial glucose levels exceeding 198 mg/dL (11 mmol/L) were randomized to an acute and chronic insulin treatment regimen versus usual care. Those randomized to the insulin arm received 24 hours or more of intravenous (IV) dextrose-insulin infusion titrated to maintain glucose levels of 126 to 180 mg/dL, initiated at 5 units/hr of IV insulin in D_{5W}, followed by subcutaneous insulin injections three times daily for the subsequent 3 months titrated to standard therapeutic targets for glucose control, to be compared with usual care. The trial enrolled 620 patients, 80% of whom had previously diagnosed diabetes. Admission glucose at study entry was 277 mg/dL in the intervention group versus 283 mg/dL in the control group. By 24 hours, those randomized to the insulin arm had achieved significantly lower glucose levels compared with the control arm (173 versus 211 mg/dL; $P < 0.0001$), although average glucose values remained significantly elevated in both groups; the differences between the groups were smaller by hospital discharge but remained statistically significant (148 versus 162 mg/dL; $P < 0.01$). Despite this early contrast in glucose levels between the groups, no significant differences in fasting glucose values were observed at any subsequent timepoint throughout the follow-up extending over 12 months from enrollment; however, hemoglobin A1c (HbA1c) levels were significantly lower in the intervention versus control group at 3 months (7.0 versus 7.5%, $P < 0.01$). Also of note, hypoglycemia (not explicitly defined in the initial study reports) was observed in 15% of the insulin infusion patients compared with none in the usual care group, and in 10% of participants resulted in discontinuation of the protocol treatment. For the primary endpoint of all-cause mortality at 3 months, there was no significant difference between the randomized groups (38 versus 49 deaths), with the respective P value reported as "not significant".[34] Therefore, from a "purist" perspective, based on failure to achieve statistical significance in the primary endpoint, DIGAMI was a negative trial. However, subsequent analyses of mortality at both 1 year and 3.5 years of follow-up showed clinically and statistically significant reductions in all-cause mortality in the insulin-treated group versus control (at 1 year: 18.6% versus 26.1%, $P = 0.027$; at 3.5 years: 33% versus 44%, $P = 0.011$, respectively).[34,35] If one accepts the validity

of the mortality reduction observed in the longer-term analyses, the relative contributions of the various aspects of the trial remain uncertain, including the effects of the acute dextrose-insulin infusion and the effects of multidose insulin injection in the outpatient setting. Therefore, although the DIGAMI data are the most compelling in the field of targeted glucose control for the treatment of ACS, the relative attribution of improved survival to acute, in-hospital glucose lowering remains uncertain.

Beyond DIGAMI, a few other studies satisfy some (but not all) of the proposed parameters of validity and generalizability with regard to targeted glycemic control in the ACS setting. The Hyperglycemia: Intensive Insulin Infusion in Infarction (HI-5) trial was designed to assess the effect of dextrose-insulin infusion versus usual care in patients with MI and hyperglycemia on arrival. Similar to DIGAMI, the therapeutic target for the insulin arm was 72 to 180 mg/dL, and IV dextrose was infused with the insulin (either D_{5W} or D_{10W}); however, the insulin dose was much lower in HI-5 at 2 units/hr (contrasted with 5 units/hr used both in DIGAMI and in most trials of GIK therapy).[36] The HI-5 trial was terminated early because of slow enrollment and failed to achieve a statistically significant difference in glucose values between the intensive and conventional glucose groups (149 versus 162 mg/dL 24 hours postrandomization, $P = NS$).[18] Mortality assessments at hospital discharge, 30 days, and 6 months all numerically favored usual care over targeted glucose control with insulin treatment, although none of these comparisons were statistically significant because of very low numbers of events (6 months: 10 versus 7 deaths; $P = 0.62$).

The DIGAMI-2 multicenter study attempted to determine whether potential survival benefit seen with targeted glucose control in the original DIGAMI study was primarily attributable to acute or chronic glucose lowering with insulin.[37] In DIGAMI-2, 1253 patients with acute MI and diabetes or admission glucose above 198 mg/dL were randomized to one of the three subgroups: (1) 24-hour insulin-glucose infusion targeting glucose of 126 to 180 mg/dL, followed by a subcutaneous insulin-based long-term glucose control regimen (group 1, identical to the original DIGAMI intervention group); (2) same 24-hour insulin-glucose infusion, but followed by standard glucose control (group 2); and (3) routine glucose management (group 3). Of note, the trial planned to recruit 3000 patients and was stopped prematurely because of slow recruitment. Glucose levels on arrival were similar among the three arms (approximately 229 mg/dL). At 24 hours postrandomization the glucose levels were modestly lower in the two groups assigned to acute glucose lowering versus control (164 versus 180 mg/dL, $P < 0.01$). This difference, although statistically significant, was clinically small and considerably less than expected; it was also much smaller than what was observed in the original DIGAMI study. There was no difference in either glucose or HbA1c levels among the three groups at any other timepoint, with up to 3 years of follow up. It is important to note that patients in group 1 failed to achieve the targeted fasting glucose range of 90 to 126 mg/dL during the outpatient management phase. Mortality over 2 years was not statistically different among the three groups (23.4% versus 21.2% and 17.9% in groups 1, 2, and 3, respectively; $P = 0.83$ for group 1 versus group 2, and $P = 0.16$ for group 1 versus group 3). Because of its limitations (primarily lack of substantial contrast in glucose levels among the three

TABLE 20-1 Clinical Trials of Glucose Control in Acute Coronary Syndrome*

TRIAL	TARGETED GLUCOSE CONTROL	ELEVATED BG ON ENTRY	GLUCOSE TARGETS SPECIFIED	BG CONTRAST ACHIEVED	CLINICAL ENDPOINTS	RESULTS
DIGAMI (1995)	+/−	+ Approximately 280 mg/dL	+ 126-180 mg/dL versus usual care acutely, 90-126 mg/dL fasting BG versus usual care afterward	+/− 173 versus 211 mg/dL during first 24 hr; difference in HbA1c but not fasting BG afterward	+	+/− Mortality neutral at 3 months (primary endpoint), improved survival in glucose control arm by 1 year
DIGAMI-2 (2005)	+/−	+ 229 mg/dL	+ 126-180 mg/dL in-hospital versus usual care acutely, 90-126 mg/dL fasting BG (group 1 only) versus usual care afterward	+/− 164 versus 180 mg/dL at 24 hr, no difference afterward	+	− Mortality neutral among three groups
HI-5 (2006)	+/−	+ Approximately 198 mg/dL	+ 72-180 mg/dL versus usual care	− 149 versus 162 mg/dL (P=NS) during first 24 hr	+	− Mortality neutral in hospital, at 3 and 6 months
Marfella et al (2009)	+	+ ≥140 mg/dL	+ 80-140 versus 180-200 mg/dL	+ 163 versus 192 mg/dL	−	+/− Higher ejection fraction, less oxidative stress, less inflammation and apoptosis in the intensive versus standard group
Marfella et al (2012)	+	+ ≥140 mg/dL	+ 80-140 versus 180-200 mg/dL or GIK	+ 161 versus 194 versus 182 mg/dL	−	+/− More regenerative potential in the peri-infarcted areas in the intensive versus conventional and GIK groups
Marfella et al (2013, myocardial salvage)	+	+ ≥140 mg/dL	+ 80-140 versus 180-200 mg/dL	+ 144 versus 201 mg/dL	−	+/− Greater myocardial salvage in the intensive versus standard group
Marfella et al (2013, ISR)	+	+ ≥140 mg/dL	+ 80-140 versus 180-200 mg/dL	+ 145 versus 191 mg/dL	−	+/− Lower ISR in the intensive versus standard group
RECREATE pilot (2012)	+	+ ≥144 mg/dL	+ 90-117 mg/dL versus usual care	+ 117 versus 143 mg/dL	−	+/− Significant difference in glucose between intensive and standard groups (primary endpoint) No difference in mortality (small number of events)
BIOMArCS-2 (2013)	+	+ ≥140 mg/dL	+ 85-110 mg/dL during day, 85-139 mg/dL at night versus <288 mg/dL	+ 112 mg/dL versus approximately 130 mg/dL	+	− No difference in infarct size by high-sensitive troponin; composite of in-hospital death and reinfarction higher in the intensive versus standard group (very small number of events)

*Full clinical trials names represented by acronyms are as follows:
 · DIGAMI—Diabetes Insulin-Glucose in Acute Myocardial Infarction
 · HI-5—Hyperglycemia: Intensive Insulin Infusion in Infarction
 · RECREATE—Researching Coronary Reduction by Appropriately Targeting Euglycemia
 · BIOMArCS-2—Biomarker Study to Identify the Acute Risk of a Coronary Syndrome 2
+=Yes, −=No.
BG=Blood glucose; GIK=glucose-insulin-potassium; ISR=in-stent restenosis.

groups), the DIGAMI-2 study did not provide a definitive answer on whether targeted glucose lowering (whether acute or chronic) has any clinical value in patients with AMI.

Several additional, smaller randomized clinical trials of intensive versus conventional glucose control in AMI have primarily tested mechanistic hypotheses, as well as the effectiveness of streamlined insulin infusion protocol in lowering glucose compared with usual care, and feasibility of its implementation internationally (including in resource-limited areas).[27,38–41] Marfella and colleagues randomized 50 patients with AMI and hyperglycemia (admission blood glucose [BG] ≥140 mg/dL) who had coronary angiography and were subsequently referred for coronary bypass surgery to either intensive or conventional glucose control for 3 days preoperatively; AMI patients requiring coronary artery bypass grafting (CABG) who had normal admission glucose levels served as controls.[27] Two-dimensional echocardiography was performed on patient admission and after achievement of glucose treatment goals. All patients underwent myocardial biopsy of peri-infarcted areas; specimens were subjected to a variety of immunohistochemical and biochemical analyses. Patients in the intensive treatment group achieved greater reduction in glucose values (78 versus 10 mg/dL reductions), but also had higher hypoglycemia rates. Compared with the conventional treatment group, patients in the intensive group had higher ejection fraction, less oxidative stress, and less inflammation and apoptosis in peri-infarcted specimens. However, the study was too small for clinically meaningful outcomes to be evaluated.

The same group subsequently embarked on an additional small randomized trial with almost identical design, except that patients could be randomized to three different arms: intensive glucose control, conventional control, or GIK.[39] Patients in the intensive control group exhibited more regenerative potential (as analyzed by myocyte precursor cells) in the peri-infarcted areas than those in the conventional and GIK groups. Two subsequent randomized trials by the same investigators evaluated the effect of intensive glucose control (versus conventional management) on myocardial salvage index among 106 hyperglycemic patients with STEMI undergoing PCI[38]; and on in-stent restenosis in 165 hyperglycemic patients with STEMI undergoing PCI.[40] Despite relatively small sample sizes, both studies showed clinically and statistically significant benefits of intensive versus conventional periprocedural glucose control in terms of both greater myocardial salvage (15% versus 7%, $P < 0.05$) and lower rates of in-stent restenosis at 6 months (24% versus 46%, $P < 0.05$). These clinical trials, although elegant, well conducted, and intriguing in their findings, require confirmation in larger studies before their results can be extrapolated to routine clinical care.

The International Multicentre Randomized Controlled Trial of Intensive Insulin Therapy Targeting Normoglycemia In Acute Myocardial Infarction: RECREATE (Researching Coronary Reduction by Appropriately Targeting Euglycemia) was a randomized open-label pilot study of targeted glucose control in patients with STEMI, with the main objective of testing the feasibility and safety of implementing a streamlined glucose control protocol across international sites, many in resource-limited environments.[41] A total of 287 patients with STEMI and initial glucose values equal to or above 144 mg/dL were randomly assigned to either intensive glucose control with a streamlined IV insulin infusion protocol or usual care. Patients in the intensive arm were treated with IV infusion of insulin glulisine for at least 24 hours and for as long as critical care unit (CCU)–level care was required, with a target glucose range of 90-117 mg/dL. Once transferred to the ward, patients in the intensive arm were switched to insulin glargine and continued this treatment for a total duration of 30 days postrandomization. Patients in the control arm received usual care for AMI, according to local practice of each participating center. Because RECREATE was a pilot study designed to demonstrate the feasibility of targeted glucose control in STEMI with a simplified insulin infusion protocol, the primary endpoint

was 24-hour difference in mean glucose between the two study groups. At 24 hours, mean glucose was significantly lower in the intervention arm versus the standard care arm (117 versus 143 mg/dL); however, at 30 days HbA1c was similar between the groups. Although the overall rates of hypoglycemia (<70 mg/dL) were significantly higher in the intensive versus the standard group (22.7 versus 4.4%, $P < 0.05$), there was only one episode of severe hypoglycemia (<50 mg/dL). The rates of mortality at 90 days were not different in the intensive versus the standard group (12 versus 13 events); however, the study lacked statistical power to provide definitive answers with regard to clinical outcomes. The RECREATE pilot demonstrated that paper-based glucose control protocols can be effectively implemented across multiple centers, including those in resource-limited environments, with very low rates of severe hypoglycemia. However, given its limited sample size, it did not address the question of whether better glucose control can reduce adverse events in patients with AMI.

The most recent study of glucose control in AMI was the randomized Biomarker Study to Identify the Acute Risk of a Coronary Syndrome 2 (BIOMArCS-2).[42] BIOMArCS-2 was a prospective, single-center, open-label clinical trial that randomized 294 patients with ACS (280 patients in the final analytic dataset; 82% with STEMI) and admission glucose level from 140 to 288 mg/dL to either intensive glucose control for 48 hours (target glucose of 85 to 110 mg/dL during the day; 85 to 139 mg/dL at night) or conventional management (target glucose <288 mg/dL). Primary outcome measure was high-sensitivity troponin T value 72 hours postadmission (hsTropT72, as a marker of infarct size). The extent of myocardial injury was also measured at 6 weeks with myocardial perfusion scintigraphy (myocardial perfusion imaging using single photon emission computed tomography [MPI-SPECT]). Glucose values were significantly lower in the intensive versus the conventional group at 6, 12, 24, and 36 hours, and equalized by 72 hours. Severe hypoglycemia (<50 mg/dL) occurred in 13 patients (9%) randomized to the intensive glucose control group. There was no significant difference in hsTropT72 between the groups (1197 versus 1354 ng/L, $P = 0.41$). The median extent of myocardial injury as revealed by MPI-SPECT was numerically lower in the intensive versus the conventional group, but this difference did not reach statistical significance (2% versus 4% respectively, $P = 0.07$). The number of in-hospital deaths and recurrent MIs was very small (nine events in total), but these events occurred more frequently in the intensive versus the conventional group (eight events versus one event, respectively, $P = 0.04$). The results of the BIOMArCS-2 study suggest that intensive glucose control after AMI does not reduce infarct size as measured by high-sensitivity troponin essay, but increases the risk of hypoglycemia and, possibly, composite of in-hospital death and recurrent MI. However, given that the number of events in the study was very small; that it had a single-center and open-label design; that the findings conflict with those of other small clinical trials that showed reduction in infarct size with intensive versus conventional glucose control[38]; and that no difference in mortality was found between the groups (despite the higher number of events in the intervention arm),[41] the results of BIOMArCS-2 are difficult to interpret.

The remaining trials evaluating the effects of insulin infusion on clinical outcomes in the ACS setting have

TABLE 20-2 Clinical Trials of Glucose-Insulin-Potassium (GIK) Therapy in Acute Coronary Syndrome*

TRIAL	TARGETED GLUCOSE CONTROL	ELEVATED BG ON ENTRY	GLUCOSE TARGETS SPECIFIED	BG CONTRAST ACHIEVED	CLINICAL ENDPOINTS	RESULTS
Pol-GIK (1999)	−	124 mg/dL	−	N/A 106 versus 112 mg/dL in intervention versus control arms	+	Significantly higher mortality in intervention versus control arm at 35 days
CREATE-ECLA (2005)	−	+ 162 mg/dL	−	N/A Glucose higher in intervention arm versus control (187 versus 148 mg/dL)	+	Mortality neutral
IMMEDIATE (2012)	−	Not specified	−	N/A	+	No difference in progression to AMI, 30-day mortality, or HF. Composite of in-hospital mortality or cardiac arrest lower in the GIK versus placebo group

*Full clinical trials names represented by acronyms are as follows:
· Pol-GIK—Poland Glucose-Insulin-Potassium trial
· CREATE-ECLA—Clinical Trial of Reviparin and Metabolic Modulation in Acute Myocardial Infarction Treatment and Evaluation—Estudios Cardiológicos Latinoamérica
· IMMEDIATE—Immediate Myocardial Metabolic Enhancement During Initial Assessment and Treatment in Emergency Care
+=Yes, −=No.
AMI=Acute myocardial infarction; BG=blood glucose; HF=heart failure.

predominantly tested the GIK hypothesis (i.e., hyperinsulinemic, hyperglycemic therapy), as summarized in published quantitative analyses,[43] and have little to do with target-driven glucose control (**Table 20-2**). Studies such as the Glucose-Insulin-Potassium (GIPS) trial[44] or the much larger Clinical Trial of Reviparin and Metabolic Modulation in Acute Myocardial Infarction Treatment and Evaluation—Estudios Cardiológicos Latinoamérica (CREATE-ECLA) and the Organization to Assess Strategies for Ischemic Syndromes (OASIS) 6 trials (which in total randomized almost 23,000 participants)[19] assigned patients to fixed-dose GIK infusion regardless of their initial glucose values or diabetes status, and did not prespecify targets for glucose control. In these studies, as dictated by the infusion protocols, high-dose delivery of insulin was supported by IV glucose administration to affect modest hyperglycemia, defined by protocol as a range of 126 to 198 mg/dL. For example, in the CREATE-ECLA trial, which enrolled more than 20,000 patients with acute MI and demonstrated no discernible treatment benefit with GIK therapy,[19] 6-hour postrandomization glucose values were significantly higher in the GIK group than in the control group (187 versus 148 mg/dL). Thus, the GIK studies were not designed to evaluate targeted glucose control with insulin, and their findings should not be used in guiding decisions about glucose management in ACS.

The Poland Glucose-Insulin-Potassium (Pol-GIK) trial randomized 954 patients with acute MI to either to fixed low-dose GIK, which included a much lower rate of insulin infusion (0.8 to 1.3 units/hr) than typical GIK regimens, versus normal saline infusion.[45] Although not a typical GIK trial, insofar as it used a much lower insulin dose, Pol-GIK cannot be considered a study of targeted glucose control either. First, it randomized patients who were on average normoglycemic at study entry (initial glucose level of approximately 124 mg/dL in both groups). It is therefore not entirely surprising that excess hypoglycemia was observed in the intervention arm, which required lowering of the fixed insulin dose during the conducting of the trial from 1.3 to 0.8 units/hour. Second, and similar to other GIK studies, no glucose goals were prespecified or aimed for in this study and the dose of GIK infusion was fixed and not adjusted to maintain a certain range of glucose values. As a result, there was no significant difference in glucose levels 24 hours postrandomization (106 mg/dL in GIK versus 112 mg/dL in the control arm). The study was stopped prematurely because of excess mortality in the GIK arm at 35 days (8.9% versus 4.8% in the control arm, $P=0.01$). However, as a result of the serious limitations of interpretation stemming from the intent of the trial to evaluate the effect of fixed-dose administration of insulin rather than a targeted glucose control hypothesis, no valuable lessons can be learned about glucose lowering and patient outcomes in AMI based on its results.

The Immediate Myocardial Metabolic Enhancement During Initial Assessment and Treatment in Emergency Care (IMMEDIATE) trial was a National Institutes of Health–sponsored randomized, placebo-controlled, double-blinded, multicenter clinical trial of GIK infusion (1.5 ml/kg/hr, continuous infusion for a total of 12 hours) versus matching placebo administered as early as possible in the setting of suspected ACS in the prehospital emergency medical service (EMS) setting. The IMMEDIATE trial was specifically designed to test the GIK hypothesis and was not a study of targeted glucose control in ACS. Similar to previous GIK trials, the presence of hyperglycemia was not required as an inclusion criterion, and there were no prespecified goals for glucose control. The primary hypothesis was that early GIK administration would prevent progression of suspected ACS to AMI within 24 hours, as determined by biomarker and electrocardiographic evidence of myocardial necrosis. Major secondary hypotheses were that GIK infusion would reduce mortality (at 30 days and 1 year), reduce prehospital or in-hospital cardiac arrest and in-hospital mortality, and reduce hospitalizations for heart failure. A small biologic cohort substudy also evaluated the impact of GIK infusion on infarct size.

A total of 871 patients (411 in the GIK group, 460 in the placebo group) were evaluated in the final analysis. There was no significant difference between the GIK and placebo groups in progression to AMI (48.7 versus 52.6%, $P=0.28$), 30-day mortality (4.4 versus 6.1%, $P=0.27$), or 30-day heart failure (1.5 versus 2.2%, $P=0.43$).[46] The rates of prespecified composite of cardiac arrest or in-hospital mortality were significantly lower in the GIK group (4.4 versus 8.7%, $P=0.01$); however, evaluation of secondary endpoints did not include statistical adjustment for multiple comparisons. The results were similar when tested among patients with STEMI. In a small biologic mechanism cohort (110 patients in total), GIK significantly reduced infarct size compared with placebo (2% versus 10% of left ventricular [LV] mass, respectively; $P = 0.01$), and significantly reduced the level of free fatty acids. Although the results from this small substudy of IMMEDIATE are intriguing, they are hypothesis generating only, and would need to be tested in a larger randomized clinical trial. Overall, the results of IMMEDIATE showed no significant clinical benefit of early GIK administration in patients with suspected ACS.

In summary, no definitive clinical trial of targeted glucose control in ACS has been performed, and the data from the existing small studies are conflicting and inconclusive. In this context, one might be tempted to look for more definitive answers in the broader critical care field of patients in other clinical settings. In 2001, van den Berghe and colleagues reported marked beneficial effects associated with normalization of blood glucose through use of an insulin infusion compared with usual care among patients hospitalized in a surgical intensive care unit (SICU).[47] These observations fueled enthusiasm among clinicians and professional societies to endorse a strategy of targeted glucose control across critically ill hospitalized populations.[48] However, in the 8 years that followed, several additional randomized trials in various ICU patient populations failed to reproduce these beneficial results.[49–53] Key among these more recent trials include the same investigators at the same institution, using the same protocol as in the SICU trial, testing intensive glucose lowering in medical intensive care unit (ICU) patients, and demonstrating lower morbidity, but no difference in the trial primary endpoint of mortality with intensive glucose lowering versus usual care.[53] In addition, the Normoglycemia in Intensive Care Evaluation—Survival Using Glucose Algorithm Regulation (NICE-SUGAR) trial, which was the largest trial of targeted glucose control in critically ill patients across ICU settings, demonstrated significantly higher mortality with intensive versus more conservative glucose control.[50] These results have substantially tempered enthusiasm for aggressive glucose lowering in the ICU setting. However, the results of NICE-SUGAR need to be interpreted in the context of the study design; NICE-SUGAR compared "very intensive" glucose control to "good" glucose control, not to "usual care." Specifically, an IV insulin protocol was used in more than two thirds of patients in the control arm, producing an average glucose level of approximately 142 mg/dL. This degree of glucose control is more intensive than what was achieved in control groups of other critical care studies, lower than what was achieved in the intensive arm of many ACS studies, and much lower than what is typically seen in routine clinical care. Thus the most appropriate conclusion from the NICE-SUGAR study is that "moderate" glucose control (with values ranging from 140 to 180 mg/dL) is sufficient, and more aggressive glucose lowering provides no additive benefit, and may even be harmful.

Regardless, extrapolation of observations from trials outside the ACS setting is problematic. Specifically, the findings from patients hospitalized with surgical illness, trauma, and sepsis cannot be simply extended to those with ACS. The pathophysiology of these conditions is different, and the treatment thresholds and targets may be distinct as well. Prior studies have shown that the relationship between glucose values and mortality may vary significantly across various cardiovascular conditions[7,54]; thus it can also vary substantially between cardiac and noncardiac disease states.

THE RELATIONSHIP BETWEEN GLUCOSE VARIABILITY AND PATIENT OUTCOMES DURING ACUTE CORONARY SYNDROME

Although mean and admission glucose levels are associated with higher risk of mortality during ACS, these metrics do not capture the variability in glucose values during hospitalization. Physiologic studies have suggested several mechanisms through which glucose variability may adversely affect prognosis in the setting of ACS, including oxidative stress and cytokine release, among others.[55,56] In addition, glucose variability has been associated with adverse events in other critically ill patient populations.[57–59] Several recent studies have examined the association of various glucose variability metrics with prognosis in patients with ACS. In the analysis of over 18,000 patients hospitalized with ACS across 61 U.S. hospitals, five different metrics of glucose variability were evaluated for their association with in-hospital mortality.[60] Although greater glucose variability was associated with increased risk of in-hospital mortality in unadjusted analyses, it was no longer independently predictive (regardless of the metric used) after multiple patient factors were controlled for, including mean blood glucose levels. In contrast, mean blood glucose remained an important independent predictor of survival. These findings suggest that glucose variability does not provide additional prognostic value above and beyond already recognized risk factors for mortality during ACS; the findings were further validated by the recent analysis of the DIGAMI-2 study, which also showed no relationship between glucose variability and survival.[61]

THE PROGNOSTIC IMPORTANCE OF HYPOGLYCEMIA IN PATIENTS WITH ACUTE CORONARY SYNDROME

Because therapy for hyperglycemia in the hospital necessitates the use of insulin, it is expected that glucose lowering in the inpatient setting will produce excess hypoglycemia. Several studies have suggested that glucose values in the hypoglycemic range may adversely affect mortality in ACS (93% increase in the adjusted odds of 2-year mortality in one study)[25,62] and have demonstrated a J-shaped relationship between average glucose values during hospitalization and in-hospital mortality (see **Fig. 20-1**).[21] Whether hypoglycemia is directly harmful in patients with ACS or whether it is simply a marker for the most critically ill patients was evaluated in a large observational study.[63] The authors showed that the risk associated with low blood glucose was confined to those who developed hypoglycemia spontaneously, most likely as the result of severe underlying illness. In contrast, hypoglycemia that occurred after insulin initiation was not associated with worse survival. Two subsequent analyses of data from the DIGAMI-2 and CREATE-ECLA trials also found no significant association between hypoglycemia and mortality, after adjustment for confounders.[64,65] These findings suggest that hypoglycemia is a marker of severe illness rather than a direct cause of adverse outcomes. Although continuous efforts to avoid hypoglycemia are certainly warranted, these studies cast some doubt on the

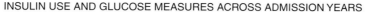

INSULIN USE AND GLUCOSE MEASURES ACROSS ADMISSION YEARS

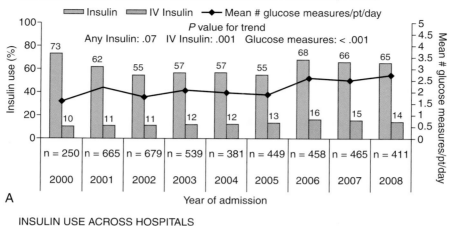

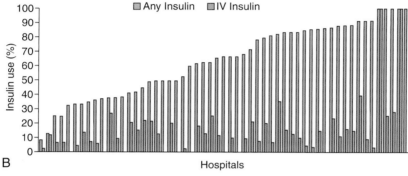

Insulin use among patients hospitalized for AMI with severe persistent hyperglycemia **A,** Overall cohort. **B,** Across hospitals.

FIGURE 20-3 The rates of treatment with insulin in patients hospitalized with ACS across mean hospitalization glucose levels. *(Modified from Venkitachalam L, McGuire DK, Gosch K, et al: Temporal trends and hospital variation in the management of severe hyperglycemia among patients with acute myocardial infarction in the United States,* Am Heart J *166:315-324, 2013.)*

assumption that the lack of clinical benefit from intensive glycemic control in clinical trials is simply a consequence of excess hypoglycemia.

CURRENT PATTERNS OF GLUCOSE CONTROL IN ACUTE CORONARY SYNDROME

The current practice of glucose management in the United States is highly variable.[28] Large proportions of ACS patients with hyperglycemia do not receive glucose-lowering therapy, even in the setting of marked hyperglycemia; this is particularly evident among those without known diabetes.[7,26] A study from the United Kingdom showed that 64% of patients without diabetes with admission glucose of 11 mmol/L (approximately 200 mg/dL) or higher received no glucose-lowering treatments during hospitalization.[66] Similar findings were observed in the recent analysis of 4297 admissions of patients with ACS and mean hospitalization glucose of 200 mg/dL or higher; insulin was used 63% of the time, and IV insulin infusion was used in only 13% of these admissions, with substantial variation among hospitals that did not change over 10 years of observation (**Fig. 20-3**).[67] Many factors contribute to this inconsistency of clinical practice, such as the lack of convincing clinical outcomes data; concerns about hypoglycemia; institutional barriers; and clinical inertia, underscoring the critical importance of continued investigation with regard to the efficacy and safety of glucose management in the setting of ACS.

SUMMARY AND RECOMMENDATIONS

There is a clear and urgent need for well-designed, large-scale clinical outcomes trials of target-driven glucose control in ACS with sufficient statistical power to detect a clinically important difference in mortality and other adverse clinical outcomes. Until such trials are completed, any specific recommendations with regard to glucose management in ACS are based on epidemiologic observations, mechanistic hypotheses, and expert consensus, and not grounded in solid clinical evidence.

Reflecting this uncertainty, in 2008 the AHA published an update on its position regarding glucose targets for ACS-MI patients, which substantially liberalized previous recommendations.[22] This AHA position advocates for a glucose treatment threshold of higher than 180 mg/dL. A similar position was adopted by the 2009 focused update of STEMI guidelines[68] and the 2012 focused update of NSTEMI guidelines[69] and was also endorsed by the revised American Association of Clinical Endocrinologists (AACE) and American Diabetes Association (ADA) guidelines.[70] These guidelines now recommend the same glucose threshold for therapeutic intervention in critically ill patients—higher than 180 mg/dL—with a suggested therapeutic target of glucose control specified at 140 to 180 mg/dL, a substantially more liberal approach than proposed in prior documents.[48] Although even these targets represent an expert consensus, it is likely the most prudent approach in the presence of the accumulated data.

Until more information becomes available, several practical suggestions are reasonable with regard to glucose management during ACS hospitalization:

1. Assessment of glucose values at the time of admission and glucose monitoring during hospitalization will provide useful information with regard to risk stratification and prognosis. Thus such assessment and monitoring should be pursued regardless of whether treatment is being considered.

2. If targeted glucose control is being considered, several precautions should be observed:

   a. Conservative treatment initiation thresholds and glucose targets (as outlined earlier) should be used, in line with the recommendations of professional societies. Very aggressive glucose lowering, including "normalization of blood glucose" as previously recommended, does not clearly offer additional benefit and may be harmful.

   b. Evidence-based protocols should be used when and if glucose control strategies are implemented. Such protocols should:

      i. have demonstrated effectiveness and safety with regard to targeted glucose control in the variety of clinical settings

      ii. incorporate the rate of change in glucose values as well as insulin sensitivity in determination of insulin infusion rates and adjustments

      iii. provide specific directions regarding the frequency of glucose testing and hypoglycemia management

Last, and most important, continued efforts are necessary for the design and execution of definitive clinical trials assessing glucose control targets, therapies, and timing, so that more evidence-based recommendations may be provided to clinicians with regard to glucose management in patients with ACS.

References

1. Datey K, Nanda N: Hyperglycemia after acute myocardial infarction: its relation to diabetes mellitus, N Engl J Med 262–265, 1967.
2. Capes SE, Hunt D, Malmberg K, et al: Stress hyperglycaemia and increased risk of death after myocardial infarction in patients with and without diabetes: a systematic overview, Lancet 355:773–778, 2000.
3. Foo K, Cooper J, Deaner A, et al: A single serum glucose measurement predicts adverse outcomes across the whole range of acute coronary syndromes, Heart 89:512–516, 2003.
4. Hadjadj S, Coisne D, Mauco G, et al: Prognostic value of admission plasma glucose and HbA in acute myocardial infarction, Diabet Med 21:305–310, 2004.
5. Ishihara M, Inoue I, Kawagoe T, et al: Impact of acute hyperglycemia on left ventricular function after reperfusion therapy in patients with a first anterior wall acute myocardial infarction, Am Heart J 146:674–678, 2003.
6. Kadri Z, Danchin N, Vaur L, et al: Major impact of admission glycaemia on 30 day and one year mortality in non-diabetic patients admitted for myocardial infarction: results from the nationwide French USIC 2000 study, Heart 92:910–915, 2006.
7. Kosiborod M, Rathore SS, Inzucchi SE, et al: Admission glucose and mortality in elderly patients hospitalized with acute myocardial infarction: implications for patients with and without recognized diabetes, Circulation 111:3078–3086, 2005.
8. Meier JJ, Deifuss S, Klamann A, et al: Plasma glucose at hospital admission and previous metabolic control determine myocardial infarct size and survival in patients with and without type 2 diabetes: the Langendreer Myocardial Infarction and Blood Glucose in Diabetic Patients Assessment (LAMBDA), Diabetes Care 28:2551–2553, 2005.
9. Stranders I, Diamant M, van Gelder RE, et al: Admission blood glucose level as risk indicator of death after myocardial infarction in patients with and without diabetes mellitus, Arch Intern Med 164:982–988, 2004.
10. Wahab NN, Cowden EA, Pearce NJ, et al: Is blood glucose an independent predictor of mortality in acute myocardial infarction in the thrombolytic era? J Am Coll Cardiol 40:1748–1754, 2002.
11. Yudkin JS, Oswald GA: Stress hyperglycemia and cause of death in non-diabetic patients with myocardial infarction, BMJ 294:773, 1987.
12. Aronson D, Hammerman H, Kapeliovich MR, et al: Fasting glucose in acute myocardial infarction: incremental value for long-term mortality and relationship with left ventricular systolic function, Diabetes Care 30:960–966, 2007.
13. Mak KH, Mah PK, Tey BH, et al: Fasting blood sugar level: a determinant for in-hospital outcome in patients with first myocardial infarction and without glucose intolerance, Ann Acad Med Singapore 22:291–295, 1993.
14. O'Sullivan JJ, Conroy RM, Robinson K, et al: In-hospital prognosis of patients with fasting hyperglycemia after first myocardial infarction, Diabetes Care 14:758–760, 1991.
15. Porter A, Assali AR, Zahalka A, et al: Impaired fasting glucose and outcomes of ST-elevation acute coronary syndrome treated with primary percutaneous intervention among patients without previously known diabetes mellitus, Am Heart J 155:284–289, 2008.
16. Suleiman M, Hammerman H, Boulos M, et al: Fasting glucose is an important independent risk factor for 30-day mortality in patients with acute myocardial infarction: a prospective study, Circulation 111:754–760, 2005.
17. Verges B, Zeller M, Dentan G, et al: Impact of fasting glycemia on short-term prognosis after acute myocardial infarction, J Clin Endocrinol Metab 92:2136–2140, 2007.
18. Cheung NW, Wong VW, McLean M: The Hyperglycemia: Intensive Insulin Infusion in Infarction (HI-5) study: a randomized controlled trial of insulin infusion therapy for myocardial infarction, Diabetes Care 29:765–770, 2006.
19. Diaz R, Goyal A, Mehta SR, et al: Glucose-insulin-potassium therapy in patients with ST-segment elevation myocardial infarction, JAMA 298:2399–2405, 2007.
20. Goyal A, Mehta SR, Gerstein HC, et al: Glucose levels compared with diabetes history in the risk assessment of patients with acute myocardial infarction, Am Heart J 157:763–770, 2009.
21. Kosiborod M, Inzucchi SE, Krumholz HM, et al: Glucometrics in patients hospitalized with acute myocardial infarction: defining the optimal outcomes-based measure of risk, Circulation 117:1018–1027, 2008.
22. Deedwania P, Kosiborod M, Barrett E, et al: Hyperglycemia and acute coronary syndrome: a scientific statement from the American Heart Association Diabetes Committee of the Council on Nutrition, Physical Activity, and Metabolism, Circulation 117:1610–1619, 2008.
23. Goyal A, Mahaffey KW, Garg J, et al: Prognostic significance of the change in glucose level in the first 24 h after acute myocardial infarction: results from the CARDINAL study, Eur Heart J 27:1289–1297, 2006.
24. Kosiborod M, Inzucchi SE, Krumholz HM, et al: Glucose normalization and outcomes in patients with acute myocardial infarction, Arch Intern Med 169:438–446, 2009.
25. Svensson AM, McGuire DK, Abrahamsson P, et al: Association between hyper- and hypoglycaemia and 2 year all-cause mortality risk in diabetic patients with acute coronary events, Eur Heart J 26:1255–1261, 2005.
26. Kosiborod M, Inzucchi S, Clark B, et al: National patterns of glucose control among patients hospitalized with acute myocardial infarction, J Am Coll Cardiol 49:1018–1183, 2007, 283A.
27. Marfella R, Di Filippo C, Portoghese M, et al: Tight glycemic control reduces heart inflammation and remodeling during acute myocardial infarction in hyperglycemic patients, J Am Coll Cardiol 53:1425–1436, 2009.
28. Kosiborod M, Inzucchi S, Clark B, et al: Variability in the hospital use of insulin to control sustained hyperglycemia among acute myocardial infarction patients, J Am Coll Cardiol 49:1018–1186, 2007, 284A.
29. Iwakura K, Ito H, Ikushima M, et al: Association between hyperglycemia and the no-reflow phenomenon in patients with acute myocardial infarction, J Am Coll Cardiol 41:1–7, 2003.
30. Kosiborod MMP, Rao S, Inzucchi SE, et al: Hyperglycemia and risk of acute kidney injury after coronary angiography in patients hospitalized with acute myocardial infarction, J Am Coll Cardiol 53:1028, 2009, A382.
31. Naruse H, Ishii J, Hashimoto T, et al: Pre-procedural glucose levels and the risk for contrast-induced acute kidney injury in patients undergoing emergency coronary intervention, Circ J 76:1848–1855, 2012.
32. Krinsley JS, Egi M, Kiss A, et al: Diabetic status and the relation of the three domains of glycemic control to mortality in critically ill patients: an international multicenter cohort study, Crit Care 17: R37, 2013.
33. Conaway DG, O'Keefe JH, Reid KJ, et al: Frequency of undiagnosed diabetes mellitus in patients with acute coronary syndrome, Am J Cardiol 96:363–365, 2005.
34. Malmberg K, Ryden L, Efendic S, et al: Randomized trial of insulin-glucose infusion followed by subcutaneous insulin treatment in diabetic patients with acute myocardial infarction (DIGAMI study): effects on mortality at 1 year, J Am Coll Cardiol 26:57–65, 1995.
35. Malmberg K: Prospective randomised study of intensive insulin treatment on long term survival after acute myocardial infarction in patients with diabetes mellitus. DIGAMI (Diabetes Mellitus, Insulin Glucose Infusion in Acute Myocardial Infarction) Study Group, BMJ 314:1512–1515, 1997.
36. Gnaim CI, McGuire DK: Glucose-insulin-potassium therapy for acute myocardial infarction: what goes around comes around, Am Heart J 148:924–930, 2004.
37. Malmberg K, Ryden L, Wedel H, et al: Intense metabolic control by means of insulin in patients with diabetes mellitus and acute myocardial infarction (DIGAMI 2): effects on mortality and morbidity, Eur Heart J 26:650–661, 2005.
38. Marfella R, Rizzo MR, Siniscalchi M, et al: Peri-procedural tight glycemic control during early percutaneous coronary intervention up-regulates endothelial progenitor cell level and differentiation during acute ST-elevation myocardial infarction: effects on myocardial salvage, Int J Cardiol 2013.
39. Marfella R, Sasso FC, Cacciapuoti F, et al: Tight glycemic control may increase regenerative potential of myocardium during acute infarction, J Clin Endocrinol Metab 97:933–942, 2012.
40. Marfella R, Sasso FC, Siniscalchi M, et al: Peri-procedural tight glycemic control during early percutaneous coronary intervention is associated with a lower rate of in-stent restenosis in patients with acute ST-elevation myocardial infarction, J Clin Endocrinol Metab 97:2862–2871, 2012.
41. Nerenberg KA, Goyal A, Xavier D, et al: Piloting a novel algorithm for glucose control in the coronary care unit: the RECREATE (REsearching Coronary REduction by Appropriately Targeting Euglycemia) trial, Diabetes Care 35:19–24, 2012.
42. Stranders I, Diamant M, van Gelder RE, et al: Intensive glucose regulation in hyperglycemic acute coronary syndrome: results of the randomized BIOMarker study to identify the acute risk of a coronary syndrome-2 (BIOMArCS-2) glucose trial, JAMA Intern Med 2013.
43. Fath-Ordoubadi F, Beatt KJ: Glucose-insulin-potassium in acute myocardial infarction, Lancet 353:1968, 1999.
44. van der Horst IC, Zijlstra F, van't Hof AW, et al: Glucose-insulin-potassium infusion inpatients treated with primary angioplasty for acute myocardial infarction: the glucose-insulin-potassium study: a randomized trial, J Am Coll Cardiol 42:784–791, 2003.
45. Ceremuzynski L, Budaj A, Czepiel A, et al: Low-dose glucose-insulin-potassium is ineffective in acute myocardial infarction: results of a randomized multicenter Pol-GIK trial, Cardiovasc Drugs Ther 13:191–200, 1999.
46. Selker HP, Beshansky JR, Sheehan PR, et al: Out-of-hospital administration of intravenous glucose-insulin-potassium in patients with suspected acute coronary syndromes: the IMMEDIATE randomized controlled trial, JAMA 307:1925–1933, 2012.
47. van den Berghe G, Wouters P, Weekers F, et al: Intensive insulin therapy in the critically ill patients, N Engl J Med 345:1359–1367, 2001.
48. Garber AJ, Moghissi ES, Bransome ED Jr, et al: American College of Endocrinology position statement on inpatient diabetes and metabolic control, Endocr Pract 10:77–82, 2004.
49. Brunkhorst FM, Engel C, Bloos F, et al: Intensive insulin therapy and pentastarch resuscitation in severe sepsis, N Engl J Med 358:125–139, 2008.
50. Finfer S, Chittock DR, Su SY, et al: Intensive versus conventional glucose control in critically ill patients, N Engl J Med 360:1283–1297, 2009.
51. Gandhi GY, Nuttall GA, Abel MD, et al: Intensive intraoperative insulin therapy versus conventional glucose management during cardiac surgery: a randomized trial, Ann Intern Med 146:233–243, 2007.
52. Gray CS, Hildreth AJ, Sandercock PA, et al: Glucose-potassium-insulin infusions in the management of post-stroke hyperglycaemia: the UK Glucose Insulin in Stroke Trial (GIST-UK), Lancet Neurol 6:397–406, 2007.
53. Van den Berghe G, Wilmer A, Hermans G, et al: Intensive insulin therapy in the medical ICU, N Engl J Med 354:449–461, 2006.

54. Kosiborod M, Inzucchi SE, Spertus JA, et al: Elevated admission glucose and mortality in elderly patients hospitalized with heart failure, *Circulation* 119:1899–1907, 2009.

55. Esposito K, Nappo F, Marfella R, et al: Inflammatory cytokine concentrations are acutely increased by hyperglycemia in humans: role of oxidative stress, *Circulation* 106:2067–2072, 2002.

56. Monnier L, Mas E, Ginet C, et al: Activation of oxidative stress by acute glucose fluctuations compared with sustained chronic hyperglycemia in patients with type 2 diabetes, *JAMA* 295:1681–1687, 2006.

57. Krinsley JS: Glycemic variability: a strong independent predictor of mortality in critically ill patients, *Crit Care Med* 36:3008–3013, 2008.

58. Krinsley JS: Glycemic variability and mortality in critically ill patients: the impact of diabetes, *J Diabetes Sci Technol* 3:1292–1301, 2009.

59. Krinsley JS: Glycemic variability in critical illness and the end of Chapter 1, *Crit Care Med* 38:1206–1208, 2010.

60. Lipska KJ, Venkitachalam L, Gosch K, et al: Glucose variability and mortality in patients hospitalized with acute myocardial infarction, *Circ Cardiovasc Qual Outcomes* 5:550–557, 2012.

61. Mellbin LG, Malmberg K, Ryden L, et al: The relationship between glycaemic variability and cardiovascular complications in patients with acute myocardial infarction and type 2 diabetes: a report from the DIGAMI 2 trial, *Eur Heart J* 34:374–379, 2013.

62. Pinto DS, Skolnick AH, Kirtane AJ, et al: U-shaped relationship of blood glucose with adverse outcomes among patients with ST-segment elevation myocardial infarction, *J Am Coll Cardiol* 46:178–180, 2005.

63. Kosiborod M, Inzucchi SE, Goyal A, et al: Relationship between spontaneous and iatrogenic hypoglycemia and mortality in patients hospitalized with acute myocardial infarction, *JAMA* 301:1556–1564, 2009.

64. Goyal A, Mehta SR, Diaz R, et al: Differential clinical outcomes associated with hypoglycemia and hyperglycemia in acute myocardial infarction, *Circulation* 120:2429–2437, 2009.

65. Mellbin LG, Malmberg K, Waldenstrom A, et al: Prognostic implications of hypoglycaemic episodes during hospitalisation for myocardial infarction in patients with type 2 diabetes: a report from the DIGAMI 2 trial, *Heart* 95:721–727, 2009.

66. Weston C, Walker L, Birkhead J: Early impact of insulin treatment on mortality for hyperglycaemic patients without known diabetes who present with an acute coronary syndrome, *Heart* 93:1542–1546, 2007.

67. Venkitachalam L, McGuire DK, Gosch K, et al: Temporal trends and hospital variation in the management of severe hyperglycemia among patients with acute myocardial infarction in the United States, *Am Heart J* 166:315–324 e1, 2013.

68. Kushner FG, Hand M, Smith SC Jr, et al: 2009 focused updates: ACC/AHA guidelines for the management of patients with ST-elevation myocardial infarction (updating the 2004 guideline and 2007 focused update) and ACC/AHA/SCAI guidelines on percutaneous coronary intervention (updating the 2005 guideline and 2007 focused update): a report of the American College of Cardiology Foundation/American Heart Association Task Force on Practice Guidelines, *Circulation* 120:2271–2306, 2009.

69. Jneid H, Anderson JL, Wright RS, et al: 2012 ACCF/AHA focused update of the guideline for the management of patients with unstable angina/Non-ST-elevation myocardial infarction (updating the 2007 guideline and replacing the 2011 focused update): a report of the American College of Cardiology Foundation/American Heart Association Task Force on practice guidelines, *Circulation* 126:875–910, 2012.

70. Moghissi ES, Korytkowski MT, Dinardo M, et al: American Association of Clinical Endocrinologists and American Diabetes Association consensus statement on inpatient glycemic control, *Endocr Pract* 15:1–17, 2009.

21 Antiplatelet and Antithrombotic Therapy in Diabetic Patients with Acute Coronary Syndrome

Stefan K. James and Lars Wallentin

Patients with diabetes mellitus (DM) and acute coronary syndrome (ACS) are at particularly high risk for recurrent cardiovascular events and death. The reason for this increased risk is multifactorial, including a higher risk profile, higher platelet reactivity, and underuse of evidence-based medications in these patients.[1] This chapter includes a summary and review of antiplatelet and antithrombotic therapies that are approved in the United States and in Europe for clinical use in patients with ACS.

PLATELET AGGREGATION

Patients with diabetes, particularly those with type 2 diabetes (T2DM), exhibit increased platelet reactivity and a reduced inhibition in response to platelet inhibitors. There is also evidence that platelet activation is directly affected by hyperglycemia and insulin resistance. Platelets are affected by insulin because of the presence of insulin receptor subtypes on the platelet surface.[2] Activation of these receptors leads to suppression of cyclic adenosine monophosphate (cAMP), resulting in inhibition of P2Y12 receptors and decreased calcium influx, thus inhibiting platelet activity. In case of insulin resistance, platelets display increased calcium influx and thereby activation of the P2Y12 receptor.[3] High platelet reactivity (HPR) is well documented in patients with diabetes[4] and may contribute to the high incidence of cardiovascular disease and poor outcomes in this population. Thromboxane A_2 (TXA$_2$), the most potent vasoconstrictor that is secreted from platelets after activation, is circulating in higher amounts in patients with T2DM.[5] Another abnormality of platelets in patients with T2DM is an increased platelet expression of P-selectin and of the glycoprotein IIb/IIIa receptor (GP IIb/IIIa) (**Fig. 21-1**).[6]

Platelet adhesion, activation, and aggregation play a pivotal role in atherothrombosis in patients with and without DM. Intracoronary atherothrombosis is the most common cause of the development of ACS and plays a central role in complications occurring around percutaneous coronary intervention (PCI), including recurrent ACS, procedure-related myocardial infarction (MI), and stent thrombosis.[7] Inhibition of platelet aggregation by medical treatment impairs formation and progression of thrombotic processes and is therefore of great importance in the prevention of complications after ACS or associated with PCI (**Fig. 21-2**).[8,9]

PLATELET INHIBITION

Antiplatelet agents include cyclooxygenase (COX) inhibitors such as aspirin, which block the production of TXA$_2$; GP IIb/IIIa receptor blockers such as abciximab, eptifibatide, and tirofiban, which inhibit fibrin-mediated platelet activation; and thienopyridines such as clopidogrel, prasugrel, cangrelor, ticagrelor, and ticlopidine, which bind to and antagonize P2Y12 receptors. Optimizing dual antiplatelet therapy (DAT) with combinations of agents from these classes may improve cardiovascular disease outcomes in patients with diabetes and ACS events (**Tables 21-1** and **21-2**).

Aspirin

The mechanism of action of aspirin occurs through permanent inactivation of the COX activity of prostaglandin H synthase 1 (PGH$_1$) and PGH$_2$ (also referred to as COX-1 and COX-2) (**Fig. 21-3**).[10] These isoenzymes catalyze the conversion of arachidonic acid to PGH$_2$. PGH$_2$ is in turn a substrate for several tissue-specific isomerases that generate several bioactive prostanoids, including TXA$_2$ and prostacyclin (prostaglandin I$_2$ [PGI$_2$]). Low levels of aspirin predominately inhibit COX-1, whereas higher levels are needed to also inhibit COX-2.[11] TXA$_2$ is mainly derived from COX-1, and PGE$_1$ mainly from COX-2 (see **Fig. 21-3**).

Aspirin has been considered the mainstay of treatment of all patients with ACS and is recommended with a high level of evidence in current international guidelines.[12,13]

In the setting of ACS, long-term low-dose aspirin treatment (75 to 100 mg/day) is recommended, with support from a meta-analysis.[14] Although a recent small study suggested that more frequent administration would be beneficial in patients with DM,[15] the large Clopidogrel and Aspirin Optimal Dose Usage to Reduce Recurrent Events—Seventh Organization to Assess Strategies in Ischemic Syndromes (CURRENT-OASIS 7) trial including almost 6000 patients with DM was not able to show that a high dose of aspirin was superior to a low dose.[16] More recent trials have also shown that modifications of clinical care based on the use of platelet function testing for aspirin responsiveness do not improve outcome.[17] The optimal dose of aspirin when used in combination with other platelet inhibitors in the setting of acute and long-term treatment of patients with ACS, with stable coronary artery disease, or after PCI with or without DM has not yet been clearly defined from large randomized controlled trials. Based on published data and tablet availability, the recommended dose should be 75 to 100 mg in patients with or without DM.

ADP Receptor Blockers

An essential part in the platelet activation process is the interaction of adenosine diphosphate (ADP) with the platelet P2Y12 receptor (see also **Chapter 16**).[7] The P2Y12 receptor is the predominant receptor involved in the ADP-stimulated

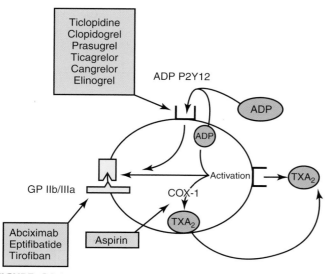

FIGURE 21-1 Platelet activation. ADP=Adenosine diphosphate; COX-1=cyclooxygenase 1. (Modified from Capodanno D, Corrado T, Angiolillo D: Update on novel P2Y12 inhibitors: focus on prasugrel, ticagrelor, cangrelor and elinogrel. E-Journal of the European Society of Cardiology Council for Cardiology Practice, 8(21), February 10, 2010. Available at: www.escardio.org/communities/councils/ccp/e-journal/volume8/Pages/P2Y12-inhibitors-Capodanno.aspx#.UxejcPldVyw.)

activation of the GP IIb/IIIa receptor.[10] Activation of the GP IIb/IIIa receptor results in enhanced platelet degranulation and thromboxane production and prolonged platelet aggregation.[11] Thienopyridines and non-thienopyridine ADP receptor blockers inhibit the platelet activation and aggregation by antagonizing the thrombocyte P2Y12 receptor. This prevents the binding of ADP to the receptor, which attenuates platelet aggregation and reaction of thrombocytes to stimuli of thrombus aggregation such as thrombin (**Table 21-3**).[4]

Clopidogrel

Although clopidogrel combined with aspirin has been used successfully to prevent thrombotic events in patients with ACS, patients with DM, when compared with those without, have consistently been shown to have higher on-treatment platelet reactivity and worse clinical outcomes. The mechanisms leading to poor response to clopidogrel in patients with DM are not fully elucidated but are likely multifactorial, including genetic, metabolic, cellular, and clinical factors. Clopidogrel, a prodrug, requires a two-step hepatic cytochrome P-450 (CYP450) metabolic activation to produce the active metabolite that inhibits the platelet P2Y12 receptor.[13] Before intestinal absorption, 85% of the prodrug is hydrolyzed by esterases to an inactive carboxylic acid derivate. Because of these pharmacodynamic characteristics of clopidogrel, several hours pass between ingestion and attainment of therapeutic levels. This results in suboptimal platelet aggregation inhibition during acute PCI for ACS and a higher risk for acute stent thrombosis. Moreover, the longer period up to therapeutic levels may raise the bleeding risk during acute coronary artery bypass grafting (CABG), if necessary based on coronary anatomy. In addition, there is substantial variability in clopidogrel response among patients. Accumulating evidence shows that a suboptimal response to clopidogrel is associated with worse clinical outcomes such as coronary ischemia or stent thrombosis.[14–17] This suboptimal therapeutic response is particularly salient

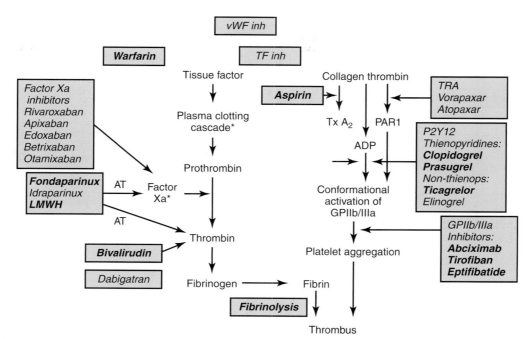

FIGURE 21-2 Targets for antithrombotic treatment. Agents approved for ACS treatment are shown in bold. AT=Antithrombotic treatment; LMWH=low molecular weight heparin; PAR1=protease receptor activator 1; TF = tissue factor; TRA = thrombin receptor antagonist; vWF=von Willebrand factor.

TABLE 21-1 Approved Agents for Acute Coronary Syndromes

AGENT	ANTITHROMBOTIC ACTION	MECHANISM OF ACTION	TYPE OR FAMILY	MODE OF ADMINISTRATION
Aspirin	Antiplatelet	Cyclooxygenase inhibitor		Oral
Clopidogrel	Antiplatelet	P2Y12 receptor inhibitor	Thienopyridine	Oral
Prasugrel	Antiplatelet	P2Y12 receptor inhibitor	Thienopyridine	Oral
Ticagrelor	Antiplatelet	P2Y12 receptor inhibitor	Cyclopentyl-triazolo-pyrimidine	Oral
Abciximab	Antiplatelet	GP IIb/IIIa inhibitor	Monoclonal antibody	Intravenous
Tirofiban	Antiplatelet	GP IIb/IIIa inhibitor	Peptide	Intravenous
Eptifibatide	Antiplatelet	GP IIb/IIIa inhibitor	Nonpeptide	Intravenous
Unfractionated heparin	Anticoagulant	Antithrombin (IIa) potentiator		Intravenous or subcutaneous
Enoxaparin	Anticoagulant	Xa/IIa (antithrombin) inhibitor		Intravenous or subcutaneous
Fondaparinux	Anticoagulant	Xa inhibitor		Intravenous or subcutaneous
Bivalirudin	Anticoagulant	Thrombin inhibitor		Intravenous
Warfarin	Anticoagulant	Vitamin K antagonist		Oral

TABLE 21-2 Common Oral Antiplatelet Agents and Doses in Patients with Acute Coronary Syndrome (ACS)

ANTIPLATELET AGENT	LOADING DOSE	WHEN TO GIVE	REGULAR DOSE	SPECIAL SITUATIONS
Aspirin	300 mg oral; 80-150 mg IV	Before or at cath	75-100 mg daily oral	
Clopidogrel	600 mg oral	Before or at cath	75 mg daily oral	
Prasugrel	60 mg	After cath for NSTE-ACS Before or at cath for STE-ACS	10 mg daily oral	Only age older than 75, weight <60 kg (consider 5 mg daily regular dose); contraindicated if history of stroke or TIA
Ticagrelor	180 mg	Before or at cath	90 mg bid oral	

cath = Catheterization; *NSTE-ACS* = non–ST-elevation acute coronary syndrome; *STE-ACS* = ST-elevation acute coronary syndrome; *TIA* = transient ischemic attack.

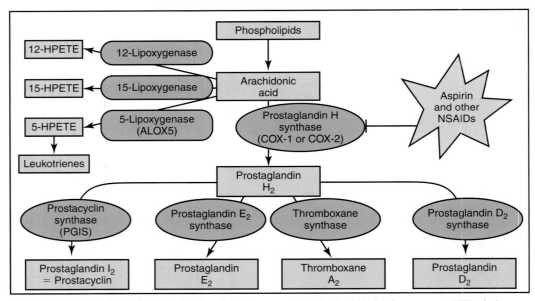

FIGURE 21-3 Mechanism of action of aspirin is through inhibition of COX enzymes. ALOX5 = Arachidonic 5-lipoxygenase; HPETE = hydroperoxyeicosatetraenoic acid; NSAIDs = nonsteroidal anti-inflammatory drugs. *(Modified from Ulrich and colleagues, 2006; Gupta and DuBois, 2001.)*

in patients with diabetes. A reduced generation of the active clopidogrel metabolite may contribute to poor clopidogrel responsiveness in patients with DM.[18] A large part of the variability in the clopidogrel response is a consequence of the variation in the *CYP* gene.[18] This gene codes for the CYP-450 enzymes involved in the biotransformation of the prodrug clopidogrel to the active metabolite. Particularly, polymorphisms in the CYP2C19 allele are associated with a reduced activity of clopidogrel. Poor response based on CYP2C19 genotype can be partly reversed by a higher dose.[19]

PCI. Fondaparinux has the highest level of recommendation in the recently released NSTEMI guidelines from the ESC.[20] None of these trials has shown any interaction by diabetes status for efficacy on clinical outcomes.

Bivalirudin

Bivalirudin is a direct thrombin inhibitor, and in contrast to heparins, it also inhibits clot-bound thrombin. Because of a very short plasma half-life of 25 minutes and a preferential renal elimination of its inactive metabolites, accumulation in case of renal failure and subsequently the bleeding risk is lower compared with heparins. In contrast to UFH, bivalirudin is not neutralized by platelet factor 4, a mechanism that is responsible for heparin-induced thrombocytopenia, and therefore not associated with this serious drug-related adverse effect. The dosage of bivalirudin is weight dependent. Bivalirudin has been investigated in patients undergoing elective PCI as well as in ACS (NSTEMI and STEMI) patients.[54-57] Bivalirudin with provisional use of UFH and GP IIb/IIIa inhibitors had similar anti-ischemic properties compared with standard treatment with GP IIb/IIIa inhibitors plus UFH, but with significantly lower bleeding risk. In the long term, the bivalirudin strategy also reduced mortality rates.[58] However, bivalirudin was associated with an increased risk for acute stent thrombosis in the early phase of treatment after primary PCI. Because T2DM is a significant predictor of early stent thrombosis,[59] a longer duration of bivalirudin administration after PCI (up to 4 hours) in the setting of ACS and especially in patients with diabetes is proposed.

SUMMARY

Patients with diabetes versus those without diabetes who experience an ACS event have a worse prognosis. Despite several new therapeutic agents that have gradually improved treatment of ACS in patients with diabetes, patients with diabetes still have a higher mortality risk compared with patients without diabetes. More research is needed to identify the optimal antithrombotic strategy and duration of therapy. Patients with diabetes have the same relative benefit from all recommended antithrombotic therapies as patients without diabetes; but when one considers the high absolute event rate, the absolute benefit is considerably greater, translating into a lower "number needed to treat" for derivation of benefit. Therefore, more attention should be focused on implementing therapies that have been shown to lower clinical events and mortality in this high-risk population.

References

1. Norhammar A, Malmberg K, Rydén L, et al: Under utilisation of evidence-based treatment partially explains for the unfavourable prognosis in diabetic patients with acute myocardial infarction, Eur Heart J 24:838–844, 2003.
2. Hunter RW, Hers I: Insulin/IGF-1 hybrid receptor expression on human platelets: consequences for the effect of insulin on platelet function, J Thromb Haemost 7:2123–2130, 2009.
3. Baldi S, Natali A, Buzzigoli G, et al: In vivo effect of insulin on intracellular calcium concentrations: relation to insulin resistance, Metabolism 45:1402–1407, 1996.
4. Angiolillo DJ, Fernandez-Ortiz A, Bernardo E, et al: Platelet function profiles in patients with type 2 diabetes and coronary artery disease on combined aspirin and clopidogrel treatment, Diabetes 54:2430–2435, 2005.
5. Davi G, Catalano I, Averna M, et al: Thromboxane biosynthesis and platelet function in type II diabetes mellitus, N Engl J Med 322:1769–1774, 1990.
6. Schneider DJ, Hardison RM, Lopes N, et al: Association between increased platelet p-selectin expression and obesity in patients with type 2 diabetes: A BARI 2D (Bypass Angioplasty Revascularization Investigation 2 Diabetes) substudy, Diabetes Care 32:944–949, 2009.
7. Jennings LK: Mechanisms of platelet activation: need for new strategies to protect against platelet-mediated atherothrombosis, Thromb Haemost 102:248–257, 2009.
8. Task Force on the management of ST-segment elevation acute myocardial infarction of the European Society of Cardiology (ESC), Steg PG, James SK, et al: ESC guidelines for the management of acute myocardial infarction in patients presenting with ST segment elevation, Eur Heart J 33:2569–2619, 2012.
9. Task Force on Myocardial Revascularization of the European Society of Cardiology (ESC) and the European Association for Cardio-Thoracic Surgery (EACTS), European Association for Percutaneous Cardiovascular Interventions (EAPCI), Wijns W, et al: Guidelines on myocardial revascularization, Eur Heart J 31:2501–2555, 2010.
10. Roth GJ, Stanford N, Majerus PW: Acetylation of prostaglandin synthase by aspirin, Proc Natl Acad Sci U S A 72:3073–3076, 1975.
11. Cipollone F, Patrignani P, Greco A, et al: Differential suppression of thromboxane biosynthesis by indobufen and aspirin in patients with unstable angina, Circulation 96:1109–1116, 1997.
12. Hamm CW, Bassand JP, Agewall S, et al: ESC guidelines for the management of acute coronary syndromes in patients presenting without persistent ST-segment elevation: the Task Force for the management of acute coronary syndromes (ACS) in patients presenting without persistent ST-segment elevation of the European Society of Cardiology (ESC), Eur Heart J 32:2999–3054, 2011.
13. Task Force on the management of ST-segment elevation acute myocardial infarction of the European Society of Cardiology (ESC), Steg PG, James SK, et al: ESC guidelines for the management of acute myocardial infarction in patients presenting with ST-segment elevation, Eur Heart J 33:2569–2619, 2012.
14. Antithrombotic Trialists' Collaboration: Collaborative meta-analysis of randomised trials of antiplatelet therapy for prevention of death, myocardial infarction, and stroke in high risk patients, BMJ 324:71–86, 2002.
15. Dillinger JG, Drissa A, Sideris G, et al: Biological efficacy of twice daily aspirin in type 2 diabetic patients with coronary artery disease, Am Heart J 164:600–606, 2012.
16. CURRENT-OASIS 7 Investigators, Mehta SR, Bassand JP, et al: Dose comparisons of clopidogrel and aspirin in acute coronary syndromes, N Engl J Med 363:930–942, 2010.
17. Collet JP, Cuisset T, Rangé G, et al: Bedside monitoring to adjust antiplatelet therapy for coronary stenting, N Engl J Med 367:2100–2109, 2012.
18. Brandt JT, Payne CD, Wiviott SD, et al: A comparison of prasugrel and clopidogrel loading doses on platelet function: magnitude of platelet inhibition is related to active metabolite formation, Am Heart J 153:66 e9–16, 2007.
19. Mega JL, Hochholzer W, Frelinger AL 3rd, et al: Dosing clopidogrel based on CYP2C19 genotype and the effect on platelet reactivity in patients with stable cardiovascular disease, JAMA 306:2221–2228, 2011.
20. Albers GW, Amarenco P, Easton JD, et al: Antithrombotic and thrombolytic therapy for ischemic stroke: American College of Chest Physicians evidence-based clinical practice guidelines (8th edition), Chest 133:630S–669S, 2008.
21. Hirsch AT, Haskal ZJ, Hertzer NR, et al: ACC/AHA 2005 guidelines for the management of patients with peripheral arterial disease (lower extremity, renal, mesenteric, and abdominal aortic): Executive summary a collaborative report from the American Association for Vascular Surgery/Society for Vascular Surgery, Society for Cardiovascular Angiography and Interventions, Society for Vascular Medicine and Biology, Society of Interventional Radiology, and the ACC/AHA Task Force on Practice Guidelines (writing committee to develop guidelines for the management of patients with peripheral arterial disease) endorsed by the American Association of Cardiovascular and Pulmonary Rehabilitation; National Heart, Lung, and Blood Institute; Society for Vascular Nursing; Transatlantic Inter-Society Consensus; and Vascular Disease Foundation, J Am Coll Cardiol 47:1239–1312, 2006.
22. CAPRIE Steering Committee: A randomised, blinded, trial of Clopidogrel Versus Aspirin in Patients at Risk of Ischaemic Events (CAPRIE), Lancet 348:1329–1339, 1996.
23. Yusuf S, Zhao F, Mehta SR, et al: Effects of clopidogrel in addition to aspirin in patients with acute coronary syndromes without ST-segment elevation, N Engl J Med 345:494–502, 2001.
24. Bhatt DL, Fox KA, Hacke W, et al: Clopidogrel and aspirin versus aspirin alone for the prevention of atherothrombotic events, N Engl J Med 354:1706–1717, 2006.
25. Angiolillo DJ, Shoemaker SB, Desai B, et al: Randomized comparison of a high clopidogrel maintenance dose in patients with diabetes mellitus and coronary artery disease: results of the Optimizing Antiplatelet Therapy In Diabetes Mellitus (OPTIMUS) study, Circulation 115:708–716, 2007.
26. Wiviott SD, Braunwald E, McCabe CH, et al: Prasugrel versus clopidogrel in patients with acute coronary syndromes, N Engl J Med 357:2001–2015, 2007.
27. Wiviott SD, Braunwald E, Angiolillo DJ, et al: Greater clinical benefit of more intensive oral antiplatelet therapy with prasugrel in patients with diabetes mellitus in the trial to assess improvement in therapeutic outcomes by optimizing platelet inhibition with prasugrel—Thrombolysis in Myocardial Infarction 38, Circulation 118:1626–1636, 2008.
28. Gurbel PA, Bliden KP, Butler K, et al: Response to ticagrelor in clopidogrel nonresponders and responders and effect of switching therapies: the respond study, Circulation 121:1188–1199, 2010.
29. Inhibition of the platelet glycoprotein IIb/IIIa receptor with tirofiban in unstable angina and non-Q-wave myocardial infarction. Platelet Receptor Inhibition in Ischemic Syndrome Management in Patients Limited by Unstable Signs and Symptoms (PRISM-PLUS) Study Investigators, N Engl J Med 338:1488–1497, 1998.
30. James S, Angiolillo DJ, Cornel JH, et al: Ticagrelor vs. Clopidogrel in patients with acute coronary syndromes and diabetes: a substudy from the Platelet Inhibition and Patient Outcomes (PLATO) trial, Eur Heart J 31:3006–3016, 2010.
31. Roe MT, Armstrong PW, Fox KA, et al: Prasugrel versus clopidogrel for acute coronary syndromes without revascularization, N Engl J Med 367:1297–1309, 2012.
32. Use of a monoclonal antibody directed against the platelet glycoprotein IIb/IIIa receptor in high-risk coronary angioplasty. The EPIC Investigation, N Engl J Med 330:956–961, 1994.
33. Randomized placebo controlled trial of abciximab before and during coronary intervention in refractory unstable angina: the CAPTURE Study, Lancet 349:1429–1435, 1997.
34. EPILOG Investigators: Platelet glycoprotein IIb/IIIa receptor blockade and low-dose heparin during percutaneous coronary revascularization, N Engl J Med 336:1689–1696, 1997.
35. Adgey AA: An overview of the results of clinical trials with glycoprotein IIb/IIIa inhibitors, Eur Heart J (19 Suppl D):D10–D21, 1998.
36. Boersma E, Harrington RA, Moliterno DJ, et al: Platelet glycoprotein IIb/IIIa inhibitors in acute coronary syndromes: a meta-analysis of all major randomised clinical trials, Lancet 359:189–198, 2002.
37. Topol EJ, Mark DB, Lincoff AM, et al: Outcomes at 1 year and economic implications of platelet glycoprotein IIb/IIIa blockade in patients undergoing coronary stenting: results from a multicentre randomised trial. EPISTENT Investigators Evaluation of Platelet IIb/IIIa Inhibitor for Stenting, Lancet 354:2019–2024, 1999.
38. International, randomized, controlled trial of lamifiban (a platelet glycoprotein IIb/IIIa inhibitor), heparin, or both in unstable angina. The PARAGON Investigators. Platelet IIb/IIIa Antagonism for the Reduction of Acute coronary syndrome events in a Global Organization Network, Circulation 97:2386–2395, 1998.
39. Theroux P, Kouz S, Roy L, et al: Platelet membrane receptor glycoprotein IIb/IIIa antagonism in unstable angina. The Canadian lamifiban study, Circulation 94:899–905, 1996.
40. Boersma E, Akkerhuis KM, Theroux P, et al: Platelet glycoprotein IIb/IIIa receptor inhibition in non-ST-elevation acute coronary syndromes: early benefit during medical treatment only, with additional protection during percutaneous coronary intervention, Circulation 100:2045–2048, 1999.
41. Hamm CW, Heeschen C, Goldmann B, et al: Benefit of abciximab in patients with refractory unstable angina in relation to serum troponin T levels. c7E3 Fab Antiplatelet Therapy in Unstable Refractory Angina (CAPTURE) Study Investigators, N Engl J Med 340:1623–1629, 1999.

42. Heeschen C, Hamm CW, Goldmann B, et al: Troponin concentrations for stratification of patients with acute coronary syndromes in relation to therapeutic efficacy of tirofiban. PRISM Study Investigators Platelet Receptor Inhibition in Ischemic Syndrome Management, *Lancet* 354:1757–1762, 1999.

43. Boersma E, Pieper KS, Steyerberg EW, et al: Predictors of outcome in patients with acute coronary syndromes without persistent ST-segment elevation. Results from an international trial of 9461 patients. The PURSUIT investigators, *Circulation* 101:2557–2567, 2000.

44. Ronner E, Boersma E, Akkerhuis KM, et al: Patients with acute coronary syndromes without persistent ST elevation undergoing percutaneous coronary intervention benefit most from early intervention with protection by a glycoprotein IIb/IIIa receptor blocker, *Eur Heart J* 23:239–246, 2002.

45. Roffi M, Chew DP, Mukherjee D, et al: Platelet glycoprotein IIb/IIIa inhibitors reduce mortality in diabetic patients with non-ST-segment-elevation acute coronary syndromes, *Circulation* 104:2767–2771, 2001.

46. Marso SP, Lincoff AM, Ellis SG, et al: Optimizing the percutaneous interventional outcomes for patients with diabetes mellitus: results of the EPISTENT (Evaluation of platelet IIb/IIIa inhibitor for stenting trial) diabetic substudy, *Circulation* 100:2477–2484, 1999.

47. Boden G, Vaidyula VR, Homko C, et al: Circulating tissue factor procoagulant activity and thrombin generation in patients with type 2 diabetes: effects of insulin and glucose, *J Clin Endocrinol Metab* 92:4352–4358, 2007.

48. Weitz JI: Low-molecular-weight heparins, *N Engl J Med* 337:688–698, 1997.

49. Wallentin L: Low molecular weight heparins: a valuable tool in the treatment of acute coronary syndromes, *Eur Heart J* 17:1470–1476, 1996.

50. Montalescot G, Zeymer U, Silvain J, et al: Intravenous enoxaparin or unfractionated heparin in primary percutaneous coronary intervention for ST-elevation myocardial infarction: the international randomised open-label ATOLL trial, *Lancet* 378:693–703, 2011.

51. Fifth Organization to Assess Strategies in Acute Ischemic Syndromes Investigators, Yusuf S, Mehta SR, et al: Comparison of fondaparinux and enoxaparin in acute coronary syndromes, *N Engl J Med* 354:1464–1476, 2006.

52. Yusuf S, Mehta SR, Chrolavicius S, et al: Effects of fondaparinux on mortality and reinfarction in patients with acute ST-segment elevation myocardial infarction: the OASIS-6 randomized trial, *JAMA* 295:1519–1530, 2006.

53. Oldgren J, Wallentin L, Afzal R, et al: Effects of fondaparinux in patients with ST-segment elevation acute myocardial infarction not receiving reperfusion treatment, *Eur Heart J* 29:315–323, 2008.

54. Stone GW, Witzenbichler B, Guagliumi G, et al: Bivalirudin during primary PCI in acute myocardial infarction, *N Engl J Med* 358:2218–2230, 2008.

55. Stone GW, White HD, Ohman EM, et al: Bivalirudin in patients with acute coronary syndromes undergoing percutaneous coronary intervention: a subgroup analysis from the Acute Catheterization and Urgent Intervention Triage strategy (ACUITY) trial, *Lancet* 369:907–919, 2007.

56. Kastrati A, Neumann FJ, Schulz S, et al: Abciximab and heparin versus bivalirudin for non-ST-elevation myocardial infarction, *N Engl J Med* 365:1980–1989, 2011.

57. White HD, Chew DP, Hoekstra JW, et al: Safety and efficacy of switching from either unfractionated heparin or enoxaparin to bivalirudin in patients with non-ST-segment elevation acute coronary syndromes managed with an invasive strategy: results from the ACUITY (Acute Catheterization and Urgent Intervention Triage Strategy) trial, *J Am Coll Cardiol* 51:1734–1741, 2008.

58. Stone GW, Witzenbichler B, Guagliumi G, et al: Heparin plus a glycoprotein IIb/IIIa inhibitor versus bivalirudin monotherapy and paclitaxel-eluting stents versus bare-metal stents in acute myocardial infarction (HORIZONS-AMI): final 3-year results from a multicentre, randomised controlled trial, *Lancet* 377:2193–2204, 2011.

59. Lagerqvist B, Carlsson J, Frobert O, et al: Stent thrombosis in Sweden: a report from the Swedish coronary angiography and angioplasty registry, *Circulation Cardiovascular interventions* 2:401–408, 2009.

22 Role of Primary Invasive Strategy and Revascularization in Diabetic Patients with Acute Coronary Syndromes

Franz-Josef Neumann

In patients with diabetes mellitus, the risk of developing coronary artery disease is increased by twofold to fourfold compared with patients without diabetes.[1,2] Moreover, patients with diabetes are more likely to present with acute coronary syndromes (ACSs) than people without diabetes mellitus.[2] In the contemporary INTERHEART study, the presence of diabetes more than doubled the risk of myocardial infarction.[3] Similarly, a large proportion of patients presenting with ACSs have diabetes. In large registries of patients with ACSs—such as the Euro Heart Survey on ACS, Can Rapid Risk Stratification of Unstable Angina Patients Suppress Adverse Outcomes with Early Implementation of the ACC/AHA Guidelines (CRUSADE), and the Global Registry of Acute Coronary Events (GRACE)—the prevalence of known diabetes mellitus has ranged from 23% to 34%.[4–6] Moreover, the Euro Heart Survey on Diabetes and the Heart demonstrated that in patients with ACS, an oral glucose tolerance test reveals impaired glucose tolerance in 32% and diabetes mellitus in 22% of the patients without previously known diabetes.[7] Thus, it can be estimated that more than half of the patients presenting with ACSs have either impaired glucose tolerance or diabetes mellitus.

DIABETES MELLITUS AS A MAJOR RISK FACTOR IN ACUTE CORONARY SYNDROMES

Diabetic patients are more likely to present with atypical symptoms, and in both ST-segment elevation and non–ST-segment elevation myocardial infarction the delay from onset of pain to clinical presentation is longer than in non-diabetic patients.[5,8,9] Moreover, diabetic patients presenting with ACSs are older, more often female, more often obese, and have more comorbidities, specifically hypertension and renal failure.[6,10,11] They also exhibit more complex coronary artery disease than patients without diabetes. In an analysis of the Euro Heart Survey on percutaneous coronary intervention (PCI), the number of patients with severely stenosed segments (>70%) was significantly higher in patients with diabetes compared with patients without ACS.[11] There was also a higher proportion of patients with left main disease and triple vessel disease as well as more type C lesions in patients with versus without diabetes.[11]

Moreover, compared with nondiabetic ACS patients, those with diabetes exhibit increased short-term and long-term mortality.[6,9,11–16] In the Organization to Assess Strategies for Ischemic Syndromes (OASIS) registry, diabetes independently predicted 2-year mortality (relative risk 1.52, 95% confidence interval [95% CI] 1.38-1.81, $P < 0.001$). Subsequently, GRACE reported odds ratios (ORs) for in-hospital death in patients with versus without diabetes of 1.48 (95% CI 1.03-2.31) for ST-segment elevation myocardial infarction (STEMI), 1.14 (95% CI 0.85-1.52) for non–ST-segment elevation myocardial infarction (NSTEMI), and 1.14 (95% CI 1.02-1.95) for unstable angina. Similar results were obtained in a pooled analysis of 62,036 patients of 11 independent ACS trials of the Thrombolysis in Myocardial Infarction (TIMI) study group. In this analysis, diabetes was significantly and independently associated with 30-day and 1-year mortality, both in NSTEMI ACSs and STEMI (hazard ratios [95% CI] 1.65 [1.30-2.10] and 1.12 [1.08-1.38], respectively).[13] The association of diabetes mellitus with poor survival after ACSs is stronger in women than in men.[10]

Hyperglycemia on admission for ACSs also strongly predicts mortality independent of the presence or absence of diabetes mellitus.[17–20] Thorough analyses of the GRACE trial have suggested that fasting glucose levels were better predictors for in-hospital and 6-month survival than the presence or absence of diabetes.[17] Hyperglycemia on admission has been considered to be a strong reflection of an acute stress response.[7] The close relation between glucose metabolism and outcome of ACSs is also reflected by the recent demonstration of an independent association of hemoglobin A1c (HbA1c) with long-term (3.3 ± 1.5 years) mortality after PCI in STEMI.[21]

The association between impaired glucose tolerance and survival after ACSs is less clear. Whereas an earlier study demonstrated an association between impaired glucose tolerance and poor survival,[22] a more recent analysis of the Euro Heart Survey on diabetes and the heart did not find any significant independent predictive value of impaired glucose tolerance with respect to survival.[23]

In addition to its impact on mortality, the presence of diabetes also increases the risk of heart failure as well as renal failure during the in-hospital phase by approximately twofold in patients presenting with STEMI or NSTEMI ACSs, as shown by the GRACE study,[6] and the risk of bleeding complications by approximately one quarter, as shown by the CRUSADE trial.[24] The risk of recurrent myocardial infarction and heart failure is also increased during long-term follow-up.[14,25,26] Moreover, in a large Danish registry, target lesion revascularization after PCI for ACSs was more often needed in patients with versus without diabetes (adjusted hazard ratio 1.55, 95% CI 1.14-2.11).[14] Even more important, an analysis from the Harmonizing Outcomes with Revascularization and Stents in Acute Myocardial Infarction (HORIZONS-AMI) trial revealed that the risk of stent thrombosis after placement of a drug-eluting stent in acute myocardial infarction was tripled in patients with diabetes.[27] In the Acute Catheterization and Urgent Intervention Triage Strategy (ACUITY) trial, patients with stent thrombosis more frequently had insulin-requiring diabetes than patients without stent thrombosis, with similar outcomes for drug-eluting and bare metal stents.[28]

BENEFITS OF A PRIMARY INVASIVE STRATEGY

ST-Segment Elevation Myocardial Infarction

In acute myocardial infarction, fibrinolysis compared with conservative treatment reduces the mortality by 18% as shown by a meta-analysis of randomized trials in this setting.[29] In addition to this benefit, coronary reperfusion by primary PCI reduces in-hospital mortality by an additional 37%.[30] Moreover, PCI compared with fibrinolysis reduces the risk of reinfarction and stroke, particularly of hemorrhagic stroke.[31] The initial benefit has been maintained during a long-term follow-up.[31]

The specific role of primary PCI compared with fibrinolysis for myocardial infarction in diabetes mellitus was addressed by a pooled analysis of individual patient data (N = 6315) from 19 trials comparing primary PCI with fibrinolysis.[32] As compared with fibrinolysis, the benefit of primary PCI with respect to 30-day survival was numerically larger in patients with versus without diabetes (**Fig. 22-1**).[32] Nevertheless, a statistically significant P value for interaction was not achieved ($P_{int} = .24$). The ORs comparing primary PCI with fibrinolysis with regard to death and recurrent myocardial infarction were similar in patients with and without diabetes (OR [95% CI] 0.52 [0.35-0.77] and 0.51 [0.42-0.61], respectively), whereas those for stroke were numerically more favorable in patients with diabetes (ORs [95% CI] 0.40 [0.16-0.99] and 0.58 [0.39-0.86], respectively), yet without reaching a significant interaction P value.[32] Because the incidence of death, recurrent myocardial infarction, and stroke was higher in patients with versus without diabetes irrespective of the treatment modality, similar risk ratios resulted in larger absolute risk reductions. In summary, this meta-analysis demonstrates that primary PCI in patients with diabetes is at least as safe and efficacious as in patients without diabetes and may even confer a larger absolute benefit over fibrinolysis than in patients without diabetes.[32] Nevertheless, the

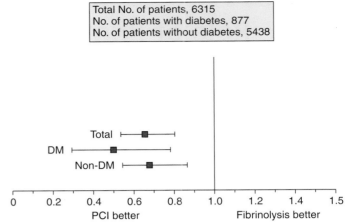

Total No. of patients, 6315
No. of patients with diabetes, 877
No. of patients without diabetes, 5438

FIGURE 22-1 Adjusted odds ratios and 95% confidence intervals for the risk of 30-day mortality according to the method of reperfusion therapy in patients with and without diabetes. Results from a pooled analysis of individual patient data (N = 6315) from 19 trials.[32] DM = Diabetes mellitus. *(Modified from Timmer JR, Ottervanger JP, de Boer MJ, et al: Primary percutaneous coronary intervention compared with fibrinolysis for myocardial infarction in diabetes mellitus: results from the primary coronary angioplasty vs thrombolysis-2 trial, Arch Intern Med 167:1353-1359, 2007.)*

increased mortality associated with diabetes remained.[32] This may be attributed to differences in baseline patient characteristics, but possibly also to less effective microvascular reperfusion. Analyses of the Enhanced Myocardial Efficacy and Removal by Aspiration of Liberated Debris (EMERALD) trial suggested impaired microvascular reperfusion despite similar vessel patency in patients with versus without diabetes.[33] This was evidenced by significantly inferior ST resolution and a significantly lower proportion of patients achieving a myocardial blush grade of 2 or 3 among the diabetes subset of patients.[33]

Non–ST-Segment Elevation Acute Coronary Syndromes

For high- to intermediate-risk patients with NSTEMI ACSs, current guidelines recommend an invasive strategy that involves coronary angiography and revascularization irrespective of the primary success of medical treatment.[34,35] This recommendation is supported by a number of trials. A meta-analysis published in 2005 concluded that the invasive strategy, although increasing the risk of in-hospital death and myocardial infarction (early hazard), significantly reduced death and myocardial infarction by 18% (95% CI 2%-42%) during the entire follow-up, ranging from 6 months to 2 years in various studies.[36] Some of the studies included in this meta-analysis, however, were not contemporary because of marginal use of stents and low-level use of antiplatelet therapy. Nevertheless, a more recent meta-analysis of eight randomized controlled trials with contemporary management strategies demonstrated that the invasive strategy compared with the conservative strategy significantly reduced the composite of death, myocardial infarction, and rehospitalization because of ACSs at 1 year.[37] Long-term benefits of the invasive strategy over 5 years were addressed by the FIR collaboration, who performed a meta-analysis of individual patient data from three major trials: Fragmin and Fast Revascularization During Instability of Coronary Artery Disease (FRISC II), Invasive Versus Conservative Treatment in Unstable Coronary Syndromes (ICTUS), and Randomized trial of a conservative treatment strategy versus an Interventional Treatment strategy in patients with unstable Angina (RITA 3).[38] They found a significant reduction in the 5-year incidence of cardiovascular death and myocardial infarction (hazard ratio [95% CI] 0.81 [0.71-0.93], $P=0.02$), which comprised a significant reduction in the incidence of myocardial infarctions (hazard ratio [95% CI] 0.77 [0.65-0.90], $P=0.01$) and a trend toward decrease in cardiovascular death (hazard ratio [95% CI] 0.83 [0.68-0.01], $P=0.068$).[38] The FIR collaboration also stratified their meta-analysis cohort according to the extent of baseline cardiovascular risk into three groups with low, intermediate, and high risk. As shown in **Figure 22-2**, the benefit of routine invasive strategy versus conservative strategy increased substantially with increasing risk, with an only minor benefit in low-risk patients, but a substantial, more than 10% absolute reduction in the 5-year incidence of death and myocardial infarction in high-risk patients.[38] Among the variables included in this risk stratification, diabetes was the strongest multivariable predictor of risk, with a hazard ratio of 2.06 (95% CI 1.75-2.41).[38]

Extending these findings by specifically addressing the role of diabetes mellitus, a collaborative meta-analysis of nine randomized trials comprising 9904 patients with non–ST-elevation ACSs, of whom 1798 (18.1%) had diabetes, was performed.[39] In this meta-analysis, an invasive strategy was associated with a comparable relative reduction in death, myocardial infarction, or rehospitalization because of ACSs in patients with or without diabetes ($P_{interaction} =.83$) (**Fig. 22-3**).[39] In diabetic patients, the meta-analysis revealed a significant reduction in the 1-year incidence of nonfatal myocardial infarction by the invasive as compared with the conservative strategy (relative risk [95% CI] 0.71 [0.55-0.92]) and of rehospitalization (relative risk [95% CI] 0.75 [0.61-0.92]).[39] The efficacy of the invasive strategy in reducing recurrent nonfatal myocardial infarction and readmissions for ACSs even appeared to be larger in diabetic patients than in nondiabetic patients. Taken together, the results of this meta-analysis and the results of the FIR collaboration suggest that diabetic patients represent a subset of patients with NSTEMI ACSs who derive particular benefit from an invasive strategy.

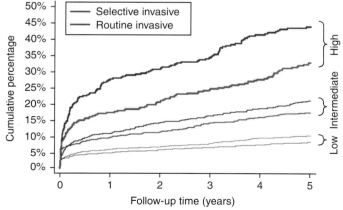

FIGURE 22-2 Cumulative risk of cardiovascular death or myocardial infarction by risk group in the pooled analysis of patients with non–ST-elevation acute coronary syndromes from FRISC, RITA 3, and ICTUS.[38] *(Modified from Fox KA, Clayton TC, Damman P, et al: Long-term outcome of a routine versus selective invasive strategy in patients with non–ST-segment elevation acute coronary syndrome: a meta-analysis of individual patient data,* J Am Coll Cardiol *55:2435-2445, 2010.)*

TIMING OF INTERVENTION

ST-Segment Elevation Myocardial Infarction

For minimization of myocardial necrosis, reperfusion therapy in acute myocardial infarction should be instituted as soon as possible. Three independent studies have indicated that a delay of up to approximately 2 hours for PCI as compared with immediate fibrinolysis maintains the survival benefit of PCI over fibrinolysis.[30,40,41] It must be kept in mind, however, that the largest benefit of PCI over fibrinolytic therapy was achieved when the delay to PCI was less than an hour.[30] Although fibrinolysis is more effective within the first 1 to 3 hours after onset of symptoms than after larger delays,[42,43] the benefit from PCI as compared with fibrinolysis is largely independent of the time from onset of symptoms to intervention, as shown by meta-analysis of earlier trials.[30] More recently, the Strategic Reperfusion Early after Myocardial Infarction (STREAM) study specifically addressed patients with STEMI who presented within 3 hours after symptom onset and who were unable to undergo primary PCI within 1 hour.[44] This trial did not show any advantage of fibrinolysis followed by systematic angiography over primary PCI, but a higher risk of stroke with fibrinolysis was reported.[44] The findings of STREAM concur with earlier studies showing no benefit of upstream administration of fibrinolysis[45] and/or abciximab[46] for facilitation of subsequent PCI.

With respect to timing of primary PCI in STEMI, there are no data suggesting that patients with diabetes mellitus need to be managed differently from nondiabetic patients.

Non–ST-Segment Elevation Acute Coronary Syndromes

There is general consensus that among patients with NSTEMI ACSs, those with refractory angina, severe heart failure, life-threatening ventricular arrhythmia, or hemodynamic instability may have an evolving large myocardial infarction and should be taken to coronary angiography and intervention immediately.[34,35]

In most patients presenting with NSTEMI ACSs, however, timing of the intervention is less critical. Nevertheless, intervention should not be intentionally delayed for stabilization and antithrombotic pretreatment (cooling-off strategy).[47,48] Such delay is of no benefit and, specifically, does not reduce the risk of peri-interventional myocardial infarctions.[47] A recent meta-analysis summarized the results of four trials on timing of intervention in NSTEMI ACSs: Timing of Intervention in Patients with Acute Coronary Syndromes (TIMACS), Angioplasty to Blunt the Rise of Troponin in Acute Coronary Syndrome Randomized for an Immediate or Delayed Intervention (ABOARD), Early or Late Intervention in Unstable Angina (ELISA), and Intracoronary Stenting with Antithrombotic Regimen Cooling-Off (ISAR-COOL).[49] In this meta-analysis, the median time from admission or randomization to coronary angiography ranged from 1.2 to 14 hours in the early and from 21 to 86 hours in the delayed group.[49] The early invasive approach significantly reduced the length of hospital stay by 28% (95% CI 22%-35%, $P<0.001$) and also reduced the incidence of recurrent ischemia (relative risk [95% CI] 0.57 [0.44-0.74]).[49] There also was a trend favoring the early invasive approach toward a lower composite risk of death, myocardial infarction, or stroke (relative risk [95% CI] 0.91 [0.82-0.01]) and lower risk of major bleeding (relative risk [95% CI] 0.78 [0.57-1.07]).[49]

Diabetes mellitus	Event rates (n/N)		RR (95% CI)
	Invasive	Conservative	
TIMI IIIB	42.9% (24/56)	43.1% (25/58)	0.99 (0.65–1.52)
MATE	50.0% (6/12)	37.5% (9/24)	1.33 (0.62–2.87)
VANQWISH	40.0% (46/115)	41.6% (52/125)	0.96 (0.71–1.30)
FRISC II	27.1% (39/144)	41.8% (56/134)	0.65 (0.46–0.91)
TACTICS-TIMI 18	21.7% (68/313)	28.3% (85/300)	0.77 (0.58–1.01)
RITA 3	20.8% (27/130)	27.2% (31/114)	0.76 (0.49–1.20)
VINO	11.8% (2/17)	35.7% (5/14)	0.33 (0.08–1.45)
ICTUS	31.4% (27/86)	28.8% (23/80)	1.09 (0.69–1.74)
OASIS 5 Substudy	42.1% (8/19)	25.9% (7/27)	1.62 (0.71–3.71)
OVERALL	**27.7% (247/892)**	**33.4% (293/876)**	**0.87 (0.73–1.03)**

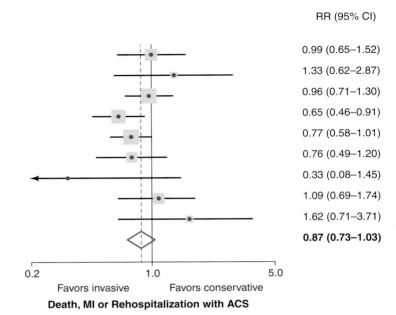

Favors invasive   Favors conservative

Death, MI or Rehospitalization with ACS

No Diabetes	Event rates (n/N)		RR (95% CI)
	Invasive	Conservative	
TIMI IIIB	30.7% (105/342)	35.6% (116/326)	0.86 (0.70–1.07)
MATE	21.2% (21/99)	19.7% (13/66)	1.08 (0.58–2.00)
VANQWISH	29.2% (101/346)	22.8% (76/333)	1.28 (0.99–1.65)
FRISC II	16.5% (157/949)	27.5% (266/968)	0.60 (0.51–0.72)
TACTICS-TIMI 18	14.6% (117/801)	16.9% (136/806)	0.87 (0.69–1.09)
RITA 3	12.4% (95/765)	17.5% (140/801)	0.71 (0.56–0.90)
VINO	6.4% (3/47)	26.4% (14/53)	0.24 (0.07–0.79)
ICTUS	21.2% (110/518)	20.0% (103/516)	1.06 (0.84–1.35)
OASIS 5 Substudy	17.8% (13/73)	15.4% (10/65)	1.16 (0.54–2.46)
OVERALL	**18.3% (722/3940)**	**22.2% (874/3934)**	**0.86 (0.70–1.06)**

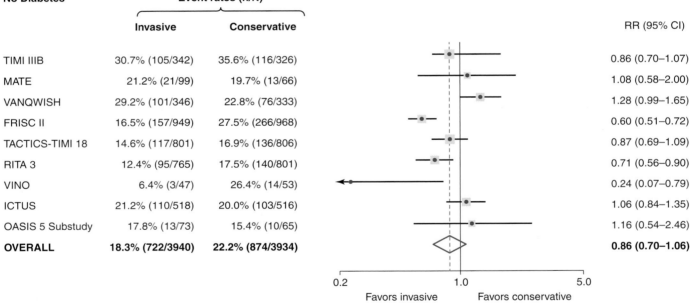

Favors invasive   Favors conservative

Death, MI or Rehospitalization with ACS

FIGURE 22-3 Benefit of an invasive strategy by diabetes mellitus status. The relative risk (RR) of death, myocardial infarction (MI), or rehospitalization with ACS with an invasive versus conservative treatment strategy stratified by the presence *(top)* or absence *(bottom)* of diabetes mellitus. Results from a meta-analysis of nine randomized trials comprising 9904 patients with non–ST-segment elevation ACSs.[39] Number of patients in denominators reflects those with ascertainment for the composite endpoint. *(Modified from O'Donoghue ML, Vaidya A, Afsal R, et al: An invasive or conservative strategy in patients with diabetes mellitus and non–ST-segment elevation acute coronary syndromes: a collaborative meta-analysis of randomized trials,* J Am Coll Cardiol *60:106-111, 2012.)*

More detailed insight was obtained from the TIMACS trial, which was the largest study addressing the timing of intervention in NSTEMI ACSs.[50] In TIMACS the cohort was stratified into low- and high-risk subsets according to a GRACE risk score above 140.[50] The GRACE risk score, derived from the GRACE study, is a score to predict mortality in ACSs; it comprises a number of clinical variables including, among others, age, electrocardiographic changes, and cardiac enzymes. In high-risk patients, TIMACS found a significant 38% reduction in death, myocardial infarction, or stroke at 6 months with early (≤24 hours) intervention as compared with delayed intervention (≥36 hours), whereas in the low-risk subsets timing did not matter (**Fig. 22-4**).[50] Based on these findings, it is recommended that patients with high-risk features in general should undergo coronary angiography within 24 hours after admission for a NSTEMI ACS (**Fig. 22-5**).[35] Specifically, this pertains to patients with diabetes mellitus and other high-risk features, even though dedicated studies addressing the timing of intervention in this subset are missing.

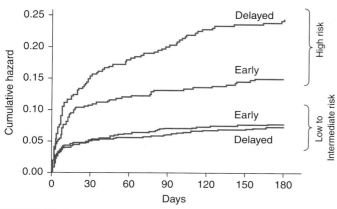

FIGURE 22-4 Kaplan-Meier cumulative risk of death, myocardial infarction, or stroke, stratified according to GRACE risk score at baseline in patients undergoing early versus delayed intervention in the TIMACS trial.[50] Patients who had a GRACE risk score higher than 140 (high risk) benefited more from early intervention than did patients with a score of 140 or lower (low to intermediate risk). *(Modified from Mehta SR, Granger CB, Boden WE, et al: Early versus delayed invasive intervention in acute coronary syndromes, N Engl J Med 360:2165-2175, 2009.)*

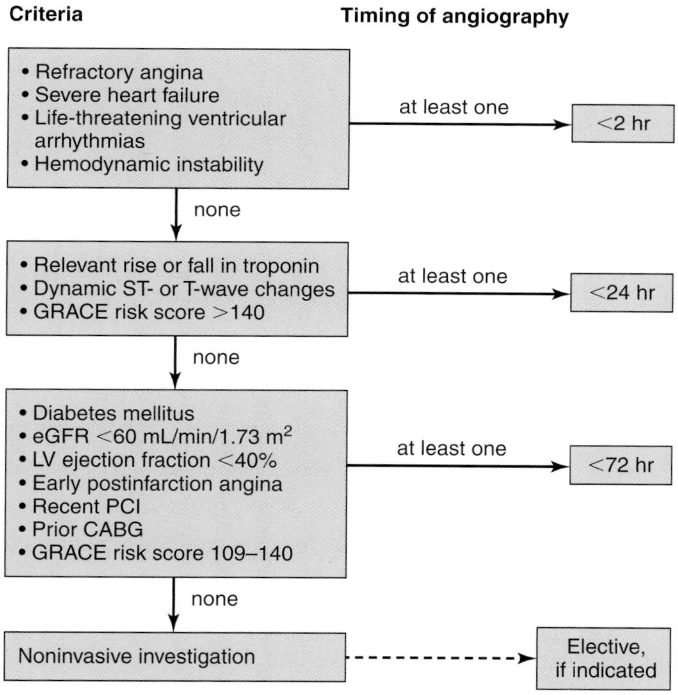

Criteria   **Timing of angiography**

- Refractory angina
- Severe heart failure
- Life-threatening ventricular arrhythmias
- Hemodynamic instability

→ at least one → <2 hr

↓ none

- Relevant rise or fall in troponin
- Dynamic ST- or T-wave changes
- GRACE risk score >140

→ at least one → <24 hr

↓ none

- Diabetes mellitus
- eGFR <60 mL/min/1.73 m²
- LV ejection fraction <40%
- Early postinfarction angina
- Recent PCI
- Prior CABG
- GRACE risk score 109–140

→ at least one → <72 hr

↓ none

Noninvasive investigation - - - → Elective, if indicated

FIGURE 22-5 Suggested algorithm for timing of coronary angiography in non–ST-segment elevation acute coronary syndromes. CABG = coronary artery bypass grafting; eGRF = estimated glomerular filtration rate; LV = left ventricular. *(Modified from Hamm CW, Bassand JP, Agewall S, et al: ESC guidelines for the management of acute coronary syndromes in patients presenting without persistent ST-segment elevation: the Task Force for the Management of Acute Coronary Syndromes (ACS) in Patients Presenting Without Persistent ST-Segment Elevation of the European Society Of Cardiology (ESC), Eur Heart J 32:2999-3054, 2011.)*

Because the risk of contrast-induced nephropathy is increased in patients with diabetes (OR [95% CI] 1.73 [1.48-2.02]),[51] adequate pretreatment is particularly mandatory in patients with diabetes and impaired renal function before they undergo coronary angiography.[52] Usually this can be achieved by intravenous infusion of isotonic saline for 12 hours before and 24 hours after the intervention.[53–56] In addition, iso-osmolar contrast medium reduces the risk of contrast-induced nephropathy compared with low-osmolar

medium.[57] In patients with severely decreased glomerular filtration rate (<30 mL/min/1.73 m²), prophylactic hemofiltration before PCI followed by hemofiltration for 24 hours after the procedure may be considered.[58] Pretreatment for prevention of contrast-induced nephropathy should not unduly delay coronary intervention for NSTEMI ACSs in diabetic patients with impaired renal function. These patients have a distinctly increased risk of coronary events of more than two-fold compared with patients with diabetes with normal renal function.[59]

Delayed coronary angiography is not required with use of metformin.[34] In contemporary clinical trials[60] and cohort studies[61] of patients with diabetes, the dreaded lactic acidosis was exceedingly rare (five or fewer cases per 100,000 patient-years), and its incidence did not differ between patients on metformin and those on other oral antidiabetic drugs. The most recent ESC guidelines recommend that renal function should be carefully monitored after coronary angiography/PCI in all patients on metformin. In addition, if renal function deteriorates in patients on metformin undergoing coronary angiography/PCI it is recommended to withhold treatment for 48 hours or until renal function has returned to its initial level.[62]

REVASCULARIZATION STRATEGY

ST-Segment Elevation Myocardial Infarction

Acute STEMI is an established prognostic indication for PCI. Compared with PCI, coronary artery bypass grafting (CABG) delays reperfusion and is associated with a high perioperative risk.[63,64] Nevertheless, CABG may be indicated as the primary reperfusion strategy for complex coronary anatomy, particularly when the culprit lesion cannot be identified with certainty. Also, CABG may be needed as treatment for failed PCI or as part of repair of mechanical complications after infarction. In the Primary Angioplasty in Myocardial Infarction (PAMI-2) study, 5.3% of the patients underwent CABG as the primary reperfusion strategy, and 6.1% as a secondary intervention.[65] More recently in the Thrombus Aspiration During Percutaneous Coronary Intervention in Acute Myocardial Infarction Study (TAPAS), the corresponding percentages for CABG were substantially lower, 0.65% and 4.86%, respectively.[66] Because of more complex coronary disease, diabetic patients in PAMI-2 were more likely to undergo in-hospital cardiac surgery after STEMI than patients without diabetes (OR [95% CI] 1.96 [1.21-3.10]). In PAMI-2, early and late survival free of reinfarction adjusted for baseline risk factors were similar in patients undergoing versus patients not undergoing in-hospital cardiac surgery.[65] Nevertheless, early complications, such as bleeding and recurrent ischemia, were frequent in surgical patients.[65] TAPAS yielded similar results: Despite a higher incidence of surgical complications, surgical management during the acute and subacute phase was associated with excellent 30-day and 1-year survival.[66]

Non–ST-Segment Elevation Acute Coronary Syndromes

In NSTEMI ACSs, revascularization by CABG carries a substantially increased risk,[67,68] particularly if myocardial marker proteins are elevated.[69] Treatment of the culprit lesion in NSTEMI is therefore generally considered to be the domain of PCI.

Yet, dedicated studies addressing the optimal revascularization strategy in NSTEMI ACSs are lacking. Thus, treatment decisions need to be based on individual considerations, taking into account the location of the culprit lesion and the amount of the jeopardized downstream myocardium, the ischemic damage that has already occurred, the extent of coronary artery disease outside the culprit lesion, and the specific risks of PCI and CABG in this setting. Depending on the culprit lesion and the extent of myocardial ischemia, the treatment strategy needs to follow the same principles as in STEMI. In most patients, however, the criteria derived from studies in stable angina may guide the choice of revascularization modality, as recommended by contemporary guidelines.[34,35]

Whereas single-vessel disease may be safely and efficiently treated with PCI,[34] decision making is more complex in multivessel disease. The recently published findings of the Future Revascularization Evaluation in Patients with Diabetes Mellitus: Optimal Management of Multivessel Disease (FREEDOM) trial compared the 5-year outcome of CABG with that of PCI in diabetic patients under optimal medical therapy.[70] The study enrolled 1900 patients, of whom 31% presented with a recent ACS. The primary outcome, the 5-year composite incidence of death from any cause, nonfatal myocardial infarction, or nonfatal stroke, occurred more frequently in the PCI group ($P = 0.05$) with rates of 26.6% after PCI and 18.7% after CABG (**Fig. 22-6**).[70] There was a substantial 5-year survival benefit of CABG (10.9% versus 16.3%; $P = 0.049$), and the 5-year incidence of myocardial infarction was also lower after CABG than after PCI (6.0% versus 13.9%; $P < 0.01$) (see **Fig. 22-6**).[70] The benefit of CABG was similar in two-vessel and three-vessel disease (**Fig. 22-7**).[70] The authors also quantified the extent and complexity of coronary artery disease by the Synergy Between Percutaneous Coronary Intervention with Taxus and Cardiac Surgery (SYNTAX) score, which accounts for the number of lesions, their location, and the angiographic characteristics associated with poor outcome. A subgroup analysis was performed according to low (≤ 22), intermediate (23 to 32), and high (≥ 33) SYNTAX scores. These thresholds were derived from the previously published SYNTAX trial.[71] In the low range of SYNTAX scores, the hazard ratio comparing CABG with PCI was close to unity and statistically insignificant, whereas at SYNTAX scores of 23 and above, a substantial and statistically significant benefit of CABG was found (see **Fig. 22-7**).[70] These findings are, however, difficult to interpret because the P value for interaction did not reach statistical significance ($P_{int} = .485$).[70]

Additional evidence is presented by the SYNTAX trial, which compared CABG with PCI with the paclitaxel-eluting stent in patients with three-vessel disease or left main coronary artery disease with or without distal coronary artery stenoses. In SYNTAX, 1800 patients underwent randomization; 28% presented with unstable angina.[71] Results from the diabetic subgroup, comprising 453 randomized patients, were published recently.[72] Among diabetic patients, the 5-year incidence of the primary endpoint, the composite of all-cause death, myocardial infarction, stroke, and repeat revascularization, was significantly lower after CABG than after PCI (29.0% versus 46.5%; $P < 0.001$), which was largely driven by a significant difference in the need for repeat revascularization (16.4 versus 35.3%; $P < 0.001$).[72] Consistent with FREEDOM, there also was a trend toward better survival after CABG compared with PCI (mortality 12.9% versus

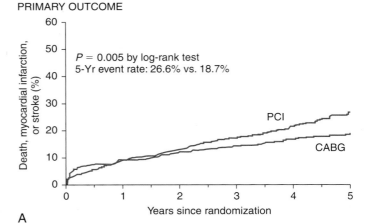

PRIMARY OUTCOME

$P = 0.005$ by log-rank test
5-Yr event rate: 26.6% vs. 18.7%

A

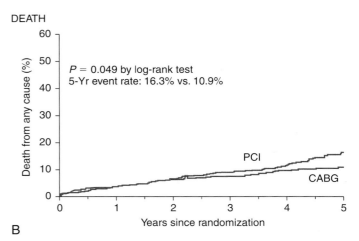

DEATH

$P = 0.049$ by log-rank test
5-Yr event rate: 16.3% vs. 10.9%

B

FIGURE 22-6 Kaplan-Meier estimates of the composite primary outcome and death in the FREEDOM trial comparing PCI with CABG in diabetic patients with coronary multivessel disease.[70] Shown are rates of the composite primary outcome of death, myocardial infarction, or stroke **(A)** and death from any cause **(B)** truncated at 5 years after randomization. The P value was calculated by means of the log-rank test on the basis of all available follow-up data. *(Modified from Farkouh ME, Domanski M, Sleeper LA, et al: Strategies for multivessel revascularization in patients with diabetes,* N Engl J Med *367:2375-2384, 2012.)*

19.5%; $P = 0.065$), which included a significant difference in the incidence of cardiac death (6.5% versus 12.7%; $P = 0.034$).[72] The difference in survival between CABG and PCI was largely the result of a high cardiac mortality in insulin-treated patients undergoing PCI. At low SYNTAX scores, the 5-year incidence of death, myocardial infarction, and stroke was similar after CABG or PCI; yet the need for repeat revascularization remained higher after PCI than after CABG even at low SYNTAX scores (**Fig. 22-8**).[72]

Although subgroup analyses for patients with ACSs from FREEDOM or SYNTAX have not been reported yet, the available 5-year data strongly suggest that in diabetic patients presenting with ACSs, CABG is the treatment of choice for complex multivessel coronary disease.[62] In less complex cases, PCI may be considered, too.

PROCEDURAL ASPECTS OF PERCUTANEOUS CORONARY INTERVENTION AND CORONARY ARTERY BYPASS GRAFTING

Completeness of Revascularization

Several independent studies have demonstrated that incomplete as compared with complete revascularization

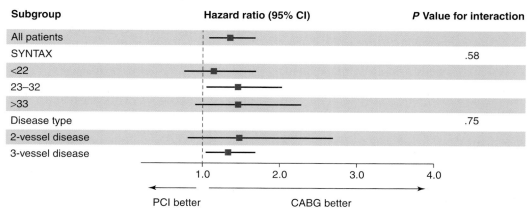

FIGURE 22-7 Primary composite outcome, according to subgroup of the FREEDOM trial comparing PCI with CABG in diabetic patients with coronary multivessel disease.[70] Subgroup analyses were performed with the use of Cox proportional-hazards regression. Five-year composite event rates for death, myocardial infarction, or stroke are shown. *(Modified from Farkouh ME, Domanski M, Sleeper LA, et al: Strategies for multivessel revascularization in patients with diabetes,* N Engl J Med *367:2375-2384, 2012.)*

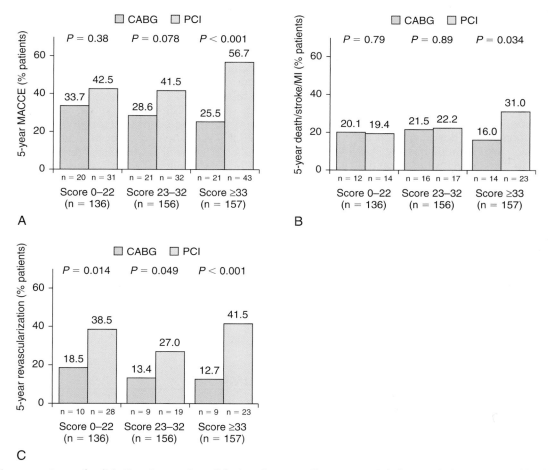

FIGURE 22-8 Five-year outcomes for diabetic patients and nondiabetic patients according to anatomic lesion complexity, as measured by the SYNTAX score. Results from the SYNTAX trial comparing CABG with PCI in patients with three-vessel disease or left main coronary artery disease with or without distal coronary artery stenosis. Shown are binary event rates of **(A)** major adverse cardiac or cerebrovascular events (MACCE); **(B)** the composite endpoint of all-cause death, stroke, and myocardial infarction; and **(C)** repeat revascularization in diabetic patients. Rates are separated according to SYNTAX score tertiles, indicating low (0 to 22), intermediate (23 to 32), and high (≥33) anatomic lesion complexity. CABG, blue bars; PCI, pink bars. *(Modified from Kappetein AP, Head SJ, Morice MC, et al. Treatment of complex coronary artery disease in patients with diabetes: 5-year results comparing outcomes of bypass surgery and percutaneous coronary intervention in the syntax trial,* Eur J Cardiothorac Surg *43:1006-1013, 2013.)*

is associated with inferior survival, both after PCI[73] and after CABG.[74,75] In a recent subanalysis of the SYNTAX trial, the incompleteness of revascularization after PCI was quantitated by the residual SYNTAX score—the SYNTAX score calculated after PCI. A progressively higher residual SYNTAX score was shown to be associated with increased 5-year mortality. Patients with complete revascularization (and therefore low residual SYNTAX scores) had a 5-year mortality of 8.5%, whereas in those with a residual SYNTAX score above 8, 5-year mortality rose to 35.3% (*P* < 0.01). These results were consistent across various subsets including patients with diabetes.

Specifically addressing patients with diabetes, an analysis from the Bypass Angioplasty Revascularization Investigation 2 Diabetes (BARI 2D) study revealed that diabetic patients with less complete revascularization had more long-term cardiovascular events than those with more complete revascularization, irrespective of whether they had been treated with PCI or CABG.[76] Earlier, the Bypass Angioplasty Revascularization Investigation (BARI) also suggested the relevance of complete revascularization in patients with diabetes. In BARI, the more complete revascularization of diabetic patients by CABG, especially when an arterial conduit was used for the LAD, as compared with plain balloon angioplasty[77] was considered to be a major cause for the survival benefit of CABG seen in this trial (see also Chapter 18).[78]

Staged Revascularization for Multivessel Coronary Disease

Given the importance of complete revascularization, there is continued debate about whether this should be achieved during the same procedure as for the culprit lesion (single-step approach) or whether a superior method is a staged procedure that involves initial treatment of the culprit lesion and subsequent treatment of the other lesions after further stabilization. Dedicated adequately powered randomized studies comparing the single-step approach with the staged approach are currently missing. A relevant retrospective analysis in this respect is based on the HORIZONS-AMI trial.[79] In a factorial design, this trial primarily compared bivalirudin versus heparin plus a glycoprotein (GP) IIB/IIIa inhibitor[79] and paclitaxel-eluting stents versus bare metal stents[80] in patients undergoing PCI for STEMI. In this trial, 668 patients underwent PCI of culprit and nonculprit lesions for multivessel disease.[81] Staged PCI was associated with significantly lower 1-year mortality than single-step PCI (9.2% versus 3.2%; $P < 0.001$).[81] Even after adjustment for differences in baseline characteristics, the difference in all-cause mortality favoring staged PCI over single-step PCI remained statistically significant at 30 days and at 1 year.[81] This analysis did not address the role of diabetes mellitus, specifically.

In a network meta-analysis of 15 studies, long-term mortality after staged PCI was significantly lower than after single-step multivessel PCI (OR 0.34 [95% CI 0.20-0.58]).[82] Staged PCI also conferred a significant benefit compared with single-step culprit-only PCI (OR 0.56 [95% CI 0.34-0.87]).[82] A more recent small (N=465) randomized study found a benefit of single-step multivessel PCI over culprit-only PCI, but did not address staged multivessel PCI.[83] Therefore in the absence of definite proof, staged PCI may still be considered to be a reasonable approach for unselected patient cohorts with STEMI. However, to what extent patients with STEMI and cardiogenic shock may benefit from single-step multivessel PCI is still a matter of debate.

The limited clinical experience with respect to the comparison of staged versus single-step PCI for multivessel disease in ACSs is derived from mixed populations comprising patients both with and without diabetes. There is, however, no indication that patients with diabetes are in special need of single-step multivessel PCI in this setting.

Percutaneous Coronary Intervention with Drug-Eluting Stents

Dedicated clinical studies on the optimal choice of stent type in diabetic patients undergoing PCI for ACSs are missing. There is, however, extensive literature on the choice of stent type in myocardial infarction (irrespective of the presence or absence of diabetes) and in patients with diabetes (irrespective of the presence or absence of ACSs). As discussed in Chapter 17, drug-eluting stents compared with bare metal stents substantially reduce the need for target lesion reinterventions in patients with diabetes mellitus. The absolute reduction in the risk of target lesion revascularization by drug-eluting stents is even larger in patients with diabetes than in patients without diabetes, although relative risk reductions are similar. Moreover, even in patients with diabetes, drug-eluting stents are at least as safe as bare metal stents, provided that adequate dual antiplatelet therapy is administered.

Concerning the choice of stent type in ACSs, it is now generally accepted that in the absence of contraindications to extended dual antiplatelet therapy, drug-eluting stents are the treatment of choice for PCI in this setting.[34,84] This concept is based on a number of studies that showed increased efficacy of drug-eluting stents in acute myocardial infarction without any safety issue, as summarized by two independent meta-analyses.[85,86] The largest randomized study in this setting is HORIZONS-AMI.[80] Notably, HORIZONS-AMI identified three independent risk factors for restenosis after PCI in STEMI: insulin-treated diabetes mellitus (hazard ratio 3.12 [95% CI 1.23-7.87]), baseline reference vessel diameter 3.0 mm or smaller (hazard ratio 2.89 [95% CI 1.56-5.34]), and total lesion length of 30 mm or greater (hazard ratio 2.49 [95% CI 1.33-4.68]).[87] Underscoring the particular benefit of drug-eluting stents in patients with diabetes with STEMI, the reduction in restenosis by the paclitaxel-eluting stent compared with the bare metal stent increased substantially with increasing number of risk factors for restenosis (Fig. 22-9).[87] There was no safety issue associated with the paclitaxel-eluting stent. On the contrary, in patients with two or more risk factors for restenosis, there was trend toward lower 12-month cardiac mortality after paclitaxel-eluting stents compared with bare metal stents (2.4% versus 6.2%; $P = 0.08$).[87]

SUMMARY

More than half of all patients with ACSs have either diabetes mellitus or impaired glucose tolerance. Patients with diabetes are more likely to present with atypical symptoms, and in both STEMI and NSTEMI, the delay from onset of pain to clinical presentation is longer than in patients without diabetes. Because of more frequent comorbidities and more complex coronary artery disease, patients with diabetes exhibit an increased short-term and long-term mortality after ACS compared with patients without diabetes. In addition to its impact on mortality, the presence of diabetes also increases the risk of heart failure and renal failure during the in-hospital phase, as well as the risk of bleeding complications.

In STEMI, primary PCI is at least as safe and efficacious in patients with diabetes as in patients without diabetes and may even confer a larger absolute benefit over fibrinolysis. Primary PCI must be performed as soon as possible, preferably within the first hour after first medical contact. In any

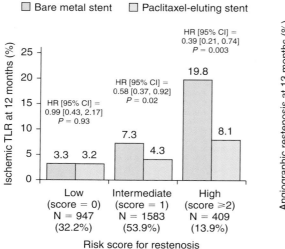
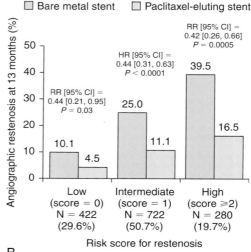

FIGURE 22-9 Rates of 12-month ischemic target lesion revascularization (TLR; A) and 13-month angiographic restenosis (B) in patients randomly allocated to paclitaxel-eluting stents (pink bars) or to bare metal stents (blue bars) according to the risk strata for restenosis. Results from the HORIZONS-AMI trial comparing paclitaxel-eluting stents with bare metal stents in patients undergoing PCI for ST-elevation myocardial infarction. RR = relative risk. *(Modified from Stone GW, Parise H, Witzenbichler B, et al: Selection criteria for drug-eluting versus bare-metal stents and the impact of routine angiographic follow-up: 2-year insights from the HORIZONS-AMI (Harmonizing Outcomes with Revascularization and Stents in Acute Myocardial Infarction) trial, J Am Coll Cardiol 56:1597-1604, 2010.)*

case, the delay for PCI compared with fibrinolysis may not exceed 2 hours to maintain the survival benefit of PCI over fibrinolysis. In multivessel disease, staged revascularization is the preferred approach in the absence of cardiogenic shock, based on currently available inconclusive evidence. Although PCI is the primary treatment of choice, CABG may be indicated for complex coronary anatomy.

In NSTEMI ACSs with high to intermediate risk, an invasive strategy that involves coronary angiography and revascularization irrespective of the primary success of medical treatment reduces the long-term risk of death and myocardial infarction. Patients with diabetes represent a subset of patients with NSTEMI ACSs who derive particular benefit from an invasive strategy. Although timing of the intervention is less critical in NSTEMI ACSs than in STEMI, intervention should not be intentionally delayed for stabilization and antithrombotic pretreatment (cooling-off strategy). In general, patients with high-risk features should undergo coronary angiography within 24 hours after admission with a NSTEMI ACS. Metformin does not require delayed coronary angiography. Yet pretreatment for prevention of contrast-induced nephropathy should be considered in patients with diabetes and impaired renal function unless the clinical setting does not allow for such delay.

Dedicated studies addressing the optimal revascularization strategy in NSTEMI ACSs are lacking. Thus, treatment decisions need to be based on individual considerations, taking into account the location of the culprit lesion and the amount of the jeopardized downstream myocardium, the ischemic damage that has already occurred, the extent of coronary artery disease outside the culprit lesion, and the specific risks of PCI and CABG in this setting. In general, the primary treatment of the culprit lesion will be PCI. It has to be considered, however, that in multivessel coronary disease, patients with diabetes are more likely to derive a larger benefit from CABG as compared with PCI than are patients without diabetes. Irrespective of the treatment modality, complete revascularization should be achieved. If the choice is PCI, drug-eluting stents are preferred in both NSTEMI ACSs and STEMI.

References

1. Resnick HE, Shorr RI, Kuller L, et al: Prevalence and clinical implications of American diabetes association-defined diabetes and other categories of glucose dysregulation in older adults: the health, aging and body composition study, *J Clin Epidemiol* 54:869–876, 2001.
2. Beckman JA, Creager MA, Libby P: Diabetes and atherosclerosis: epidemiology, pathophysiology, and management, *JAMA* 287:2570–2581, 2002.
3. Mente A, Yusuf S, Islam S, et al: Metabolic syndrome and risk of acute myocardial infarction a case-control study of 26,903 subjects from 52 countries, *J Am Coll Cardiol* 55:2390–2398, 2010.
4. Mandelzweig L, Battler A, Boyko V, et al: The second euro heart survey on acute coronary syndromes: characteristics, treatment, and outcome of patients with ACS in Europe and the Mediterranean basin in 2004, *Eur Heart J* 27:2285–2293, 2006.
5. Ting HH, Chen AY, Roe MT, et al: Delay from symptom onset to hospital presentation for patients with non–ST-segment elevation myocardial infarction, *Arch Intern Med* 170:1834–1841, 2010.
6. Franklin K, Goldberg RJ, Spencer F, et al: Implications of diabetes in patients with acute coronary syndromes. The global registry of acute coronary events, *Arch Intern Med* 164:1457–1463, 2004.
7. Bartnik M, Ryden L, Ferrari R, et al: The prevalence of abnormal glucose regulation in patients with coronary artery disease across Europe. The euro heart survey on diabetes and the heart, *Eur Heart J* 25:1880–1890, 2004.
8. Ting HH, Bradley EH, Wang Y, et al: Factors associated with longer time from symptom onset to hospital presentation for patients with ST-elevation myocardial infarction, *Arch Intern Med* 168:959–968, 2008.
9. Hasin T, Hochadel M, Gitt AK, et al: Comparison of treatment and outcome of acute coronary syndrome in patients with versus patients without diabetes mellitus, *Am J Cardiol* 103:772–778, 2009.
10. Dotevall A, Hasdai D, Wallentin L, et al: Diabetes mellitus: clinical presentation and outcome in men and women with acute coronary syndromes. Data from the Euro Heart Survey ACS, *Diabet Med* 22:1542–1550, 2005.
11. Bauer T, Mollmann H, Weidinger F, et al: Impact of diabetes mellitus status on coronary pathoanatomy and interventional treatment: insights from the Euro Heart Survey PCI registry, *Catheter Cardiovasc Interv* 78:702–709, 2011.
12. Malmberg K, Yusuf S, Gerstein HC, et al: Impact of diabetes on long-term prognosis in patients with unstable angina and non–Q-wave myocardial infarction: results of the OASIS (Organization to Assess Strategies for Ischemic Syndromes) registry, *Circulation* 102:1014–1019, 2000.
13. Donahoe SM, Stewart GC, McCabe CH, et al: Diabetes and mortality following acute coronary syndromes, *JAMA* 298:765–775, 2007.
14. Jensen LO, Maeng M, Thayssen P, et al: Influence of diabetes mellitus on clinical outcomes following primary percutaneous coronary intervention in patients with ST-segment elevation myocardial infarction, *Am J Cardiol* 109:629–635, 2012.
15. Brener SJ, Mehran R, Dressler O, et al: Diabetes mellitus, myocardial reperfusion, and outcome in patients with acute st-elevation myocardial infarction treated with primary angioplasty (from Horizons AMI), *Am J Cardiol* 109:1111–1116, 2012.
16. Canto JG, Kiefe CI, Rogers WJ, et al: Atherosclerotic risk factors and their association with hospital mortality among patients with first myocardial infarction (from the National Registry of Myocardial Infarction), *Am J Cardiol* 110:1256–1261, 2012.
17. Sinnaeve PR, Steg PG, Fox KA, et al: Association of elevated fasting glucose with increased short-term and 6-month mortality in ST-segment elevation and non–ST-segment elevation acute coronary syndromes: the global registry of acute coronary events, *Arch Intern Med* 169:402–409, 2009.
18. Kolman L, Hu YC, Montgomery DG, et al: Prognostic value of admission fasting glucose levels in patients with acute coronary syndrome, *Am J Cardiol* 104:470–474, 2009.
19. Hoebers LP, Damman P, Claessen BE, et al: Predictive value of plasma glucose level on admission for short and long term mortality in patients with ST-elevation myocardial infarction treated with primary percutaneous coronary intervention, *Am J Cardiol* 109:53–59, 2012.
20. Goyal A, Mehta SR, Gerstein HC, et al: Glucose levels compared with diabetes history in the risk assessment of patients with acute myocardial infarction, *Am Heart J* 157:763–770, 2009.
21. Timmer JR, Hoekstra M, Nijsten MW, et al: Prognostic value of admission glycosylated hemoglobin and glucose in nondiabetic patients with ST-segment-elevation myocardial infarction treated with percutaneous coronary intervention, *Circulation* 124:704–711, 2011.
22. DECODE i Glucose tolerance and mortality: comparison of WHO and American Diabetes Association diagnostic criteria. The decode study group. European Diabetes Epidemiology Group. Diabetes epidemiology: collaborative analysis of diagnostic criteria in Europe, *Lancet* 354:617–621, 1999.

23. Lenzen M, Ryden L, Ohrvik J, et al: Diabetes known or newly detected, but not impaired glucose regulation, has a negative influence on 1-year outcome in patients with coronary artery disease: a report from the Euro Heart Survey on Diabetes and the Heart, Eur Heart J 27: 2969–2974, 2006.

24. Subherwal S, Bach RG, Chen AY, et al: Baseline risk of major bleeding in non–ST-segment-elevation myocardial infarction: the CRUSADE (Can Rapid Risk Stratification of Unstable Angina Patients Suppress Adverse Outcomes with Early Implementation of the ACC/AHA Guidelines) bleeding score, Circulation 119:1873–1882, 2009.

25. Farkouh ME, Aneja A, Reeder GS, et al: Usefulness of diabetes mellitus to predict long-term outcomes in patients with unstable angina pectoris, Am J Cardiol 104:492–497, 2009.

26. Palmerini T, Genereux P, Caixeta A, et al: A new score for risk stratification of patients with acute coronary syndromes undergoing percutaneous coronary intervention: the ACUITY-PCI (Acute Catheterization and Urgent Intervention Triage Strategy—Percutaneous Coronary Intervention) risk score, JACC Cardiovasc Interv 5:1108–1116, 2012.

27. Dangas GD, Caixeta A, Mehran R, et al: Frequency and predictors of stent thrombosis after percutaneous coronary intervention in acute myocardial infarction, Circulation 123: 1745–1756, 2011.

28. Aoki J, Lansky AJ, Mehran R, et al: Early stent thrombosis in patients with acute coronary syndromes treated with drug-eluting and bare metal stents: the Acute Catheterization and Urgent Intervention Triage Strategy trial, Circulation 119:687–698, 2009.

29. Fibrinolytic, Therapy, (FTT) T, Collaborative, Group: Indications for fibrinolytic therapy in suspected acute myocardial infarction: Collaborative overview of early mortality and major morbidity results from all randomised trials of more than 1000 patients. Fibrinolytic Therapy Trialists' (FTT) Collaborative Group, Lancet 343:311–322, 1994.

30. Boersma E: The primary coronary angioplasty vs. Thrombolysis group: Does time matter? A pooled analysis of randomized clinical trials comparing primary percutaneous coronary intervention and in-hospital fibrinolysis in acute myocardial infarction patients, Eur Heart J 27:779–788, 2006.

31. Keeley EC, Boura JA, Grines CL: Primary angioplasty versus intravenous thrombolytic therapy for acute myocardial infarction: a quantitative review of 23 randomised trials, Lancet 361:13–20, 2003.

32. Timmer JR, Ottervanger JP, de Boer MJ, et al: Primary percutaneous coronary intervention compared with fibrinolysis for myocardial infarction in diabetes mellitus: results from the primary coronary angioplasty vs thrombolysis-2 trial, Arch Intern Med 167:1353–1359, 2007.

33. Marso SP, Miller T, Rutherford BD, et al: Comparison of myocardial reperfusion in patients undergoing percutaneous coronary intervention in ST-segment elevation acute myocardial infarction with versus without diabetes mellitus (from the EMERALD trial), Am J Cardiol 100:206–210, 2007.

34. Wijns W, Kolh P, Danchin N, et al: Guidelines on myocardial revascularization, Eur Heart J 31:2501–2555, 2010.

35. Hamm CW, Bassand JP, Agewall S, et al: Esc guidelines for the management of acute coronary syndromes in patients presenting without persistent ST-segment elevation: the Task Force for the Management of Acute Coronary Syndromes (ACS) in patients presenting without persistent ST-Segment elevation of the European Society of Cardiology (ESC), Eur Heart J 32:2999–3054, 2011.

36. Mehta SR, Cannon CP, Fox KA, et al: Routine vs selective invasive strategies in patients with acute coronary syndromes: a collaborative meta-analysis of randomized trials, JAMA 293:2908–2917, 2005.

37. O'Donoghue M, Boden WE, Braunwald E, et al: Early invasive vs conservative treatment strategies in women and men with unstable angina and non–ST-segment elevation myocardial infarction: a meta-analysis, JAMA 300:71–80, 2008.

38. Fox KA, Clayton TC, Damman P, et al: Long-term outcome of a routine versus selective invasive strategy in patients with non–ST-segment elevation acute coronary syndrome a meta-analysis of individual patient data, J Am Coll Cardiol 55:2435–2445, 2010.

39. O'Donoghue ML, Vaidya A, Afsal R, et al: An invasive or conservative strategy in patients with diabetes mellitus and non–ST-segment elevation acute coronary syndromes: a collaborative meta-analysis of randomized trials, J Am Coll Cardiol 60:106–111, 2012.

40. Betriu A, Masotti M: Comparison of mortality rates in acute myocardial infarction treated by percutaneous coronary intervention versus fibrinolysis, Am J Cardiol 95:100–101, 2005.

41. Pinto DS, Kirtane AJ, Nallamothu BK, et al: Hospital delays in reperfusion for ST-elevation myocardial infarction: implications when selecting a reperfusion strategy, Circulation 114:2019–2025, 2006.

42. Schömig A, Ndrepepa G, Mehilli J, et al: Therapy-dependent influence of time-to-treatment interval on myocardial salvage in patients with acute myocardial infarction treated with coronary artery stenting or thrombolysis, Circulation 108:1084–1088, 2003.

43. Schömig A, Ndrepepa G, Kastrati A: Late myocardial salvage: time to recognize its reality in the reperfusion therapy of acute myocardial infarction, Eur Heart J 27:1900–1907, 2006.

44. Armstrong PW, Gershlick AH, Goldstein P, et al: Fibrinolysis or primary PCI in ST-segment elevation myocardial infarction, N Engl J Med 368:1379–1387, 2013.

45. ASSENT-4: Primary versus tenecteplase-facilitated percutaneous coronary intervention in patients with ST-segment elevation acute myocardial infarction (ASSENT-4 PCI): randomised trial, Lancet 367:569–578, 2006.

46. Ellis SG, Tendera M, de Belder MA, et al: Facilitated PCI in patients with ST-elevation myocardial infarction, N Engl J Med 358:2205–2217, 2008.

47. Neumann FJ, Kastrati A, Pogatsa-Murray G, et al: Evaluation of prolonged antithrombotic pretreatment ("cooling-off" strategy) before intervention in patients with unstable coronary syndromes: a randomized controlled trial, JAMA 290:1593–1599, 2003.

48. Giugliano RP, White JA, Bode C, et al: Early versus delayed, provisional eptifibatide in acute coronary syndromes, N Engl J Med 360:2176–2190, 2009.

49. Katritsis DG, Siontis GC, Kastrati A, et al: Optimal timing of coronary angiography and potential intervention in non–ST-elevation acute coronary syndromes, Eur Heart J 32:32–40, 2011.

50. Mehta SR, Granger CB, Boden WE, et al: Early versus delayed invasive intervention in acute coronary syndromes, N Engl J Med 360:2165–2175, 2009.

51. Mehran R, Aymong ED, Nikolsky E, et al: A simple risk score for prediction of contrast-induced nephropathy after percutaneous coronary intervention: development and initial validation, J Am Coll Cardiol 44:1393–1399, 2004.

52. Goldenberg I, Matetzky S: Nephropathy induced by contrast media: pathogenesis, risk factors and preventive strategies, CMAJ 172:1461–1471, 2005.

53. Mueller C, Buerkle G, Buettner HJ, et al: Prevention of contrast media-associated nephropathy: randomized comparison of 2 hydration regimens in 1620 patients undergoing coronary angioplasty, Arch Intern Med 162:329–336, 2002.

54. Trivedi HS, Moore H, Nasr S, et al: A randomized prospective trial to assess the role of saline hydration on the development of contrast nephrotoxicity, Nephron Clin Pract 93:C29–C34, 2003.

55. Bader BD, Berger ED, Heede MB, et al: What is the best hydration regimen to prevent contrast media-induced nephrotoxicity? Clin Nephrol 62:1–7, 2004.

56. Klima T, Christ A, Marana I, et al: Sodium chloride vs. Sodium bicarbonate for the prevention of contrast medium-induced nephropathy: a randomized controlled trial, Eur Heart J 33:2071–2079, 2012.

57. Aspelin P, Aubry P, Fransson SG, et al: Nephrotoxic effects in high-risk patients undergoing angiography, N Engl J Med 348:491–499, 2003.

58. Marenzi G, Marana I, Lauri G, et al: The prevention of radiocontrast-agent-induced nephropathy by hemofiltration, N Engl J Med 349:1333–1340, 2003.

59. Tonelli M, Muntner P, Lloyd A, et al: Risk of coronary events in people with chronic kidney disease compared with those with diabetes: a population-level cohort study, Lancet 380: 807–814, 2012.

60. Salpeter SR, Greyber E, Pasternak GA, Salpeter EE: Risk of fatal and nonfatal lactic acidosis with metformin use in type 2 diabetes mellitus, Cochrane Database Syst Rev 2010, CD002967.

61. Bodmer M, Meier C, Krahenbuhl S, et al: Metformin, sulfonylureas, or other antidiabetes drugs and the risk of lactic acidosis or hypoglycemia: a nested case-control analysis, Diabetes Care 31:2086–2091, 2008.

62. Ryden L, Grant PJ, Anker SD, et al: ESC guidelines on diabetes, pre-diabetes, and cardiovascular diseases developed in collaboration with the easd: the Task Force on diabetes, pre-diabetes, and cardiovascular diseases of the European Society of Cardiology (ESC) and developed in collaboration with the European Association for the Study of Diabetes (EASD), Eur Heart J 34:3035–3087, 2013.

63. Lee DC, Oz MC, Weinberg AD, Ting W: Appropriate timing of surgical intervention after transmural acute myocardial infarction, J Thorac Cardiovasc Surg 125:115–119, 2003, discussion 119–120.

64. Weiss ES, Chang DD, Joyce DL, et al: Optimal timing of coronary artery bypass after acute myocardial infarction: a review of California discharge data, J Thorac Cardiovasc Surg 135:503–511, 2008, 511 e501–e503.

65. Stone GW, Brodie BR, Griffin JJ, et al: Role of cardiac surgery in the hospital phase management of patients treated with primary angioplasty for acute myocardial infarction, Am J Cardiol 85:1292–1296, 2000.

66. Gu YL, van der Horst IC, Douglas YL, et al: Role of coronary artery bypass grafting during the acute and subacute phase of ST-elevation myocardial infarction, Neth Heart J 18:348–354, 2010.

67. O'Connor GT, Plume SK, Olmstead EM, et al: A regional prospective study of in-hospital mortality associated with coronary artery bypass grafting. The Northern New England Cardiovascular Disease Study Group, JAMA 266:803–809, 1991.

68. Fortescue EB, Kahn K, Bates DW: Development and validation of a clinical prediction rule for major adverse outcomes in coronary bypass grafting, Am J Cardiol 88:1251–1258, 2001.

69. Hochholzer W, Buettner HJ, Trenk D, et al: Percutaneous coronary intervention versus coronary artery bypass grafting as primary revascularization in patients with acute coronary syndrome, Am J Cardiol 102:173–179, 2008.

70. Farkouh ME, Domanski M, Sleeper LA, et al: Strategies for multivessel revascularization in patients with diabetes, N Engl J Med 367:2375–2384, 2012.

71. Serruys PW, Morice MC, Kappetein AP, et al: Percutaneous coronary intervention versus coronary-artery bypass grafting for severe coronary artery disease, N Engl J Med 360:961–972, 2009.

72. Kappetein AP, Head SJ, Morice MC, et al: Treatment of complex coronary artery disease in patients with diabetes: 5-year results comparing outcomes of bypass surgery and percutaneous coronary intervention in the SYNTAX trial, Eur J Cardiothorac Surg 43:1006–1013, 2013.

73. Hannan EL, Racz M, Holmes DR, et al: Impact of completeness of percutaneous coronary intervention revascularization on long-term outcomes in the stent era, Circulation 113:2406–2412, 2006.

74. Cosgrove DM, Loop FD, Lytle BW, et al: Determinants of 10-year survival after primary myocardial revascularization, Ann Surg 202:480–490, 1985.

75. Bell MR, Gersh BJ, Schaff HV, et al: Effect of completeness of revascularization on long-term outcome of patients with three-vessel disease undergoing coronary artery bypass surgery. A report from the Coronary Artery Surgery Study (CASS) registry, Circulation 86:446–457, 1992.

76. Schwartz L, Bertolet M, Feit F, et al: Impact of completeness of revascularization on long-term cardiovascular outcomes in patients with type 2 diabetes mellitus: results from the Bypass Angioplasty Revascularization Investigation 2 Diabetes (BARI 2D), Circ Cardiovasc Interv 5:166–173, 2012.

77. Kip KE, Alderman EL, Bourassa MG, et al: Differential influence of diabetes mellitus on increased jeopardized myocardium after initial angioplasty or bypass surgery: bypass angioplasty revascularization investigation, Circulation 105:1914–1920, 2002.

78. Bari I: Seven-year outcome in the Bypass Angioplasty Revascularization Investigation (BARI) by treatment and diabetic status, J Am Coll Cardiol 35:1122–1129, 2000.

79. Stone GW, Witzenbichler B, Guagliumi G, et al: Bivalirudin during primary PCI in acute myocardial infarction, N Engl J Med 358:2218–2230, 2008.

80. Stone GW, Lansky AJ, Pocock SJ, et al: Paclitaxel-eluting stents versus bare-metal stents in acute myocardial infarction, N Engl J Med 360:1946–1959, 2009.

81. Kornowski R, Mehran R, Dangas G, et al: Prognostic impact of staged versus "one-time" multivessel percutaneous intervention in acute myocardial infarction: analysis from the HORIZONS-AMI (Harmonizing Outcomes with Revascularization and Stents in Acute Myocardial Infarction) trial, J Am Coll Cardiol 58:704–711, 2011.

82. Vlaar PJ, Mahmoud KD, Holmes DR Jr, et al: Culprit vessel only versus multivessel and staged percutaneous coronary intervention for multivessel disease in patients presenting with st-segment elevation myocardial infarction: A pairwise and network meta-analysis, J Am Coll Cardiol 58:692–703, 2011.

83. Wald DS, Morris JK, Wald NJ, et al: Randomized trial of preventive angioplasty in myocardial infarction, N Engl J Med 369:1115–1123, 2013.

84. Steg PG, James SK, Atar D, et al: Esc guidelines for the management of acute myocardial infarction in patients presenting with ST-segment elevation, Eur Heart J 33:2569–2619, 2012.

85. Kastrati A, Dibra A, Spaulding C, et al: Meta-analysis of randomized trials on drug-eluting stents vs. Bare-metal stents in patients with acute myocardial infarction, Eur Heart J 28:2706–2713, 2007.

86. De Luca G, Dirksen MT, Spaulding C, et al: Drug-eluting vs bare-metal stents in primary angioplasty: a pooled patient-level meta-analysis of randomized trials, Arch Intern Med 172:611–621, 2012, discussion 621–612.

87. Stone GW, Parise H, Witzenbichler B, et al: Selection criteria for drug-eluting versus bare-metal stents and the impact of routine angiographic follow-up: 2-year insights from the HORIZONS-AMI (Harmonizing Outcomes with Revascularization and Stents in Acute Myocardial Infarction) trial, J Am Coll Cardiol 56:1597–1604, 2010.

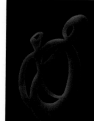

23 Epidemiology of Heart Failure in Diabetes

David Aguilar

Multiple epidemiologic studies have demonstrated that diabetes mellitus (DM) is associated with increased risk for the development of heart failure (HF). The mechanisms contributing to this greater risk are likely multifactorial and include the often accelerated comorbid conditions such as obesity, hypertension, and coronary artery disease (CAD). In addition, diabetes may contribute to cardiac dysfunction through other pathways related to insulin resistance, including lipotoxicity, abnormal calcium handling, mitochondrial dysfunction, increased reactive oxygen species, abnormalities in autophagy, and changes in adipokines (see also Chapter 24). It is important to note that the coexistence of diabetes and HF in a patient is associated with increased morbidity and mortality. This chapter reviews the epidemiology of diabetes and HF.

ASSOCIATION OF DIABETES AND INCIDENT HEART FAILURE

Multiple epidemiologic studies have demonstrated that diabetes increases the risk for the development of HF (**Table 23-1**). In the first 20 years of follow-up in the Framingham Heart Study, diabetes was associated with an almost twofold increased risk of HF in men and a fourfold increased risk in women independent of other risk factors (age, systolic blood pressure, tobacco use, cholesterol, and left ventricular (LV) hypertrophy).[1] Multivariable analyses revealed that diabetes had a high population attributable risk for HF in the Framingham Heart Study, accounting for 6% of cases in men and 12% in women.[2] In the Multi-Ethnic Study of Atherosclerosis (MESA) study of 6814 individuals free of symptomatic cardiovascular disease (CVD) at baseline, diabetes was associated with an almost twofold increased risk for the development of HF, independent of other established risk factors, including baseline LV function (hazard ratio [HR] 1.99, 95% confidence interval [CI] 1.08-3.68).[3]

In the National Health and Nutrition Examination Survey (NHANES) Epidemiologic Follow-up Study, the multivariable adjusted relative risk associated with diabetes for the development of HF was 1.85 (95% CI 1.51-2.28; $P < 0.001$), and the population attributable risk for diabetes was 3.1%.[4] Several other epidemiologic studies have also confirmed that DM is associated with a 2-fold to 3.5-fold increased risk for the development of incident HF compared with the risk in people without diabetes in the general population.[5–7]

Other studies in populations with greater baseline risk of developing HF have also demonstrated that diabetes is independently associated with incident HF. For example, in the Cardiovascular Health Study of people 65 years of age or older, the multivariable adjusted relative risk of HF in people with diabetes compared with those without diabetes was 1.74 (95% CI 1.38-2.19).[8] In the Cardiovascular Health Study, the incidence rates of HF in men and women with diabetes were 44.6 and 32.5/1000 person-years, respectively, and were markedly greater than in those without diabetes (see **Table 23-1**).[8] In patients with established CAD, diabetes also remains a powerful risk factor for incident HF. In the Heart and Soul Study of 839 individuals with stable CAD, individuals with diabetes had a threefold increased risk of HF compared with those without diabetes (adjusted HR 3.34, 95% CI 1.65-6.76).[9] The incidence rate of HF in the Heart and Soul Study was 36.6/1000 person-years and 17.9/1000 person-years in individuals with and without diabetes, respectively.[9] Diabetes was associated with a more-than-doubled risk of development of HF in patients with stable CAD enrolled in the PEACE clinical trial (HR 2.16, 95% CI 1.67-2.79).[10] Finally, among 2391 women with established CAD who were free of HF at baseline and who were enrolled in the Heart and Estrogen/Progestin Replacement Study (HERS), diabetes was the strongest risk factor for the development of HF (adjusted HR 3.1, 95% CI 2.3-4.2).[11]

TABLE 23-1 Incidence of Heart Failure (HF) in Individuals With and Without Diabetes in Select Epidemiologic Studies

STUDY	SAMPLE	FOLLOW-UP (TIME)	HF EVENTS (INCIDENCE)	RISK FOR HF COMPARED WITH RISK IN PATIENTS WITHOUT DIABETES (ADJUSTED)	POPULATION ATTRIBUTABLE FRACTION
Framingham[1]	5209 individuals	20 yr	DM (men): 7.6/1000 person-yr (age-adjusted) No DM (men): 3.5/1000 person-yr (age-adjusted) DM (women): 11.4/1000 person-yr (age-adjusted) No DM (women): 2.2/1000 person-yr (age-adjusted)	RR (men): 1.82 RR (women): 3.75	Men 7.7% Women 18.6%
Cardiovascular Health Study[8]	5888 individuals older than 65 yr	Average 5.5 yr	DM (men): 44.6/1000 person-yr No DM (men): 22.9/100 person-yr DM (women): 32.5/1000 person-yr No DM (women): 12.1/1000 person-yr	RR: 1.74 (95% CI 1.38-2.19)	8.3%
Heart and Soul Study[9]	839 participants with stable CAD	Mean 4.1 years	DM: 36.6/1000 person-yr No DM: 17.9/1000 person-yr	HR: 3.34 (95% CI 1.65-6.76).	N/A

CI = Confidence interval; HR = hazard ratio; RR = relative risk.

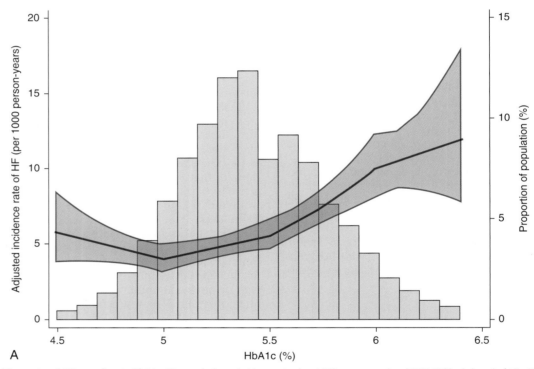

A

FIGURE 23-1 Incident rates of HF according to HbA1c. The graph shows incidence rates (per 1000 person-years) and 95% CI (shaded area) of HF with spline terms of A1c (knots at 5.0%, 5.5%, and 6.0%). *(Modified from Matsushita K, Blecker S, Pazin-Filho A, et al: The association of hemoglobin a1c with incident heart failure among people without diabetes: the Atherosclerosis Risk in Communities study, Diabetes 59:2020-2026, 2010.)*

In addition to overt diabetes, epidemiologic studies have also demonstrated that milder abnormalities of glucose regulation (below the diagnostic threshold for diabetes) are associated with increased rates of HF. In a community-based, observational cohort of 1187 elderly men without congestive heart failure (CHF) and valvular disease at baseline, parameters of insulin resistance (clamp glucose disposal rate and fasting proinsulin level) predicted CHF incidence independently of established risk factors including clinical diabetes.[12] Similarly, in participants without diabetes or HF at baseline in the Atherosclerosis Risk in Communities (ARIC) study, incident HF rates increased in a stepwise manner with increasing hemoglobin A1c

(HbA1c) when compared with the reference group (HbA1c 5.0% to 5.4%) (**Fig. 23-1**).[13]

Risk factors for incident HF in patients with diabetes are similar to those in individuals without diabetes (see also Chapter 25). Cohort studies of individuals with diabetes have shown that risk factors for the development of HF include older age, the presence of ischemic heart disease and CAD, peripheral vascular disease, nephropathy and renal insufficiency, metabolic complications of diabetes, retinopathy, diabetes duration, obesity, and hypertension.[7,11,14] In addition, multiple studies have demonstrated that worsened glycemic control is associated with greater risk for the development of HF in individuals with diabetes. Several

TABLE 23-3 Mortality in Patients with Diabetes and Established Heart Failure (HF) in Selected Population-Based Studies and Clinical Trials

STUDY	YEAR OF PUBLICATION	SAMPLE SIZE	MULTIVARIATE ADJUSTED RISK FOR DEATH (COMPARED WITH INDIVIDUALS WITHOUT DM)	COMMENT
Population-Based Studies				
Framingham[71]	1993	9405	Women: HR 1.70 (95% CI 1.21-2.38) Men: HR 0.99 (95% CI 0.70-1.40)	
Rotterdam[70]	2001	5540	Age-adjusted HR 3.19 (95% CI 1.80-2.26)	
Olmsted County[44]	2006	665	RR 1.33 (95% CI 1.07-1.66)	DM and no CAD: RR 1.79 (95% CI 1.33 to 2.41) DM and CAD: RR 1.11 (95% CI 0.81 to 1.15)
United Kingdom[69]	2013	1091	HR 1.72 (95% CI 1.29-2.28)	Association between DM and increased mortality is similar in those with ischemic and nonischemic CMP.
Clinical Trials				
SOLVD[73]	1991	6797 (reduced LVEF)	RR: 1.37 (95% CI 1.21-1.55) in those with ischemic CMP RR 0.98 (95% CI 0.76-1.32) in those without ischemic CMP	
DIAMOND[74]	2004	5491	RR 1.5 (95% CI 1.3-1.8) total cohort RR 1.4 (95% CI 1.3-1.6) men RR 1.7 (95% CI 1.4-1.9) women	Excess mortality associated with DM was greater in women than in men.
VALIANT[48]	2004	14,703 (acute MI and HF)	HR 1.43 (95% CI 1.29-1.59) with previously diagnosed DM HR 1.50 (95% CI 1.21-1.85) with newly diagnosed DM	Individuals with newly diagnosed DM had similar mortality at 1-year compared with individuals with previously diagnosed DM.
CHARM[50,72]	2006	7500	HR (DM, no insulin): 1.60 (95% CI 1.34-1.68) HR (DM, on insulin): 1.80 (95% CI 1.56-2.08) HR (DM, preserved EF): 1.84 (95% CI 1.51-2.26) HR (DM, reduced EF): 1.55 (95% CI 1.38-1.74)	The association between DM and increased mortality was similar between HF patients with reduced LVEF and those with preserved LVEF. The association between DM and mortality was not modified by gender or cause of HF.
I-PRESERVE[75]	2011	4128 (HF with preserved EF)	HR 1.43 (1.2, 1.60)	

CMP = Cardiomyopathy; DIAMOND = Danish Investigations of Arrhythmia and Mortality on Dofetilide; I-PRESERVE = Irbesartan in Heart Failure with Preserved Ejection Fraction; SOLVD = Studies of Left Ventricular Dysfunction.

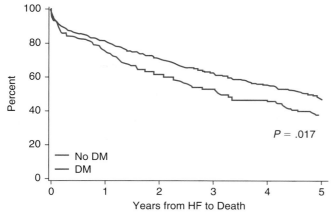

FIGURE 23-7 Kaplan-Meier survival estimates in HF patients with and without DM. *(Modified from From AM, Leibson CL, Bursi F, et al: Diabetes in heart failure: prevalence and impact on outcome in the population, Am J Med 119:591-599, 2006.)*

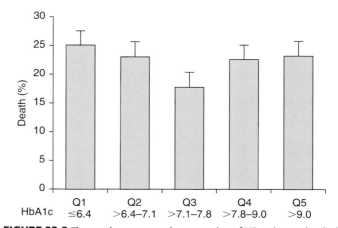

FIGURE 23-8 The graph represents the proportion of HF patients who died during 2-year follow-up by quintiles (Q) of glycosylated hemoglobin (HbA1c). Global chi-square, $P=0.001$. Error bars indicate 95% CI. *(Modified from Aguilar D, Bozkurt B, Ramasubbu K, Deswal A: Relationship of hemoglobin A1c and mortality in heart failure patients with diabetes, J Am Coll Cardiol 54:422-428, 2009.)*

In populations with established HF, the excess risk in diabetic patients may be particularly prominent in women,[74] although this finding has not been consistently observed.[50] In a meta-analysis of more than 40,000 patients with HF, DM was a strong, independent predictor of mortality in both men and women, but the presence of diabetes attenuated the protective effect of female sex on overall prognosis in women with established HF.[43]

Etiology of Heart Failure

Although some studies have suggested that diabetes may have greater prognostic significance in individuals with HF because of the presence of ischemic heart disease,[49,73] these findings have not been confirmed in other studies.[44,50,69]

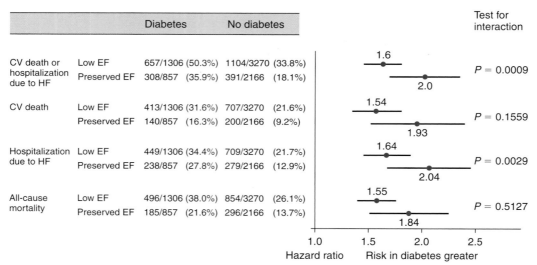

FIGURE 23-9 **Adjusted HR of different outcomes associated with diabetes.** Horizontal bars represent 95% CI. *(Modified from MacDonald MR, Petrie MC, Varyani F, et al: Impact of diabetes on outcomes in patients with low and preserved ejection fraction heart failure: an analysis of the Candesartan in Heart failure: Assessment of Reduction in Mortality and morbidity (CHARM) programme,* Eur Heart J *29:1377-1385, 2008.)*

Heart Failure with Preserved Left Ventricular Ejection Fraction

As previously described, abnormalities of increased LV mass, increased left atrial size, and diastolic Doppler abnormalities are commonly present in individuals with diabetes, and these diastolic abnormalities are associated with greater rates of HF (see **Fig. 23-4**).[41] In the Framingham Heart Study, diabetes was a risk factor for both systolic HF and HF with preserved EF.[84] In patients with HF with preserved EF, the presence of diabetes is associated with increased mortality,[47,50,75] and the increased mortality risk associated with diabetes is similar in HF patients with preserved LVEF compared with patients with reduced LVEF.[47,50] Diabetes does appear to confer a greater risk for HF hospitalization in HF patients with preserved LVEF compared with those with low EF. In the CHARM program, the adjusted HR for HF hospitalization in diabetic versus nondiabetic patients was 1.64 (95% CI 1.44-1.86) in patients with low EF and 2.014 (95% CI 1.68-2.07) in patients with preserved EF (**Fig. 23-9**).[50]

SUMMARY

Multiple studies have demonstrated that DM is associated with increased risk for the development of HF in a variety of populations. The prevalence of HF in individuals with type 2 diabetes is greater than estimates in the general population, and prevalence rates increase with age and other comorbid conditions. In patients with established HF, diabetes may be present in 12% to 40%, and its occurrence may be even higher in populations such as those with acute decompensated HF. The prevalence of diabetes in HF patients may be even higher when systematic screening for diabetes is performed. It is important to note that the coexistence of diabetes and HF is associated with increased mortality and morbidity compared with HF patients without diabetes or compared with diabetic patients without HF. This increased hazard is seen throughout the spectrum of HF, including HF with preserved EF and HF with reduced EF.

References

1. Kannel WB, McGee DL: Diabetes and cardiovascular disease. The Framingham study, *JAMA* 241:2035–2038, 1979.
2. Levy D, Larson MG, Vasan RS, et al: The progression from hypertension to congestive heart failure, *JAMA* 275:1557–1562, 1996.
3. Bahrami H, Bluemke DA, Kronmal R, et al: Novel metabolic risk factors for incident heart failure and their relationship with obesity: the MESA (Multi-Ethnic Study of Atherosclerosis) study, *J Am Coll Cardiol* 51:1775–1783, 2008.
4. He J, Ogden LG, Bazzano LA, et al: Risk factors for congestive heart failure in US men and women: NHANES I epidemiologic follow-up study, *Arch Intern Med* 161:996–1002, 2001.
5. Agarwal SK, Chambless LE, Ballantyne CM, et al: Prediction of incident heart failure in general practice: the Atherosclerosis Risk in Communities (ARIC) Study, *Circ Heart Fail* 5:422–429, 2012.
6. Goyal A, Norton CR, Thomas TN, et al: Predictors of incident heart failure in a large insured population: a one million person-year follow-up study, *Circ Heart Fail* 3:698–705, 2010.
7. Nichols GA, Gullion CM, Koro CE, et al: The incidence of congestive heart failure in type 2 diabetes: an update, *Diabetes Care* 27:1879–1884, 2004.
8. Gottdiener JS, Arnold AM, Aurigemma GP, et al: Predictors of congestive heart failure in the elderly: the Cardiovascular Health Study, *J Am Coll Cardiol* 35:1628–1637, 2000.
9. van Melle JP, Bot M, de Jonge P, et al: Diabetes, glycemic control, and new-onset heart failure in patients with stable coronary artery disease: data from the heart and soul study, *Diabetes Care* 33:2084–2089, 2010.
10. Lewis EF, Solomon SD, Jablonski KA, et al: Predictors of heart failure in patients with stable coronary artery disease: a PEACE study, *Circ Heart Fail* 2:209–216, 2009.
11. Bibbins-Domingo K, Lin F, Vittinghoff E, et al: Predictors of heart failure among women with coronary disease, *Circulation* 110:1424–1430, 2004.
12. Ingelsson E, Sundstrom J, Arnlov J, et al: Insulin resistance and risk of congestive heart failure, *JAMA* 294:334–341, 2005.
13. Matsushita K, Blecker S, Pazin-Filho A, et al: The association of hemoglobin A1c with incident heart failure among people without diabetes: the Atherosclerosis Risk in Communities study, *Diabetes* 59:2020–2026, 2010.
14. Bertoni AG, Hundley WG, Massing MW, et al: Heart failure prevalence, incidence, and mortality in the elderly with diabetes, *Diabetes Care* 27:699–703, 2004.
15. Iribarren C, Karter AJ, Go AS, et al: Glycemic control and heart failure among adult patients with diabetes, *Circulation* 103:2668–2673, 2001.
16. Pazin-Filho A, Kottgen A, Bertoni AG, et al: HbA 1c as a risk factor for heart failure in persons with diabetes: the Atherosclerosis Risk in Communities (ARIC) study, *Diabetologia* 51:2197–2204, 2008.
17. Stratton IM, Adler AI, Neil HA, et al: Association of glycaemia with macrovascular and microvascular complications of type 2 diabetes (UKPDS 35): prospective observational study, *BMJ* 321:405–412, 2000.
18. Kannel WB, Hjortland M, Castelli WP: Role of diabetes in congestive heart failure: the Framingham study, *Am J Cardiol* 34:29–34, 1974.
19. Gerstein HC, Bosch J, Dagenais GR, et al: Basal insulin and cardiovascular and other outcomes in dysglycemia, *N Engl J Med* 367:319–328, 2012.
20. Intensive blood-glucose control with sulphonylureas or insulin compared with conventional treatment and risk of complications in patients with type 2 diabetes (UKPDS 33). UK Prospective Diabetes Study (UKPDS) Group, *Lancet* 352:837–853, 1998.
21. Kaul S, Bolger AF, Herrington D, et al: Thiazolidinedione drugs and cardiovascular risks: a science advisory from the American Heart Association and American College Of Cardiology Foundation, *J Am Coll Cardiol* 55:1885–1894, 2010.
22. Lago RM, Singh PP, Nesto RW: Congestive heart failure and cardiovascular death in patients with prediabetes and type 2 diabetes given thiazolidinediones: a meta-analysis of randomised clinical trials, *Lancet* 370:1129–1136, 2007.
23. Erdmann E, Charbonnel B, Wilcox RG, et al: Pioglitazone use and heart failure in patients with type 2 diabetes and preexisting cardiovascular disease: data from the PROactive study (PROactive 08), *Diabetes Care* 30:2773–2778, 2007.
24. Komajda M, McMurray JJ, Beck-Nielsen H, et al: Heart failure events with rosiglitazone in type 2 diabetes: data from the RECORD clinical trial, *Eur Heart J* 31:824–831, 2010.
25. Guan Y, Hao C, Cha DR, et al: Thiazolidinediones expand body fluid volume through PPARgamma stimulation of ENaC-mediated renal salt absorption, *Nat Med* 11:861–866, 2005.
26. Narang N, Armstead SI, Stream A, et al: Assessment of cardiac structure and function in patients without and with peripheral oedema during rosiglitazone treatment, *Diab Vasc Dis Res* 8:101–108, 2011.

27. Gerstein HC, Miller ME, Byington RP, et al: Effects of intensive glucose lowering in type 2 diabetes, *N Engl J Med* 358:2545–2559, 2008.

28. Frye RL, August P, Brooks MM, et al: A randomized trial of therapies for type 2 diabetes and coronary artery disease, *N Engl J Med* 360:2503–2515, 2009.

29. Pfeffer MA, Burdmann EA, Chen CY, et al: A trial of darbepoetin alfa in type 2 diabetes and chronic kidney disease, *N Engl J Med* 361:2019–2032, 2009.

30. Go AS, Mozaffarian D, Roger VL, et al: Heart disease and stroke statistics–2013 update: a report from the American Heart Association, *Circulation* 127:e6–e245, 2013.

31. Thrainsdottir IS, Aspelund T, Thorgeirsson G, et al: The association between glucose abnormalities and heart failure in the population-based Reykjavik study, *Diabetes Care* 28:612–616, 2005.

32. Nichols GA, Hillier TA, Erbey JR, et al: Congestive heart failure in type 2 diabetes: prevalence, incidence, and risk factors, *Diabetes Care* 24:1614–1619, 2001.

33. Boonman-de Winter LJ, Rutten FH, Cramer MJ, et al: High prevalence of previously unknown heart failure and left ventricular dysfunction in patients with type 2 diabetes, *Diabetologia* 2012.

34. Wang TJ, Levy D, Benjamin EJ, et al: The epidemiology of "asymptomatic" left ventricular systolic dysfunction: implications for screening, *Ann Intern Med* 138:907–916, 2003.

35. Wang TJ, Evans JC, Benjamin EJ, et al: Natural history of asymptomatic left ventricular systolic dysfunction in the community, *Circulation* 108:977–982, 2003.

36. Devereux RB, Bella JN, Palmieri V, et al: Left ventricular systolic dysfunction in a biracial sample of hypertensive adults: the Hypertension Genetic Epidemiology Network (HyperGEN) Study, *Hypertension* 38:417–423, 2001.

37. Devereux RB, Roman MJ, Paranicas M, et al: Impact of diabetes on cardiac structure and function: the strong heart study, *Circulation* 101:2271–2276, 2000.

38. Galderisi M: Diastolic dysfunction and diabetic cardiomyopathy: evaluation by Doppler echocardiography, *J Am Coll Cardiol* 48:1548–1551, 2006.

39. Palmieri V, Bella JN, Arnett DK, et al: Effect of type 2 diabetes mellitus on left ventricular geometry and systolic function in hypertensive subjects: Hypertension Genetic Epidemiology Network (HyperGEN) study, *Circulation* 103:102–107, 2001.

40. Rutter MK, Parise H, Benjamin EJ, et al: Impact of glucose intolerance and insulin resistance on cardiac structure and function: sex-related differences in the Framingham Heart Study, *Circulation* 107:448–454, 2003.

41. From AM, Scott CG, Chen HH: The development of heart failure in patients with diabetes mellitus and pre-clinical diastolic dysfunction a population-based study, *J Am Coll Cardiol* 55:300–305, 2010.

42. MacDonald MR, Petrie MC, Hawkins NM, et al: Diabetes, left ventricular systolic dysfunction, and chronic heart failure, *Eur Heart J* 29:1224–1240, 2008.

43. Martinez-Selles M, Doughty RN, Poppe K, et al: Gender and survival in patients with heart failure: interactions with diabetes and aetiology. Results from the MAGGIC individual patient meta-analysis, *Eur J Heart Fail* 14:473–479, 2012.

44. From AM, Leibson CL, Bursi F, et al: Diabetes in heart failure: prevalence and impact on outcome in the population, *Am J Med* 119:591–599, 2006.

45. Adams KF Jr, Fonarow GC, Emerman CL, et al: Characteristics and outcomes of patients hospitalized for heart failure in the United States: rationale, design, and preliminary observations from the first 100,000 cases in the Acute Decompensated Heart Failure National Registry (ADHERE), *Am Heart J* 149:209–216, 2005.

46. Klapholz M, Maurer M, Lowe AM, et al: Hospitalization for heart failure in the presence of a normal left ventricular ejection fraction: results of the New York Heart Failure Registry, *J Am Coll Cardiol* 43:1432–1438, 2004.

47. Owan TE, Hodge DO, Herges RM, et al: Trends in prevalence and outcome of heart failure with preserved ejection fraction, *N Engl J Med* 355:251–259, 2006.

48. Aguilar D, Solomon SD, Kober L, et al: Newly diagnosed and previously known diabetes mellitus and 1-year outcomes of acute myocardial infarction: the VALsartan In Acute myocardial iNfarcTion (VALIANT) trial, *Circulation* 110:1572–1578, 2004.

49. Domanski M, Krause-Steinrauf H, Deedwania P, et al: The effect of diabetes on outcomes of patients with advanced heart failure in the BEST trial, *J Am Coll Cardiol* 42:914–922, 2003.

50. MacDonald MR, Petrie MC, Varyani F, et al: Impact of diabetes on outcomes in patients with low and preserved ejection fraction heart failure: an analysis of the Candesartan in Heart failure: Assessment of Reduction in Mortality and morbidity (CHARM) programme, *Eur Heart J* 29:1377–1385, 2008.

51. Martin DT, McNitt S, Nesto RW, et al: Cardiac resynchronization therapy reduces the risk of cardiac events in patients with diabetes enrolled in the multicenter automatic defibrillator implantation trial with cardiac resynchronization therapy (MADIT-CRT), *Circ Heart Fail* 4:332–338, 2011.

52. Murcia AM, Hennekens CH, Lamas GA, et al: Impact of diabetes on mortality in patients with myocardial infarction and left ventricular dysfunction, *Arch Intern Med* 164:2273–2279, 2004.

53. Shindler DM, Kostis JB, Yusuf S, et al: Diabetes mellitus, a predictor of morbidity and mortality in the Studies of Left Ventricular Dysfunction (SOLVD) Trials and Registry, *Am J Cardiol* 77:1017–1020, 1996.

54. Egstrup M, Schou M, Gustafsson I, et al: Oral glucose tolerance testing in an outpatient heart failure clinic reveals a high proportion of undiagnosed diabetic patients with an adverse prognosis, *Eur J Heart Fail* 13:319–326, 2011.

55. Preiss D, Zetterstrand S, McMurray JJ, et al: Predictors of development of diabetes in patients with chronic heart failure in the Candesartan in Heart Failure Assessment of Reduction in Mortality and Morbidity (CHARM) program, *Diabetes Care* 32:915–920, 2009.

56. Preiss D, van Veldhuisen DJ, Sattar N, et al: Eplerenone and new-onset diabetes in patients with mild heart failure: results from the Eplerenone in Mild Patients Hospitalization and Survival Study in Heart Failure (EMPHASIS-HF), *Eur J Heart Fail* 14:909–915, 2012.

57. Centers for Disease Control and Prevention. Diabetes Data and Trends. (Accessed April 5, 2012, at www.cdc.gov/diabetes/statistics/incidence/fig3.htm.).

58. Torp-Pedersen C, Metra M, Charlesworth A, et al: Effects of metoprolol and carvedilol on pre-existing and new onset diabetes in patients with chronic heart failure: data from the Carvedilol Or Metoprolol European Trial (COMET), *Heart* 93:968–973, 2007.

59. Tenenbaum A, Motro M, Fisman EZ, et al: Functional class in patients with heart failure is associated with the development of diabetes, *Am J Med* 114:271–275, 2003.

60. Ashrafian H, Frenneaux MP, Opie LH: Metabolic mechanisms in heart failure, *Circulation* 116:434–448, 2007.

61. Shimizu I, Yoshida Y, Katsuno T, et al: p53-induced adipose tissue inflammation is critically involved in the development of insulin resistance in heart failure, *Cell Metab* 15:51–64, 2012.

62. Nasir S, Aguilar D: Congestive heart failure and diabetes mellitus: balancing glycemic control with heart failure improvement, *Am J Cardiol* 110:50B–57B, 2012.

63. Sarma S, Mentz RJ, Kwasny MJ, et al: Association between diabetes mellitus and post-discharge outcomes in patients hospitalized with heart failure: findings from the EVEREST trial, *Eur J Heart Fail* 15:194–202, 2013.

64. Shah AM, Uno H, Kober L, et al: The inter-relationship of diabetes and left ventricular systolic function on outcome after high-risk myocardial infarction, *Eur J Heart Fail* 12:1229–1237, 2010.

65. Shah AM, Shin SH, Takeuchi M, et al: Left ventricular systolic and diastolic function, remodelling, and clinical outcomes among patients with diabetes following myocardial infarction and the influence of direct renin inhibition with aliskiren, *Eur J Heart Fail* 14:185–192, 2012.

66. Solomon SD, St John Sutton M, Lamas GA, et al: Ventricular remodeling does not accompany the development of heart failure in diabetic patients after myocardial infarction, *Circulation* 106:1251–1255, 2002.

67. Kapoor JR, Fonarow GC, Zhao X, et al: Diabetes, quality of care, and in-hospital outcomes in patients hospitalized with heart failure, *Am Heart J* 162:480–486 e3, 2011.

68. McEwen LN, Karter AJ, Waitzfelder BE, et al: Predictors of mortality over 8 years in type 2 diabetic patients: Translating Research Into Action for Diabetes (TRIAD), *Diabetes Care* 35:1301–1309, 2012.

69. Cubbon RM, Adams B, Rajwani A, et al: Diabetes mellitus is associated with adverse prognosis in chronic heart failure of ischaemic and non-ischaemic aetiology, *Diab Vasc Dis Res* 10(4):330–336, 2013 Jul.

70. Mosterd A, Cost B, Hoes AW, et al: The prognosis of heart failure in the general population: The Rotterdam Study, *Eur Heart J* 22:1318–1327, 2001.

71. Ho KK, Anderson KM, Kannel WB, et al: Survival after the onset of congestive heart failure in Framingham Heart Study subjects, *Circulation* 88:107–115, 1993.

72. Pocock SJ, Wang D, Pfeffer MA, et al: Predictors of mortality and morbidity in patients with chronic heart failure, *Eur Heart J* 27:65–75, 2006.

73. Dries DL, Sweitzer NK, Drazner MH, et al: Prognostic impact of diabetes mellitus in patients with heart failure according to the etiology of left ventricular systolic dysfunction, *J Am Coll Cardiol* 38:421–428, 2001.

74. Gustafsson I, Brendorp B, Seibaek M, et al: Influence of diabetes and diabetes-gender interaction on the risk of death in patients hospitalized with congestive heart failure, *J Am Coll Cardiol* 43:771–777, 2004.

75. Komajda M, Carson PE, Hetzel S, et al: Factors associated with outcome in heart failure with preserved ejection fraction: findings from the Irbesartan in Heart Failure with Preserved Ejection Fraction Study (I-PRESERVE), *Circ Heart Fail* 4:27–35, 2011.

76. Smooke S, Horwich TB, Fonarow GC: Insulin-treated diabetes is associated with a marked increase in mortality in patients with advanced heart failure, *Am Heart J* 149:168–174, 2005.

77. Aguilar D, Bozkurt B, Ramasubbu K, et al: Relationship of hemoglobin A1C and mortality in heart failure patients with diabetes, *J Am Coll Cardiol* 54:422–428, 2009.

78. Eshaghian S, Horwich TB, Fonarow GC: An unexpected inverse relationship between HbA1c levels and mortality in patients with diabetes and advanced systolic heart failure, *Am Heart J* 151:91, 2006.

79. Tomova GS, Nimbal V, Horwich TB: Relation between hemoglobin A(1c) and outcomes in heart failure patients with and without diabetes mellitus, *Am J Cardiol* 2012.

80. Gerstein HC, Swedberg K, Carlsson J, et al: The hemoglobin A1c level as a progressive risk factor for cardiovascular death, hospitalization for heart failure, or death in patients with chronic heart failure: an analysis of the Candesartan in Heart Failure: Assessment of Reduction in Mortality and Morbidity (CHARM) program, *Arch Intern Med* 168:1699–1704, 2008.

81. Henry RM, Kamp O, Kostense PJ, et al: Left ventricular mass increases with deteriorating glucose tolerance, especially in women: independence of increased arterial stiffness or decreased flow-mediated dilation: the Hoorn study, *Diabetes Care* 27:522–529, 2004.

82. Bertoni AG, Goff DC Jr, D'Agostino RB Jr, et al: Diabetic cardiomyopathy and subclinical cardiovascular disease: the Multi-Ethnic Study of Atherosclerosis (MESA), *Diabetes Care* 29:588–594, 2006.

83. Lee M, Gardin JM, Lynch JC, et al: Diabetes mellitus and echocardiographic left ventricular function in free-living elderly men and women: The Cardiovascular Health Study, *Am Heart J* 133:36–43, 1997.

84. Lee DS, Gona P, Vasan RS, et al: Relation of disease pathogenesis and risk factors to heart failure with preserved or reduced ejection fraction: insights from the Framingham Heart Study of the National Heart, Lung, and Blood Institute, *Circulation* 119:3070–3077, 2009.

24 Diabetic Cardiomyopathy
Mediators and Mechanisms

Pavan K. Battiprolu, Zhao V. Wang, and Joseph A. Hill

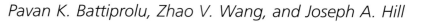

SCOPE OF THE PROBLEM

Heart disease is the greatest noninfectious health hazard ever to confront the human race. Rampant for some years in the developed world, this epidemic is spreading rapidly around the globe. As one prominent example, it is estimated that 5 million Americans have heart failure (HF), a syndrome with a 5-year mortality of approximately 50%.[1] Indeed, HF has remained the leading cause of death in industrialized nations for several years. Accordingly, HF, the end result of disease-related remodeling of the myocardium, is responsible for a huge societal burden of morbidity, mortality, and cost.

Numerous events contribute to the rise in HF, but the increasing prevalence of diabetes is a significant contributor. For one, cardiovascular disease, including HF, is the leading cause of morbidity and mortality in patients with diabetes (see also **Chapter 23**). Although the underlying causes of diabetes-associated heart disease are multifactorial, the importance of ventricular dysfunction independent of coronary artery disease (CAD) or hypertension, a condition termed *diabetic cardiomyopathy*, has been emphasized.[2–4] The diabetes and cardiovascular communities embraced the concept of diabetic cardiomyopathy as a distinct entity in the early 1970s when autopsy specimens from diabetic patients with nephropathy revealed a myopathic process in the absence of epicardial CAD.[5] Over the years, substantial evidence has accumulated that a specific, discrete diabetic cardiomyopathy, distinct from ischemic injury, does indeed exist. The exact prevalence, nature, and cause of cardiac dysfunction directly attributable to diabetes per se have given rise to considerable debate, inasmuch as the disease is associated with numerous comorbidities, including hypertension, coronary atherosclerosis, and microvascular dysfunction.

Constant and unremitting metabolic stress on the heart leads over time to progressive deterioration of myocardial structure and function. This suggests that therapeutic interventions early in the disease, targeting specific metabolic and structural derangements, may be required. This is especially relevant because rigid control of hyperglycemia, however central to treatment, has not fulfilled hopes of meaningful morbidity and mortality benefit.[6] Recent and ongoing research into mechanisms of metabolic control, insulin resistance, and diabetes-associated derangements portend novel therapies designed to benefit the rapidly expanding cohort of patients with diabetes, a benefit with tremendous societal impact. Current therapies are insufficient to arrest the progression of HF. Developing new therapies will require greater understanding of molecular events underlying pathologic cardiac remodeling. Substantial work will be required to elucidate the role(s) of specific molecular mechanisms in the pathogenesis of diabetes-induced remodeling. It is our hope that insights gleaned from such studies will lead to identification of therapeutic targets with clinical relevance.

EPIDEMIOLOGICAL EVIDENCE

The incidence and prevalence of diabetes mellitus (DM) are both rising rapidly (see also **Chapter 1**).[7] DM affects 350 million people around the world, and the World Health Organization (WHO) has projected that diabetes-related deaths will double between 2005 and 2030 (www.who.int/diabetes/en/). Within this burgeoning health care problem of worldwide proportions, obesity-related type 2 diabetes mellitus (T2DM) accounts for more than 90% of all diagnosed diabetes in adults.[8] Furthermore, more than 60% of patients who present with symptomatic chronic heart disease have abnormal glucose homeostasis (see also **Chapter 23**).[9–11] Patients with DM and established cardiovascular disease have an unfavorable prognosis. In fact, diabetes and insulin resistance are powerful predictors of cardiovascular morbidity and mortality, and each is an independent risk factor for death in patients with established HF.[12]

The term *diabetic cardiomyopathy*, although admittedly vague, refers to the multifactorial manifestations of diabetes-related left ventricular (LV) failure characterized by both systolic and diastolic function (**Box 24-1**).[13] The Framingham Heart Study showed that men with diabetes

BOX 24-1 Diabetic Cardiomyopathy: Hallmark Features

Structural and Morphologic
Near-normal end-diastolic volume
Elevated left ventricular mass relative to chamber volume
Elevated wall thickness to chamber radius
Myocardial hypertrophy
Myocardial fibrosis
Intramyocyte lipid accumulation

Functional
Abnormal left ventricular diastolic function (observed in 75% of asymptomatic diabetic patients)[146]
Compromised left ventricular systolic function
Reduced ventricular elasticity
Clinical heart failure

Data from Boudina S, Abel ED: Diabetic cardiomyopathy revisited, *Circulation* 115:3213-3223, 2007.

are twice as likely to develop HF as their nondiabetic counterparts, and women with diabetes have a fivefold increase in the rate of HF. The clinical spectrum of HF ranges from asymptomatic to overt symptoms at rest. Diabetes complicated by hypertension represents a particularly high-risk group for the development of HF.[14] Diastolic dysfunction is common (>50% prevalence in some studies) and can sometimes be linked to diabetes in the absence of concomitant hypertension.

Echocardiographic studies confirm that diastolic abnormalities occur in young diabetic patients who have no known diabetic complications.[15] One study reported that patients with diabetes manifest early findings of systolic dysfunction preceding echocardiographically detectable changes in LV ejection fraction.[15] Patients with diabetes who are also hypertensive have increased LV mass when compared with their nondiabetic counterparts, and LV function may in fact be hyperdynamic.[15]

PATHOPHYSIOLOGY AND MOLECULAR MECHANISMS

A number of molecular mechanisms have been proposed to contribute to the pathogenesis of diabetic cardiomyopathy.[16–20] However, evidence for a direct, causal link between insulin resistance, a hallmark of type 2 diabetes,

and ventricular dysfunction has not been established. The natural history of diabetic cardiomyopathy has been broadly divided into two phases (**Table 24-1**).[19] Although the first phase represents short-term, physiologic adaptation to the metabolic alterations of diabetes, the second phase involves degenerative changes that the myocardium is unable to repair and that ultimately culminate in irreversible pathologic remodeling.

The hormone insulin is central to the control of intermediary metabolism, orchestrating substrate usage for storage or oxidation in all cells.[21] As a result, insulin has profound effects on both carbohydrate and lipid metabolism throughout the body, as well as significant influences on protein metabolism. Consequently, derangements in insulin signaling have widespread and devastating effects in numerous tissues, including the cardiovascular system. Insulin is the main hormone for regulation of blood glucose, and, in general, normoglycemia is maintained by precisely tuned insulin secretion. It is important to note that the normal pancreatic beta cell can adapt to changes in requirements for circulating insulin; when the downstream actions of insulin are hampered (e.g., in insulin resistance), the pancreas compensates by upregulating beta cell function (hyperinsulinemia). Relative insulin resistance occurs when the biologic actions of insulin are inadequate for both glucose disposal in peripheral tissues and suppression of hepatic glucose production.[22]

T2DM is typified by hyperglycemia, hyperinsulinemia, and obesity, and insulin resistance is a cardinal feature.[2] The disease itself arises from a variety of causes,[24] including dysregulated glucose sensing or insulin secretion (maturity-onset diabetes of the young), autoimmune-mediated beta cell destruction (type 1 diabetes mellitus [T1DM]), or insufficient compensatory insulin secretion in the setting of peripheral insulin resistance or T2DM, which accounts for 90% of diabetes. These events, acting through a variety of mediators such as altered intracellular calcium, increased reactive oxygen species (ROS), ceramides, hexosamines, and advanced glycation end products (AGEs), contribute to the pathogenesis of the disorder.[3] In addition, the interplay between dysregulated function of endothelial cells and fibroblasts contributes, highlighting the multifactorial etiology of diabetic cardiomyopathy. Recent studies have highlighted that transcriptional and metabolic derangements within the

TABLE 24-1 Natural History of Diabetic Cardiomyopathy

PHASE		MOLECULAR AND CELLULAR EVENTS	ALTERATIONS IN STRUCTURE AND MORPHOLOGY	MYOCARDIAL PERFORMANCE
I	Early	Metabolic disturbances: hyperglycemia, increased circulating free fatty acids, insulin resistance Altered Ca^{2+} homeostasis Endothelial dysfunction	Normal left ventricular dimensions, wall thickness, and mass	Impaired diastolic compliance with normal systolic function, or no obvious functional changes
	Middle	Cardiomyocyte injury, apoptosis, necrosis Activation of cardiac fibroblasts leading to myocardial fibrosis	Minor changes in structure: slightly increased heart mass, wall thickness, and/or ventricular dimensions Cardiomyocyte hypertrophy Insignificant myocardial vascular changes	Significant changes in diastolic and systolic function
II	Late	Hypertension Coronary artery disease Microangiopathy Cardiac autonomic neuropathy	Significant changes in structure: increased heart size, wall thickness, and mass Myocardial microvascular disease	Abnormal diastolic and systolic function

Data from Fang ZY, Prins JB, Marwick TH: Diabetic cardiomyopathy: evidence, mechanisms, and therapeutic implications, *Endocr Rev* 25:543-567, 2004.

cardiomyocyte itself are important elements in the pathogenesis of the disorder, as well.[25]

The concept of diabetic cardiomyopathy is based on the notion that the disease, DM, itself is a key factor eliciting changes at the molecular and cellular levels of the myocyte, culminating in structural and functional abnormalities in the heart. In other words, the diabetic milieu is toxic to the myocyte, above and beyond contributions from ischemia (CAD) or pressure stress (hypertension). Whereas the cause of diabetic cardiomyopathy is multifactorial and incompletely characterized, progress has been made in recent years to define underlying mechanisms (**Fig. 24-1**).[5] As a result, several novel molecular targets with potential therapeutic relevance have been proposed (**Fig. 24-2**).

Cardiomyocytes are capable of metabolizing a spectrum of substrates. The myocardium as a "metabolic omnivore" normally relies on metabolism of fatty acids (FAs) and glucose, and to a lesser extent lactate and ketone bodies, to produce adenosine triphosphate (ATP).[26] These substrates, however, are unable to enter the cardiomyocyte by simple diffusion and must be taken up by facilitated transport. FA uptake is mediated by FAT (fatty acid translocase; also known as cluster of differentiation 36 [CD36]), and

glucose intake is accomplished by both GLUT-1 and GLUT-4 (glucose transporter types 1 and 4). In response to availability of nutrients or increased cardiac work, plasma insulin concentrations rise.[27] This, in turn, provokes translocation of both GLUT-4 and FAT to the myocyte sarcolemma. To date, several studies have implicated signaling pathways that regulate GLUT-4 translocation with those involved in transport of FAT to the sarcolemma.[27,28] However, during the development of insulin resistance and T2DM, FAT becomes preferentially sarcolemma-localized, whereas GLUT-4 remains internalized. This reciprocal positioning of GLUT-4 and FAT is central to aberrant substrate uptake in the diabetic heart, where FA metabolism is chronically increased at the expense of glucose.[27,28] Moreover, dyslipidemia triggered by insulin resistance provokes increases in systemic free FAs, which in turn promote uptake and usage of fat in cardiomyocytes. In addition, the interplay of preferential substrate usage is affected by a variety of other mediators, as previously reviewed.[3]

Hyperglycemia and Glucotoxicity

Hyperglycemia, a consequence of combined decreased glucose clearance plus augmented hepatic gluconeogenesis, plays a central role in the pathogenesis of diabetic cardiomyopathy. In patients with T2DM, endogenous glucose production is accelerated.[29] Because this increase occurs in the presence of hyperinsulinemia, at least in the early and intermediate stages of disease, hepatic insulin resistance is a driving force of hyperglycemia.

Chronic hyperglycemia promotes glucotoxicity, which contributes to cardiac injury through multiple mechanisms, including direct and indirect effects of glucose on cardiomyocytes, cardiac fibroblasts, and endothelial cells. Chronic hyperglycemia promotes the overproduction of ROS through the electron transport chain, which can induce apoptosis[30] and activate poly (adenosine diphosphate-ribose) polymerase 1 (PARP). This enzyme mediates the direct ribosylation and inhibition of glyceraldehyde phosphate dehydrogenase (GAPDH), diverting glucose from the glycolytic pathway toward alternative biochemical cascades that participate in hyperglycemia-induced cellular injury. These include increases in AGEs and the activation of the hexosamine

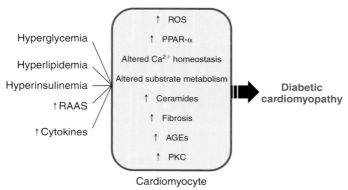

FIGURE 24-1 The cause of diabetic cardiomyopathy is multifactorial. An overview of triggers, mediators, and consequences involved in the pathogenesis of diabetic cardiomyopathy. AGEs = Advanced glycation end products; PKC = protein kinase C; PPAR-α = peroxisome proliferator-activated receptor alpha; RAAS = renin-angiotensin-aldosterone system. (*Modified from Rubler S, Dlugash J, Yuceoglu YZ, et al: New type of cardiomyopathy associated with diabetic glomerulosclerosis, Am J Cardiol 1972;30:595-602, 1972.*)

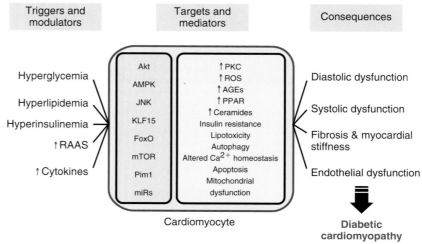

FIGURE 24-2 New molecular targets and their role in diabetic cardiomyopathy. An overview of triggers, mediators and consequences involved in the pathogenesis of diabetic cardiomyopathy. AGEs = Advanced glycation end products; FoxO = forkhead box O protein; KLF = Krüppel-like factor; mTOR = mammalian target of rapamycin; PKC = protein kinase C; PPAR = peroxisome proliferator-activated receptor; RAAS = renin-angiotensin-aldosterone system.

biosynthetic pathway, the polyol pathway, and protein kinase C.[30,31] Hyperglycemia-induced apoptosis is stimulated by ROS,[32] PARP,[33] AGEs,[34] and aldose reductase.[35] Hyperglycemia also contributes to altered cardiac structure and function through post-translational modification of extracellular matrix components (e.g., collagens) and altered expression and function of both the ryanodine receptor (RyR) and sarco(endo)plasmic reticulum Ca^{2+}-ATPase (SERCA), which in aggregate contribute to decreased systolic and diastolic function.[30]

Hyperlipidemia and Lipotoxicity

Enhanced lipid synthesis in hepatocytes and increased lipolysis in adipocytes together lead to increases in circulating FAs and triglycerides (TGs) in patients with diabetes. Also, insulin stimulates FA transport into cardiomyocytes.[36] Thus the combination of elevated circulating lipids plus hyperinsulinemia increases FA delivery to cardiac cells, which rapidly adapt by promoting FA use. However, if FA delivery overtakes the oxidative capacity of the cell, FAs accumulate intracellularly, promoting lipotoxicity.[37]

Several major mechanisms contribute to cardiac lipotoxicity.
· *ROS generation.* High rates of FA oxidation increase mitochondrial membrane potential, leading to the production of ROS, which under normal physiologic conditions are removed by molecular antioxidants and antioxidant enzymes. However, cardiomyocyte damage and death by apoptosis ensue if the generation of ROS exceeds their degradation, leading to ROS accumulation (oxidative stress).[38]
· *Ceramide production.* Accumulation of intracellular lipids can contribute directly to cell death under conditions in which FAs are not metabolized.[39] Reaction of palmitoyl CoenzymeA (CoA) with serine leads to the generation of ceramide, a sphingolipid that can trigger apoptosis through inhibition of the mitochondrial respiratory chain.[40]
· *Insulin resistance.* Diacylglycerol, ceramide, and fatty acyl-CoA can each activate a negative regulatory signaling pathway involving the atypical protein kinase C-θ and IκB kinase (IKK). Both kinases, in turn, stimulate serine phosphorylation of the insulin receptor substrate (IRS), impairing insulin signaling.[41]
· *Impaired contractility.* Intracellular FA accumulation can trigger opening of the K-ATP channel, leading to action potential shortening. This in turn diminishes the duty cycle of the L-type Ca^{2+} channel, leading to reduced sarcoplasmic reticular Ca^{2+} stores and depressed contractility.[42]

Thus, high FA uptake and metabolism not only stimulate accumulation of FA intermediates but also increase oxygen demand, provoke mitochondrial uncoupling and ROS generation, decrease ATP synthesis, induce mitochondrial dysfunction, and trigger apoptosis. Together, these events participate importantly in the pathogenesis of diabetic cardiomyopathy.

Hyperinsulinemia, Insulin Resistance, and Altered Substrate Metabolism

Early clinical studies reported an association between systemic hyperinsulinemia and development of cardiac hypertrophy.[43,44] Potential mechanisms include crosstalk between insulin-dependent signaling and pro-growth pathways in the heart. For example, the signaling cascade activated by insulin shares common elements with the

neurohormonal growth agonists insulin-like growth factor 1 (IGF-1) and angiotensin II (Ang II).[45] These pathways, in turn, activate both the ERK and phosphoinositide 3-kinase, Protein Kinase B, mammalian target of rapamycin (PI3K/PKB/Akt/mTOR) cascades, each of which is involved in regulating cell growth and protein synthesis. Activation of the PI3K/PKB/Akt/mTOR) pathway is associated with development of physiologic hypertrophy, whereas ERK signaling, along with the Protein Kinase C, PKC; Nuclear factor of activated T-cells, NFAT (PKC and calcineurin/NFAT) pathways, triggers pathologic hypertrophy.[45] Also, activation of the sympathetic nervous system (SNS) and the renin-angiotensin aldosterone system (RAAS) have each been reported in diabetes, leading to enhanced stimulation of both adrenergic and angiotensin receptor 1 (AT1).[19,46] Chronic hyperinsulinemia may augment myocardial Akt-1 indirectly through increased SNS activation[47] or by triggering the Ang II pathway.[48]

In the normal heart, approximately two thirds of the energy required for cardiac contractility derives from FA oxidation, with the remainder deriving from glucose and lactate metabolism. By contrast, in conditions of insulin resistance or diabetes, myocardial glucose use is significantly reduced, and a greater proportion of substrate usage shifts to beta-oxidation of FA.[49] Associated with the reduction in glucose use by diabetic myocardium is depletion of the glucose transporter proteins GLUT-1 and GLUT-4. Indeed, altered myocardial substrate metabolism favoring FAs over glucose as an energy source has been identified as a metabolic target of relevance. The diabetic heart relies on FA oxidation and is unable to switch to glucose, despite its lower oxygen consumption requirement. As a consequence, cardiac efficiency, the ratio of cardiac work to myocardial oxygen consumption, decreases; decreased cardiac efficiency has been reported in humans and experimental animals with diabetes (**Fig. 24-3**).[16–18,20]

Insulin resistance is defined as diminished insulin-dependent stimulation of muscle glucose uptake.[16–18,20] Underlying mechanisms include accumulation of FAs, which impairs insulin-mediated glucose uptake through inhibition of IRS and Akt. The serine protein kinases PKC-θ and IκB kinase (IKK), which elicit serine phosphorylation of IRS, are activated.[50] Phosphorylation and activation of PI3K and Akt are reduced, with significant consequences on the metabolic effects of insulin in the heart.[51]

Abnormalities in Intracellular Ca^{2+} Homeostasis

Precise control of intracellular Ca^{2+} homeostasis is central to the regulation of myocardial function and growth.[52] During each heartbeat, Ca^{2+} enters the cardiomyocyte through L-type channels. The resulting increase in intracellular Ca^{2+} triggers further Ca^{2+} release from the sarcoplasmic/endoplasmic reticulum (SR) through the RyR, raising Ca^{2+} levels around the sarcomere. Binding of Ca^{2+} to troponin C in the contractile apparatus, in turn, initiates actin-myosin cross-bridging and myocardial contraction. Ca^{2+} reuptake into the SR by sarco/endoplasmic reticulum Ca^{2+}-ATPase (SERCA) and consequent declines in cytoplasmic Ca^{2+} allow for muscle relaxation.[52] Oxidative stress, accumulation of long-chain acetylcarnitines, and abnormal membrane lipid content also contribute to abnormalities of Ca^{2+} handling in diabetic cardiomyopathy.[18] Alterations in the function or expression of

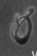

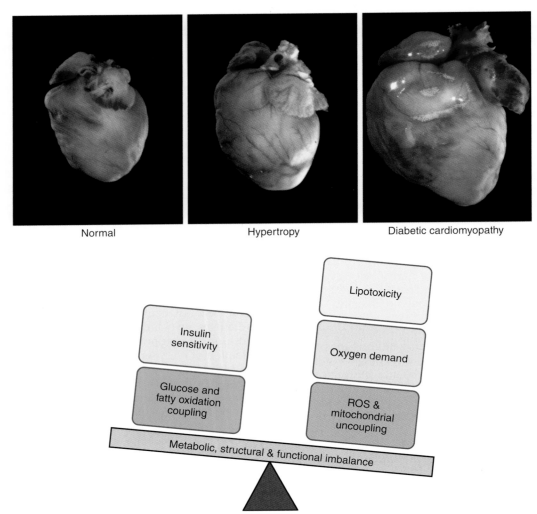

FIGURE 24-3 **Metabolic events participating in diabetic cardiomyopathy.** *Top,* Gross morphology of fixed mouse hearts collected over the course of exposure to high-fat diet. *Bottom,* Schematic depiction of key factors involved in metabolic, structural, and functional remodeling in diabetic cardiomyopathy.

SERCA, Na-K-ATPase (sodium-potassium adenosine triphosphatase), Na^+/Ca^{2+} exchanger, and RyR have each been observed in animal models of diabetes,[52–55] and cardiac overexpression of SERCA improves Ca^{2+} homeostasis and contraction in diabetic mice.[57]

Mitochondrial Dysfunction and Oxidative Stress

Mitochondrial dysfunction contributes to progression of diabetes and diabetic cardiomyopathy.[58] However, mechanisms whereby mitochondrial dysfunction contributes to diabetic cardiomyopathy are poorly understood. For one, hyperglycemia-induced mitochondrial ROS generation has been implicated.[16–18,20] Mitochondrial oxidative metabolism is the major source of ATP production in the heart. Acetyl-CoA generated from either FA oxidation or glycolysis is metabolized in the tricarboxylic acid cycle to produce nicotinamide adenine dinucleotide-reduced (NADH) and flavin adenine dinucleotide-reduced (FADH2). These electron carriers transfer electrons to the mitochondrial electron transport chain, where ATP and ROS are generated. Increased ROS generation in the setting of high FA oxidation induces pathologic accumulation of ROS and consequent oxidative stress

and cell damage.[16–18,20] Furthermore, it has been reported that p53 contributes to cardiac dysfunction in diabetes by promoting mitochondrial oxygen consumption, ROS production, and lipid accumulation.[59] The *SCO2* (synthesis of cytochrome c oxidase 2) gene is a transcriptional target of p53, and this protein plays a key role in the assembly of mitochondrial respiration complex IV. Nakamura and colleagues reported a marked increase in cardiac SCO2 expression in diabetic mice that contributed to increases in mitochondrial respiration rate.[59] This elevated mitochondrial activity triggers enhanced lipid uptake that exceeds mitochondrial oxidation capacity, leading to lipid accumulation and increased mitochondrial ROS production, together culminating in cardiac dysfunction. Reports from some studies also suggest that hyperglycemia promotes production of Rac1-mediated increases in nicotinamide adenine dinucleotide phosphate-reduced (NADPH) in addition to mitochondria-derived ROS,[60] each promoting accelerated apoptosis. The activation of NADPH oxidase by Rac1 can induce myocardial remodeling and dysfunction in diabetic mice,[61] suggesting that these two molecules are relevant therapeutic targets. Inhibition of ROS by overexpression of antioxidant enzymes protects against mitochondrial dysfunction and cardiomyopathy.[13]

Dysregulation of Renin-Angiotensin System

Involvement of the RAAS in the pathogenesis of diabetes-associated HF is increasingly recognized. For example, Ang II has diverse and widespread actions that affect cardiac function.[62] Ang II also exerts actions on other insulin-sensitive tissues, such as liver, skeletal muscle, and adipose tissue, where it has effects on the insulin receptor (IR), IRS proteins, and the downstream effectors PI3K, Akt, and GLUT-4.[63] Underlying molecular mechanisms have not been elucidated definitively, but phosphorylation of both the IR and IRS-1 proteins contributing to desensitization of insulin action is well established.[63] Ang II also has direct effects on cardiomyocytes and cardiac fibroblasts through AT1 receptors, promoting cardiac hypertrophy and fibrosis.[64] Up-regulation of the RAAS has also been described in diabetes and is associated with development of cardiac hypertrophy and fibrosis.[65,66] Furthermore, cardiac dysfunction in diabetes can be mitigated by pharmacologic inhibition of the RAAS.[46] In addition, cardiomyocytes and endothelial cells in the hearts of individuals with diabetes and end-stage HF manifest evidence of oxidative stress, apoptosis, and necrosis that correlate with RAAS activation.[67,68]

Emerging Modulators of Insulin Signaling and Cardiac Function

Adipokines

Historically, adipose tissue has been viewed largely as a repository for surplus lipids, available for mobilization and use in times of metabolic need. It is now recognized that adipocytes synthesize and secrete a number of cytokines (adipokines) that play significant roles in type 2 diabetes and insulin resistance and interact with most organs in the body. Studies to date have focused on the effects of adipokines in promoting or retarding progression from metabolic syndrome to overt T2DM. However, the effects of long-term exposure to circulating adipokines in diabetes warrant further exploration.

Leptin

The hormone leptin is largely involved in regulating food intake, via actions in the central nervous system and peripheral tissues. However, despite extensive investigation into the role of leptin in diabetic cardiomyopathy, controversy persists.[69] For one, leptin has been thought to exert largely detrimental effects on the heart, including negative inotropy (mediated by endogenously produced nitric oxide), prohypertrophy (via an autocrine response to endothelin-1 and Ang II stimulation), and decreased cardiac efficiency (mediated by increased FA oxidation and TG hydrolysis).[18] Now, emerging evidence suggests that leptin protects the heart from lipotoxicity and the relatively hypoxic milieu associated with diabetic cardiomyopathy. Administration of exogenous leptin reverses both LV dysfunction and hypertrophy and is associated with improved mortality in leptin-deficient–ob/ob mice after 4 weeks of coronary ligation.[70] Although elevated plasma leptin levels are generally predictors of poor outcome in patients with CAD and HF, leptin may protect against ischemia/reperfusion injury, possibly via ERK1/2 and PI3K-dependent mechanisms.[71] A possible explanation for these apparent contradictions is the complex interplay between the effects of provoking a central, sympathetic response and the peripheral actions of leptin. Unraveling these multifactorial actions will require both cardiac-specific inactivation of leptin receptors and elucidation of the central nervous system effects of leptin.

Adiponectin

Adiponectin is an adipose tissue–derived hormone that circulates at high levels (5 to 10 µg/mL). In both humans and rodents, plasma adiponectin levels correlate positively with insulin sensitivity and inversely with hypertension, hyperlipidemia, and insulin resistance.[72] Adiponectin stimulates beta-oxidation in muscle and suppresses glucose production in liver, which together antagonize the metabolic syndrome and maintain whole body energy homeostasis.[73] Depressed levels of circulating adiponectin have been shown to correlate with elevated risk of myocardial infarction, CAD, and HF.[74] Recently, mechanisms underlying the actions of adiponectin on the cardiovascular system have been uncovered. Shibata and colleagues reported that adiponectin elicits antihypertrophic effects during cardiac remodeling; adiponectin-deficient animals manifest an amplified hypertrophic growth response to surgical thoracic aortic constriction (TAC).[75] Conversely, adenoviral reconstitution of circulating adiponectin restores the typical hypertrophic response to TAC through activation of adenosine monophosphate–activated protein kinase (AMPK).[75] Adiponectin can mitigate ischemia/reperfusion injury to the myocardium through activation of AMPK and cyclooxygenase 2.[76] It is interesting to note that adiponectin has been detected in cardiomyocytes, raising the possibilities of both autocrine and paracrine effects within the myocardium.[77] In addition, recently it has been shown that adiponectin treatment can increase intracellular calcium levels in muscle through the adiponectin receptor 1[78]; however, the function of adiponectin in cardiomyocyte calcium homeostasis remains to be elucidated.

Resistin

Resistin is a 12-kD hormone that circulates as a high-order complex in plasma.[79] Ample evidence from animal studies points to a significant proinflammatory action of resistin to promote insulin resistance in various tissues.[80] Epidemiologic studies have revealed a positive correlation between circulating resistin levels and risk of developing HF.[81] Recent studies suggest that resistin can modulate glucose metabolism, insulin signaling, and contractile performance in the diabetic heart. Resistin has been reported to impair glucose transport in isolated murine cardiomyocytes and to be upregulated by cyclic stretch and aorta-caval shunting in rodent models, suggesting that resistin affects cardiac function.[18] Adenoviral transduction of resistin in neonatal rat cardiomyocytes triggers robust hypertrophy with increased expression of hypertrophic genes.[82] Resistin is also associated with activation of the ERK1/2-p38 MAPK pathways and with increased serine-636 phosphorylation of insulin receptor substrate 1 (IRS 1).[82] Adenoviral induction of resistin in adult myocytes reduces contractility, possibly via reduction in Ca^{2+} transients.[82] It is likely, therefore, that high levels of resistin as observed in diabetes contribute to the impairment of cardiac function, possibly through alterations in cardiac metabolism and induction of myocardial insulin resistance.

UNFOLDED PROTEIN RESPONSE

Up to 35% of cellular proteins are synthesized and assembled in the endoplasmic reticulum (ER).[83] Abnormal protein folding and the accumulation of excessive aberrantly processed molecules have been linked to pathology of various diseases including diabetic cardiomyopathy.

Cells have evolved an elaborate quality control system to ensure that only correctly folded proteins exit the cell.[84] The unfolded protein response (UPR) is an evolutionarily conserved mechanism to cope with and ameliorate stress imposed by misfolded proteins. When misfolded proteins accumulate in the ER lumen, cells react by upregulating molecular chaperones to enhance protein-folding capacity and ER-associated protein degradation to eliminate terminally unfolded molecules. In concert, protein translation is attenuated to decrease the influx of new client molecules in the ER, thereby creating a window-for-repair to reestablish homeostasis. Ultimately, if ER stress persists, the UPR may trigger cell death for the benefit of the organism.[85]

The UPR is governed by three distinct branches of signal transducers (**Fig. 24-4**).[86] When the UPR is triggered, protein kinase RNA–like endoplasmic reticulum kinase (PERK) is activated, which in turn phosphorylates E74-like factor 2alpha (eIF2α). This phosphorylation event, in turn, attenuates the translation initiation activity of eIF2α, thereby decreasing the ER workload. Activation of the second branch, inositol-requiring enzyme 1 (IRE1), stimulates unconventional splicing of X-box binding protein 1 (XBP1) to generate spliced XBP1 (XBP1s). XBP1s acts as a transcription factor to upregulate a host of molecular chaperones to aid folding within the ER. As for the third arm, activating transcription factor 6 (ATF6) is transported to the Golgi apparatus and processed and activated by protease-mediated cleavage. ATF6 then functions as a transcription factor to boost expression of genes coding for ER chaperones.

Accumulating evidence suggests that ER stress is involved in the pathogenesis of diabetic cardiomyopathy. ER stress markers, including binding protein (BiP), C/EBP homologous protein (CHOP), and PERK, are induced in the heart in animal models of diabetes.[87,88] These findings were later confirmed in several in vitro studies using H9c2 cells or neonatal cardiomyocytes in culture.[88] Mechanistically, excessive production of ROS in the diabetic heart causes protein-folding abnormalities in the ER, which leads to the UPR.[61,87,88] Some evidence suggests that antioxidant treatment can ameliorate cardiomyopathy and attenuate ER stress activation, suggesting a direct link between diabetic cardiomyopathy, ROS, and the UPR.[87]

AUTOPHAGY

Autophagy is a self-eating process that serves to sustain cell function in the setting of nutrient deprivation.[89] Basal autophagic activity is indispensable to recycle long-lived proteins and defective organelles. Dysregulation of autophagy has been implicated in various diseases, including cancer, cardiovascular disease, and the metabolic syndrome.[90]

Autophagy is an elegantly controlled and highly dynamic process (**Fig. 24-5**). To date, 32 autophagy-related proteins (ATGs) have been identified; these proteins regulate the

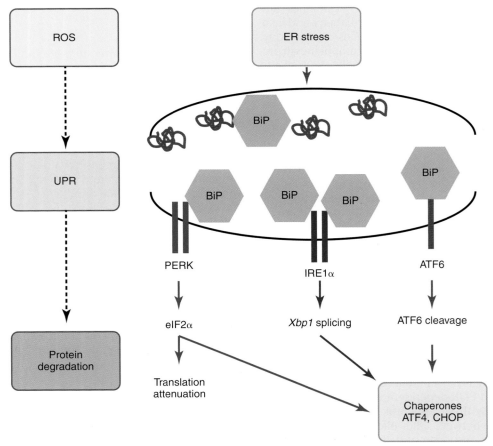

FIGURE 24-4 ER stress response. Schematic representations of three signaling transducers of the ER stress response. Under normal conditions, the ER-resident chaperone BiP (binding protein) interacts with the transducers and prevents their activation. Accumulation of misfolded protein in the ER releases BiP, triggering activation of protein kinase RNA–like endoplasmic reticulum kinase (PERK) and inositol-requiring enzyme 1 (IRE1) and activating transcription factor 6 (ATF6). CHOP = C/EBP homologous protein; eIF2a = eukaryotic initiation factor 2 alpha; Xbp1 = X-box binding protein 1.

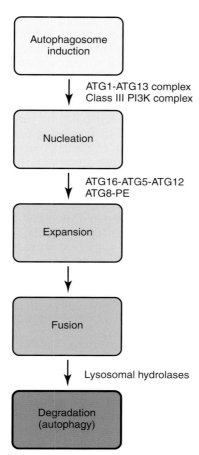

FIGURE 24-5 The autophagic process. Autophagy is an evolutionarily conserved process of intracellular protein and organelle recycling that copes with metabolic and protein-folding stress. A number of autophagy-related genes are involved in this dynamic and tightly regulated process. ATG = Autophagy-related protein; PE = phosphatidylethanolamine.

initiation and progression of autophagy.[91,92] Nutrient deprivation promotes activation of an ATG1-ATG13 kinase complex and formation of the nascent autophagic membrane, the phagophore. The subsequent expansion process is regulated by two ubiquitin-like complexes, ATG5-ATG12 and ATG8-phosphatidylethanolamine. A portion of the cytosol is engulfed within the growing membrane complex, and ultimately a double-membrane structure (autophagosome) is formed. Next, fusion of the autophagosome with a lysosome occurs, leading to hydrolysis of the engulfed contents by lysosomal enzymes. Constituent elements, including amino acids, lipids, and sugars, are released into cytosol for energy production. Finally, ATG9 is involved in retrieval of certain components of autolysosome. Although basal autophagy is essential, excessive autophagic activity has been linked to adverse effects and maladaptive responses.[93]

Autophagy has been implicated in diabetic cardiomyopathy. Early studies found that high-fructose feeding caused cardiac damage in mice, which correlated with significant upregulation of autophagy.[94] However, another study using a different animal model reported opposite findings; autophagy was decreased in diabetic OVE26 mouse hearts.[95] These investigators also showed that metformin significantly improved cardiac function and enhanced the autophagic response in heart.[95] A subsequent study from the same group found that active AMPK can disrupt the Bcl-2–Beclin 1

complex and therefore stimulate autophagy.[96] Although the role of autophagy in diabetic cardiomyopathy remains elusive, current evidence suggests that autophagy plays a role.

CURRENT TREATMENT STRATEGIES AND POTENTIAL THERAPEUTIC TARGETS

Therapy specific to diabetic cardiomyopathy does not exist. However, dissection of the pathophysiology of diabetic cardiomyopathy and disease-related metabolic remodeling in the heart has progressed considerably in recent years. As a result, several novel mechanisms and molecular targets have emerged. The central role of myocyte insulin resistance in the pathogenesis of cardiomyopathy suggests that this signaling cascade is a logical starting point for targeted treatment. For one, lifestyle changes, including diet and exercise, can reduce the incidence of T2DM and improve cardiovascular health.[97] In addition, drugs that enhance glycemic control, such as the antidiabetic drug metformin, which activates AMPK, may confer cardiovascular benefit. AMPK plays a central role in the heart-regulating metabolism and energy homeostasis, and AMPK activation can be cardioprotective during conditions of ischemic stress.[98] Incretin pathway modulators, such as glucagon-like peptide-1 (GLP-1) agonists, have been suggested to be cardioprotective,[99] but whether these effects extend to treatment of diabetic cardiomyopathy is not known. Modulators of free FA metabolism (e.g., perhexiline, trimetazidine, ranolazine, amiodarone), some originally identified as antianginal drugs, have also been suggested to be of potential benefit and may reduce lipotoxicity.[100] Resveratrol, an activator of the NAD-dependent protein deacetylase Sirt1, lowers blood glucose and increases insulin sensitivity,[101] and Sirt1 regulates the activity of FoxO transcription factors.[102] In addition, Sirt1 modulates the activity of peroxisome proliferator-activated receptor gamma coactivator 1 alpha (PGC-1α), which is involved in, among other things, mitochondrial biogenesis and function.[102] More potent activators of Sirt1 are currently being developed. Finally, cell-based therapy and genetic correction (through vector-based gene transfer) of abnormalities in cardiac excitation-contraction coupling and insulin signaling are emerging as potential strategies in the treatment of HF.[18]

Forkhead Transcription Factors

FoxO (Forkhead box-containing protein, O subfamily) proteins are emerging as important targets of insulin and other growth factor action in the myocardium.[103,104] Abundant evidence demonstrates that three members of the FoxO subfamily (FoxO1, FoxO3, FoxO4) are critical to maintenance of cardiac function and stress responsiveness.[103,104] FoxO transcription factors regulate cardiac growth and govern insulin signaling and glucose metabolism in heart.[105,106] Furthermore, recent work has implicated chronic activation of FoxOs in the pathogenesis of diabetic cardiomyopathy (**Fig. 24-6**).[25] Specifically, cardiomyocyte-specific inactivation of FoxO1 (FoxO1 KO) rescued high-fat diet (HFD)–induced myocyte hypertrophy and associated declines in cardiac function while preserving cardiomyocyte insulin responsiveness.[25] FoxO1-depleted cardiomyocytes displayed a shift in their metabolic substrate usage from free

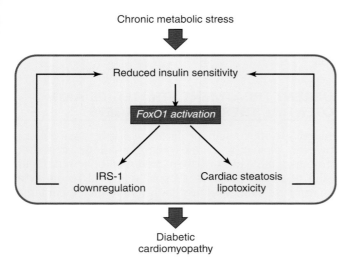

FIGURE 24-6 FoxO1. Hypothesized role of FoxO1 in the pathogenesis of diabetic cardiomyopathy. *(Modified from Battiprolu PK, Hojayev B, Jiang N, et al. Metabolic stress-induced activation of FoxO1 triggers diabetic cardiomyopathy in mice,* J Clin Invest *122:1109-1118, 2012.)*

FAs to glucose, and accumulation of myocardial lipids was reduced.[25] Furthermore, a direct causal link was demonstrated, by which FoxO1-dependent downregulation of IRS-1 resulted in blunted Akt signaling and insulin resistance. Although these findings suggest that activation of FoxO1 is a significant mechanism underlying diabetic cardiomyopathy, an in-depth understanding of specific molecular targets and the transcriptional interplay between FoxO1 and IRS-1 will be required to move this biology toward the clinic.

FoxO has emerged recently as a major mechanism governing insulin signaling and glucose metabolism in a variety of tissues, including liver.[107,108] Chronic activation of hepatic FoxO1 triggers dysregulated expression of a wide array of gluconeogenic genes, events that contribute to systemic insulin resistance.[107,108] It is interesting to note that concomitant liver-specific deletion of both Akt1/2 and FoxO1 in mice restored appropriate adaptation to the fed and fasted states, as well as normal insulin action to suppress hepatic glucose production.[107,108] Moreover, silencing of hepatic FoxO1 largely normalized gluconeogenesis gene expression, lowered the concentration of circulating glucose, and diminished the basal rate of glucose production in insulin-resistant, diabetic mice.[106–108] Thus, inhibition of FoxO1 activity might emerge as a promising strategy to ameliorate features of the metabolic syndrome, such as hyperglycemia, hyperinsulinemia, and insulin resistance.[107] However, the role of FoxO1 in hypertriglyceridemia and hepatic steatosis, which typically accompany insulin resistance and hyperglycemia, warrants further investigation.[107,108] It has also been reported that Notch1 signaling can act in a coordinated manner with FoxO1 to regulate hepatic glucose production, and pharmacologic inhibition of the Notch1 cascade enhanced insulin sensitivity in diet-induced obese mice.[110]

Mammalian Target of Rapamycin

Mammalian target of rapamycin (mTOR) is a serine/threonine protein kinase that regulates cell growth and metabolism and is dysregulated in cancer and DM.[111,112] mTOR comprises two multiprotein complexes: mTORC1, which regulates pathways involved in messenger RNA (mRNA) translation and autophagy, and mTORC2, which regulates insulin signaling and other cellular processes. Insulin and IGFs are major mTOR activators that signal through phosphoinositide 3-kinase (PI3K) and Akt.[113] Also, AMPK, which is activated on energy depletion, calorie restriction, or genotoxic damage, has been implicated in stress-responsive inhibition of mTOR.[113,114] mTOR stimulates cell growth and anabolism by increasing protein and lipid synthesis through activation of S6K (p70 ribosomal protein S6 kinase), 4E-BP (eukaryotic translation initiation factor 4E-binding protein), and SREBP (sterol response element binding protein)[113,115,116] and by decreasing autophagic catabolism through inhibition of ATG1.[115] Persistent activation of mTOR has been implicated in diverse pathologies, including cancer and obesity-related metabolic pathologies.[115] Sestrins, another group of conserved stress-responsive proteins, are increased by ROS accumulation, leading to activation of JNKs (c-Jun N-terminal kinase) and FoxOs.[117] In contrast, silencing of sestrin resulted in triglyceride accumulation, mitochondrial dysfunction, muscle degeneration, and cardiac dysfunction, suggesting involvement in negative feedback regulation of mTOR.[117]

mTOR, along with other kinases such as JNK, phosphorylate IRS-1 on serine residues, leading ultimately to IRS-1 degradation.[118] Indeed, deletion of mTOR substrates such as S6K1 is sufficient to improve insulin sensitivity and extend lifespan in mice.[119] This suggests that rapamycin, a known inhibitor of mTORC1, might act in a similar manner. Conversely, recent work suggests that chronic treatment with rapamycin impaired, rather than improved, glucose homeostasis.[120] This effect was shown to be mediated by mTORC2 inhibition, provoking insulin resistance and impaired glucose homeostasis potentially by blocking insulin-responsive Akt.[120,121] Thus, modulators of either mTOR (e.g., rapamycin) or the distinct branches of the mTOR signaling cascade and their downstream molecular targets (e.g., growth factor receptor–bound protein 10 [GRB10]),[122,123] are of interest as potential points of therapeutic attack in diabetic heart disease.

MicroRNAs

MicroRNAs (miRNAs or miRs) are naturally occurring, small noncoding single-strand RNAs that regulate gene expression, usually by targeting mRNAs for degradation or by repressing protein translation. In some circumstances, miRNAs upregulate translation of certain mRNAs, especially during cell cycle arrest or in terminally differentiated cells.[124] miRNAs have been identified as important molecular regulators participating in many biologic functions. However, their actions are complex and nuanced, as they target a wide range of transcripts, often in a cluster of processes involved in a given biologic event (e.g., fibrosis, cell death). Furthermore, miRNAs merely fine-tune, as opposed to frankly suppress, the actions of their target mRNAs.

Numerous miRNAs are altered in diabetes.[124–127] For example, miRNAs 103 and 107 (miR-103 and miR-107) are negative regulators of hepatic insulin sensitivity,[129] and both are upregulated in obesity. Silencing miR-103 and miR-107 rescues insulin sensitivity in ob/ob and diet-induced obese mice by affecting adipocyte differentiation.[129] One of the targets for miR-103 and miR-107 is the gene encoding caveolin-1, the major protein of caveolae, the distinctive lipid- and cholesterol-enriched invaginations of the plasma membrane. Caveolin-1 stabilizes caveolae and their associated IRs, promoting insulin signaling. By reducing caveolin-1 levels, miR-103 and miR-107 alter IR stability and activation.[129] However, whereas both miRNAs are strongly expressed in cardiac and skeletal muscle,[130] their potential role in insulin resistance in the heart remains unknown.

miR-223 is another miRNA that is consistently upregulated in diabetes, including in cardiac tissue.[125] miR-223 expression increases basal glucose uptake in cardiomyocytes, and exposure to insulin does not lead to further increases.[125] This enhanced glucose uptake is caused by elevated expression and preferential plasma membrane translocation of GLUT-4.[125] Because plasma membrane–localized GLUT-4 is markedly downregulated in diabetic hearts,[131] the increase in miR-223 expression in diabetic patients could be an adaptive response to restore glucose uptake.

A recent report demonstrated that the cardiac-specific miR-208a regulates systemic energy homeostasis by targeting MED13, a subunit of the mediator complex that controls transcription by nuclear hormone receptors, including the thyroid hormone receptor.[132] Pharmacologic inhibition of miR-208a or cardiac overexpression of MED13 enhanced metabolic rate, conferred resistance to obesity, improved glucose homeostasis, and lowered plasma lipid levels in mice.[132] Further research will be required to elucidate mechanisms whereby MED13 alters systemic metabolic rate.

Alterations in intracellular calcium handling and impaired SERCA2a activity are cardinal features of the failing heart. Indeed, *SERCA2a* gene therapy in failing hearts improves cardiac function and reduces arrhythmias in vivo.[133,134] It is interesting to note that elevated cytoplasmic calcium concentrations in failing cardiomyocytes promote CaMKK (calcium/calmodulin-dependent protein kinase kinase)–dependent activation of Akt, which in turn inhibits FoxO3a activity, leading to downregulation of miR-1, a FoxO3a target.[135] NCX-1 (sodium-calcium exchanger 1) mRNA is one of the main targets of miR-1, and increases in NCX-1 levels may contribute to calcium mishandling in HF. *SERCA2a* gene therapy restored calcium levels in cardiomyocytes from failing hearts, normalizing Akt and FoxO3a activity and miR-1 and NCX-1 levels.[135] Collectively, these studies raise the prospect that altering miRNA expression may provide novel opportunities for therapeutic intervention in diabetic cardiomyopathy and other cardiac diseases.

Pim-1

In addition to altered calcium homeostasis, downregulation of prosurvival signaling factors has also been implicated in diabetic cardiomyopathy.[136] Pim-1 (proviral integration site for Moloney murine leukemia virus 1) is a serine/threonine protein kinase that modulates SERCA and promotes cardiomyocyte survival and function.[136,137] Pim-1 is upregulated in failing hearts, potentially as an inefficient, last-ditch attempt to preserve cardiac function.[138] It is interesting to note that Pim-1 is downregulated in the initial phase of diabetic cardiomyopathy and continues to decline, leading to severe contractile dysfunction and HF.[136] Furthermore, Pim-1 is positively regulated by STAT3 (signal transducer and activator of transcription 3) and Akt,[137] both of which are downregulated in diabetic cardiomyopathy.[139] Both STAT3 and Akt

act as modulators of insulin and nutritional status in the heart.[140] On the other hand, Pim-1 is inactivated by protein phosphatase 2A (PP2A)[141] and is a target of miR-1.[142] It has been proposed that the increased intracellular levels of ceramide in diabetic myocardium may in part explain the upregulation of PP2A,[141] contributing to Pim-1 downregulation.

Pim-1 is also implicated in promotion of cardiomyocyte survival via activation of Bcl2 (B-cell lymphoma 2) and phosphorylation or inhibition of Bcl-2-associated death promoter (BAD) and in the maintenance of mitochondrial integrity.[137,143] Furthermore, Pim-1 increases the proliferative activity of cardiac progenitor cells by inducing c-Myc, nucleostemin, cyclin E expression, and p21 phosphorylation.[144,145] Therefore, it is tempting to speculate that the accrual of alterations in upstream Pim-1 activators[139] and the confounding upregulation of Pim-1 inhibitors, such as PP2A and miR-1, contribute to the unique features observed in hearts of diabetic mice compared with other ischemic and pressure-overload models. In addition, as noted earlier, some work suggests that cardiac-specific *Pim1* gene therapy attenuates the progression of diabetic cardiomyopathy,[136] raising yet further the prospects of targeting this interesting molecule. Finally, it is important to point out that all the studies on Pim-1 have been performed in streptozotocin-treated animals, a model used to mimic late stages of T2DM characterized by insufficient insulin action. Future studies will be required to determine the relevance of Pim-1 in T2DM or metabolic syndromes associated with hyperinsulinemia.

CONCLUSIONS AND PERSPECTIVE

Heart failure has remained a leading cause of death in industrialized nations for some years. Numerous events contribute to the rise in HF, but the increasing prevalence of DM is an important contributor. Derangements in insulin signaling have widespread and devastating effects in numerous tissues, including the cardiovascular system. The multiple, interlacing events occurring in patients with diabetes culminate in an environment that, coupled with insulin resistance, leads to diabetic cardiomyopathy. In recent years, novel insights into mechanisms that increase vulnerability of the diabetic heart to failure have emerged. Functional consequences, including diastolic dysfunction, systolic dysfunction, fibrosis, and ultimately clinical HF, correlate with glycemic control. These organ-level functional alterations are preceded by a complex array of molecular and cellular changes, many of which are present in asymptomatic diabetic individuals and experimental models of diabetes. Despite emergence of these insights, our understanding of diabetic cardiomyopathy—a disease that is at once intricate and clinically significant—remains rudimentary.

Constant and unremitting metabolic stress on the heart leads over time to progressive deterioration of myocardial structure and function. This suggests that therapeutic interventions early in the disease, targeting specific metabolic and structural derangements, may be required. This is especially relevant because rigid control of hyperglycemia, however central to treatment, has not fulfilled hopes of meaningful morbidity and mortality benefit.[6] Recent and ongoing research into mechanisms of metabolic control, insulin resistance, and diabetes-associated derangements portend novel therapies designed to benefit the rapidly expanding cohort of patients with diabetes. Continued

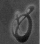
efforts to identify effective preventive strategies and treatments are essential. At the same time, there remains a growing need to identify therapies that slow, arrest, or even reverse disease progression, and ongoing research efforts suggest that such may emerge with time.

ACKNOWLEDGMENTS

This work was supported by grants from the NIH (HL-075173, JAH; HL-080144, JAH; HL-090842, JAH), AHA (0640084 N, JAH; 12POST9030041, PKB; 10POST4320009, ZVW), ADA mentor-based postdoctoral fellowship (7-08-MN-21-ADA, JAH and PKB), the AHA-Jon Holden DeHaan Foundation (0970518 N, JAH).

References

1. Go AS, Mozaffarian D, Roger VL, et al: Heart disease and stroke statistics—2013 update: a report from the American Heart Association, *Circulation* 127:e6–e245, 2013.
2. Witteles RM, Fowler MB: Insulin-resistant cardiomyopathy clinical evidence, mechanisms, and treatment options, *J Am Coll Cardiol* 51:93–102, 2008.
3. Battiprolu PK, Gillette TG, Wang ZV, et al: Diabetic cardiomyopathy: mechanisms and therapeutic targets, *Drug Discov Today Dis Mech* 7:e135–e143, 2010.
4. Turer AT, Hill JA. Elmquist JK, et al: Adipose tissue biology and cardiomyopathy: translational implications, *Circ Res* 111:1565–1577, 2012.
5. Rubler S, Dlugash J, Yuceoglu YZ, et al: New type of cardiomyopathy associated with diabetic glomerulosclerosis, *Am J Cardiol* 30:595–602, 1972.
6. Gerstein HC, Miller ME, Genuth S, et al: Long-term effects of intensive glucose lowering on cardiovascular outcomes, *N Engl J Med* 364:818–828, 2011.
7. Roger VL, Go AS, Lloyd-Jones DM, et al: Heart disease and stroke statistics—2012 update: a report from the American Heart Association, *Circulation* 125:e2–e220, 2012.
8. Roger VL, Go AS, Lloyd-Jones DM, et al: Heart disease and stroke statistics—2011 update: a report from the American Heart Association, *Circulation* 123:e18–e209, 2011.
9. Capes SE, Hunt D, Malmberg K, et al: Stress hyperglycaemia and increased risk of death after myocardial infarction in patients with and without diabetes: a systematic overview, *Lancet* 355:773–778, 2000.
10. Held C, Gerstein HC, Yusuf S, et al: Glucose levels predict hospitalization for congestive heart failure in patients at high cardiovascular risk, *Circulation* 115:1371–1375, 2007.
11. O'Keefe JH, Bell DS: Postprandial hyperglycemia/hyperlipidemia (postprandial dysmetabolism) is a cardiovascular risk factor, *Am J Cardiol* 100:899–904, 2007.
12. Kannel WB, Hjortland M, Castelli WP: Role of diabetes in congestive heart failure: the Framingham study, *Am J Cardiol* 34:29–34, 1974.
13. Boudina S, Abel ED: Diabetic cardiomyopathy revisited, *Circulation* 115:3213–3223, 2007.
14. Palmieri V, Bella JN, Arnett DK, et al: Effect of type 2 diabetes mellitus on left ventricular geometry and systolic function in hypertensive subjects: Hypertension Genetic Epidemiology Network (HyperGEN) study, *Circulation* 103:102–107, 2001.
15. Fang ZY, Yuda S, Anderson V, et al: Echocardiographic detection of early diabetic myocardial disease, *J Am Coll Cardiol* 41:611–617, 2003.
16. An D, Rodrigues B: Role of changes in cardiac metabolism in development of diabetic cardiomyopathy, *Am J Physiol Heart Circ Physiol* 291:H1489–H1506, 2006.
17. Boudina S, Abel ED: Diabetic cardiomyopathy, causes and effects, *Rev Endocr Metab Disord* 11:31–39, 2010.
18. Dobrin JS, Lebeche D: Diabetic cardiomyopathy: signaling defects and therapeutic approaches, *Expert Rev Cardiovasc Ther* 8:373–391, 2010.
19. Fang ZY, Prins JB, Marwick TH: Diabetic cardiomyopathy: evidence, mechanisms, and therapeutic implications, *Endocr Rev* 25:543–567, 2004.
20. Hayat SA, Patel B, Khattar RS, et al: Diabetic cardiomyopathy: mechanisms, diagnosis and treatment, *Clin Sci (Lond)* 107:539–557, 2004.
21. White MF: Insulin signaling in health and disease, *Science* 302:1710–1711, 2003.
22. Weyer C, Bogardus C, Mott DM, et al: The natural history of insulin secretory dysfunction and insulin resistance in the pathogenesis of type 2 diabetes mellitus, *J Clin Invest* 104:787–794, 1999.
23. Deleted in proofs; duplicate of Reference 2.
24. Stumvoll M, Goldstein BJ, van Haeften TW: Type 2 diabetes: principles of pathogenesis and therapy, *Lancet* 365:1333–1346, 2005.
25. Battiprolu PK, Hojayev B, Jiang N, et al: Metabolic stress-induced activation of FoxO1 triggers diabetic cardiomyopathy in mice, *J Clin Invest* 122:1109–1118, 2012.
26. Hue L, Taegtmeyer H: The Randle cycle revisited: a new head for an old hat, *Am J Physiol Endocrinol Metab* 297:E578–E591, 2009.
27. Schwenk RW, Luiken JJ, Bonen A, et al: Regulation of sarcolemmal glucose and fatty acid transporters in cardiac disease, *Cardiovasc Res* 79:249–258, 2008.
28. Steinbusch LK, Schwenk RW, Ouwens DM, et al: Subcellular trafficking of the substrate transporters GLUT4 and CD36 in cardiomyocytes, *Cell Mol Life Sci* 68:2525–2538, 2011.
29. Meyer C, Stumvoll M, Nadkarni V, et al: Abnormal renal and hepatic glucose metabolism in type 2 diabetes mellitus, *J Clin Invest* 102:619–624, 1998.
30. Poornima IG, Parikh P, Shannon RP: Diabetic cardiomyopathy: the search for a unifying hypothesis, *Circ Res* 98:596–605, 2006.
31. Brownlee M: Biochemistry and molecular cell biology of diabetic complications, *Nature* 414:813–820, 2001.
32. Cai L, Li W, Wang G, et al: Hyperglycemia-induced apoptosis in mouse myocardium: mitochondrial cytochrome C-mediated caspase-3 activation pathway, *Diabetes* 51:1938–1948, 2002.
33. Eliasson MJ, Sampei K, Mandir AS, et al: Poly(ADP-ribose) polymerase gene disruption renders mice resistant to cerebral ischemia, *Nat Med* 3:1089–1095, 1997.
34. Montagnani M: Diabetic cardiomyopathy: how much does it depend on AGE? *Br J Pharmacol* 154:725–726, 2008.
35. Galvez AS, Ulloa JA, Chiong M, et al: Aldose reductase induced by hyperosmotic stress mediates cardiomyocyte apoptosis: differential effects of sorbitol and mannitol, *J Biol Chem* 278:38484–38494, 2003.
36. Luiken JJ, Koonen DP, Willems J, et al: Insulin stimulates long-chain fatty acid utilization by rat cardiac myocytes through cellular redistribution of FAT/CD36, *Diabetes* 51:3113–3119, 2002.
37. Wende AR, Abel ED: Lipotoxicity in the heart, *Biochim Biophys Acta* 1801:311–319.
38. Khullar M, Al-Shudiefat AA, Ludke A, et al: Oxidative stress: a key contributor to diabetic cardiomyopathy, *Can J Physiol Pharmacol* 88:233–240, 2010.
39. Leichman JG, Lavis VR, Aguilar D, et al: The metabolic syndrome and the heart–a considered opinion, *Clin Res Cardiol* 95(Suppl 1):i134–i141, 2006.
40. Park TS, Hu YY, Noh HL, et al: Ceramide is a cardiotoxin in lipotoxic cardiomyopathy, *J Lipid Res* 49:2101–2112, 2008.
41. Zhang LY, Keung W, Samokhvalov V, et al: Role of fatty acid uptake and fatty acid beta-oxidation in mediating insulin resistance in heart and skeletal muscle, *Biochim Biophys Acta* 2010:1–22, 1801.
42. Liu GX, Hanley PJ, Ray J, et al: Long-chain acyl-coenzyme A esters and fatty acids directly link metabolism to K-ATP channels in the heart, *Circ Res* 88:918–924, 2001.
43. Iacobellis G, Ribaudo MC, Zappaterreno A, et al: Relationship of insulin sensitivity and left ventricular mass in uncomplicated obesity, *Obes Res* 11:518–524, 2003.
44. Ilercil A, Devereux RB, Roman MJ, et al: Associations of insulin levels with left ventricular structure and function in American Indians—The Strong Heart Study, *Diabetes* 51:1543–1547, 2002.
45. Heineke J, Molkentin JD: Regulation of cardiac hypertrophy by intracellular signalling pathways, *Nat Rev Mol Cell Biol* 7:589–600, 2006.
46. Privratsky JR, Wold LE, Sowers JR, et al: AT1 blockade prevents glucose-induced cardiac dysfunction in ventricular myocytes: role of the AT1 receptor and NADPH oxidase, *Hypertension* 42:206–212, 2003.
47. Morisco C, Condorelli G, Trimarco V, et al: Akt mediates the cross-talk between beta-adrenergic and insulin receptors in neonatal cardiomyocytes, *Circ Res* 96:180–188, 2005.
48. Samuelsson AM, Bollano E, Mobini R, et al: Hyperinsulinemia: effect on cardiac mass/function, angiotensin II receptor expression, and insulin signaling pathways, *Am J Physiol Heart Circ Physiol* 291:H787–H796, 2006.
49. Rodrigues B, Cam MC, McNeill JH: Metabolic disturbances in diabetic cardiomyopathy, *Mol Cell Biochem* 180:53–57, 1998.
50. Ueno M, Carvalheira JB, Tambascia RC, et al: Regulation of insulin signalling by hyperinsulinaemia: role of IRS-1/2 serine phosphorylation and the mTOR/p70 S6K pathway, *Diabetologia* 48:506–518, 2005.
51. Abel ED: Insulin signaling in heart muscle: lessons from genetically engineered mouse models, *Curr Hypertens Rep* 6:416–423, 2004.
52. Berridge MJ, Bootman MD, Roderick HL: Calcium signalling: dynamics, homeostasis and remodelling, *Nat Rev Mol Cell Biol* 4:517–529, 2003.
53. Belke DD, Swanson EA, Dillmann WH: Decreased sarcoplasmic reticulum activity and contractility in diabetic db/db mouse heart, *Diabetes* 53:3201–3208, 2004.
54. Golfman L, Dixon IM, Takeda N, et al: Cardiac sarcolemmal Na(+)-Ca2+ exchange and Na(+)-K +ATPase activities and gene expression in alloxan-induced diabetes in rats, *Mol Cell Biochem* 188:91–101, 1998.
55. Hattori Y, Matsuda N, Kimura J, et al: Diminished function and expression of the cardiac Na+-Ca2+ exchanger in diabetic rats: implication in Ca2+ overload, *J Physiol* 527(Pt 1):85–94, 2000.
56. Pereira L, Matthes J, Schuster I, et al: Mechanisms of [Ca2+]i transient decrease in cardiomyopathy of db/db type 2 diabetic mice, *Diabetes* 55:608–615, 2006.
57. Trost SU, Belke DD, Bluhm WF, et al: Overexpression of the sarcoplasmic reticulum Ca(2+)-ATPase improves myocardial contractility in diabetic cardiomyopathy, *Diabetes* 51:1166–1171, 2002.
58. Duncan JG: Mitochondrial dysfunction in diabetic cardiomyopathy, *Biochim Biophys Acta* 2011:1351–1359, 1813.
59. Nakamura H, Matoba S, Iwai-Kanai E, et al: p53 promotes cardiac dysfunction in diabetic mellitus caused by excessive mitochondrial respiration-mediated reactive oxygen species generation and lipid accumulation, *Circ Heart Fail* 5:106–115, 2012.
60. Shen E, Li Y, Shan L, et al: Rac1 is required for cardiomyocyte apoptosis during hyperglycemia, *Diabetes* 58:2386–2395, 2009.
61. Li J, Zhu H, Shen E, et al: Deficiency of Rac1 blocks NADPH oxidase activation, inhibits endoplasmic reticulum stress and reduces myocardial remodeling in type-I diabetic mice, *Diabetes* 2010.
62. Fyhrquist F, Saijonmaa O: Renin-angiotensin system revisited, *J Intern Med* 264:224–236, 2008.
63. Olivares-Reyes JA, Arellano-Plancarte A, Castillo-Hernandez JR: Angiotensin II and the development of insulin resistance: implications for diabetes, *Mol Cell Endocrinol* 302:128–139, 2009.
64. Dostal DE: The cardiac renin-angiotensin system: novel signaling mechanisms related to cardiac growth and function, *Regul Pept* 91:1–11, 2000.
65. Modesti A, Bertolozzi I, Gamberi T, et al: Hyperglycemia activates JAK2 signaling pathway in human failing myocytes via angiotensin II-mediated oxidative stress, *Diabetes* 54:394–401, 2005.
66. Neumann S, Huse K, Semrau R, et al: Aldosterone and D-glucose stimulate the proliferation of human cardiac myofibroblasts in vitro, *Hypertension* 39:756–760, 2002.
67. Dhalla NS, Liu X, Panagia V, et al: Subcellular remodeling and heart dysfunction in chronic diabetes, *Cardiovasc Res* 40:239–247, 1998.
68. Frustaci A, Kajstura J, Chimenti C, et al: Myocardial cell death in human diabetes, *Circ Res* 87:1123–1132, 2000.
69. Yang R, Barouch LA: Leptin signaling and obesity: cardiovascular consequences, *Circ Res* 101:545–559, 2007.
70. McGaffin KR, Sun CK, Rager JJ, et al: Leptin signalling reduces the severity of cardiac dysfunction and remodelling after chronic ischaemic injury, *Cardiovasc Res* 77:54–63, 2008.
71. Smith CC, Mocanu MM, Davidson SM, et al: Leptin, the obesity-associated hormone, exhibits direct cardioprotective effects, *Br J Pharmacol* 149:5–13, 2006.
72. Scherer PE: Adipose tissue: from lipid storage compartment to endocrine organ, *Diabetes* 55:1537–1545, 2006.
73. Kadowaki T, Yamauchi T, Kubota N, et al: Adiponectin and adiponectin receptors in insulin resistance, diabetes, and the metabolic syndrome, *J Clin Invest* 116:1784–1792, 2006.
74. Wang ZV, Scherer PE: Adiponectin, cardiovascular function, and hypertension, *Hypertension* 51:8–14, 2008.
75. Shibata R, Ouchi N, Ito M, et al: Adiponectin-mediated modulation of hypertrophic signals in the heart, *Nat Med* 10:1384–1389, 2004.
76. Shibata R, Sato K, Pimentel DR, et al: Adiponectin protects against myocardial ischemia-reperfusion injury through AMPK- and COX-2-dependent mechanisms, *Nat Med* 11:1096–1103, 2005.
77. Ding G, Qin Q, He N, et al: Adiponectin and its receptors are expressed in adult ventricular cardiomyocytes and upregulated by activation of peroxisome proliferator-activated receptor gamma, *J Mol Cell Cardiol* 43:73–84, 2007.
78. Iwabu M, Yamauchi T, Okada-Iwabu M, et al: Adiponectin and AdipoR1 regulate PGC-1alpha and mitochondria by Ca(2+) and AMPK/SIRT1, *Nature* 464:1313–1319, 2010.
79. Patel SD, Rajala MW, Rossetti L, et al: Disulfide-dependent multimeric assembly of resistin family hormones, *Science* 304:1154–1158, 2004.
80. Lazar MA: Resistin- and obesity-associated metabolic diseases, *Horm Metab Res* 39:710–716, 2007.
81. Frankel DS, Vasan RS, D'Agostino Sr RB, et al: Resistin, adiponectin, and risk of heart failure the Framingham offspring study, *J Am Coll Cardiol* 53:754–762, 2009.

82. Kim M, Oh JK, Sakata S, et al: Role of resistin in cardiac contractility and hypertrophy, *J Mol Cell Cardiol* 45:270–280, 2008.

83. Blobel G: Protein targeting, *Biosci Rep* 20:303–344, 2000.

84. Ron D, Walter P: Signal integration in the endoplasmic reticulum unfolded protein response, *Nat Rev Mol Cell Biol* 8:519–529, 2007.

85. Schroder M, Kaufman RJ: The mammalian unfolded protein response, *Annu Rev Biochem* 74:739–789, 2005.

86. Harding HP, Calfon M, Urano F, et al: Transcriptional and translational control in the Mammalian unfolded protein response, *Annu Rev Cell Dev Biol* 18:575–599, 2002.

87. Xu J, Wang G, Wang Y, et al: Diabetes- and angiotensin II-induced cardiac endoplasmic reticulum stress and cell death: metallothionein protection, *J Cell Mol Med* 13:1499–1512, 2009.

88. Younce CW, Wang K, Kolattukudy PE: Hyperglycaemia-induced cardiomyocyte death is mediated via MCP-1 production and induction of a novel zinc-finger protein MCPIP, *Cardiovasc Res* 87:665–674, 2010.

89. Levine B, Klionsky DJ: Development by self-digestion: molecular mechanisms and biological functions of autophagy, *Dev Cell* 6:463–477, 2004.

90. Mizushima N, Levine B, Cuervo AM, et al: Autophagy fights disease through cellular self-digestion, *Nature* 451:1069–1075, 2008.

91. Yang Z, Klionsky DJ: Mammalian autophagy: core molecular machinery and signaling regulation, *Curr Opin Cell Biol* 22:124–131, 2010.

92. Xie Z, Klionsky DJ: Autophagosome formation: core machinery and adaptations, *Nat Cell Biol* 9:1102–1109, 2007.

93. Zhu H, Tannous P, Johnstone JL, et al: Cardiac autophagy is a maladaptive response to hemodynamic stress, *J Clin Invest* 117:1782–1793, 2007.

94. Mellor KM, Bell JR, Young MJ, et al: Myocardial autophagy activation and suppressed survival signaling is associated with insulin resistance in fructose-fed mice, *J Mol Cell Cardiol* 50:1035–1043, 2011.

95. Xie Z, Lau K, Eby B, et al: Improvement of cardiac functions by chronic metformin treatment is associated with enhanced cardiac autophagy in diabetic OVE26 mice, *Diabetes* 60:1770–1778, 2011.

96. He C, Zhu H, Li H, et al: Dissociation of Bcl-2-Beclin1 complex by activated AMPK enhances cardiac autophagy and protects against cardiomyocyte apoptosis in diabetes, *Diabetes* 2012.

97. Knowler WC, Fowler SE, Hamman RF, et al: 10-year follow-up of diabetes incidence and weight loss in the Diabetes Prevention Program Outcomes Study, *Lancet* 374:1677–1686, 2009.

98. Kim AS, Miller EJ, Young LH: AMP-activated protein kinase: a core signalling pathway in the heart, *Acta Physiol (Oxf)* 196:37–53, 2009.

99. Fonseca VA, Zinman B, Nauck MA, et al: Confronting the type 2 diabetes epidemic: the emerging role of incretin-based therapies, *Am J Med* 123:S2–S10, 2010.

100. Horowitz JD, Chirkov YY, Kennedy JA, et al: Modulation of myocardial metabolism: an emerging therapeutic principle, *Curr Opin Cardiol* 25:329–334, 2010.

101. Sharma S, Misra CS, Arumugam S, et al: Antidiabetic activity of resveratrol, a known SIRT1 activator in a genetic model for type-2 diabetes, *Phytother Res* 2010.

102. Finkel T, Deng CX, Mostoslavsky R: Recent progress in the biology and physiology of sirtuins, *Nature* 460:587–591, 2009.

103. Ronnebaum SM, Patterson C: The FoxO family in cardiac function and dysfunction, *Annu Rev Physiol* 72:81–94, 2010.

104. Ferdous A, Battiprolu PK, Ni YG, et al: FoxO, autophagy, and cardiac remodeling, *J Cardiovasc Transl Res* 3:355–364, 2010.

105. Ni YG, Wang N, Cao DJ, et al: FoxO transcription factors activate Akt and attenuate insulin signaling in heart by inhibiting protein phosphatases, *Proc Natl Acad Sci U S A* 104: 20517–20522, 2007.

106. Ni YG, Berenji K, Wang N, et al: Foxo transcription factors blunt cardiac hypertrophy by inhibiting calcineurin signaling, *Circulation* 114:1159–1168, 2006.

107. Cheng Z, White MF: The AKTion in non-canonical insulin signaling, *Nat Med* 18:351–353, 2012.

108. Lu M, Wan M, Leavens KF, et al: Insulin regulates liver metabolism in vivo in the absence of hepatic Akt and Foxo1, *Nat Med* 18:388–395, 2012.

109. Dong XC, Copps KD, Guo S, et al: Inactivation of hepatic Foxo1 by insulin signaling is required for adaptive nutrient homeostasis and endocrine growth regulation, *Cell Metab* 8:65–76, 2008.

110. Pajvani UB, Shawber CJ, Samuel VT, et al: Inhibition of Notch signaling ameliorates insulin resistance in a FoxO1-dependent manner, *Nat Med* 17:961–967, 2011.

111. Laplante M, Sabatini DM: mTOR signaling at a glance, *J Cell Sci* 122:3589–3594, 2009.

112. Zoncu R, Efeyan A, Sabatini DM: mTOR: from growth signal integration to cancer, diabetes and ageing, *Nat Rev Mol Cell Biol* 12:21–35, 2011.

113. Hay N, Sonenberg N: Upstream and downstream of mTOR, *Genes Dev* 18:1926–1945, 2004.

114. Towler MC, Hardie DG: AMP-activated protein kinase in metabolic control and insulin signaling, *Circ Res* 100:328–341, 2007.

115. Wullschleger S, Loewith R, Hall MN: TOR signaling in growth and metabolism, *Cell* 124:471–484, 2006.

116. Porstmann T, Santos CR, Griffiths B, et al: SREBP activity is regulated by mTORC1 and contributes to Akt-dependent cell growth, *Cell Metab* 8:224–236, 2008.

117. Lee JH, Budanov AV, Park EJ, et al: Sestrin as a feedback inhibitor of TOR that prevents age-related pathologies, *Science* 327:1223–1228, 2010.

118. Hiratani K, Haruta T, Tani A, et al: Roles of mTOR and JNK in serine phosphorylation, translocation, and degradation of IRS-1, *Biochem Biophys Res Commun* 335:836–842, 2005.

119. Selman C, Tullet JM, Wieser D, et al: Ribosomal protein S6 kinase 1 signaling regulates mammalian life span, *Science* 326:140–144, 2009.

120. Lamming DW, Ye L, Katajisto P, et al: Rapamycin-induced insulin resistance is mediated by mTORC2 loss and uncoupled from longevity, *Science* 335:1638–1643, 2012.

121. Hughes KJ, Kennedy BK: Cell biology. Rapamycin paradox resolved, *Science* 335:1578–1579, 2012.

122. Hsu PP, Kang SA, Rameseder J, et al: The mTOR-regulated phosphoproteome reveals a mechanism of mTORC1-mediated inhibition of growth factor signaling, *Science* 332:1317–1322, 2011.

123. Yu Y, Yoon SO, Poulogiannis G, et al: Phosphoproteomic analysis identifies Grb10 as an mTORC1 substrate that negatively regulates insulin signaling, *Science* 332:1322–1326, 2011.

124. Vasudevan S, Tong Y, Steitz JA: Switching from repression to activation: microRNAs can up-regulate translation, *Science* 318:1931–1934, 2007.

125. Lu H, Buchan RJ, Cook SA: MicroRNA-223 regulates Glut4 expression and cardiomyocyte glucose metabolism, *Cardiovasc Res* 86:410–420, 2010.

126. Shen E, Diao X, Wang X, et al: MicroRNAs involved in the mitogen-activated protein cascades pathway during glucose-induced cardiomyocyte hypertrophy, *Am J Pathol* 179:639–650, 2011.

127. Greco S, Fasanaro P, Castelvecchio S, et al: MicroRNA dysregulation in diabetic ischemic heart failure patients, *Diabetes* 61:1633–1641, 2012.

128. Shantikumar S, Caporali A, Emanueli C: Role of microRNAs in diabetes and its cardiovascular complications, *Cardiovasc Res* 93:583–593, 2012.

129. Trajkovski M, Hausser J, Soutschek J, et al: MicroRNAs 103 and 107 regulate insulin sensitivity, *Nature* 474:649–653, 2011.

130. Finnerty JR, Wang WX, Hebert SS, et al: The miR-15/107 group of microRNA genes: evolutionary biology, cellular functions, and roles in human diseases, *J Mol Biol* 402:491–509, 2010.

131. Cook SA, Varela-Carver A, Mongillo M, et al: Abnormal myocardial insulin signalling in type 2 diabetes and left-ventricular dysfunction, *Eur Heart J* 31:100–111, 2010.

132. Grueter CE, van Rooij E, Johnson BA, et al: A cardiac microRNA governs systemic energy homeostasis by regulation of MED13, *Cell* 149:671–683, 2012.

133. Miyamoto MI, del Monte F, Schmidt U, et al: Adenoviral gene transfer of SERCA2a improves left-ventricular function in aortic-banded rats in transition to heart failure, *Proc Natl Acad Sci U S A* 97:793–798, 2000.

134. Lyon AR, Bannister ML, Collins T, et al: SERCA2a gene transfer decreases sarcoplasmic reticulum calcium leak and reduces ventricular arrhythmias in a model of chronic heart failure, *Circ Arrhythm Electrophysiol* 4:362–372, 2011.

135. Kumarswamy R, Lyon AR, Volkmann I, et al: SERCA2a gene therapy restores microRNA-1 expression in heart failure via an Akt/FoxO3A-dependent pathway, *Eur Heart J* 33:1067–1075, 2012.

136. Katare R, Caporali A, Zentilin L, et al: Intravenous gene therapy with PIM-1 via a cardiotropic viral vector halts the progression of diabetic cardiomyopathy through promotion of prosurvival signaling, *Circ Res* 108:1238–1251, 2011.

137. Muraski JA, Rota M, Misao Y, et al: Pim-1 regulates cardiomyocyte survival downstream of Akt, *Nat Med* 13:1467–1475, 2007.

138. Muraski JA, Fischer KM, Wu W, et al: Pim-1 kinase antagonizes aspects of myocardial hypertrophy and compensation to pathological pressure overload, *Proc Natl Acad Sci U S A* 105:13889–13894, 2008.

139. Katare RG, Caporali A, Oikawa A, et al: Vitamin B1 analog benfotiamine prevents diabetes-induced diastolic dysfunction and heart failure through Akt/Pim-1-mediated survival pathway, *Circ Heart Fail* 3:294–305, 2010.

140. Shiojima I, Yefremashvili M, Luo Z, et al: Akt signaling mediates postnatal heart growth in response to insulin and nutritional status, *J Biol Chem* 277:37670–37677, 2002.

141. Ma J, Arnold HK, Lilly MB, et al: Negative regulation of Pim-1 protein kinase levels by the B56beta subunit of PP2A, *Oncogene* 26:5145–5153, 2007.

142. Nasser MW, Datta J, Nuovo G, et al: Down-regulation of micro-RNA-1 (miR-1) in lung cancer. Suppression of tumorigenic property of lung cancer cells and their sensitization to doxorubicin-induced apoptosis by miR-1, *J Biol Chem* 283:33394–33405, 2008.

143. Borillo GA, Mason M, Quijada P, et al: Pim-1 kinase protects mitochondrial integrity in cardiomyocytes, *Circ Res* 106:1265–1274, 2010.

144. Cottage CT, Bailey B, Fischer KM, et al: Cardiac progenitor cell cycling stimulated by pim-1 kinase, *Circ Res* 106:891–901, 2010.

145. Tjwa M, Dimmeler S: A nucleolar weapon in our fight for regenerating adult hearts: nucleostemin and cardiac stem cells, *Circ Res* 103:4–6, 2008.

146. Boyer JK, Thanigaraj S, Schechtman KB, et al: Prevalence of ventricular diastolic dysfunction in asymptomatic, normotensive patients with diabetes mellitus, *Am J Cardiol* 93:870–875, 2004.

Prevention of Heart Failure in Patients with Diabetes

Yee Weng Wong and Adrian F. Hernandez

Chronic heart failure (HF) is increasing in prevalence, affecting over 5 million patients in the United States, and it is estimated that more than 20 million individuals have HF globally.[1,2] An ageing population, improved survival after myocardial infarction (MI), and a rising incidence of noncommunicable diseases such as hypertension and diabetes in developing economies have all contributed to the increased disease burden worldwide. Although studies show progress in evidence-based treatment for HF with systolic dysfunction, it often remains a progressive condition and is associated with high mortality risk.[1] In particular, these treatments are often instituted fairly late in the disease course when patients are symptomatic with significant LV dysfunction, and its impact on overall survival may be modest on a population basis. Furthermore, there have been no major discoveries in therapeutic options for patients with HF with preserved ejection fraction (HFpEF), a condition that often coexists with a diagnosis of diabetes mellitus, especially among older women. Given the irreversible nature of late-stage HF syndromes, prevention and early detection of HF should be priorities. Largely, the prevention of HF is targeted at identifying the associated risk factors for its development and intervening, especially when multiple risk factors combine, increasing the risk of both HF and its subsequent sequelae.

Diabetes has long been associated with increased risk of incident HF (see **Chapter 23**).[3–5] Longitudinal epidemiologic studies, such as the Framingham Heart Study, have shown that diabetes increases the lifetime risk of developing symptomatic HF by 2.4-fold in men and 5.0-fold in women, independent of coexisting hypertension or coronary artery disease.[5] Furthermore, higher hemoglobin A1c (HbA1c) levels are associated with an incrementally greater risk for development of HF.[6–9] Therefore, patients diagnosed with diabetes represent a critical target population for early detection and prevention of HF. In view of the poor prognosis associated with the diagnosis of HF, its prevention should be undertaken with the same seriousness as prevention of other cardiovascular (CV) complications in patients with diabetes. In this chapter we address the strategies and challenges of preventing and screening for HF among patients with diabetes and diabetes management in patients at risk of developing HF.

STRATEGIES FOR PREVENTION OF HEART FAILURE

The fundamental principle of effective preventive strategies is to be able to reliably detect individuals who are at risk of developing a disease or who exhibit evidence of pathologic processes capable of causing progression to clinical disease state. Effective interventions should reduce the risk of progression to disease, significantly delay the clinical onset of disease, or alter the trajectory of disease progression. In addition, the condition targeted by preventive strategies should carry significant morbidity and mortality risks that need to be balanced against the resources required and potential risks that may be associated either with the screening process or with any preemptive treatment. For achievement of these goals, a thorough understanding of the prevalence and natural history of both the risk factors and the disease state is crucial.

IDENTIFYING PRECURSORS OF SYMPTOMATIC HEART FAILURE

HF is a progressive disorder. Despite the heterogeneity of the etiology of HF, LV dysfunction begins in individuals with risk factors that contribute to insults to or persistent stress on the myocardium (see **Chapter 24**), which may remain asymptomatic in a significant proportion of individuals. The resultant maladaptive changes in the LV geometry (remodeling) and neurohormonal activation culminate in a failing heart, with patients experiencing dyspnea, congestion, and decreased exercise tolerance; requiring repeated hospitalizations; and having increased mortality risk. Recognizing the importance of prevention in addressing the rising prevalence of HF, international professional guidelines and scientific statements have highlighted the need for aggressive risk modification among individuals at risk of developing HF. The American College of Cardiology (ACC) and the American Heart Association (AHA) introduced an HF classification based on stages of risk and development and progression of HF.[10] The classification includes individuals with risk factors associated with increased risk of developing clinical HF without evidence of structural heart

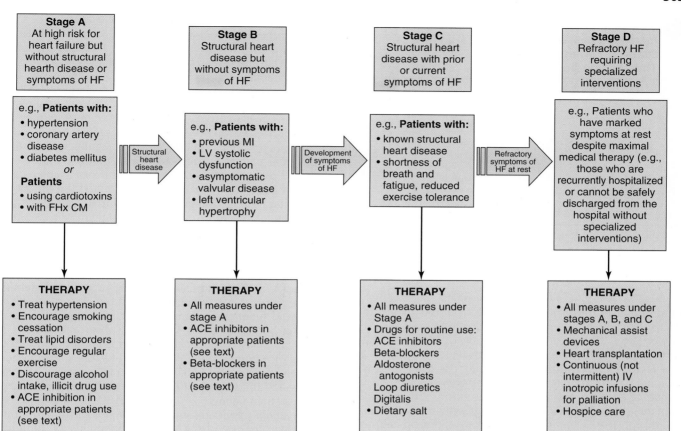

FIGURE 25-1 ACC/AHA stages of HF evolution and recommended therapy. ACE=Angiotensin-converting enzyme; FHx CM=family history of cardiomyopathy; IV=intravenous; MI=myocardial infarction. (Modified from Hunt SA, Baker DW, Chin MH, et al: ACC/AHA guidelines for the evaluation and management of chronic heart failure in the adult: executive summary. A Report of the American College of Cardiology/American Heart Association Task Force on Practice Guidelines [Committee to Revise the 1995 Guidelines for the Evaluation and Management of Heart Failure]: developed in collaboration with the International Society for Heart and Lung Transplantation; endorsed by the Heart Failure Society of America, Circulation 104:2996-3007, 2001.)

disease (stage A), patients with structural heart disease but without overt clinical symptoms (stage B), patients with clinical HF syndromes with either current or past HF symptoms (stage C); and patients with end-stage refractory HF (stage D) (**Fig. 25-1**). By incorporating those who are at increased risk for HF but do not exhibit HF symptoms (stages A and B), but who are nevertheless at significant risk of progressing to irreversible cardiac dysfunction, the ACC/AHA classification highlighted the need to target these "pre-HF" patients for preventive measures with the aim of altering the natural history progression.

Stage A Heart Failure

Among patients with diabetes, coexisting risk factors for HF such as atherosclerotic diseases, hypertension, and obesity increase the risk of developing subsequent LV dysfunction. These risk factors are highly prevalent among patients with diabetes and represent an important clustering of modifiable risk factors to consider for population-targeted intensive risk factor intervention for HF prevention. From population studies, the prevalence of stage A HF among individuals aged 45 years or older is approximately 20%.[11] The underlying assumption is that by aggressively treating these modifiable risk factors underpinning the hazard for HF, the risk of progression to overt LV dysfunction could be mitigated. As these CV risk factors often coexist and contribute to other diabetes

CV complications, lifestyle modification and pharmacologic treatments aimed at treating such risk factors may lead to multifaceted CV risk reduction, including but extending beyond risk for HF.

Stage B Heart Failure

Stage B heart failure refers to structural and functional cardiac abnormalities without overt clinical manifestations of HF, based predominantly on cardiac imaging results. For practical purposes, it has been narrowly defined as previous MI with regional dysfunction or scar, left ventricular hypertrophy (LVH), left ventricular systolic dysfunction (LVSD; or reduced ejection fraction [EF]), or structural valve disease. Based on data from cross-sectional population studies, stage B HF is estimated to affect approximately one third of the population 45 years of age or older.[11] The magnitude of this at-risk group suggests that a significant proportion of the population may benefit from early identification of abnormal LV structure and function so that preventive interventions may be applied most efficiently. This is also an important group to target for clinical trials of early pharmacologic intervention for systolic and diastolic dysfunction.

Among the subcategories of stage B HF, LVSD has been the most studied. Depending on the age of the population studied and the EF threshold chosen to characterize abnormal LV function, the prevalence of asymptomatic LVSD in

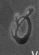
BOX 25-1 Risk Factors Associated with Increased Risk of Heart Failure (HF) in Diabetic Patients Treated with Thiazolidinediones (TZDs)

History of HF (either systolic or diastolic)
History of prior MI or symptomatic coronary artery disease
Hypertension
LVH
Significant aortic or mitral valve heart disease
Advanced age (>70 years)
Longstanding diabetes (>10 years)
Preexisting edema or current treatment with loop diuretics
Development of edema or weight gain on TZD therapy
Insulin coadministration
Chronic renal failure (creatinine >2.0 mg/dL)

Data from Nesto RW, Bell D, Bonow RO, et al: Thiazolidinedione use, fluid retention, and congestive heart failure: a consensus statement from the American Heart Association and American Diabetes Association. October 7, 2003, *Circulation* 108:2941-2948, 2003.

predominantly middle-aged and elderly adults ranges from 2% to 10%, with higher rates reported among men and older adults (**Box 25-1**).[11-20] Asymptomatic LVSD is associated with markedly increased risk of developing clinical HF and is associated with higher mortality risk compared with patients having similar risk factor profiles but without evidence of LVSD. In the Framingham cohort, 26% of participants with asymptomatic LVSD progressed to symptomatic HF during the 5-year follow-up, representing an approximately fivefold increased risk compared with subjects with normal LV function.[13] This was associated with a 60% higher mortality risk, but, more important, over half of the deaths occurred before symptomatic HF developed.[13] Although most studies examining the risk of stage B HF progressing to symptomatic HF have included predominantly older white individuals, in a large cohort of white and black young adults (18 to 30 years old at baseline), the presence of asymptomatic LVSD was a strong predictor of incident HF (greater than 30 times the rate compared with individuals with normal EF) before the age of 50 years, independent of other clinical risk factors, including blood pressure (BP).[21] Given the irrefutable evidence suggesting stage B HF as a precursor to symptomatic HF and its associated risk of mortality, targeting diabetic patients with stage B HF for aggressive preventive measures may meaningfully modify the trajectory of the disease progression into symptomatic HF.

SCREENING STRATEGIES FOR PREVENTION OF HEART FAILURE

The first step of any HF preventive strategy is to identify the patient population at risk of developing symptomatic HF. Screening may be achieved by using established clinical risk markers as mentioned earlier, complemented by biomarker- and imaging-based approaches to identify patients with subclinical abnormal cardiac structure or function on a progressive path of developing symptomatic HF. Through identification of these at-risk individuals, interventions aimed to modify and reduce the risk of development of clinical HF may be implemented and objectively assessed to determine if a given preventive strategy leads to improved outcomes.

Screening with Clinical Risk Factors

As described, several well-established clinical risk factors, including the diagnosis of diabetes, increase the risk of incident HF and should be used by clinicians to identify those at-risk patients who will benefit from aggressive risk factor modification and primary prevention. Advantages of this strategy are their broad availability and generalized feasibility for clinicians even in areas of limited health care resources. Nevertheless, despite the well-documented association of individual risk factors for HF, quantifying the magnitude of risk for an individual patient in the presence of multiple risk markers may be challenging. Validated HF risk scores, such as those derived from the Framingham Heart Study and the Health, Aging, and Body Composition (Health ABC) Study, allow both clinicians and researchers to systematically risk-stratify patients into various risk levels for development of overt HF.[22-24] Although these risk scores are not specific for patients with diabetes, diabetes and elevated fasting blood glucose have been consistently found to be independent predictors for incident HF. In addition, increased risk of HF identified by the risk scores is associated with subclinical cardiac structural and functional alterations that may lead to overt HF. Among adults 30 to 65 years old, observations from the population-based Dallas Heart Study demonstrated that the prevalence and severity of increased LV mass, LVH concentric remodeling, and LVSD identified with cardiac magnetic resonance imaging (cMRI) incrementally increased across the risk strata defined by the Health ABC risk scores.[25] These observations provided some pathophysiologic underpinnings to support the use of risk scores for identification of individuals at increased risk of incident HF.

Several limitations exist with regard to use of risk prediction scores as a screening strategy. The risk scores mentioned earlier were derived from population studies with either predominantly white participants (Framingham Heart Study) or only white and black participants (Health ABC study), and both studies included only individuals from the United States. This may limit the generalizability of these risk scores in other populations. There also remains a lack of validated risk scores derived specifically from patients with diabetes. Furthermore, despite the availability and validity of these risk scores, in practice appropriate risk stratification and implementation of risk modification interventions are often suboptimal during routine clinical encounters. Recent data from the National Health and Nutrition Examination Survey (NHANES) from 1988 to 2010 showed that although achievement of recommended treatments goals for HbA1c, BP, and low-density lipoprotein cholesterol (LDL-C) among patients with diabetes has improved during the last decade, there remains significant room for further optimization (**Fig. 25-2**).[26] Therefore, there clearly remains an unmet need to effectively translate risk prediction model results into a clinical tool to further advance efforts in prevention of HF through aggressive management of these risk factors. One potential direction is to capitalize on the evolution of integrated health systems and the increasing use of electronic health data, whereby an automated analysis and summary of documented risk elements yielding an estimation of risk could be included in the patient care fields to allow for continuous screening for risk and assessment of efficacy of relevant interventions. Such a process could also generate clinical alerts to inform screening and therapeutic modifications. (See also Chapter 31.)

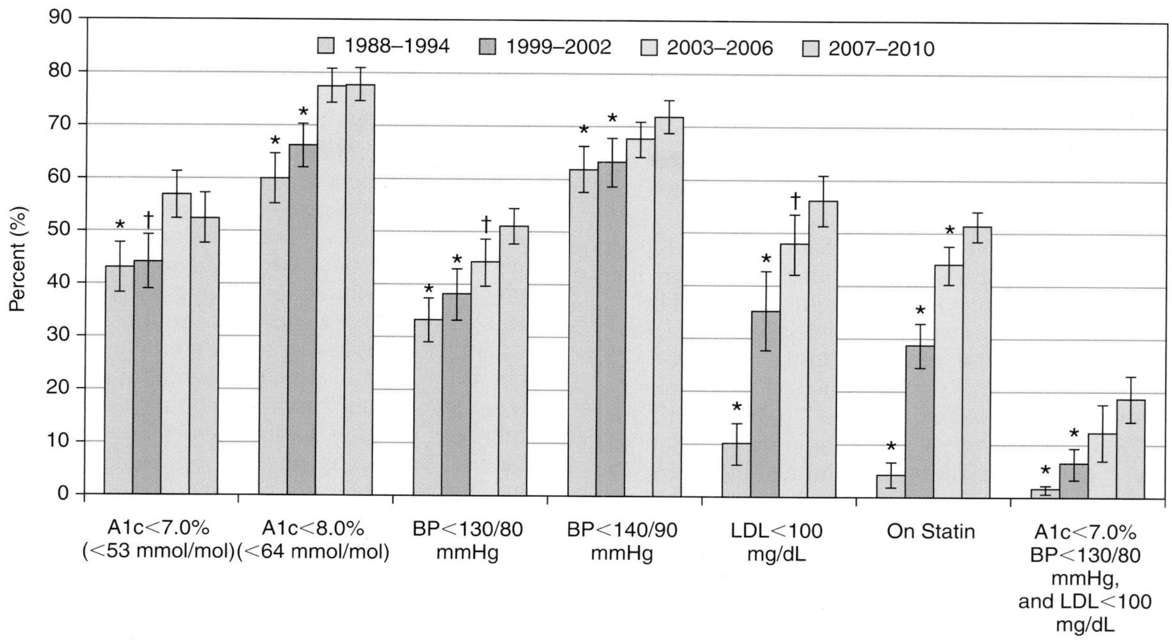

FIGURE 25-2 Prevalence of meeting Health ABC goals among adults aged 20 years of age or older with diagnosed diabetes, NHANES 1988 to 2010. Estimates are age and gender standardized to the 2007 to 2010 NHANES population with diabetes. *P<0.01, estimates are compared with those of 2007 to 2010. †P<0.05, estimates are compared with those of 2007 to 2010. LDL=Low-density lipoprotein. (Modified from Stark Casagrande S, Fradkin JE, Saydah SH, et al: The prevalence of meeting A1c, blood pressure, and LDL goals among people with diabetes, 1988-2010. Diabetes Care 36:2271-2279, 2013.)

Screening with Biomarkers

In theory, biomarkers are biologic variables that are capable of providing information about the presence, severity, and prognosis of a condition of interest. In practice, the term *biomarker* in HF is limited to circulating serum and plasma analytes that reflect various aspects of the pathophysiology of HF beyond routine hematology and biochemistry panels. To be clinically useful, a particular biomarker must be shown to provide additional information that may alter clinical decision making or guide interventions, above and beyond careful clinical assessment.

Natriuretic Peptides

Circulating levels of biologically active brain natriuretic peptide (BNP) and its biologically inert precursor N-terminal peptide (NT-proBNP) are elevated in response to high ventricular filling pressure and have been well established as important diagnostic and prognostic biomarkers among patients with signs and symptoms of overt HF. The success observed demonstrating their value in the clinical context of symptomatic HF has prompted interest in evaluation of these biomarkers as screening tools for HF risk. In population studies and in cohorts with stage A or B HF, the addition of either NT-proBNP or BNP measurements helps refine the predictive capability of traditional clinical risk factors in predicting risk for incident HF hospitalization and mortality, especially in patients with diabetes.[24,27-29] Furthermore, in population studies that included cardiac imaging, the combination of a high clinical risk score and an elevated BNP or NT-proBNP had the ideal predictive characteristics to detect subclinical LVSD, LVH, and diastolic dysfunction.[30,31] Whether the improved risk prediction and stratification may alter management strategies, and in turn improve patient outcomes, remains uncertain. Recent data suggest that a refined HF risk assessment with the use of NT-proBNP

and clinical risk factors in conjunction with multifaceted collaborative clinical care may potentially reduce the incidence of clinical HF. The St. Vincent's Screening to Prevent Heart Failure (STOP-HF) study was designed as a pragmatic, prospective randomized trial to examine the efficacy of a screening program using BNP and collaborative care in an at-risk population in reducing newly diagnosed HF and prevalence of stage B HF. The study found that patients randomized to the intervention arm (BNP screening and collaborative care) had a lower incidence of LV dysfunction with or without overt HF (odds ratio [OR], 0.55; 95% confidence interval [CI], 0.37-0.82; P=0.003). This may be mediated by better-coordinated care, increased emphasis on adherence to guideline-recommended treatments and healthy lifestyle behaviors, higher rate of screening echocardiography, and significantly more prescription of renin-angiotensin-aldosterone system (RAAS)–based therapy. Nevertheless, the proportion of patients with diabetes in the study was relatively low (less than 20%). Furthermore, the event rate in the STOP-HF study was relatively low, and whether the lower rate of HF diagnosis will indeed translate to improved clinical outcomes in the long term compared with standard care practice remains to be determined.

Cardiac Troponin

Cardiac troponins are key sarcomeric proteins responsible for the contractile function of cardiac myocytes. Detectable circulating levels, a marker of myocyte necrosis, have long been used in the diagnosis and prognostication of acute coronary syndromes,[32-35] myocarditis,[36] and HF.[37-39] The specificity of cardiac troponin as a biomarker for myocardial necrosis underpins its demonstrated adjunctive usefulness when added to clinical risk factors for risk-stratifying apparently healthy individuals to discriminate those at highest risk of developing HF.[40-43] Moreover, newer generations of cardiac troponin assays with markedly improved detection sensitivity have resulted in much larger proportions of cohorts tested having detectable levels, allowing analysis of their association with subclinical CV pathology and subsequent CV risk across the spectrum of circulating concentrations. For example, in the multiethnic, population-based Dallas Heart Study, detectable levels of high-sensitivity cardiac troponin T (hs-cTnT; lower detection limit 0.003 ng/mL) were associated with increased LVH and left ventricular end-diastolic volume (LVEDV) and modestly reduced left ventricular ejection fraction (LVEF) identified with cMRI.[40] Higher levels of hs-cTnT were also associated with increased risk of subsequent all-cause mortality from 1.9% (95% CI 1.5%- 2.6%) to 28.4% (95% CI 21.0%-37.8%) across incrementally higher quartiles of hs-cTnT levels ($P < 0.001$) during a median follow-up of 6.4 years.[40] In a separate population-based study focused on older individuals (65 years or older), higher levels of baseline hs-cTnT levels and changes in cTnT levels were significantly associated with incident HF and CV death (**Fig. 25-3**).[43] Although the overall predictive value of troponins is independent of the presence of diabetes, the magnitude of the incremental value of troponins in predicting incident HF among patients with diabetes is less defined.[44]

Because different biomarkers may reflect specific and different pathophysiologic pathways contributing to myocardial damage, incorporating multiple such biomarkers in risk prediction models may further improve risk prediction beyond that obtained using individual biomarker predictors.[45-47] Before such strategies can easily be incorporated into practice, more data on the cost-effectiveness and the impact of biomarker-based screening strategies on clinical outcomes will be needed.

Screening with Imaging

In the era of multimodality CV imaging, detecting LV systolic or diastolic dysfunction can be easily achieved with high precision. Conventional two-dimensional (2-D) or newer three-dimensional (3-D) echocardiography, cMRI, computed tomography (CT) coronary angiography with left ventriculography, and radionuclide imaging could be used to determine LV function, evaluate for the presence of obstructive coronary artery disease (CAD), determine the extent of viable myocardium, and evaluate dyssynchronous LV contraction, either as stand-alone modalities or in combination with complementary imaging techniques. Despite the technologic advances, it remains unclear if imaging-guided screening would further optimize primary prevention of HF or be cost-effective. In the Cardiovascular Health Study (CHS), a multicenter prospective observational cohort study, researchers found that of the 4137 participants without prevalent HF, 107 (2.6%) had subnormal LVEF (<45%) and 210 (5.1%) had a borderline reduced LVEF (45% to 54%) determined with baseline 2-D echocardiography. Although abnormal LVEF (<55%) was associated with increased CV mortality independent of clinical factors and NT-proBNP level, the LVEF did not provide significant incremental predictive value for incident HF when added to NT-proBNP levels and traditional clinical risk factors.[48] These findings, together with the low prevalence of asymptomatic LVSD observed in the general adult population (2% to 10%),[11-20,49] do not support the rationale of using conventional CV imaging modalities as a primary screening tool to identify those at risk of clinical HF. Furthermore, some of these modalities carry significant radiation exposure (e.g., CT and radionuclide scans) and costs (e.g., magnetic resonance imaging [MRI] and single photon emission computed tomography [SPECT]), hence limiting their usefulness as general screening tools. Preselection of a small higher-risk subset based on clinical and biomarker risk markers may improve the yield of an imaging-based screening program, but its effectiveness on improving outcomes would need to be studied.

STRATEGIES FOR RISK MODIFICATION

The ultimate goal of primary prevention of HF in patients with diabetes is to minimize adverse cardiac remodeling by reducing the risk of myocardial necrosis or stressors. This can be achieved by directly addressing prevalent risk factors among patients with diabetes such as coronary heart disease (CHD), hypertension, dyslipidemia, and obesity. Specific pharmacologic agents indicated for other diabetes microvascular and macrovascular complications might offer parallel reduction in the risk of incident HF, in addition to their primary indications. Direct evidence on the efficacy and cost-effectiveness of HF preventive measures is lacking, with most current recommendations based on either (1) observational data on associations of certain risk factors with risk of HF; or (2) secondary endpoints of randomized controlled trials in which incident HF was inconsistently measured and which often lacked adequate statistical power to detect true efficacy. Finally, special considerations regarding the diabetes treatment regimens of patients at risk of developing HF are warranted and are briefly reviewed here.

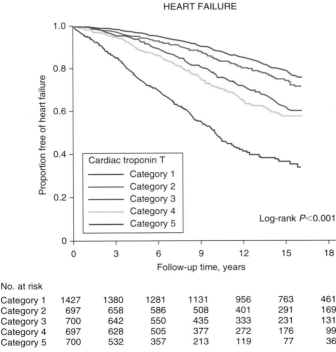

HEART FAILURE

FIGURE 25-3 Association of serial measures of cTnT using a sensitive assay with incident HF in older adults. Categories of cTnT concentrations were divided into category 1 (<3.00 pg/mL), category 2 (3.00 to 5.44 pg/mL), category 3 (5.45 to 8.16 pg/mL), category 4 (8.17 to 12.94 pg/mL), and category 5 (>12.94 pg/mL). *(Modified from deFilippi CR, de Lemos JA, Christenson RH, et al: Association of serial measures of cardiac troponin T using a sensitive assay with incident heart failure and cardiovascular mortality in older adults,* JAMA *304:2494-2502, 2010.)*

No. at risk

Category 1	1427	1380	1281	1131	956	763	461
Category 2	697	658	586	508	401	291	169
Category 3	700	642	550	435	333	231	131
Category 4	697	628	505	377	272	176	99
Category 5	700	532	357	213	119	77	36

Coronary Heart Disease and Diabetes

CHD remains the most important risk factor for incident HF among patients with diabetes (see **Chapter 7**). Compared with their nondiabetic counterparts, patients with diabetes are more likely to have CHD and to have multivessel disease when CHD is present, are at increased risk of silent myocardial ischemia, have more microvascular cardiac ischemia, and are at increased risk of restenosis after revascularization procedures. All these factors contribute to higher risks for and increased severity of MI, which in turn increases the risk of post-MI LVSD and downstream HF. Therefore, comprehensive and aggressive management, which includes pharmacologic treatments and lifestyle modifications, of this prevalent comorbidity is key to effectively reduce the risks of developing overt HF.

Despite advances in treatment of acute MI in recent decades, it remains an important cause of clinical HF, especially among patients with diabetes. However, with the exception of the intensity of antithrombotic therapies (see **Chapters 16** and **21**) and choice of coronary stents in percutaneous revascularization (see **Chapter 17**), the management of patients with acute MI is largely similar regardless of the diagnosis of diabetes (see **Chapters 20, 21,** and **22**).

Post–Myocardial Infarction Prevention of Heart Failure

In addition to the initial ischemic insult caused by an episode of acute MI, patients with diabetes are at risk of recurrent ischemic events, which will gradually deplete the remaining functional myocytes and lead to ongoing adverse remodeling and neurohormonal activation with the resultant increased risk of progression to HF. Therapies aimed at reducing post-MI adverse remodeling and future MIs will likely lead to lower risk of HF development.

The RAAS is activated immediately after MI. Angiotensin II plays a key role in early remodeling of the infarct area and mediates fibrosis via aldosterone and other fibrotic pathway mediators such as transforming growth factor beta (TGF-β), connective tissue growth factor, and tissue inhibitor of matrix metalloproteinase 1 (MMP-1). One of the first studies to demonstrate a cardiac protective effect of angiotensin-converting enzyme (ACE) inhibitors in post-MI patients with LVSD was the Survival and Ventricular Enlargement (SAVE) trial.[50] This study showed that long-term administration of captopril in post-MI patients with LVEF below 40% was associated with significant reduction in all-cause mortality, risk of recurrent MI, and incidence of severe HF (relative risk reduction 34%).[50] In a subgroup analysis, the point estimate of risk reduction among patients with diabetes was consistent with the findings of the main study. However, because of the relatively smaller sample size of the diabetes subgroup and the lack of statistical power based on few events, the treatment difference within the diabetes subset was not statistically significant.[50,51] This finding was confirmed by the Studies of Left Ventricular Dysfunction prevention trial (SOLVD-Prevention), which enrolled 4228 patients with an LVEF below 35%, of whom 83% had had an MI more than 30 days from entry. The study showed that treatment with enalapril (up to 20 mg once per day) significantly reduced the incidence of progression to overt HF and the rate of related hospitalizations.[52] In the echocardiography substudy of the SOLVD-Prevention trial, enalapril was associated with less LV dilation and LVH in patients with stage B HF.[53] Similarly, subgroup analysis of the SOLVD-Prevention study showed that the presence of diabetes was associated with an adverse prognosis; however, the treatment effect of enalapril and its impact on incident HF were similar across the risk profile of patients, which included those with diabetes.[54] In congruence with other studies, the TRACE study showed that treatment with trandolapril in the subset of enrolled patients with diabetes (237 of 1749 patients [14%]) was associated with lower risk of progression to severe HF (relative risk 0.38; 95% CI 0.21-0.67), but no significant reduction of this endpoint was seen in the nondiabetic group.[55] Similarly, in the GISSI-3 trial, treatment with lisinopril versus placebo was evaluated in patients with acute MI; the magnitude of relative risk reduction for all-cause mortality at 6 weeks favoring lisinopril was greatest in the subset of patients with versus without diabetes (**Fig. 25-4**).[56]

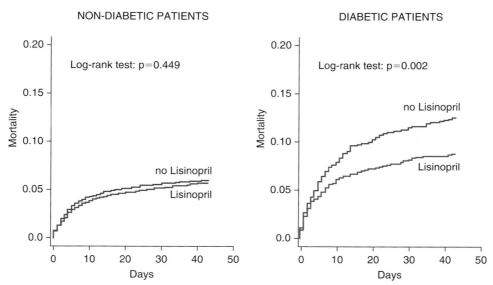

FIGURE 25-4 Differential effects of lisinopril compared with placebo on all-cause mortality in patients with or without diabetes mellitus. *(Modified from Zuanetti G, Latini R, Maggioni AP, et al: Effect of the ACE inhibitor lisinopril on mortality in diabetic patients with acute myocardial infarction: data from the GISSI-3 study,* Circulation *96:4239-4245, 1997.)*

In contrast, treatment with lisinopril versus placebo was not statistically different in either subgroup stratified by diabetes status for the combined endpoint of mortality and LV dysfunction morbidity (defined as [1] clinical HF, [2] asymptomatic LVEF of 35% or lower, or [3] LVEF above 35% but with 45% or more injured myocardial segments evaluated with 2-D echocardiography)—with diabetes, 21.6% versus 24.5% (OR 0.85, 95% CI 0.71-1.01); and without diabetes, 14.3% versus 15.5% (OR 0.91; 95% CI 0.83-1.00). The apparent paradox as compared with the primary endpoint of mortality could be explained by the lower mortality during the acute phase in patients treated with lisinopril, which consequently led to a remnant burden of morbidity for post-MI LVSD among survivors (**Fig. 25-5**).

Hypertension

Hypertension often coexists with diabetes and visceral adiposity and represents a major risk factor for both macrovascular and microvascular complications, including increased risk of incident HF among patients with diabetes. Untreated hypertension accelerates the progression of atherosclerosis, and chronic pressure overload leads to maladaptive LVH, diastolic dysfunction, and subendocardial ischemia caused by impaired microvascular perfusion, and in some patients LVSD ensues. Therefore, appropriate hypertension management is a key treatment goal in improving the overall clinical outcomes of patients with diabetes and specifically preventing progression to HF. (See also **Chapter 14**.)

The United Kingdom Prospective Diabetes Study (UKPDS) compared more intensive BP control (<150/85 mm Hg) with lesser control of BP (<180/105 mm Hg) in 1148 patients with newly diagnosed type 2 diabetes and hypertension.[57] Over a median follow-up period of approximately 10 years, more intensive BP control decreased the risk of developing HF (hazard ratio 0.44; 95% CI 0.2-0.94, $P = 0.043$). The UKPDS also demonstrated that captopril and atenolol were comparably efficacious in reducing the risk of HF and other diabetes-related complications.

The role of the angiotensin receptor blocker (ARB) losartan in reducing the risk of incident HF hospitalization among patients with diabetes has been reported from analyses of the patients with diabetes enrolled in two randomized trials: (1) diabetic cohort of the LIFE (Losartan Intervention for Endpoint Reduction in Hypertension) trial, which enrolled patients with hypertension and LVH,[58,59] and (2) the RENAAL (Reduction of Endpoints in NIDDM with the Angiotensin II Antagonist Losartan) trial of patients with diabetic nephropathy.[58,60] Although the RENAAL trial targeted enrollment of patients with nephropathy and not hypertension specifically, the baseline mean systolic BP was 153 mm Hg.[60] In both trials, losartan was associated with significantly lower incidence of first HF hospitalization, versus placebo in the RENAAL trial (39.3% versus 53.5%; HR 0.74, $P = 0.037$) and versus atenolol in the LIFE trial (10.6% versus 18.7%; Hazard ratio [HR] 0.57, $P = 0.019$) (**Fig. 25-6**).[58]

Despite the benefits associated with treatment of hypertension in patients with diabetes, the ideal target BP remains debatable (see also **Chapter 14**). Most recent management guidelines recommend that the goal BP be less than 140/90 mm Hg,[61,62] although others advocate a lower target of 130/80 mm Hg in selected patients.[63] Specific treatment goals for patients at risk of HF should be considered for the purpose of minimizing incident HF and should be individualized based on the presence of comorbidities, such as atherosclerosis or nephropathy (proteinuria), and the individual patient's ability to tolerate the antihypertensive without significant adverse effects.

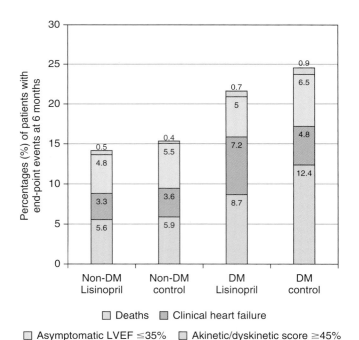

FIGURE 25-5 Effect of the ACE inhibitor lisinopril on mortality and secondary endpoints in diabetic (DM) and nondiabetic (non-DM) patients with acute MI at 6 months follow-up. *(Modified from Zuanetti G, Latini R, Maggioni AP, et al: Effect of the ACE inhibitor lisinopril on mortality in diabetic patients with acute myocardial infarction: data from the GISSI-3 study, Circulation 96:4239-4245, 1997.)*

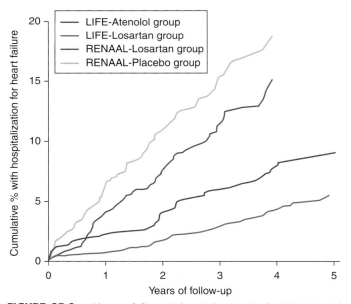

FIGURE 25-6 Incidence of first HF hospitalization in the RENAAL trial (losartan versus control) and the diabetic cohort of the LIFE trial (losartan versus atenolol). *(Modified from Carr AA, Kowey PR, Devereux RB, et al: Hospitalizations for new heart failure among subjects with diabetes mellitus in the RENAAL and LIFE studies, Am J Cardiol 96:1530-1536, 2005.)*

Glucose Lowering and Prevention of Heart Failure

Hyperglycemia is the hallmark of diabetes mellitus, and control of hyperglycemia is the primary treatment goal in managing patients with diabetes. Glycated hemoglobin, measured as HbA1c, reflects glycemic control over several months and is routinely used in monitoring treatment response clinically; it is a marker commonly used to evaluate treatment efficacy in research studies. Although reduction in HbA1c has been shown to reduce microvascular complications in diabetes, the usefulness of HbA1c as a surrogate marker for reduction in CV complications, including HF, remains questionable.[63-65] Furthermore, the impact of intensive glycemic control and glucose-lowering drugs on the prevention of HF largely remains unknown.

Impact of Glycemic Control (See also Chapter 13)

In general, there is consensus that clinicians should make every effort to control hyperglycemia, but evidence remains lacking regarding the effects (if any) of glucose control on the risk of HF.[66,67] Several studies have examined the impact of intensive glycemic control on vascular complications in diabetes, but, unfortunately, incident HF events were not uniformly collected nor independently adjudicated (see also Chapter 26). The best data regarding the role of intensive glycemic control in reducing the risk of HF come from a meta-analysis including the UKPDS,[68] the Action to Control Cardiovascular Risk in Diabetes (ACCORD) trial,[69] the Action in Diabetes and Vascular Disease: Preterax and Diamicron Modified Release Controlled Evaluation (ADVANCE) trial,[70] and the Veterans Affairs Diabetes Trial (VADT).[71] Intensive glucose control was associated with a modestly lower risk of major CV events (HR 0.91, 95% CI 0.84-0.99), driven by a 15% reduction in risk of MI (HR 0.85, 95% CI 0.76-0.94). However, there was no difference for hospitalized or fatal HF events (HR 1.00, 95% CI 0.86-1.16).[72]

Antihyperglycemic Agents and Risk of Heart Failure
Thiazolidinediones

Thiazolidinediones (TZDs), namely rosiglitazone and pioglitazone, improve insulin sensitivity by activating peroxisome proliferator-activated receptor gamma (PPAR-γ), which in turn reduces blood glucose levels.[73] Because of the efficacy in glycemic control, both as monotherapy and in combination with sulfonylureas, metformin, and insulin, the use of TZDs initially expanded rapidly worldwide after their clinical introduction in 1997. However, results from subsequent postmarketing observational studies, meta-analyses, and clinical trials raised the concern of increased risk for HF associated with TZD use.[73-79a]

The main side effects of TZDs indicating potential HF were signs of fluid retention such as pedal edema and weight gain. In the initial randomized trials, pedal edema was reported in 4.8% of patients receiving pioglitazone as monotherapy and in 6% to 7.5% when used in combinations with either metformin or sulfonylureas, compared with 1.2% to 2.5% in patients receiving either placebo or active comparators.[80] The incidence of edema is significantly higher in patients receiving concomitant insulin—15.3% of patients assigned to pioglitazone compared with 7.0% for insulin alone.[79] However, the incidence of investigator-reported edema was dramatically higher in the CV outcome trial of pioglitazone, the Prospective Pioglitazone Clinical Trial in Macrovascular Events (PROactive), which enrolled patients with long-duration

diabetes and prevalent CV disease at trial entry. In this high-risk population, edema was observed in 27.4% of pioglitazone-treated patients compared with 15.9% of placebo-treated patients ($P < 0.001$).[81,82] Similar trends were also observed with rosiglitazone, with edema observed in 4.8% of patients treated with rosiglitazone alone compared with 1.3% receiving placebo in randomized trials with rosiglitazone.[80] A higher incidence of edema has been observed with rosiglitazone use in combination with metformin or sulfonylurea (3% to 4%), compared with 1.1% to 2.2% in patients taking either comparator drug alone.[80] Similarly, concomitant use of insulin was associated with higher rates of edema, in 13.1% and 16.2% of patients taking rosiglitazone 4 or 8 mg/day, respectively, compared with 4.7% in those taking insulin alone.[83]

Pioglitazone and rosiglitazone also increase the risk of HF, as has been observed in patients with diabetes participating in major outcome trials designed to assess the CV safety of TZDs. In the PROactive trial, a significantly higher proportion of patients in the pioglitazone versus the placebo arm had an HF event (11% versus 8%; $P < 0.0001$). Of these HF events, more pioglitazone than placebo patients (5.7% versus 4.1%) had serious HF—defined by requirement for hospitalization or prolongation of a hospital stay, HF that was fatal or life-threatening, or HF that resulted in persistent significant disability or incapacity ($P = 0.007$). It is important to highlight that HF events were not prespecified endpoints in the PROactive study, but were detected as part of standard adverse event reporting and were later confirmed through adjudication of these safety events.[84] Similarly, rosiglitazone use increased the risk of HF hospitalization as observed in the Rosiglitazone Evaluated for Cardiovascular Outcomes in Oral Agent Combination Therapy for Type 2 Diabetes (RECORD) study.[79,79a] HF-related hospitalization or mortality occurred in 61 people in the rosiglitazone group and 29 in the active control group (HR 2.10, 1.35-3.27; risk difference per 1000 person-years, 2.6, 1.1-4.1) (**Fig. 25-7**).[79a]

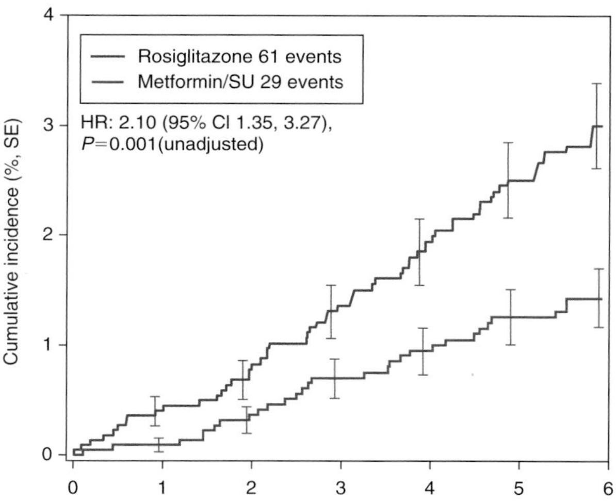

FIGURE 25-7 Kaplan-Meier plots of time to HF (fatal or nonfatal) in the RECORD study (intent-to-treat analysis). *(Modified from Komajda M, McMurray JJ, Beck-Nielsen H, et al: Heart failure events with rosiglitazone in type 2 diabetes: data from the RECORD clinical trial, Eur Heart J 31:824-831, 2010.)*

The mechanistic and causal relationship between TZDs and incident HF remains unclear. However, it is generally accepted that this is predominantly mediated by the effect of TZDs on increased fluid retention, hence unmasking underlying LV dysfunction (either diastolic or systolic), rather than direct cardiotoxicity. Nonetheless, clinicians should not discount the clinical significance of such events, because patients who developed HF events experienced high mortality rates (approximately 30%) during the follow-up period.

Earlier observations and findings from the PROactive and RECORD trials support the recommendations from the AHA and American Diabetes Association advising clinicians to assess the individual patient's risks before commencing TZDs (see **Box 25-1**) and to discontinue TZD use in patients with symptomatic HF.[79] More importantly, the experiences with TZDs highlighted the pitfall of relying on intermediate markers, such as HbA1c, in assessing the clinical effectiveness of glucose-lowering agents in the risk of macrovascular complications.

Dipeptidyl Peptidase 4 Inhibitors

Dipeptidyl peptidase 4 (DPP-4) inhibitors (saxagliptin, sitagliptin, linagliptin, alogliptin, and vildagliptin) potentiate endogenous action of glucagon-like peptide 1 (GLP-1) by inhibiting its enzymatic degradation by DPP-4. Once-daily tablets with a low risk for hypoglycemia, DPP-4 inhibitors are increasingly used for glycemic control and have generally been considered safe with regard to CV risk based on the absence of adverse CV signals from phase I to IIIa trials.

The Saxagliptin Assessment of Vascular Outcomes Recorded in Patients with Diabetes Mellitus–Thrombolysis in Myocardial Infarction 53 (SAVOR-TIMI 53) trial enrolled over 16,000 patients with type 2 diabetes with or at increased risk for CV disease complications, evaluating randomized blinded treatment with saxagliptin versus placebo with a primary trial outcome of the composite of CV death, MI, and stroke. Overall, with a median 2.1-year trial follow-up, no benefit and no harm were detected for the primary major adverse CV event endpoint, meeting the regulatory threshold to exclude an upper 95% noninferiority confidence limit (HR 1.00; 95% CI 0.89-1.12). In the present context, a safety signal of increased risk for adjudicated HF hospitalization, a predefined component of the secondary efficacy endpoint, was observed with saxagliptin (3.5% versus 2.8%; HR 1.27, 95% CI 1.07-1.51; $P=0.007$).[85] This was an unexpected finding given prior observations of favorable myocardial effects of DPP-4 inhibitors in various HF experimental models[86–90] and, if these results from secondary trial analyses are true, raises the question of whether this may be a class effect. The Examination of Cardiovascular Outcomes with Alogliptin Versus Standard of Care (EXAMINE) trial evaluated the effects of alogliptin versus placebo in 5380 patients with type 2 diabetes and a recent acute coronary syndrome event and, similar to SAVOR, demonstrated noninferiority with regard to the effect of alogliptin on the same three-point major adverse cardiovascular event (MACE) primary outcomes (HR 0.96; an upper boundary of the one-sided repeated confidence interval of 1.17)[90a] over a median follow-up of 18 months. In preliminary post hoc analyses (unpublished), a numeric increase in hospitalized HF events was observed in the alogliptin group, although this difference did not achieve statistical significance (3.9% versus 3.3%; HR 1.19, 95% CI 0.89-1.58). No mechanism has yet

been proposed to account for the possibility of increased HF risk with DPP-4 inhibitors, and unfortunately no systematic assessment of cardiac structure or function was performed in either of these two clinical trials.

Insulin

The relationship between insulin use and risk of incident HF is unclear. Mechanistically, acute insulin administration is thought to be associated with fluid retention, potentially mediated by increased renal sodium retention caused by insulin,[91] and may theoretically contribute to overt HF among at-risk patients. Furthermore, chronic insulin administration is associated with weight gain and obesity, known risk factors for incident HF. However, data from prospective randomized trials are largely lacking, with the exception of one trial that assessed the CV effects of insulin glargine versus usual care in patients with early diabetes or prediabetic impaired glucose metabolism, the Outcome Reduction with Initial Glargine Intervention (ORIGIN) trial. ORIGIN randomized individuals aged 50 years or older with CV risk factors, plus impaired fasting glucose, impaired glucose tolerance, or early type 2 diabetes, to receive insulin glargine or standard care. HF-related hospitalization was a prespecified component of the secondary composite endpoint. At median follow-up of 6.2 years (interquartile range, 5.8 to 6.7), there was no statistical difference in the risk of HF hospitalization between the study groups (HR 0.90; 95% CI 0.77-1.05; $P=0.16$).[92]

Evidence regarding the potential impact of other emerging glucose-lowering agents on risk for HF is mostly lacking, with numerous large CV outcome trials presently under way. GLP-1 agonists (exenatide, liraglutide) may have benefits for patients at risk for HF based on early studies demonstrating favorable effects on measures of cardiac function. For example, in a small study of patients with severe LV dysfunction after acute MI and reperfusion, patients treated with a 3-day GLP-1 infusion had a greater increase in LVEF (from 29% ± 2% to 39% ± 3%, $P<0.01$) compared with historical controls (28% ± 2% to 29% ± 2%).[93] GLP-1 treated patients also had a shorter length of hospital stay (6 versus 10 days, $P<0.02$). In another small randomized crossover clinical trial, patients with a low LVEF (<35%) and New York Heart Association (NYHA) Class III or IV HF symptoms, the GLP-1 agonist exenatide significantly increased cardiac index and decreased pulmonary capillary wedge pressure compared with placebo.[94]

Although there remains a lack of conclusive evidence on the long-term CVD outcomes with GLP-1 use, several studies have also shown favorable effects on CV risk factor profiles with these agents, such as lowering of systolic BP, weight loss, and possibly improvement in lipid profile, and these effects may in turn play a role in primary prevention of HF in patients with diabetes.[95]

Another class of agents that holds promise for potential benefits in preventing HF is the sodium-glucose cotransporter 2 (SGLT-2) inhibitors (canagliflozin, dapagliflozin, empagliflozin). SGLT-2 antagonists inhibit glucose reclamation from the urine by blocking SGLT-2 in the proximal tubule, causing glucosuria to occur at much lower concentrations of plasma glucose. This results in loss of 200 to 400 kcal/day and some diuresis, thereby reducing body weight and lowering BP—both potentially favorable for HF prevention and suggesting a potential role for these drugs in the management of patients with type 2 diabetes and prevalent

HF. Until further data are available from ongoing clinical trial programs across this class of medications, all such effects on HF remain speculative.

CHALLENGES IN PREVENTION OF HEART FAILURE AND FUTURE DIRECTIONS

Preventing HF is a public health priority, and creating strategies to detect and treat patients at risk for HF will be critical. Recognition of major risk factors such as diabetes is important, but there is limited evidence to indicate the best strategies to identify patients to prevent them from progressing to stage B (asymptomatic with LV dysfunction) or to stage C or D (symptomatic HF). Moving forward, prevention strategies in the population with diabetes will likely require multidimensional efforts including the management of hyperglycemia and treatment of other common comorbidities associated with the risk of HF.[96,97] However, the evidence needed will likely require large, pragmatic clinical trials that rigorously evaluate different approaches to glucose-lowering strategies and/or other care for patients with diabetes.[98]

References

1. Go AS, Mozaffarian D, Roger VL, et al: Heart disease and stroke statistics—2013 update: a report from the American Heart Association, *Circulation* 127(1):e6–e245, 2013.
2. McMurray JJ, Petrie MC, Murdoch DR, Davie AP: Clinical epidemiology of heart failure: public and private health burden, *Eur Heart J* (19 Suppl P):P9–P16, 1998.
3. Gottdiener JS, Arnold AM, Aurigemma GP, et al: Predictors of congestive heart failure in the elderly: the Cardiovascular Health Study, *J Am Coll Cardiol* 35(6):1628–1637, 2000.
4. He J, Ogden LG, Bazzano LA, et al: Risk factors for congestive heart failure in US men and women: NHANES I epidemiologic follow-up study, *Arch Intern Med* 161(7):996–1002, 2001.
5. Kannel WB, Hjortland M, Castelli WP: Role of diabetes in congestive heart failure: the Framingham study, *Am J Cardiol* 34(1):29–34, 1974.
6. Nichols GA, Gullion CM, Koro CE, et al: The incidence of congestive heart failure in type 2 diabetes: an update, *Diabetes Care* 27(8):1879–1884, 2004.
7. Stratton IM, Adler AI, Neil HA, et al: Association of glycaemia with macrovascular and microvascular complications of type 2 diabetes (UKPDS 35): prospective observational study, *BMJ* 321 (7258):405–412, 2000.
8. Iribarren C, Karter AJ, Go AS, et al: Glycemic control and heart failure among adult patients with diabetes, *Circulation* 103(22):2668–2673, 2001.
9. Vaur L, Gueret P, Lievre M, et al: Development of congestive heart failure in type 2 diabetic patients with microalbuminuria or proteinuria: observations from the DIABHYCAR (type 2 DIABetes, Hypertension, CArdiovascular Events and Ramipril) study, *Diabetes Care* 26(3):855–860, 2003.
10. Hunt SA, Baker DW, Chin MH, et al: ACC/AHA guidelines for the evaluation and management of chronic heart failure in the adult: executive summary a report of the American College of Cardiology/American Heart Association Task Force on Practice Guidelines (Committee to Revise the 1995 Guidelines for the Evaluation and Management of Heart Failure): Developed in Collaboration With the International Society for Heart and Lung Transplantation; Endorsed by the Heart Failure Society of America, *Circulation* 104(24):2996–3007, 2001.
11. Ammar KA, Jacobsen SJ, Mahoney DW, et al: Prevalence and prognostic significance of heart failure stages: application of the American College of Cardiology/American Heart Association heart failure staging criteria in the community, *Circulation* 115(12):1563–1570, 2007.
12. Abhayaratna WP, Smith WT, Becker NG, et al: Prevalence of heart failure and systolic ventricular dysfunction in older Australians: the Canberra Heart Study, *Med J Aust* 184(4):151–154, 2006.
13. Wang TJ, Evans JC, Benjamin EJ, et al: Natural history of asymptomatic left ventricular systolic dysfunction in the community, *Circulation* 108(8):977–982, 2003.
14. Redfield MM, Jacobsen SJ, Burnett JC Jr, et al: Burden of systolic and diastolic ventricular dysfunction in the community: appreciating the scope of the heart failure epidemic, *JAMA* 289 (2):194–202, 2003.
15. Devereux RB, Roman MJ, Paranicas M, et al: A population-based assessment of left ventricular systolic dysfunction in middle-aged and older adults: the Strong Heart Study, *Am Heart J* 141 (3):439–446, 2001.
16. Davies M, Hobbs F, Davis R, et al: Prevalence of left-ventricular systolic dysfunction and heart failure in the Echocardiographic Heart of England Screening study: a population based study, *Lancet* 358(9280):439–444, 2001.
17. Mosterd A, Hoes AW, de Bruyne MC, et al: Prevalence of heart failure and left ventricular dysfunction in the general population; The Rotterdam Study, *Eur Heart J* 20(6):447–455, 1999.
18. Schunkert H, Broeckel U, Hense HW, et al: Left-ventricular dysfunction, *Lancet* 351(9099):372, 1998.
19. McDonagh TA, Morrison CE, Lawrence A, et al: Symptomatic and asymptomatic left-ventricular systolic dysfunction in an urban population, *Lancet* 350(9081):829–833, 1997.
20. Gardin JM, Siscovick D, Anton-Culver H, et al: Sex, age, and disease affect echocardiographic left ventricular mass and systolic function in the free-living elderly. The Cardiovascular Health Study, *Circulation* 91(6):1739–1748, 1995.
21. Bibbins-Domingo K, Pletcher MJ, Lin F, et al: Racial differences in incident heart failure among young adults, *N Engl J Med* 360(12):1179–1190, 2009.
22. Kannel WB, D'Agostino RB, Silbershatz H, et al: Profile for estimating risk of heart failure, *Arch Intern Med* 159(11):1197–1204, 1999.
23. Butler J, Kalogeropoulos A, Georgiopoulou V, et al: Incident heart failure prediction in the elderly: the health ABC heart failure score, *Circ Heart Fail* 1(2):125–133, 2008.
24. Kalogeropoulos A, Psaty BM, Vasan RS, et al: Validation of the Health ABC heart failure model for incident heart failure risk prediction: the Cardiovascular Health Study, *Circ Heart Fail* 3 (4):495–502, 2010.
25. Gupta S, Berry JD, Ayers CR, et al: Association of Health, Aging, and Body Composition (ABC) heart failure score with cardiac structural and functional abnormalities in young individuals, *Am Heart J* 159(5):817–824, 2010.
26. Stark Casagrande S, Fradkin JE, Saydah SH, et al: The prevalence of meeting A1C, blood pressure, and LDL goals among people with diabetes, 1988-2010, *Diabetes Care* 2013.
27. McKie PM, Cataliotti A, Lahr BD, et al: The prognostic value of N-terminal pro–B-type natriuretic peptide for death and cardiovascular events in healthy normal and stage A/B heart failure subjects, *J Am Coll Cardiol* 55(19):2140–2147, 2010.
28. Onodera M, Nakamura M, Tanaka F, et al: Plasma B-type natriuretic peptide is useful for cardiovascular risk assessment in community-based diabetes subjects: comparison with albuminuria, *Int Heart J* 53(3):176–181, 2012.
29. Wang TJ, Larson MG, Levy D, et al: Plasma natriuretic peptide levels and the risk of cardiovascular events and death, *N Engl J Med* 350(7):655–663, 2004.
30. Gupta S, Rohatgi A, Ayers CR, et al: Risk scores versus natriuretic peptides for identifying prevalent stage B heart failure, *Am Heart J* 161(5):923–930 e2, 2011.
31. McGrady M, Reid CM, Shiel L, et al: N-terminal B-type natriuretic peptide and the association with left ventricular diastolic function in a population at high risk of incident heart failure: results of the SCReening Evaluation of the Evolution of New-Heart Failure Study (SCREEN-HF), *Eur J Heart Fail* 15(5):573–580, 2013.
32. Thygesen K, Alpert JS, Jaffe AS, et al: Third universal definition of myocardial infarction, *J Am Coll Cardiol* 60(16):1581–1598, 2012.
33. Reichlin T, Hochholzer W, Bassetti S, et al: Early diagnosis of myocardial infarction with sensitive cardiac troponin assays, *N Engl J Med* 361(9):858–867, 2009.
34. Keller T, Zeller T, Peetz D, et al: Sensitive troponin I assay in early diagnosis of acute myocardial infarction, *N Engl J Med* 361(9):868–877, 2009.
35. Newby LK, Roe MT, Chen AY, et al: Frequency and clinical implications of discordant creatine kinase-MB and troponin measurements in acute coronary syndromes, *J Am Coll Cardiol* 47 (2):312–318, 2006.
36. Lauer B, Niederau C, Kühl U, et al: Cardiac troponin T in patients with clinically suspected myocarditis, *J Am Coll Cardiol* 30(5):1354–1359, 1997.
37. Peacock WF 4th, De Marco T, Fonarow GC, et al: Cardiac troponin and outcome in acute heart failure, *N Engl J Med* 358(20):2117–2126, 2008.
38. Del Carlo CH, Pereira-Barretto AC, Cassaro-Strunz C, et al: Serial measure of cardiac troponin T levels for prediction of clinical events in decompensated heart failure, *J Card Fail* 10(1):43–48, 2004.
39. Latini R, Masson S, Anand IS, et al: Prognostic value of very low plasma concentrations of troponin T in patients with stable chronic heart failure, *Circulation* 116(11):1242–1249, 2007.
40. de Lemos JA, Drazner MH, Omland T, et al: Association of troponin T detected with a highly sensitive assay and cardiac structure and mortality risk in the general population, *JAMA* 304 (22):2503–2512, 2010.
41. Saunders JT, Nambi V, de Lemos JA, et al: Cardiac troponin T measured by a highly sensitive assay predicts coronary heart disease, heart failure, and mortality in the Atherosclerosis Risk in Communities Study, *Circulation* 123(13):1367–1376, 2011.
42. Sundström J, Ingelsson E, Berglund L, et al: Cardiac troponin-I and risk of heart failure: a community-based cohort study, *Eur Heart J* 30(7):773–781, 2009.
43. de Filippi CR, de Lemos JA, Christenson RH, et al: Association of serial measures of cardiac troponin T using a sensitive assay with incident heart failure and cardiovascular mortality in older adults, *JAMA* 304(22):2494–2502, 2010.
44. Hallén J, Johansen OE, Birkeland KI, et al: Determinants and prognostic implications of cardiac troponin T measured by a sensitive assay in type 2 diabetes mellitus, *Cardiovasc Diabetol* 9:52, 2010.
45. Velagaleti RS, Gona P, Larson MG, et al: Multimarker approach for the prediction of heart failure incidence in the community, *Circulation* 122(17):1700–1706, 2010.
46. Nambi V, Liu X, Chambless LE, et al: Troponin T and N-terminal pro-B-type natriuretic peptide: a biomarker approach to predict heart failure risk—the atherosclerosis risk in communities study, *Clin Chem* 59(12):1802–1810, 2013.
47. de Antonio M, Lupon J, Galan A, et al: Combined use of high-sensitivity cardiac troponin T and N-terminal pro-B type natriuretic peptide improves measurements of performance over established mortality risk factors in chronic heart failure, *Am Heart J* 163(5):821–828, 2012.
48. deFilippi CR, Christenson RH, Kop WJ, et al: Left ventricular ejection fraction assessment in older adults: an adjunct to natriuretic peptide testing to identify risk of new-onset heart failure and cardiovascular death? *J Am Coll Cardiol* 58(14):1497–1506, 2011.
49. Senni M, Tribouilloy CM, Rodeheffer RJ, et al: Congestive heart failure in the community: a study of all incident cases in Olmsted County, Minnesota, in 1991, *Circulation* 98(21):2282–2289, 1998.
50. Pfeffer MA, Lamas GA, Vaughan DE, et al: Effect of captopril on progressive ventricular dilatation after anterior myocardial infarction, *N Engl J Med* 319(2):80–86, 1988.
51. Moyé LA, Pfeffer MA, Wun CC, et al: Uniformity of captopril benefit in the SAVE Study: subgroup analysis. Survival and Ventricular Enlargement Study, *Eur Heart J* (15 Suppl B):2–8, 1994, discussion 26–30.
52. Effect of enalapril on mortality and the development of heart failure in asymptomatic patients with reduced left ventricular ejection fractions. The SOLVD Investigators, *N Engl J Med* 327 (10):685–691, 1992.
53. Greenberg B, Quinones MA, Koilpillai C, et al: Effects of long-term enalapril therapy on cardiac structure and function in patients with left ventricular dysfunction. Results of the SOLVD echocardiography substudy, *Circulation* 91(10):2573–2581, 1995.
54. Parker AB, Yusuf S, Naylor CD: The relevance of subgroup-specific treatment effects: the Studies of Left Ventricular Dysfunction (SOLVD) revisited, *Am Heart J* 144(6):941–947, 2002.
55. Gustafsson I, Torp-Pedersen C, Køber L, et al: Effect of the angiotensin-converting enzyme inhibitor trandolapril on mortality and morbidity in diabetic patients with left ventricular dysfunction after acute myocardial infarction. Trace Study Group, *J Am Coll Cardiol* 34(1):83–89, 1999.
56. Zuanetti G, Latini R, Maggioni AP, et al: Effect of the ACE inhibitor lisinopril on mortality in diabetic patients with acute myocardial infarction: data from the GISSI-3 study, *Circulation* 96 (12):4239–4245, 1997.
57. Tight blood pressure control and risk of macrovascular and microvascular complications in type 2 diabetes: UKPDS 38. UK Prospective Diabetes Study Group, *BMJ* 317(7160):703–713, 1998.
58. Carr AA, Kowey PR, Devereux RB, et al: Hospitalizations for new heart failure among subjects with diabetes mellitus in the RENAAL and LIFE studies, *Am J Cardiol* 96(11):1530–1536, 2005.
59. Dahlöf B, Devereux RB, Kjeldsen SE, et al: Cardiovascular morbidity and mortality in the Losartan Intervention For Endpoint reduction in hypertension study (LIFE): a randomised trial against atenolol, *Lancet* 359(9311):995–1003, 2002.
60. Brenner BM, Cooper ME, de Zeeuw D, et al: Effects of losartan on renal and cardiovascular outcomes in patients with type 2 diabetes and nephropathy, *N Engl J Med* 345(12):861–869, 2001.
61. James PA, Oparil S, Carter BL, et al: 2014 evidence-based guideline for the management of high blood pressure in adults: report from the panel members appointed to the Eighth Joint National Committee (JNC 8), *JAMA* 311(5):507–520, 2014.
62. Mancia G, Fagard R, Narkiewicz K, et al: 2013 ESH/ESC guidelines for the management of arterial hypertension: the Task Force for the management of arterial hypertension of the European Society of Hypertension (ESH) and of the European Society of Cardiology (ESC), *J Hypertens* 31 (7):1281–1357, 2013.
63. American Diabetes Association: Standards of medical care in diabetes—2014, *Diabetes Care* (37 Suppl 1):S14–S80, 2014.
64. Hennekens CH, Hebert PR, Schneider WR, et al: Academic perspectives on the United States Food and Drug Administration's guidance for industry on diabetes mellitus, *Contemp Clin Trials* 31(5):411–413, 2010.

65. Drucker DJ, Goldfine AB: Cardiovascular safety and diabetes drug development, *Lancet* 377 (9770):977–979, 2011.

66. Yancy CW, Jessup M, Bozkurt B, et al: 2013 ACCF/AHA guideline for the management of heart failure: executive summary: a report of the American College of Cardiology Foundation/American Heart Association Task Force on practice guidelines, *Circulation* 128(16):1810–1852, 2013.

67. Rydén L, Grant PJ, Anker SD, et al: ESC guidelines on diabetes, pre-diabetes, and cardiovascular diseases developed in collaboration with the EASD: the Task Force on diabetes, pre-diabetes, and cardiovascular diseases of the European Society of Cardiology (ESC) and developed in collaboration with the European Association for the Study of Diabetes (EASD), *Eur Heart J* 34 (39):3035–3087, 2013.

68. Intensive blood-glucose control with sulphonylureas or insulin compared with conventional treatment and risk of complications in patients with type 2 diabetes (UKPDS 33). UK Prospective Diabetes Study (UKPDS) Group, *Lancet* 352(9131):837–853, 1998.

69. Action to Control Cardiovascular Risk in Diabetes Study Group, Gerstein HC, Miller ME, et al: Effects of intensive glucose lowering in type 2 diabetes, *N Engl J Med* 358(24):2545–2559, 2008.

70. ADVANCE Collaborative Group, Patel A, MacMahon S, et al: Intensive blood glucose control and vascular outcomes in patients with type 2 diabetes, *N Engl J Med* 358(24):2560–2572, 2008.

71. Duckworth W, Abraira C, Moritz T, et al: Glucose control and vascular complications in veterans with type 2 diabetes, *N Engl J Med* 360(2):129–139, 2009.

72. Control Group, Turnbull FM, Abraira C, et al: Intensive glucose control and macrovascular outcomes in type 2 diabetes, *Diabetologia* 52(11):2288–2298, 2009.

73. Yki-Jarvinen H: Thiazolidinediones, *N Engl J Med* 351(11):1106–1118, 2004.

74. Masoudi FA, Inzucchi SE, Wang Y, et al: Thiazolidinediones, metformin, and outcomes in older patients with diabetes and heart failure: an observational study, *Circulation* 111(5):583–590, 2005.

75. Dargie HJ, Hildebrandt PR, Riegger GA, et al: A randomized, placebo-controlled trial assessing the effects of rosiglitazone on echocardiographic function and cardiac status in type 2 diabetic patients with New York Heart Association Functional Class I or II Heart Failure, *J Am Coll Cardiol* 49(16):1696–1704, 2007.

76. Delea TE, Edelsberg JS, Hagiwara M, et al: Use of thiazolidinediones and risk of heart failure in people with type 2 diabetes: a retrospective cohort study, *Diabetes Care* 26(11):2983–2989, 2003.

77. Singh S, Loke YK, Furberg CD: Thiazolidinediones and heart failure: a teleo-analysis, *Diabetes Care* 30(8):2148–2153, 2007.

78. Lago RM, Singh PP, Nesto RW: Congestive heart failure and cardiovascular death in patients with prediabetes and type 2 diabetes given thiazolidinediones: a meta-analysis of randomised clinical trials, *Lancet* 370(9593):1129–1136, 2007.

79. Home PD, Pocock SJ, Beck-Nielsen H, et al: Rosiglitazone evaluated for cardiovascular outcomes in oral agent combination therapy for type 2 diabetes (RECORD): a multicentre, randomised, open-label trial, *Lancet* 373(9681):2125–2135, 2009.

79a. Komajda M, McMurray JJ, Beck-Nielsen H, et al: Heart failure events with rosiglitazone in type 2 diabetes: data from the RECORD clinical trial, *Eur Heart J* 31(7):824–831, 2010a.

80. Nesto RW, Bell D, Bonow RO, et al: Thiazolidinedione use, fluid retention, and congestive heart failure: a consensus statement from the American Heart Association and American Diabetes Association. October 7, 2003, *Circulation* 108(23):2941–2948, 2003.

81. Holman RR, Retnakaran R, Farmer A, et al: PROactive study, *Lancet* 367(9504):25–26, 2006, author reply 26-7.

82. Erdmann E, Charbonnel B, Wilcox RG, et al: Pioglitazone use and heart failure in patients with type 2 diabetes and preexisting cardiovascular disease: data from the PROactive study (PROactive 08), *Diabetes Care* 30(11):2773–2778, 2007.

83. Raskin P, Rendell M, Riddle MC, et al: A randomized trial of rosiglitazone therapy in patients with inadequately controlled insulin-treated type 2 diabetes, *Diabetes Care* 24(7):1226–1232, 2001.

84. Ryden L, Thrainsdottir I, Swedberg K: Adjudication of serious heart failure in patients from PROactive, *Lancet* 369(9557):189–190, 2007.

85. Scirica BM, Bhatt DL, Braunwald E, et al: Saxagliptin and cardiovascular outcomes in patients with type 2 diabetes mellitus, *N Engl J Med* 369(14):1317–1326, 2013.

86. Gomez N, Touihri K, Matheeussen V, et al: Dipeptidyl peptidase IV inhibition improves cardiorenal function in overpacing-induced heart failure, *Eur J Heart Fail* 14(1):14–21, 2012.

87. Shigeta T, Aoyama M, Bando YK, et al: Dipeptidyl peptidase-4 modulates left ventricular dysfunction in chronic heart failure via angiogenesis-dependent and -independent actions, *Circulation* 126(15):1838–1851, 2012.

88. Lourenço P, Friões F, Silva N, et al: Dipeptidyl peptidase IV and mortality after an acute heart failure episode, *J Cardiovasc Pharmacol* 62(2):138–142, 2013.

89. Scheen AJ: Cardiovascular effects of gliptins, *Nat Rev Cardiol* 10(2):73–84, 2013.

90. Takahashi A, Asakura M, Ito S, et al: Dipeptidyl-peptidase IV inhibition improves pathophysiology of heart failure and increases survival rate in pressure-overloaded mice, *Am J Physiol Heart Circ Physiol* 304(10):H1361–H1369, 2013.

90a. White WB, Cannon CP, Heller SR, et al: Alogliptin after acute coronary syndrome in patients with type 2 diabetes, *N Engl J Med* 369(14):1327–1335, 2013.

91. DeFronzo RA, Cooke CR, Andres R, et al: The effect of insulin on renal handling of sodium, potassium, calcium, and phosphate in man, *J Clin Invest* 55(4):845–855, 1975.

92. ORIGIN Trial Investigators, Gerstein HC, Bosch J, et al: Basal insulin and cardiovascular and other outcomes in dysglycemia, *N Engl J Med* 367(4):319–328, 2012.

93. Nikolaidis LA, Mankad S, Sokos GG, et al: Effects of glucagon-like peptide-1 in patients with acute myocardial infarction and left ventricular dysfunction after successful reperfusion, *Circulation* 109 (8):962–965, 2004.

94. Nathanson D, Ullman B, Löfström U, et al: Effects of intravenous exenatide in type 2 diabetic patients with congestive heart failure: a double-blind, randomised controlled clinical trial of efficacy and safety, *Diabetologia* 55(4):926–935, 2012.

95. Mundil D, Cameron-Vendrig A, Husain M: GLP-1 receptor agonists: a clinical perspective on cardiovascular effects, *Diab Vasc Dis Res* 9(2):95–108, Apr 2012.

96. Ledwidge M, Gallagher J, Conlon C, et al: Natriuretic peptide-based screening and collaborative care for heart failure: the STOP-HF randomized trial, *JAMA* 310(1):66–74, 2013.

97. Heidenreich PA, Albert NM, Allen LA, et al: Forecasting the impact of heart failure in the United States: a policy statement from the American Heart Association, *Circ Heart Fail* 6(3):606–619, 2013.

98. Hernandez AF: Preventing heart failure, *JAMA* 310(1):44–45, 2013.

26 Treatment of Heart Failure in Diabetes: Systolic Dysfunction, Diastolic Dysfunction, and Post-Acute Coronary Syndrome

John J.V. McMurray, Mark C. Petrie, and B. Miles Fisher

Diabetes and heart failure commonly occur together in a patient.[1] Up to a quarter of patients with diabetes also have heart failure, and approximately a third of patients with heart failure also have diabetes.[1] In this chapter we review the evidence-based medications device, and surgical treatment of heart failure. The primary focus is on patients with chronic heart failure, but when it exists, evidence about the treatment of patients with heart failure, left ventricular (LV) systolic dysfunction, or both after acute myocardial infarction is also reviewed. For each treatment we summarize the evidence base and, when possible, describe whether there is evidence specifically in patients with diabetes. As will become apparent, there is good evidence that the key pharmacologic and device therapies are as beneficial in patients with diabetes as in those without. Consequently, evidence-based guidelines on the treatment of heart failure apply to both those with and those without diabetes.[2]

TREATMENT OF HEART FAILURE IN PATIENTS WITH DIABETES MELLITUS

The landmark clinical trials providing the evidentiary basis for guidelines on the treatment of heart failure included a large proportion of patients with diabetes (**Table 26-1**). Consequently, we can make reasonable assumptions about the efficacy of most of the key treatments based on subgroup analyses. Unfortunately, the evidence base (**Table 26-2**) for patients with and without diabetes is confined to heart failure and reduced ejection fraction (HF-REF), and there is currently no proven treatment for heart failure and preserved ejection fraction (HF-PEF).[2]

Pharmacologic Therapy
Angiotensin-Converting Enzyme Inhibitors
Two key randomized controlled trials (RCTs), the Cooperative North Scandinavian Enalapril Survival Study (CONSENSUS) and the treatment arm of the Studies of Left Ventricular Dysfunction (SOLVD-Treatment) assigned approximately 2800 patients with mild to severely symptomatic heart failure

to placebo or enalapril.[3,4] Most patients were also treated with a diuretic and digoxin, but only approximately 10% of patients in each trial were treated with a beta blocker. In CONSENSUS, which enrolled patients with severely symptomatic heart failure, 53% of patients were treated with spironolactone.[3] Each trial showed that angiotensin-converting enzyme (ACE) inhibitor treatment reduced mortality (relative risk reduction [RRR] 27% in CONSENSUS and 16% in SOLVD-Treatment). In SOLVD-Treatment there was also an RRR of 26% in heart failure hospitalization.[4] The absolute risk reduction (ARR) in mortality in patients with mild to moderately symptomatic heart failure (SOLVD-Treatment) was 4.5%, equating to a number needed to treat (NNT) of 22 to postpone one death (over an average of 41 months).[2] The equivalent figures for severely symptomatic heart failure (CONSENSUS) were 14.6% for ARR and 7 for NNT (over an average of 6 months).[2] These findings are supported by a meta-analysis of smaller, short-term, placebo-controlled trials, which showed a clear reduction in mortality within only 3 months.[5] These trials also showed that ACE inhibitor treatment improves symptoms, quality of life, and functional capacity.

CONSENSUS had too few patients with diabetes (n = 253) to justify subgroup analysis. It is surprising to note that no diabetes subgroup analysis of SOLVD-Treatment has been published. However, the effectiveness of ACE inhibitors in patients with both diabetes and heart failure or postinfarction LV systolic dysfunction has been examined in a large meta-analysis of seven RCTs including SOLVD.[6] Of the 12,586 patients included in that analysis, 2398 had diabetes. For the endpoint of all-cause mortality, ACE inhibitors had a similar treatment benefit in patients with and without diabetes: hazard ratio (HR) 0.84 (95% CI 0.70-1.00) and 0.85 (95% CI 0.78-0.92), respectively.

Although detailed reports of adverse events in SOLVD have been published, these do not describe the subgroup of patients with diabetes.

The only large ACE inhibitor trial in HF-REF (n = 3164 patients) to provide detailed information on patients with diabetes (n = 611) was the Assessment of Treatment with

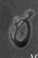
TABLE 26-1 Prevalence of Diabetes Mellitus in Key Trials in Patients with Heart Failure and Reduced Ejection Fraction

	NUMBER OF PATIENTS	PERCENT WITH DIABETES
CONSENSUS[3]	253	23
SOLVD-Treatment[4]	2569	26
CIBIS-2[29]	2647	12
MERIT-HF[31]	3991	24
COPERNICUS[30]	2289	26
SENIORS[32]	2128	26
Val-HeFT[15]	5010	25
CHARM-Alternative[14]	2028	27
CHARM-Added[18]	2548	30
RALES[40]	1663	25
EMPHASIS-HF[41]	2737	31
V-HeFT I	459	21
A-HeFT[46]	1050	41
DIG[52]	6800	28
GISSI-HF[48]	6975	28
SHIFT[47]	6558	31
COMPANION[57]	1520	41
CARE-HF[58]	813	26
MADIT-CRT[63]	1820	30
RAFT[60]	1798	34
SCD-HeFT[53]	1676	31
REMATCH	129	NR
STICH[64]	1212	40
HF-ACTION[66]	2331	32

Lisinopril and Survival (ATLAS) trial, which compared low-dose (2.5 to 5.0 mg daily) with high-dose (32.5 to 35.0 mg daily) lisinopril.[7,8] Overall, this trial showed no difference in the primary outcome of all-cause mortality over the median follow-up of 46 months but did show a significant reduction in a number of other endpoints including the composite of all-cause mortality or hospitalization for heart failure: HR 0.85 (0.78-0.93), $P < 0.001$.[7] These findings, in addition to those of the Heart Failure Endpoint Evaluation of Angiotensin II Antagonist Losartan (HEAAL) trial, discussed later, suggest that higher doses of renin-angiotensin-aldosterone system (RAAS) blockers are better than lower doses.[9] In ATLAS, the greater relative benefit of high-dose lisinopril was similar in patients with and without diabetes, but because patients with diabetes were at greater risk, the absolute benefit of high-dose lisinopril was larger in patients with diabetes (**Figs. 26-1** and **26-2**). Overall, hypotension, renal dysfunction, and hyperkalemia were slightly more frequent in the high-dose group than in the low-dose group, but hypokalemia and cough were less common in the high-dose group.[8] The rate of study drug discontinuation was not greater in the high-dose group (17% versus 18% in the low-dose group). The occurrence of adverse effects with high-dose lisinopril was similar in those with and without diabetes with respect to hypotension and dizziness (35% versus 32%, respectively), renal dysfunction and hyperkalemia (29% versus 22%), and cough (12% versus 10%).[8]

Additional support for the use of ACE inhibitors comes from a trial in patients with a low ejection fraction (EF) but no symptoms of HF ("asymptomatic LV systolic dysfunction")—that is, the prevention arm of SOLVD (SOLVD-Prevention)—and three large (5966 patients in total) placebo-controlled, randomized, outcome trials in patients with heart failure, LV systolic dysfunction, or both after acute myocardial infarction.[10,11]

In the SOLVD-Prevention trial (which randomized 4228 patients with asymptomatic LV systolic dysfunction), there was a 20% RRR in death or heart failure hospitalization.[10] Although 15% of patients in SOLVD-Prevention had diabetes, outcomes in this subgroup were not reported.

In myocardial infarction trials that evaluated captopril (Survival and Ventricular Enlargement [SAVE]), ramipril (Acute Infarction Ramipril Efficacy [AIRE]), and trandolapril (Trandolapril Cardiac Evaluation [TRACE]), there was a 26% RRR in death and a 27% RRR in death or HF hospitalization.[11] The meta-analysis of these trials did not report a subgroup analysis according to baseline diabetes status.

In a subgroup analysis of SAVE, the RRR in all-cause mortality with captopril 50 mg three times daily in patients with diabetes was 12% (-21% to 36%) compared with 20% (2% to 35%) in those without.[12] For the composite outcome of cardiovascular (CV) mortality, heart failure requiring either ACE inhibitor treatment or hospitalization, or the occurrence of recurrent infarction, these reductions were 17% (-6% to 36%) and 26% (12% to 37%), respectively. In a later report describing a multivariable analysis, captopril was reported to decrease all-cause mortality (HR 0.81; 95% confidence interval [CI] 0.68-0.96) as well as CV mortality or morbidity (HR 0.75; 95% CI 0.65-0.86). The benefit of captopril was similar among patients with (HR 0.83; 95% CI 0.63-0.87) and without (HR 0.80; 95% CI 0.64-0.94) diabetes (interaction $P = 0.45$).[13]

Angiotensin Receptor Blockers

More patients were randomized into large angiotensin receptor blocker (ARB) outcome trials than ACE inhibitor trials.

An ARB was examined as an alternative to an ACE inhibitor in the Candesartan in Heart Failure: Assessment of Reduction in Mortality and Morbidity (CHARM-Alternative), which was a placebo-controlled RCT with candesartan in 2028 patients with a left ventricular ejection fraction (LVEF) of 40% or lower who were intolerant of an ACE inhibitor.[14] Treatment with candesartan resulted in an RRR of CV or heart failure hospitalization of 23% (ARR 7%, NNT 14, over 34 months of follow-up). Valsartan was also beneficial in the subset of 366 patients in the Valsartan Heart Failure Trial (Val-HeFT) not treated with an ACE inhibitor.[15] Another trial, the Evaluation of Losartan in the Elderly (ELITE II), failed to show that losartan 50 mg daily was as effective as captopril 50 mg three times daily.[16] However, a subsequent RCT, the HEAAL trial,[9] showed that 150 mg daily of losartan (n = 1927) was superior to 50 mg daily (n = 1919), supporting the similar findings of the ATLAS trial with the ACE inhibitor lisinopril (see earlier).[7] In HEAAL, there was a RRR of 10% in death or HF hospitalization in the high-dose losartan group (P = 0.027) over a median follow-up of 4.7 years.[9]

The efficacy and safety of adding an ARB to an ACE inhibitor has been studied. Two key placebo-controlled RCTs, Val-HeFT[17] and CHARM-Added,[18] randomized approximately 7600 patients with mild to severely symptomatic heart failure to placebo or an ARB (valsartan and candesartan), added to an ACE inhibitor (in 93% of patients in Val-HeFT and all patients

TABLE 26-2 Key Randomized Controlled Trials[a] in Symptomatic Heart Failure with Reduced Ejection Fraction

TREATMENT, TRIAL, AND YEAR PUBLISHED	N	SEVERITY OF HEART FAILURE SYMPTOMS	BACKGROUND TREATMENT[b]	TREATMENT ADDED	TRIAL DURATION (YEARS)	PRIMARY ENDPOINT	RELATIVE RISK REDUCTION (%)[c]	EVENTS PREVENTED PER 1000 PATIENTS TREATED[d]		
								Death	HF Hospitalization	Death or HF Hospitalization
ACE Inhibitors										
CONSENSUS, 1987	253	End stage	Spiro	Enalapril 20 mg bid	0.54[e]	Death	40	146	—	—
SOLVD-T, 1991	2569	Mild to severe	—	Enalapril 20 mg bid	3.5	Death	16	45	96	108
BBs										
CIBIS-2, 1999	2647	Moderate to severe	ACE inhibitor	Bisoprolol 10 mg qd	1.3[e]	Death	34	55	56	—
MERIT-HF, 1999	3991	Mild to severe	ACE inhibitor	Metoprolol CR/XL 200 mg qd	1.0[e]	Death	34	36	46	63
COPERNICUS, 2001	2289	Severe	ACE inhibitor	Carvedilol 25 mg bid	0.87[e]	Death	35	55	65	81
SENIORS, 2005	2128	Mild to severe	ACE inhibitor +spiro	Nebivolol 10 mg qd	1.75	Death or CV hospitalization	14	23	0	—
ARBs										
Val-HeFT, 2001	5010	Mild to severe	ACE inhibitor	Valsartan 160 mg bid	1.9	CV death or morbidity	13	0	35	33[f]
CHARM-Alternative, 2003	2028	Mild to severe	BB	Candesartan 32 mg qd	2.8	CV death or HF hospitalization	23	30	31	60
CHARM-Added, 2003	2548	Moderate to severe	ACE inhibitor+BB	Candesartan 32 mg qd	3.4	CV death or HF hospitalization	15	28	47	39
MRAs										
RALES, 1999	1663	Moderate to severe	ACE inhibitor	Spiro 25-50 mg qd	2.0[e]	Death	30	113	95	—
EMPHASIS-HF, 2011	2737	Mild	ACE inhibitor+BB	Eplerenone 25-50 mg qd	1.75[e]	CV death or HF hospitalization	37	30	64	66
H-ISDN										
V-HeFT-1, 1986	459	Mild to severe	—	Hydralazine 75 mg tid-qid ISDN 40 mg qid	2.3	Death	34	52	0	—
A-HeFT, 2004	1050	Moderate to severe	ACE inhibitor–BB +spiro	Hydralazine 75 mg tid ISDN 40 mg tid	0.83[e]	Composite	—	40	80	—
Digitalis Glycoside										
DIG, 1997	6800	Mild to severe	ACE inhibitor	Digoxin	3.1	Death	0	0	79	73
n-3 PUFA										
GISSI-HF, 2008	6975	Mild to severe	ACE inhibitor–BB– spiro	n-3 PUFA 1 g qd	3.9	Death Death or CV hospitalization	8	—	—	—
CRT										
COMPANION, 2004	925	Moderate to severe	ACE inhibitor+BB +spiro	CRT	1.35[e]	Death or any hospitalization	19	38	—	87
CARE-HF, 2005	813	Moderate to severe	ACE inhibitor+BB +spiro	CRT	2.45	Death or CV hospitalization	37	97	151	184

TABLE 26-2 Key Randomized Controlled Trials[a] in Symptomatic Heart Failure with Reduced Ejection Fraction—cont'd

TREATMENT, TRIAL, AND YEAR PUBLISHED	N	SEVERITY OF HEART FAILURE SYMPTOMS	BACKGROUND TREATMENT[b]	TREATMENT ADDED	TRIAL DURATION (YEARS)	PRIMARY ENDPOINT	RELATIVE RISK REDUCTION (%)[c]	EVENTS PREVENTED PER 1000 PATIENTS TREATED[d]		
								Death	HF Hospitalization	Death or HF Hospitalization
CRT-D										
COMPANION, 2004	903	Moderate to severe	ACE inhibitor+BB +spiro	CRT-ICD	1.35[e]	Death or any hospitalization	20	74	—	114
MADIT-CRT, 2009	1820	Mild	ACE inhibitor+BB +spiro+ICD	CRT-ICD	2.4[e]	Death or HF event[g]	34	5	—	—
RAFT, 2011	1798	Mild to moderate	ACE inhibitor+BB +spiro+ICD	CRT-ICD	3.23	Death or HF hospitalization	25	53	66	70
ICD										
SCD-HeFT, 2005	1676	Mild to severe	ACE inhibitor+BB	ICD	3.8	Death	23	—	—	—
VAD										
REMATCH, 2001	129	End stage	ACE inhibitor +spiro	LVAD	1.8	Death	48	282	—	—
CABG										
STICH, 2011	1212	Mild to severe	ACE inhibitor+BB +spiro	CABG	4.67	Death	14	48	—	63
Exercise Training										
HF-ACTION, 2009	2331	Mild to severe	ACE inhibitor+BB +spiro	Exercise training	2.5	Death or any hospitalization	7	6	—	—

HF hospitalization = patients with at least one hospital admission for worsening HF; some patients had multiple admissions.

ACE = Angiotensin-converting enzyme; ARB = angiotensin receptor blocker; BB = beta blocker; CABG = coronary artery bypass grafting; CR/XL = controlled release/extended release; CRT = cardiac resynchronization therapy (biventricular pacing); CRT-D = CRT device that also defibrillates; CV = cardiovascular; HF = heart failure; H-ISDN = combination of hydralazine and isosorbide dinitrate; ICD = implantable cardioverter defibrillator; ISDN = isosorbide dinitrate; LVAD = left ventricular assist device; n-3 PUFA = omega-3 polyunsaturated fatty acid; MRA = mineralocorticoid receptor antagonist; spiro = spironolactone; VAD = ventricular assist device.

[a]Excluding active controlled trials.

[b]In more than one third of patients: ACE inhibitor+BB means ACE inhibitors used in almost all patients and BB in the majority. Most patients also taking diuretics, and many digoxin (except in DIG). Spironolactone was used at baseline in 5% Val-HeFT, 8% MERIT-HF, 17% CHARM-Added, 19% SCD-HeFT, 20% COPERNICUS, and 24% CHARM-Alternative.

[c]Relative risk reduction in primary endpoint.

[d]Individual trials may not have been designed or powered to evaluate effect of treatment on these outcomes.

[e]Stopped early for benefit.

[f]Primary endpoint also included treatment of HF with intravenous medications for 4 hours or more without admission and resuscitated cardiac arrest (both added small numbers).

[g]Heart failure hospitalization or heart failure treated with intravenous therapy as an out patient.

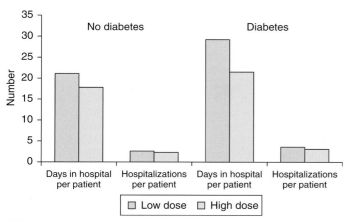

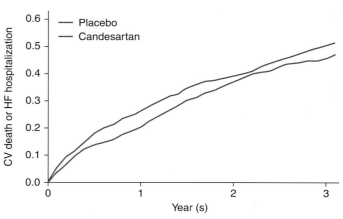

FIGURE 26-1 Effect of high-dose compared with low-dose lisinopril in patients with HF-REF in the ATLAS trial.

FIGURE 26-3 Effect of candesartan compared with placebo in patients with HF-REF and diabetes in the CHARM program: CV mortality or heart failure hospitalization.

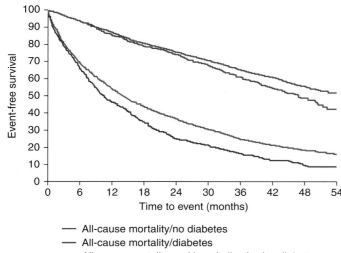

FIGURE 26-2 Effect of high-dose compared with low-dose lisinopril in patients with HF-REF in the ATLAS trial: all-cause mortality and all-cause mortality or hospitalization. Comparison of patients with and without diabetes.

$P<0.001$) and all-cause mortality (HR 0.84; 95% CI 0.79-0.98; $P=0.018$).[19] The effect of treatment was not statistically different in patients with and without diabetes (interaction $P=0.12$). The effect of candesartan in patients with HF-REF and diabetes in the CHARM program is shown in **Figure 26-3**. In Val-HeFT the effect of valsartan was not statistically different in the subgroup of patients with diabetes (interaction P value not provided).

In HEAAL the treatment effect of high-dose compared with low-dose losartan was not different in the subgroup of patients with diabetes (HR 0.96; 95% CI 0.82-1.12; $P=0.35$). However, in all three reports, the point estimate for the HR was less favorable in patients with diabetes than in those without.

There is little information about the tolerability of ARBs in diabetes. In the overall CHARM program, patients with diabetes had double the risk of developing hyperkalemia on candesartan compared with those without diabetes.[20]

Additional support for the use of ARBs comes from the Valsartan in Acute Myocardial Infarction (VALIANT) trial, a trial in which 14,703 patients with heart failure, LV systolic dysfunction, or both after acute myocardial infarction were assigned to treatment with captopril 50 mg three times daily, valsartan 160 mg twice daily, or the combination.[21] Valsartan was found to be noninferior to captopril overall, but combination therapy was not better than monotherapy. The effect of valsartan relative to captopril was not significantly different in patients with and without diabetes, either for all-cause mortality (interaction $P=0.10$) or CV mortality and morbidity (interaction $P=0.12$).

In the Optimal Therapy in Myocardial Infarction with the Angiotensin II Antagonist Losartan (OPTIMAAL) trial,[22] losartan 50 mg once daily did not demonstrate noninferiority when compared with captopril 50 mg three times daily, which, considered in conjunction with the findings of ELITE II and HEAAL, suggests that 50 mg of losartan daily is a suboptimal dose.

Direct Renin Inhibitors

Recently, a third approach to blocking the renin-angiotensin system has been tested in heart failure. In the Aliskiren Trial on Acute Heart Failure Outcomes (ASTRONAUT) trial, patients with an LVEF of 40% or lower, elevated natriuretic peptides, and signs and symptoms of fluid overload who had been admitted on an emergency basis to a hospital for the treatment of heart failure were randomized, when stabilized (a median 5 days after admission), to 12 months of

in CHARM-Added). In addition, approximately a third of patients in Val-HeFT and just over half in CHARM-Added were treated with a beta blocker, but few patients were taking a mineralocorticoid receptor antagonist (MRA). Each of these two trials showed that ARB treatment reduced the risk of heart failure hospitalization (RRR 24% in Val-HeFT and 17% in CHARM-Added). There was a 16% RRR in the risk of CV death with candesartan in CHARM-Added, but CV death was not reduced by valsartan in Val-HeFT.[17,18] The ARR in the primary composite mortality-morbidity endpoint in patients with mild to moderately severe symptoms was 4.4%, equating to an NNT (for an average of 41 months to postpone one event) of 23 in CHARM-Added. The equivalent figures for Val-HeFT were ARR 3.3% and NNT 30 (over an average of 23 months). The CHARM trials and Val-HeFT also showed that ARBs improve symptoms and quality of life. Other trials showed that these agents improve exercise capacity.

Pooling the two CHARM HF-REF trials (CHARM-Alternative and CHARM-Added)[19] showed that treatment with candesartan reduced the risk of CV death or heart failure hospitalization with an HR of 0.82 (95% CI 0.74-0.90, treatment with the direct renin inhibitor (DRI) aliskiren 150 mg daily (increased to 300 mg as tolerated) or placebo daily. The study drug was given in addition to standard therapy, which included diuretics (96%), beta blockers (83%), ACE inhibitors or ARBs (84%), and MRAs (57%). The main endpoint was the composite of CV death or heart failure rehospitalization at 6 months (the main secondary endpoint was this composite at 12 months). In total, 1639 patients were randomized and 1615 patients included in the final efficacy analysis cohort (808 aliskiren, 807 placebo). The mean age was 65 years, LVEF was 28%, and estimated glomerular filtration rate (eGFR) was 67 mL/min/1.73 m^2; 41% of patients had diabetes mellitus. Overall, 24.9% of patients receiving aliskiren (77 CV deaths, 153 HF rehospitalizations) and 26.5% of patients receiving placebo (85 CV deaths, 166 HF rehospitalizations) experienced the primary endpoint at 6 months (HR 0.92, 95% CI 0.76-1.12; $P = 0.41$). At 12 months, the rates were 35.0% for aliskiren (126 CV deaths, 212 HF rehospitalizations) and 37.3% in the placebo group (137 CV deaths, 224 HF rehospitalizations); HR 0.93, 95% CI 0.79-1.09; $P = 0.36$. The rates of hypotension, renal dysfunction, and hyperkalemia were higher in the aliskiren group compared with placebo.

Although there was no evidence for heterogeneity of treatment effect for any subgroup with respect to the primary endpoint, there was a significant interaction between treatment and diabetes status at baseline (patients with diabetes: HR 1.16, 95% CI 0.91-1.47; no diabetes group: HR 0.80, 95% CI 0.64-0.99; $P = 0.03$ for interaction). There was also an interaction for all-cause mortality at 1 year—diabetes patients: HR 1.64, 95% CI 1.15-2.33; no diabetes group: HR 0.69, 95% CI 0.50-0.94; $P = 0.001$ for interaction). Among patients with a history of diabetes, 24.1% of patients died in the aliskiren group compared with 17.4% of patients in the placebo group, whereas the rates of death in patients without diabetes were 15.3% and 20.0% in the two treatment groups, respectively.

Whereas subgroup findings may arise by chance and are normally only considered hypothesis generating, similar findings of increased risks of hypotension, renal dysfunction, and hyperkalemia in the Aliskiren Trial in Type 2 Diabetes Using Cardiorenal Endpoints (ALTITUDE) convinced regulatory agencies to declare that aliskiren is contraindicated in patients with diabetes who are receiving an ARB or ACE inhibitor and in patients with an eGFR below 60 mL/min/1.73 m^2. In Europe this prohibition was extended to monotherapy with aliskiren in patients with diabetes or chronic kidney disease, which resulted in patients with diabetes having study drug discontinued in the ongoing Aliskiren Trial of Minimizing Outcomes for Patients with Heart Failure (ATMOSPHERE) comparing aliskiren (up to 300 mg once daily), enalapril (10 mg twice daily), and the combination of aliskiren and enalapril in over 7000 patients with chronic HF-REF. Despite this, ATMOSPHERE is expected to remain adequately powered and to run to its planned completion.[23-27]

Beta Blockers

There is more evidence showing the benefit of a beta blocker in HF-REF than any other pharmacologic therapy, yet patients with diabetes are less likely to receive this type of treatment than those without diabetes.[28]

Three key trials—the Cardiac Insufficiency Bisoprolol Study II (CIBIS II),[29] Carvedilol Prospective Randomized Cumulative Survival trial (COPERNICUS),[30] and Metoprolol CR/XL Randomised Intervention Trial in Congestive Heart Failure (MERIT-HF)[31]— randomized almost 9000 patients with mild to severely symptomatic heart failure to placebo or a beta blocker (bisoprolol, carvedilol, or metoprolol succinate CR/XL). More than 90% of the patients were on background treatment with an ACE inhibitor or an ARB. Each of these three trials showed that beta blocker treatment reduced mortality (RRR approximately 34% in each trial) and heart failure hospitalization (RRR 28% to 36%) within approximately a year of starting treatment. The ARR in mortality (after 1 year of treatment) in patients with mild to moderate symptoms (CIBIS II and MERIT-HF combined) was 4.3%, equating to an NNT for 1 year to postpone one death of 23. The equivalent figures for severely symptomatic patients (COPERNICUS) were ARR 7.1% and NNT 14. These findings are supported by another placebo-controlled trial, the Study of Effects of Nebivolol Intervention on Outcomes and Rehospitalization in Seniors with Heart Failure (SENIORS)[32] in 2128 elderly (70 years or older) patients, 36% of whom had an EF below 35%. Treatment with nebivolol resulted in an RRR of 14% in the primary composite endpoint of death or CV hospitalization but did not reduce mortality. The findings of these trials are also supported by an earlier program of studies with carvedilol (U.S. carvedilol studies).

Several subgroup analyses from these trials and meta-analyses have shown the efficacy and safety of beta blockers specifically in patients with HF-REF and diabetes. In a meta-analysis of six trials, Haas and colleagues[33] found that beta blocker therapy reduced all-cause mortality in patients with diabetes (n = 3230; HR 0.84, 95% CI 0.73-0.96) and those without diabetes (n = 9899; HR 0.72, 95% CI 0.65-0.79). Shekelle, and colleagues[6] analyzed data from three trials (CIBIS-II, MERIT-HF, and COPERNICUS) that gave a relative risk of 0.77 (95% CI 0.61, 0.96) in patients with diabetes (n = 1883) and 0.65 (95% CI 0.57, 0.74) in patients without diabetes (n = 7042). A third meta-analysis focused on seven trials in which carvedilol was used,[34] including a postinfarction trial, which collectively enrolled 1411 patients with diabetes (24.5% of total patients). In all randomized patients, carvedilol reduced all-cause mortality (RRR 34%, 95% CI 23%-44%; $P < 0.0001$). In patients with diabetes the RRR was 28% (95% CI 3% to 46%; $P = 0.029$), and it was 37% (95% CI 22% to 48%; $P < 0.0001$) in patients without diabetes (interaction $P = 0.25$). The NNT for 1 year to prevent one death was 23 (95% CI 17-36) for all patients, 25 (14-118) in patients with diabetes and 23 (95% CI 17-37) in those without diabetes.

The MERIT-HF investigators published a detailed analysis of both the efficacy and the safety of metoprolol succinate compared with placebo in patients with (n = 985) and without (n = 3006) diabetes.[35] It is important to note that this analysis also reports key nonfatal outcomes (and fatal or nonfatal composites) and shows that these too were reduced by beta blocker therapy in patients with diabetes (**Figs. 26-4** and **26-5**). Patients with diabetes were more likely to experience adverse events (in either treatment group) compared with patients without diabetes. However, patients receiving metoprolol succinate were less likely to experience adverse events than those treated with placebo, both patients with and those without diabetes, and were less likely to discontinue the study drug. The average dose of metoprolol succinate taken during the trial was similar in patients with (162 mg at the last follow-up visit) and without (156 mg) diabetes. There was no difference between metoprolol succinate and placebo in relation to adverse events indicating impaired glycemic control.

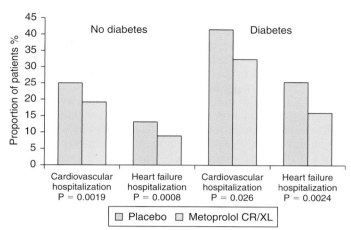

FIGURE 26-4 Effect of metoprolol succinate in patients with HF-REF in the MERIT-HF trial.

Hypoglycemia is a particular concern in patients with diabetes treated with insulin or sulfonylureas. Theoretically, beta blockers could alter awareness of hypoglycemia by decreasing palpitations and tremor and could prolong recovery from hypoglycemia by blocking beta$_2$ receptors, which partly control glucose production in the liver.

However, among patients with diabetes in MERIT-HF, only three (0.6%) in the placebo group and four (0.8%) in the metoprolol succinate group had an adverse event related to hypoglycemia (in each case in patients taking insulin).

Another trial, the Carvedilol or Metoprolol European Trial (COMET),[36,37] showed that carvedilol reduced mortality compared with short-acting metoprolol tartrate (different from the long-acting succinate formulation used in MERIT-HF). In COMET, both patients with and those without diabetes had similar risk reductions for mortality on carvedilol compared with metoprolol: relative risk 0.85, 95% CI 0.69-1.06, $P = 0.147$ for those with diabetes; and RR 0.82, 95% CI 0.71-0.94, $P = 0.006$ for patients without diabetes (interaction $P = 0.77$).

Of note, in a trial in patients with hypertension and diabetes, carvedilol had a favorable effect on glycated hemoglobin (and insulin sensitivity) compared with metoprolol tartrate.[38]

The benefit of beta blockers in heart failure is supported by a placebo-controlled trial in 1959 patients with an LVEF of 40% or lower after acute myocardial infarction—the Carvedilol Post-Infarct Survival Control in Left Ventricular Dysfunction (CAPRICORN) trial,[39] in which the RRR in

mortality with carvedilol was 23% during a mean follow-up of 1.3 years. Among the 437 patients with diabetes in CAPRICORN, the placebo-carvedilol HR for all-cause mortality was 0.93 (95% CI 0.61-1.44) compared with HR 0.71 (95% CI 0.53-0.96) in those without diabetes (n = 1522). The corresponding figures for the composite of death or CV hospitalization were HR 0.88 (95% CI 0.80-1.13) and HR 0.95 (95% CI 0.66-1.16), respectively.

In summary, beta blockers in patients with diabetes and heart failure lead to significant improvements in morbidity and mortality associated with heart failure, benefits that far outweigh the theoretical risks related to hypoglycemia and minor changes in glycated hemoglobin and lipids.

Mineralocorticoid Receptor Antagonists

In the Randomized Aldactone Evaluation Study (RALES),[40] 1663 patients with an EF of 35% or lower and in New York Heart Association (NYHA) functional class III (if in class IV within the past 6 months) or IV were randomized to placebo or spironolactone 25 to 50 mg once daily, added to conventional treatment. When this trial was conducted, beta blockers were not widely used to treat heart failure, and only 11% of patients were treated with a beta blocker. Treatment with spironolactone led to an RRR in all-cause mortality of 30% and an RRR in heart failure hospitalization of 35%. The ARR in mortality (after a mean of 2 years of treatment) was 11.4%, equating to an NNT (for 2 years to postpone one death) of 9. More recently, the Eplerenone in Mild Patients Hospitalization and Survival Study in Heart Failure (EMPHASIS-HF) trial[41] enrolled 2737 patients aged 55 years or older with NYHA functional class II symptoms and an EF of 30% or lower (≤35% if the QRS duration was >130 milliseconds). Patients had to have either a CV hospitalization within the previous 6 months or an elevated plasma natriuretic peptide concentration and to have been treated with an ACE inhibitor, ARB, or both, and a beta blocker. Treatment with eplerenone (up to 50 mg once daily) for an average of 21 months led to a RRR of 37% in CV death or heart failure hospitalization. There were also reductions in the risk of death from any cause (24%), CV death (24%), all-cause hospitalization (23%), and heart failure hospitalization (42%). The ARR in the primary composite mortality-morbidity endpoint was 7.7%, equating to an NNT (for an average of 21 months to postpone one event) of 13. The ARR in all-cause mortality was 3%, equating to an NNT of 33.

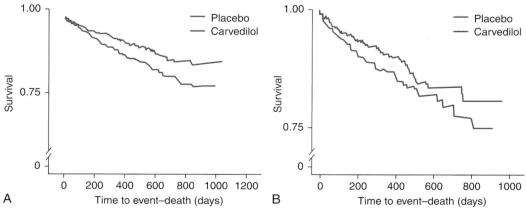

FIGURE 26-5 Effect of carvedilol on all-cause mortality in heart failure patients without (A) and with (B) diabetes.

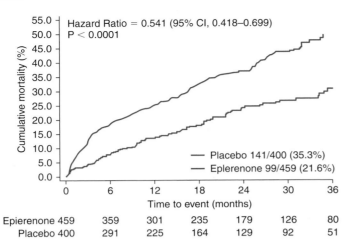

FIGURE 26-6 Effect of eplerenone on all-cause mortality in patients with HF-REF and diabetes in EMPHASIS-HF.

Epierenone 459	359	301	235	179	126	80	
Placebo 400	291	225	164	129	92	51	

In RALES, the mortality benefit was similar in patients with and without diabetes, with HR of 0.70 (95% CI 0.52-0.94) and HR 0.70 (95% CI 0.60-0.82), respectively.[42] In EMPHASIS-HF, the treatment benefit was consistent in patients with and without diabetes (interaction $P=0.10$; **Fig. 26-6**).

The finding that MRAs are beneficial in patients with chronic HF-REF is supported by another trial, the Eplerenone Post–Acute Myocardial Infarction Heart Failure Efficacy and Survival Study (EPHESUS),[43] which enrolled 6632 patients with an EF of 40% or lower and HF or diabetes 3 to 14 days after acute myocardial infarction. Patients were randomized to placebo or eplerenone 25 to 50 mg once daily added to conventional treatment including an ACE inhibitor or ARB and a beta blocker. Treatment with eplerenone reduced all-cause mortality (RR 0.85, 95% CI 0.75-0.96; $P=0.008$), and reduced the rate of the other co-primary endpoint, a composite of death from CV causes or hospitalization for CV events (RR 0.87, 95% CI 0.79-0.95; $P=0.002$).[31]

A subgroup analysis for the 1483 patients with diabetes in EPHESUS has been published.[44] The eplerenone-placebo relative risk of death from any cause in these patients was RR 0.85 (95% CI 0.68-1.05). The relative risk of death from CV causes or hospitalization for CV events was RR 0.83 (95% CI 0.71-0.98).

Hyperkalemia has been a particular concern with MRAs, and it has been suggested that this risk may be greater in patients with diabetes. There was an increase in the incidence of a potassium concentration exceeding 5.5 mmol/L with eplerenone in patients with diabetes—63 (14.1%) compared with 33 (8.5%) on placebo, $P=0.01$. However, the proportion with a serum potassium level above 6.0 mmol/L was not statistically different between the groups (17 [3.8%] compared with 8 [2.1%] on placebo, $P=0.16$), and there was no increase in the rate of discontinuation of eplerenone for hyperkalemia in those with diabetes compared with those without (interaction $P=0.12$). Similar findings we reported in EPHESUS. Among patients with diabetes in EPHESUS, hypoglycemia was reported as an adverse event in 11 patients (1.5%) treated with eplerenone and 11 patients (2.6%) treated with placebo ($P=0.14$).[44]

Some investigators believe that eplerenone may have more favorable metabolic effects than spironolactone in patients with diabetes.[45]

Nitrates and Hydralazine

The African-American Heart Failure Trial (A-HeFT)[46] examined the safety and efficacy of fixed-dose combination therapy with isosorbide dinitrate and hydralazine hydrochloride, added to an ACE inhibitor or ARB, beta blocker, and MRA in African Americans with NYHA class III or IV heart failure.[46] The trial had an unusual composite outcome including survival, hospitalization, and quality of life but was stopped early because treatment with this medication combination led to a 43% reduction in all-cause death (HR 0.57, 95% CI 0.37-0.89; $P=0.01$). There was also a 33% reduction in first hospitalization for heart failure ($P=0.001$). A very large proportion (41%) of patients in the study had diabetes. The treatment effect on mortality was similar in patients with (HR 0.56 [95% CI 0.28-1.15]) and without (HR 0.59 [95% CI 0.34-1.03]) diabetes.

Ivabradine

The Systolic Heart Failure Treatment with the I_f Inhibitor Ivabradine Trial (SHIFT)[47] enrolled 6588 patients in NYHA functional class II to IV, sinus rhythm with a rate of 70 beats/min or greater, and an EF of 35% or lower. Patients were also required to have had an HF hospitalization in the previous 12 months. They were randomized to ivabradine (uptitrated to a maximal dosage of 7.5 mg twice daily) or placebo, added to a diuretic and an ACE inhibitor or ARB, a beta blocker, and an MRA. Only 26% of patients were, however, on full-dose beta blocker. The median follow-up was 23 months. The RRR in the primary composite outcome of CV death or HF hospitalization was 18% (HR 0.82, 95% CI 0.75-0.90; $P<0.0001$); the reduction in CV death (or all-cause death) was not significant, but the RRR in HF hospitalization was 26%. Ivabradine also improved LV function and quality of life. In the 1979 patients with diabetes, the HR for the primary composite endpoint was 0.81 (95% CI 0.69-0.95), and in those without diabetes ($n=4526$) it was 0.83 (95% CI 0.74-0.93).

Omega-3 Polyunsaturated Fatty Acids

The Gruppo Italiano per lo Studio della Sopravvivenza nell'Infarto Miocardico–Heart Failure (GISSI-HF)[48] trial examined the effect of omega-3 polyunsaturated fatty acids (n-3 PUFAs) in 6975 patients with NYHA class II to IV symptoms and an EF of 40% or lower (or if not ≤40%, HF hospitalization in the previous year). Patients were randomized to placebo or 1 g daily of an n-3 PUFA preparation added to background treatment with an ACE inhibitor or ARB beta blocker and an MRA. The median follow-up was 3.9 years; n-3 PUFA treatment led to an hazard reduction of 8% (HR 0.92, 95% CI 0.85-1.00) in the co-primary composite outcome of death or CV hospitalization in an adjusted analysis (adjusted $P=0.009$). There was no reduction in heart failure hospitalization, but there was a 9% RRR in all-cause mortality, the other co-primary endpoint (adjusted $P=0.041$), a 10% RRR in CV mortality (adjusted $P=0.045$), and 7% RRR in CV hospitalization (adjusted $P=0.026$). In patients with diabetes, the HR for the composite outcome of death or CV hospitalization was 0.89 (95% CI 0.80-0.99), and in those without diabetes it was 0.96 (95% CI 0.89-1.04).

The findings in GISSI-HF are supported by one post–myocardial infarction RCT (GISSI-Prevenzione)[49,50] but not by another (OMEGA),[51] although neither of these trials was specifically conducted with patients with LV systolic dysfunction or heart failure. In GISSI-Prevenzione, 11,324 patients enrolled after a recent (within 3 months) myocardial infarction received placebo or 1 g daily of n-3 PUFA. n-3 PUFA reduced the risk of the primary composite outcome of death, myocardial infarction, or stroke by 10% (95% CI 1-18%) by two-way analysis, and by 15% (95% CI 2-26%) by four-way analysis. This benefit was attributable to a decrease in the risk of all-cause mortality (14% [95% CI 3-24%] by two-way analysis, 20% [95% CI 6-33%] by four-way analysis) and CV mortality (17% [95% CI 3-29%] by two-way analysis, 30% [95% CI 13-44%] by four-way analysis). In a follow-up paper, the GISSI-Prevenzione[49,50] investigators reported that the adjusted RR for all-cause mortality in patients with diabetes was 0.72 (95% CI 0.52-0.99) and in those without diabetes RR was 0.82 (95% CI 0.67-1.01), interaction $P=0.50$.

OMEGA randomized 3851 patients 3 to 14 days after acute myocardial infarction to placebo or 1 g n-3 PUFA daily for 1 year.[51] Outcomes did not differ between treatment groups.

Digoxin
A single large morbidity-mortality trial, the Digitalis Investigation Group (DIG) trial,[52] was conducted in 6800 patients with an EF of 45% or lower and in NYHA functional class II to IV. Patients were randomized to placebo or digoxin (mostly 0.25 mg once daily), added to a diuretic and an ACE inhibitor (DIG was performed before beta blockers were widely used for heart failure), and treated for an average of 3 years. Digoxin did not reduce all-cause mortality, the primary endpoint, but did lead to a RRR of 28% (RR 0.72, 95% CI 0.66-0.79; $P<0.001$) in heart failure hospitalization. The ARR was 7.9%, equating to an NNT (for 3 years to postpone one patient admission) of 13. We are not aware of any specific data from randomized trials of digitalis glycosides reporting the effect of treatment separately in patients with diabetes.

Diuretics
Diuretics are usually required to treat the symptoms and signs of fluid overload in patients with heart failure. There are no clinical trials examining their efficacy specifically in patients with both diabetes and heart failure. Theoretically thiazide diuretics can lead to increased insulin resistance and subsequent worsening of glycemic control.

Devices and Surgery
Implantable Cardioverter Defibrillators
Approximately half of the deaths in patients with HF-REF, especially in those with milder symptoms, occur suddenly and are usually caused by a ventricular arrhythmia. Prevention of sudden death is therefore an important goal in HF. Although the key neurohumoral antagonists mentioned earlier reduce the risk of sudden death, they do not abolish it. Antiarrhythmic medications do not decrease this risk at all (and may even increase it). Consequently, implantable cardioverter defibrillator (ICDs) have an important role to play in reducing the risk of death from ventricular arrhythmias either alone or combined with cardiac resynchronization therapy (CRT). An ICD should be considered in any patient with an unprovoked, sustained, symptomatic ventricular arrhythmia.[2] ICDs also have a role in the primary prevention of arrhythmic death. The Sudden Cardiac Death in Heart Failure Trial (SCD-HeFT)[53] enrolled 2521 patients with nonischemic dilated cardiomyopathy or ischemic heart failure, no prior symptomatic ventricular arrhythmia, and an EF of

35% or lower who were in NYHA functional class II or III. These patients were randomized to placebo, amiodarone, or an ICD, in addition to receiving conventional treatment including an ACE or ARB and a beta blocker; MRA use was not reported. ICD treatment led to an RRR in death of 23% (RR 0.77, 95% CI 0.62-0.96; $P=0.007$) over a median follow-up of 45.5 months. Amiodarone did not reduce mortality. The ARR in mortality with an ICD was 6.9%, equating to an NNT (for 45.5 months to postpone one death) of 14.

Use of ICDs in patients with a reduced EF is supported by the findings of the Multicenter Automatic Defibrillator Implantation Trial II (MADIT-II),[54] an RCT in which 1232 patients with a prior myocardial infarction and an EF of 30% or lower (59% of whom were in NYHA class II or III) were assigned to receive either conventional treatment or conventional treatment plus an ICD. Use of an ICD led to a 31% RRR in mortality (HR 0.69, 95% CI 0.51-0.93; $P=0.016$). Two other trials showed no benefit in patients treated with an ICD early (within 40 days) after myocardial infarction. This is why ICD use in patients with coronary heart disease receives level of evidence A in guidelines, but only in patients 40 days or more after acute myocardial infarction. There is less evidence in patients with nonischemic heart failure, with one moderate-sized trial, Defibrillators in Non-Ischemic Cardiomyopathy Treatment Evaluation (DEFINITE, n=458)[55] showing only a nonsignificant trend to a reduction in mortality—hence the evidence level of B in guidelines for patients with nonischemic HF-REF.

The control versus ICD HR in patients with diabetes in SCD-HeFT was 0.95 (95% CI 0.68-1.33), and 0.67 (95% CI 0.50-0.90) in those without. However, in MADIT-II,[56] the HR in patients with diabetes (n=489) was 0.61 (95% CI 0.38-0.98) and in those without diabetes was 0.71 (95% CI 0.49-1.05), with no evidence of interaction.

ICD implantation should be considered only after a sufficient period of optimization of medical therapy (at least 3 months) and only if the EF remains persistently low.

ICD therapy is not indicated in patients in NYHA class IV with severe, medication-refractory symptoms who are not candidates for cardiac resynchronization therapy (CRT), a ventricular assist device, or cardiac transplantation (because such patients have a very limited life expectancy and are more likely to die from pump failure).

Cardiac Resynchronization Therapy
There is little doubt that patients expected to survive with good functional status for longer than 1 year should receive CRT if they are in sinus rhythm, their EF is low ($\leq$30%), the QRS duration is markedly prolonged ($\geq$150 milliseconds), and an electrocardiogram (ECG) shows a left bundle branch morphology, irrespective of symptom severity.[2] There is less consensus about patients with right bundle branch block or interventricular conduction delay (subgroup analyses suggest little benefit or even harm) and those in atrial fibrillation (AF) (because most trials excluded these patients and because a high ventricular rate will prevent resynchronization).[2]

Evidence is available in moderately to severely symptomatic patients. Two key placebo-controlled RCTs—the Comparison of Medical Therapy, Pacing, and Defibrillation in Heart Failure (COMPANION) trial[57] and the Cardiac Resynchronization in Heart Failure (CARE-HF) study[58]—randomized 2333 patients with moderate to severely symptomatic HF (NYHA class III or IV) to either optimal medical therapy or optimal medical therapy plus CRT. Patients in

COMPANION were required to be in sinus rhythm, to have an EF of 35% or lower, to have a QRS duration of at least 120 milliseconds, and to have had a heart failure hospitalization or the equivalent in the preceding year. Patients in CARE-HF were required to be in sinus rhythm and to have an EF of 35% or lower, a QRS duration of 120 milliseconds or longer (if the QRS duration was 120 to 149 milliseconds, other echocardiographic criteria for dyssynchrony had to be met), and an LV end-diastolic dimension of at least 30 mm (indexed to height). Each of these two trials showed that CRT reduced the risk of death from any cause and hospital admission for worsening heart failure—an RRR in death of 24% with a CRT-pacemaker (CRT-P) and of 36% with a CRT-defibrillator (CRT-D) in COMPANION and of 36% with CRT-P in CARE-HF. In CARE-HF, the RRR in HF hospitalization with CRT-P was 52%. The ARR with CRT-D in the composite outcome of CV death or CV hospitalization in COMPANION was 8.6%, equating to an NNT (over a median duration of follow-up of approximately 16 months) to postpone one event of 12. The corresponding figures for CRT-P in CARE-HF (over a mean follow-up of 29 months) were an ARR of 16.6% and an NNT of 6. These trials also showed that CRT improves symptoms, quality of life, and ventricular function. Other trials showed that these devices improve exercise capacity. A subgroup analysis according to diabetes status has been published from both trials (see later).

Evidence is also available in mild to moderately symptomatic patients. Two key placebo-controlled RCTs randomized 3618 patients with mild symptoms (MADIT-CRT[59]—15% NYHA class I and 85% NYHA class II) or moderate symptoms (the Resynchronization-Defibrillation for Ambulatory Heart Failure Trial [RAFT][60]—80% NYHA class II and 20% NYHA class III) to either optimal medical therapy plus an ICD, or optimal medical therapy plus CRT-D. Patients in MADIT-CRT were required to have an EF of 30% or lower, to have a QRS duration of 130 milliseconds of longer, and to be in sinus rhythm. Patients in RAFT were required to have an EF of 30% or lower and a QRS duration of 120 milliseconds or longer (13% of enrolled patients had AF with a well-controlled ventricular rate). Each of these two trials showed that CRT reduced the risk of the primary composite endpoint of death or heart failure hospitalization ("heart failure event" in MADIT-CRT)—RRR of 34% in MADIT-CRT and 25% in RAFT. There was a 25% reduction in all-cause mortality in RAFT ($P = 0.003$), but mortality was not reduced in MADIT-CRT. It is important to note that these benefits were in addition to those gained from conventional treatment, including a diuretic, digoxin, an ACE inhibitor, a beta blocker, an MRA, and an ICD. The ARR in the primary composite mortality-morbidity endpoint in MADIT-CRT was 8.1%, equating to an NNT (for an average of 2.4 years to postpone one event) of 12. The equivalent figures for RAFT were ARR 7.1% and NNT 14 (over an average of 40 months). These trials also showed that CRT improves symptoms, quality of life, and ventricular function. Both MADIT-CRT and RAFT showed a significant treatment-by-subgroup interaction whereby QRS duration modified the treatment effect (CRT appeared more effective in patients with a QRS of 150 milliseconds or longer), and patients with left bundle branch block also seemed to obtain more benefit than those with right bundle branch block or an interventricular conduction defect.

The COMPANION, CARE-HF, and MADIT-CRT investigators have each published subgroup analyses in relation to the baseline diabetes status of the patients in their trials.

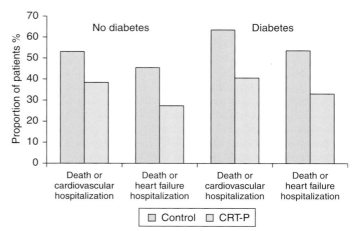

FIGURE 26-7 Effect of CRT in patients with HF-REF in the CARE-HF trial.

In the two trials in patients with moderate to severe symptoms, CRT was at least as effective in reducing death and hospitalization in patients with diabetes as in those without (**Fig. 26-7**). In particular, among patients with diabetes, CRT reduced the risk of death from any cause by 37% in COMPANION.[61] In COMPANION, CRT also improved 6-minute walk distance, NYHA class, and quality-of-life score (all significantly), compared with optimal medical therapy, in patients with diabetes. Similar benefits were reported in CARE-HF.[62]

There were 552 patients with diabetes, HF-REF, a QRS duration of 130 milliseconds or longer, and mild symptoms in MADIT-CRT.[63] CRT-D treatment, compared with optimal medical therapy and an ICD, led to a significant reduction in the risk of the primary endpoint of death from any cause or a heart failure event in patients with diabetes (adjusted HR 0.56, 95% CI 0.40-0.79; $P < 0.001$) and in those without (0.67, 95% CI 0.51-0.87; $P = 0.003$). The unadjusted Kaplan-Meier estimate of the NNT over 2 years to prevent one death or heart failure event was 6.9 (95% CI 4.5-15.0%) for patients with diabetes compared with 17.5% (10.0-73.5%) for patients without diabetes ($P = 0.054$).

Although not published as a separate paper, subgroup analysis of RAFT showed that the benefit of CRT-D was similar in patients with and without diabetes.[60]

Patients with diabetes did not experience a higher rate of complications related to device implantation, including infection. There were similar CRT-related improvements in LV volumes and EF in those with and without diabetes.

Coronary Artery Bypass Grafting

Coronary revascularization, preferably surgical revascularization (see also **Chapter 18**), is indicated for the relief of angina pectoris in patients with HF-REF (and HF-PEF) and diabetes. Surgical coronary revascularization is indicated for prognostic reasons in other patients with severe coronary artery disease (CAD), particularly those with three-vessel disease or left main coronary artery stenosis.[2] The detailed indications for coronary revascularization are covered elsewhere (see **Chapters 17** and **18**). This section focuses on recent developments relevant to heart failure.

The Surgical Treatment for Ischemic Heart Failure (STICH)[64] trial addressed the broader role of surgical revascularization in patients with HF-REF and less severe CAD. Patients with an EF of 35% or lower and CAD who were suitable for surgery were randomized to coronary artery bypass grafting (CABG) plus medical therapy or medical therapy alone. The patients enrolled were young (average age 60 years), predominantly male (88%), and in NYHA class I (11%), II (52%), or III (34%). Their Canadian Cardiovascular Society angina class was 0 in 36%, I in 16%, II in 43%, III in 4%, and IV in 1%. Most patients had two-vessel (31%) or three-vessel (60%) CAD, and 68% had a severe proximal left anterior descending coronary artery stenosis; very few (2%) had a left main coronary artery stenosis. The primary outcome (all-cause death) was not reduced by CABG. CABG did, however, reduce the secondary outcomes of CV death (RRR 19%) and death from any cause or CV hospitalization (RRR 26%).

The STICH investigators reported a subgroup analysis by diabetes status for the outcome of death from any cause. For the 478 patients with diabetes, the control versus CABG HR was 0.92 (95% CI 0.70-1.22), and for the 734 patients without diabetes HR was 0.83 (95% CI 0.65-1.05); interaction $P=0.6$.

This trial may therefore extend the indication for CABG to "STICH-like" patients with two-vessel CAD, including a left anterior descending coronary artery stenosis, who are otherwise suitable for surgery and expected to survive for longer than 1 year with good functional status. Many physicians and surgeons also assess "myocardial viability" in addition to coronary anatomy before making a decision about the potential benefits and risks of coronary revascularization (see **Chapters 17** and **18**).

Ventricular Assist Devices and Transplantation

Microvascular complications other than nonproliferative retinopathy are usually considered a relative contraindication to both cardiac transplantation and mechanical circulatory support.[65,66] Patients with advanced diabetes have poorer long-term survival than other candidates for transplantation, and this also seems to be the case with mechanical circulatory support. Good glycemic control (glycated hemoglobin below 7.5%) should be established before surgery.[65,66]

EXERCISE PRESCRIPTION

Meta-analyses of small studies have shown that physical conditioning by exercise training improves exercise tolerance and health-related quality of life and possibly reduces hospitalization in patients with heart failure. A single large trial—Heart Failure: A Controlled Trial Investigating Outcomes of Exercise Training (HF-ACTION)[66]—investigated the effects of exercise training in 2331 relatively young (mean age 59 years) medically stable patients with mild to moderately severe symptoms (NYHA class II 63% and class III 35%) and an EF of 35% or lower. The intervention comprised 36 supervised sessions in the initial 3 months followed by home-based training.[67] The median follow-up was 30 months. In an adjusted analysis, exercise training led to a 7% unadjusted ($P=0.13$) and 11% adjusted ($P=0.03$) reduction in the primary composite outcome of all-cause mortality or all-cause hospitalization. There was also a 13% unadjusted ($P=0.06$) and 15% adjusted ($P=0.03$) RRR in a secondary composite outcome of CV death or heart failure hospitalization. There was no reduction in mortality, and there were no safety concerns. Adherence to exercise declined substantially after the period of supervised training.

Collectively, the evidence suggests that physical training is beneficial in heart failure, although typical elderly patients were not enrolled in many studies and the optimum exercise

prescription is uncertain. Furthermore, the only large trial, HF-ACTION, showed a borderline treatment effect that was obtained only with a very intensive intervention that may not be practical to deliver in every center.

Although 32% of patients in HF-ACTION had diabetes, the effect of the intervention has not been reported in this subgroup.

TREATMENT OF DIABETES IN PATIENTS WITH HEART FAILURE

The overall goal of glucose management is to prevent the development of microvascular and macrovascular complications while avoiding treatment side effects. Control of glycemia is more effective at reducing microvascular than macrovascular complications. Current guidelines focus on multiple risk factor modification to reduce global CV risk, with lifestyle modification and pharmacologic therapy to improve glycemic control. Most clinical trials examining the pharmacologic treatment of diabetes have disappointingly excluded patients with heart failure. Our knowledge of the treatment of diabetes in heart failure is limited to that extrapolated from trials in patients with diabetes but without heart failure or from observational studies.

There are a number of different classes of glucose-lowering medications, each with a different mechanism of action. Initial treatment of diabetes is with lifestyle modification plus medication monotherapy. Patients who fail to reach glycemic targets are moved on to two medication combinations, then three medication combinations, then more complex insulin regimens. Heart failure is an insulin-resistant state, and control of glycemia can be very difficult. Patients may not respond to oral glucose-lowering medications and even large doses of insulin may result in only limited reductions in glycemia. We will deal with each of the main medication classes in turn and summarize the current evidence for each in patients with heart failure.

Metformin

Though it previously was, metformin is a biguanide. It appears to mediate its effect on blood glucose via a number of different mechanisms: reducing hepatic gluconeogenesis, increasing insulin sensitivity, increasing peripheral glucose uptake, and decreasing gut absorption of glucose. Metformin is considered first-line therapy in patients with diabetes, particularly in obese patients, because it slightly reduces weight, and in a small subgroup of the United Kingdom Prospective Diabetes Study (UKPDS) it was associated with a reduction in myocardial infarctions when started as initial monotherapy.[68,69]

Though it previously was, metformin is no longer contraindicated in patients with heart failure (see also **Chapter 17**). In 2006, the U.S. Food and Drug Administration (FDA) withdrew its previous recommendation that metformin should not be used in patients with heart failure, allowing product label modification for all metformin products. Metformin had been a victim of unwarranted "guilt by association." An earlier member of the biguanide family called *phenformin* was withdrawn from the market in the 1970s following its association with lactic acidosis. Two large observational studies in patients with heart failure and diabetes and one meta-analysis demonstrated no link between metformin and lactic acidosis.[70–74]

There is no large RCT examining the use of metformin in patients with diabetes and heart failure. Observational studies suggest benefit rather than harm. Two large retrospective cohort studies in the United States and Canada have examined the use of metformin in patients with both diabetes and heart failure.[72,74] Both used multivariable analyses to adjust for confounding variables. The Canadian cohort study examined outcomes in 1833 patients and demonstrated that use of metformin either as monotherapy or combined with a sulfonylurea was associated with a lower 1-year mortality when compared with sulfonylurea monotherapy.[72] The U.S. study examined 16,417 people hospitalized with heart failure. In that study, use of metformin was associated with a lower 1-year mortality when compared with treatment with insulin or sulfonylurea (24.7% versus 36%, $P < 0.0001$).[74] Metformin was also associated with a lower all-cause hospitalization and heart failure hospitalization. The use of metformin in diabetic patients with heart failure has been associated with better outcomes in several other cohort studies from the United States, the United Kingdom, Spain, and Denmark.[70-74]

Although metformin is no longer considered to be contraindicated in patients with heart failure, there are still certain patient subgroups in whom its use is contraindicated (see also **Chapter 17**).[75,76] It should not be used in patients at increased risk of developing lactic acidosis—that is, those with significant renal dysfunction (e.g., as suggested by serum creatinine levels ≥ 1.5 mg/dL in men or ≥ 1.4 mg/dL in women or reduced creatinine clearance) or in patients with acute heart failure or myocardial infarction, shock, or sepsis. If a patient is admitted to the hospital with acute heart failure, metformin should be temporarily withheld until his or her condition has stabilized.

Although metformin does not appear to be harmful in patients with heart failure and may even be associated with mortality benefit, we must stress that this impression is solely based on observational studies, which are often misleading. It is possible that metformin could simply have been a marker for patients with less severe disease. Despite this caveat, for all patients with type 2 diabetes, whether or not that patient has heart failure, metformin should be considered as the first-line medication to treat hyperglycemia. In routine clinical practice, however, its use is limited by a high incidence of gastrointestinal side effects.

Sulfonylureas

Sulfonylureas act by increasing insulin release from the beta cells of the pancreas (see also **Chapter 17**). Because heart failure is an insulin-resistant state, this is not an attractive method of achieving blood glucose control, as it may have limited efficacy. Despite this, sulfonylureas remain the most commonly prescribed glucose-lowering medications in patients with heart failure.

No randomized trial has examined the use of a sulfonylurea in patients with both heart failure and diabetes. Existing evidence is primarily from retrospective cohort studies, and this does not suggest that sulfonylureas are harmful in patients with heart failure. A large retrospective observational U.S. cohort study involving more than 16,000 patients with diabetes and heart failure found no link between sulfonylurea use and mortality (HR 0.99 (95% CI 0.91-1.08).[74] A Canadian retrospective cohort study of patients with diabetes and heart failure compared metformin use with sulfonylurea use.[72] One-year mortality in patients treated with

metformin was lower than in patients treated with sulfonylureas (adjusted HR 0.66 (95% CI 0.44-0.97). This suggests that use of a sulfonylurea should be considered only if metformin is contraindicated or not tolerated, or when being given in combination with metformin.

Thiazolidinediones

Thiazolidinediones (TZDs) are peroxisome proliferator-activated receptor gamma (PPAR-γ) agonists (see also **Chapter 17**). They improve insulin sensitivity, lipid profile, and blood glucose control. They cause weight gain and fluid retention by increasing fluid reabsorption in the renal collecting duct, which is of concern for patients with heart failure. This is particularly seen when TZDs are used in conjunction with insulin. In patients with diabetes, it has also been suggested that rosiglitazone may increase the risk of myocardial infarction, although this association has not been proven definitively.[72] Several RCTs, cohort studies, and meta-analyses have demonstrated that TZDs increase the incidence of fluid retention and heart failure in patients with diabetes.[77-79] The extent to which TZDs cause simple fluid retention or symptomatic heart failure is not clear from the literature. Most of the trials did not measure LV function or natriuretic peptides prospectively. Randomized trials suggest that although TZDs have no effect on LV function they may be associated with an increase in B-type natriuretic peptide.[80,81] It is likely that at least in a proportion of patients, TZDs cause fluid retention that converts a patient with subclinical LV dysfunction into one with symptomatic heart failure.

Most RCTs examining the safety and efficacy of TZDs in diabetes have excluded patients with heart failure. A systematic review and meta-analysis on the subject suggests that treatment with TZDs leads to an increased risk of heart failure hospitalization (pooled odds ratio 1.13 (95% CI 1.04-1.22]).[82] In the Rosiglitazone Evaluated for Cardiovascular Outcomes in Oral Agent Combination Therapy for Type 2 Diabetes (RECORD) trial, heart failure hospitalization in the rosiglitazone group had the same adverse prognostic consequence as in the placebo group.[78]

According to the FDA, TZDs are contraindicated in patients with symptomatic heart failure (NYHA III or IV). Caution is also advised in their use in patients with NYHA class I or II heart failure. Our view is that these agents should not be used in patients with heart failure or LV systolic dysfunction.

Insulin

Insulin is indicated when oral treatments have failed to provide adequate glycemic control (see also **Chapter 17**). Insulin has been shown to dilate arteries in skeletal muscle in patients with heart failure, so some have postulated that it may be an attractive glucose-lowering medication for this patient group. Insulin, however, causes weight gain and increases sodium retention, which is a concern, and there are occasional case reports of heart failure in patients starting insulin treatment. However, the CV safety of insulin glargine was tested in the recent Outcome Reduction with Initial Glargine Intervention (ORIGIN) trial in people aged 50 years or older with impaired fasting glucose, impaired glucose tolerance, or early type 2 diabetes in addition to other CV risk factors. Overall, 88% of patients in ORIGIN had diabetes and their condition had been present for a mean duration of

5.4 years; 6% had a new diagnosis and 23% were receiving no pharmacologic therapy before randomization. The median trial follow-up was 6.2 years. The rate of hospital admission for heart failure was 0.85/100 patient-years in the insulin group compared with 0.95/100 patient-years in the control group. Although these findings are reassuring, patients in ORIGIN had diabetes for a relatively short duration (or no diabetes at all), and those with longer-duration diabetes are at greater risk of heart failure and may be at greater risk of medication-induced heart failure.[83]

No large RCT has specifically examined the effect of insulin in patients with heart failure. Several post hoc analyses from clinical trials and cohort studies have identified that patients treated with insulin are at greater risk of death than patients treated with other glucose-lowering medications.[84,85] It is likely that insulin is a marker for diabetes of greater duration and the presence of extensive macrovascular disease rather than insulin being directly responsible for this association.

Despite the association of insulin with poorer outcomes in patients with heart failure, this does not mean that insulin should not be used. Prospective trials would be welcome.

Modulators of the Incretin System

In recent years a large number of new compounds have been developed for the treatment of diabetes (see also Chapter 17). For patients with both heart failure and diabetes, the most interesting group of compounds consists of modulators of the incretin system. Incretins are gut peptides excreted in response to a meal that act to reduce postprandial hyperglycemia. Glucagon-like peptide 1 (GLP-1) is an incretin peptide that stimulates insulin secretion by the beta cells of the pancreas in a glucose-dependent fashion—that is, it stimulates insulin secretion only if blood glucose crosses a threshold level. It also acts to decrease glucagon secretion, delay gastric emptying, and suppress appetite. Patients with type 2 diabetes have reduced GLP-1 secretion in response to a meal. Incretin peptides are rapidly broken down in the body by dipeptidyl peptidase 4 (DPP-4). Currently available compounds acting on the incretin system are the oral inhibitors of DPP-4, sitagliptin, vildagliptin, saxagliptin, alogliptin, and linagliptin, which act to increase endogenous GLP-1, and injectable GLP-1 receptor agonists exenatide, liraglutide, albiglutide, and lixisenatide. DPP-4 inhibitors and GLP-1 receptor agonists reduce hemoglobin A1c (HbA1c) without increasing the risk of hypoglycemia and are generally well tolerated by patients. GLP-1 receptor agonists appear to be marginally more efficacious at reducing HbA1c and have the added benefit of promoting weight loss, whereas DPP-4 inhibitors are weight neutral.

Modulators of the incretin system are of particular interest in patients with heart failure, given the potentially beneficial effects of GLP-1 on the CV system. Small studies in both animals and humans with heart failure indicate that short-term treatment with GLP-1 can lead to improvements in ventricular function and hemodynamics.[86] In one recent small study, 6 hours of intravenous exenatide increased cardiac index, reduced pulmonary capillary wedge pressure, and was reasonably well tolerated in patients with type 2 diabetes and congestive heart failure (CHF) (NYHA class III or IV).[87] It should be noted, however, that heart rate increased with exenatide, generally an unfavorable finding in heart failure.

The first long-term outcome study with an incretin-based therapy used the DPP-4 inhibitor saxagliptin. The Saxagliptin

Assessment of Vascular Outcomes Recorded in Patients with Diabetes Mellitus–Thrombolysis In Myocardial Infarction 53 (SAVOR-TIMI 53) trial randomized 16,492 patients with type 2 diabetes and established CV disease, or risk factors for CV disease, who were followed for a median of 2.1 years. Compared with placebo, saxagliptin increased the risk of hospitalization for heart failure (3.5% versus 2.8%, $P = 0.007$). More details regarding the type of heart failure patients developed and the outcomes in these patients are awaited.[88] A second trial, Examination of Cardiovascular Outcomes with Alogliptin Versus Standard of Care in Patients with Type 2 Diabetes Mellitus and Acute Coronary Syndrome (EXAMINE), evaluated the CV safety of a second DPP-4 inhibitor in patients with type 2 diabetes and a recent acute coronary syndrome. In EXAMINE, patients were randomly assigned to receive alogliptin or placebo in addition to standard-of-care medications for diabetes and CV disease. A total of 5380 patients were followed for a median of 18 months. Although the occurrence of heart failure was not reported in the primary publication from this trial, data on this outcome were presented at the 2013 congress of the European Association for the Study of Diabetes.[89] The composite outcome of CV death or heart failure hospitalization occurred in 201 alogliptin-treated patients (7.4%) and 201 placebo patients (7.5%) (HR 0.98, 95% CI 0.82-1.20). The components of this composite (first events only) included 95 CV deaths (3.5%) and 106 heart failure hospitalizations (3.9%) in the alogliptin group and 112 (4.2%) and 89 (3.3%), respectively, in the placebo group (CV death HR 0.84, 95% CI 0.64-1.10; and heart failure hospitalization HR 1.19, 95% CI 0.90-1.58). Although even less is known about heart failure in this trial, the HR and 95% CI for heart failure hospitalization appear consistent with the findings of SAVOR-TIMI 53.

Whether this completely unexpected finding reflects the play of chance, is medication specific, is a DPP-4 class-effect, or even is an issue for other incretin-based therapies (e.g., GLP-1 analogues) is unknown at this point. The findings are clearly at odds with the observation that heart failure is characterized by high DPP-4 activity and that reducing this activity with DPP-4 inhibitors has beneficial effects in experimental models of heart failure. Clearly, much more information is needed on the safety of incretin-based therapies in patients with diabetes and heart failure.[90-94]

Other Glucose-Lowering Medications

Alpha-glucosidase inhibitors inhibit the enteric enzyme alpha-glucosidase, preventing the breakdown of complex carbohydrates to glucose (see also Chapter 17). This leads to a reduction in blood glucose levels. They are associated with modest reductions in HbA1c, and the reduction in glycemia is less than with other medication classes. They can be used as monotherapy or in combination with other glucose-lowering medications. Frequent gastrointestinal side effects limit the use of these medications in the United States and Europe, but they are widely used in Asia. There is no evidence available examining their pros and cons in patients with diabetes and heart failure.

A sustained-release formulation of bromocriptine has been approved for use in diabetes by the FDA. The mechanism of reduction in HbA1c is not well understood; the medication may act centrally to reduce insulin resistance. In a 1-year safety study it was demonstrated to reduce CV events.[95] Exclusion criteria included NYHA class III or IV heart failure, and separate data have not been provided for patients with heart failure at baseline. The number of total events in the study was small, and the findings require confirmation in a longer study.

Colesevelam, a bile acid sequestrant, is associated with modest reductions in HbA1c and so far has limited use as a treatment for type 2 diabetes. Pramlintide, an amylin mimetic, is an injected therapy that reduces glucagon secretion in type 1 diabetes and has to given along with insulin. Reductions in HbA1c are also modest, with nausea and vomiting as side effects, and overall use has been limited. There are no specific data on use in diabetic patients with heart failure for either of these treatments.

Sodium-glucose cotransporter 2 (SGLT-2) inhibitors are a new class of medications that inhibit the reabsorbtion of glucose in the kidney, promoting glycosuria. This leads to a decrease in blood glucose levels and a reduction in weight. A slight reduction in blood pressure has been observed and may be related to renal sodium loss. These agents can be used as monotherapy or in combination with other glucose-lowering medications including in combination with insulin. There is currently no evidence available examining their pros and cons in patients with diabetes and heart failure. Theoretically, the slight loss of fluid might improve symptoms of heart failure, whereas caution might be required in fluid-depleted patients.

Intensity of Glucose-Lowering

Three large clinical trials set out to address whether or not more intensive glycemic control versus contemporary standard care would reduce the risk of CV events in patients with type 2 diabetes, and their results have recently been published: ACCORD (Action to Control Cardiovascular Risk in Diabetes), ADVANCE (Action in Diabetes and Vascular Disease: Preterax and Diamicron Modified Release Controlled Evaluation), and VADT (Veteran Affairs Diabetes Trial) (see also **Chapter 17**).[96-98] All three studies demonstrated that intensive reduction of HbA1c (to levels below currently recommended) did not translate into reductions of CV outcomes. In fact, ACCORD was stopped early because of an excess number of deaths in the intensive therapy group. How does this new evidence apply to patients with both heart failure and diabetes? It should be noted that few patients in these studies had heart failure; in ACCORD only 4.8% had a history of heart failure. Also, the pharmacologic strategies used in these studies may not have been the ideal choice for heart failure patients; in the ACCORD trial there was very high use of TZDs, and in the ADVANCE trial there was much greater use of insulin sulfonylureas than metformin. Meta-analysis of intensive glycemic control has shown no impact on the risk of heart failure in type 2 diabetes, but longer studies or follow-up may be required to show reductions in heart failure outcomes, and off-target effects of the treatments used, such as fluid retention with TZDs,[98] may have offset beneficial effects of improved glycemic control. Prospective clinical trials in patients with both diabetes and heart failure, using agents with favorable CV risk profiles, are warranted.

SUMMARY

The evidence presented here regarding the treatment of diabetes in patients with heart failure must not be over-interpreted. These results are not based on evidence from randomized controlled trials specifically designed to assess outcomes in patients with diabetes and heart failure. They are predominantly based on data from retrospective cohort studies. From the available evidence, metformin appears to be the initial glucose-lowering medication of choice in patients with type 2 diabetes and heart failure. After metformin, physicians must weigh the pros and cons of alternative agents and tailor therapy to the individual. The future may be brighter for glucose management, with many new agents in development. Some of these are reported to have beneficial effects on myocardial metabolism. The FDA now requires these new agents to undergo rigorous prospective assessment to ensure CV safety.

Large numbers of patients worldwide have both diabetes and heart failure. The two conditions when present together lead to significantly increased morbidity and mortality. Unfortunately, most clinical trials examining diabetic treatments have excluded patients with heart failure. The management of diabetes in patients with heart failure must follow standard guidelines for both heart failure and diabetes. Physicians must be aware that metformin is not contraindicated in patients with heart failure, and it should be considered as first-line therapy. Clinical trials examining the safety and efficacy of novel glucose-lowering agents in patients with heart failure are under way.

REFERENCES

1. MacDonald MR, Petrie MC, Hawkins NM, et al: Diabetes, left ventricular systolic dysfunction and chronic heart failure, *Eur Heart J* 29:1224–1240, 2008.
2. McMurray JJV, Adamopoulos S, Anker SD, et al: ESC guidelines for the diagnosis and treatment of acute and chronic heart failure 2012; The Task Force for the Diagnosis and Treatment of Acute and Chronic Heart Failure 2012 of the European Society of Cardiology. Developed in collaboration with the Heart Failure Association (HFA) of the ESC, *Eur J Heart Fail* 14:803–869, 2012.
3. The CONSENSUS Trial Study Group: Effects of enalapril on mortality in severe congestive heart failure- results of the Cooperative North Scandinavian Enalapril Survival Study (CONSENSUS), *N Engl J Med* 316:1429–1435, 1987.
4. The SOLVD Investigators: Effect of enalapril on survival in patients with reduced left ventricular ejection fractions and congestive heart failure, *N Engl J Med* 325:293–302, 1991.
5. Garg R, Yusuf S, for the Collaborative Group on ACE Inhibitor Trials: Overview of randomized trials of angiotensin-converting enzyme inhibitors on mortality and morbidity in patient with heart failure, *JAMA* 273:1450–1456, 1995.
6. Shekelle PG, Rich MW, Morton SC, et al: Efficacy of angiotensin-converting enzyme inhibitors and beta-blockers in the management of left ventricular systolic dysfunction according to race, gender, and diabetic status. A meta-analysis of major clinical trials, *J Am Coll Cardiol* 41:1529–1538, 2003.
7. Packer M, Poole-Wilson PA, Armstrong PW, et al: on behalf of the ATLAS Study Group: Comparative effects of low and high doses of the angiotensin-converting enzyme inhibitor, lisinopril, on morbidity and mortality in chronic heart failure. ATLAS Study Group, *Circulation* 100:2312–2318, 1999.
8. Ryden L, Armstrong PW, Cleland JGF, et al: on behalf of the ATLAS Study Group: Efficacy and safety of high-dose lisinopril in chronic heart failure patients at high cardiovascular risk, including those with diabetes mellitus. Results from the ATLAS trial, *Eur Heart J* 21:1967–1978, 2000.
9. Konstam MA, Neaton JD, Dickstein K, et al: for the HEAAL Investigators: Effects of high-dose versus low-dose losartan on clinical outcomes in patients with heart failure (HEAAL study): a randomised, double-blind trial, *Lancet* 374:1840–1848, 2009.
10. The SOLVD Investigators: Effect of enalapril on mortality and the development of heart failure in asymptomatic patients with reduced left ventricular ejection fractions, *N Engl J Med* 327:685–691, 1992.
11. Flather MD, Yusuf S, Kober L, et al: for the ACE-Inhibitor Myocardial Infarction Collaborative Group: Long-term ACE-inhibitor therapy in patients with heart failure or left-ventricular dysfunction: a systematic overview of data from individual patients. ACE-Inhibitor Myocardial Infarction Collaborative Group, *Lancet* 355:1575–1581, 2000.
12. Moye LA, Pfeffer MA, Wun CC, et al: for the SAVE investigators: Uniformity of captopril benefit in the SAVE Study: subgroup analysis. Survival and Ventricular Enlargement Study, *Eur Heart J* 15 (Suppl):2–8, 1994.
13. Murcia AM, Hennekens CH, Lamas GA, et al: Impact of diabetes on mortality in patients with myocardial infarction and left ventricular dysfunction, *Arch Intern Med* 164:2273–2279, 2004.
14. Granger CB, McMurray JJ, Yusuf S, et al: Effects of candesartan in patients with chronic heart failure and reduced left-ventricular systolic function intolerant to angiotensin-converting-enzyme inhibitors: the CHARM-Alternative trial, *Lancet* 362:772–776, 2003.
15. Maggioni AP, Anand I, Gottlieb SO, et al: On behalf of the Val-HeFT Investigators: Effects of valsartan on morbidity and mortality in patients with heart failure not receiving angiotensin-converting enzyme inhibitors, *J Am Coll Cardiol* 40:1414–1421, 2002.
16. Pitt B, Poole-Wilson PA, Segal R, et al: Effect of losartan compared with captopril on mortality in patients with symptomatic heart failure: randomised trial—the Losartan Heart Failure Survival Study ELITE II, *Lancet* 355:1582–1587, 2000.
17. Cohn JN, Tognoi G: Valsartan Heart Failure Trial Investigators: A randomized trial of the ARB valsartan in chronic heart failure, *N Engl J Med* 345:1667–1675, 2001.
18. McMurray JJ, Ostergren J, Swedberg K, et al: Effects of candesartan in patients with chronic heart failure and reduced left-ventricular systolic function taking angiotensin-converting-enzyme inhibitors: the CHARM-Added trial, *Lancet* 362:767–771, 2003.
19. Young JB, Dunlap ME, Pfeffer MA, et al: for the Candesartan in Heart failure Assessment of Reduction in Mortality and morbidity (CHARM) Investigators and Committees: Mortality and morbidity reduction with Candesartan in patients with chronic heart failure and left ventricular systolic dysfunction: results of the CHARM low-left ventricular ejection fraction trials, *Circulation* 110:2618–2626, 2004.

20. Desai AS, Swedberg K, McMurray JJV, et al: on behalf of the CHARM Program Investigators: Incidence and predictors of hyperkalemia in patients with heart failure: an analysis of the CHARM Program, *J Am Coll Cardiol* 50:1959–1966, 2007.
21. Pfeffer MA, McMurray JJV, Velazquez EJ, et al: for the Valsartan in Acute Myocardial Infarction Trial Investigators: *N Engl J Med* 349:1893–1906, 2003.
22. Dickstein K, Kjekshus J: Effects of losartan and captopril on mortality and morbidity in high-risk patients after acute myocardial infarction: the OPTIMAAL randomised trial. Optimal Trial in Myocardial Infarction with Angiotensin II Antagonist Losartan, *Lancet* 360:752–760, 2002.
23. Krum H, Massie B, Abraham WT, et al: ATMOSPHERE Investigators: Direct renin inhibition in addition to or as an alternative to angiotensin converting enzyme inhibition in patients with chronic systolic heart failure: rationale and design of the Aliskiren Trial to Minimize OutcomeS in Patients with HEart failuRE (ATMOSPHERE) study, *Eur J Heart Fail* 13:107–114, 2011.
24. McMurray JJ, Abraham WT, Dickstein K, et al: Aliskiren, ALTITUDE, and the implications for ATMOSPHERE, *Eur J Heart Fail* 14:341–343, 2012.
25. Parving HH, Brenner BM, McMurray JJ, et al: ALTITUDE Investigators: Cardiorenal end points in a trial of aliskiren for type 2 diabetes, *N Engl J Med* 367:2204–2213, 2012.
26. Maggioni AP, Greene SJ, Fonarow GC, et al: ASTRONAUT Investigators and Coordinators: Effect of aliskiren on post-discharge outcomes among diabetic and non-diabetic patients hospitalized for heart failure: insights from the ASTRONAUT trial, *Eur Heart J* 34:3117–3127, 2013.
27. Gheorghiade M, Böhm M, Greene SJ, et al: ASTRONAUT Investigators and Coordinators: Effect of aliskiren on postdischarge mortality and heart failure readmissions among patients hospitalized for heart failure: the ASTRONAUT randomized trial, *JAMA* 309:1125–1135, 2013.
28. Gupta R, Tang WH, Young JB: Patterns of beta-blocker utilization in patients with chronic heart failure: experience from a specialized outpatient heart failure clinic, *Am Heart J* 147:79–83, 2004.
29. The Cardiac Insufficiency Bisoprolol Study II (CIBIS-II): a randomised trial, *Lancet* 353:9–13, 1999.
30. Packer M, Fowler MB, Roecker EB, et al: Effect of carvedilol on the morbidity of patients with severe chronic heart failure: results of the carvedilol prospective randomized cumulative survival (COPERNICUS) study, *Circulation* 106:2194–2199, 2002.
31. Effect of metoprolol CR/XL in chronic heart failure: Metoprolol CR/XL Randomised Intervention Trial in Congestive Heart Failure (MERIT-HF), *Lancet* 353:2001–2007, 1999.
32. Flather MD, Shibata MC, Coats AJ, et al: Randomized trial to determine the effect of nebivolol on mortality and cardiovascular hospital admission in elderly patients with heart failure (SENIORS), *Eur Heart J* 26:215–225, 2005.
33. Haas SJ, Vos T, Gilbert RE, Krum H: Are β-blockers as efficacious in patients with diabetes mellitus as in patients without diabetes mellitus who have chronic heart failure: a meta-analysis of large-scale clinical trials, *Am Heart J* 146:848–853, 2003.
34. Bell DS, Lukas MA, Holdbrook FK, et al: The effect of carvedilol on mortality risk in heart failure patients with diabetes: results of a meta-analysis, *Curr Med Res Opin* 22:287–296, 2006.
35. Deedwania PC, Giles TD, Klibaner M, et al: on behalf of the MERIT-HF Study Group: Efficacy, safety and tolerability of metoprolol CR/XL in patients with diabetes and chronic heart failure: experiences from MERIT-HF, *Am Heart J* 149:159–167, 2005.
36. Poole-Wilson PA, Swedberg K, Cleland JG, et al: Comparison of carvedilol and metoprolol on clinical outcomes in patients with chronic heart failure in the Carvedilol Or Metoprolol European Trial (COMET): randomised controlled trial, *Lancet* 362:7–13, 2003.
37. Torp-Pedersen C, Metra M, Charlesworth A, et al: for the COMET investigators: Effects of metoprolol and carvedilol on pre-existing and new onset diabetes in patients with chronic heart failure: data from the Carvedilol Or Metoprolol European Trial (COMET), *Heart* 93:968–973, 2007.
38. Bakris GL, Fonseca V, Katholi RE, et al: for the GEMINI Investigators: Metabolic effects of carvedilol vs metoprolol in patients with type 2 diabetes mellitus and hypertension: a randomized controlled trial, *JAMA* 292:2227–2236, 2004.
39. Dargie HJ: Effect of carvedilol on outcome after myocardial infarction in patients with left-ventricular dysfunction: the CAPRICORN randomised trial, *Lancet* 357:1385–1390, 2001.
40. Pitt B, Zannad F, Remme WJ, et al: The effect of spironolactone on morbidity and mortality in patients with severe heart failure. Randomized Aldactone Evaluation Study Investigators, *N Engl J Med* 341:709–717, 1999.
41. Zannad F, McMurray JJ, Krum H, et al: Eplerenone in patients with systolic heart failure and mild symptoms, *N Engl J Med* 364:11–21, 2011.
42. Pitt B, Perez A, et al: for the Randomized Aldactone Evaluation Study Investigators: Spironolactone in patients with heart failure, *N Engl J Med* 342:132–134, 2000.
43. Pitt B, Remme W, Zannad F, et al: for the Eplereonone Post-Acute Myocardial Infarction Heart Failure Efficacy and Survival Study Investigators: *N Engl J Med* 348:1309–1321, 2003.
44. O'Keefe JH, Abuissa H, Pitt B: Eplerenone improves prognosis in postmyocardial infarction diabetic patients with heart failure: results from EPHESUS, *Diabetes Obes Metabol* 10:492–497, 2008.
45. Yamaji M, Tsutamoto T, Kawahara C, et al: Effect of eplerenone versus spironolactone on cortisol and hemoglobin A1(c) levels in patients with chronic heart failure, *Am Heart J* 160:915–921, 2010.
46. Taylor AL, Ziesche S, Yancy C, et al: Combination of isosorbide dinitrate and hydralazine in blacks with heart failure, *N Engl J Med* 351:2049–2057, 2004.
47. Swedberg K, Komajda M, Bohm M, et al: Ivabradine and outcomes in chronic heart failure (SHIFT): a randomised placebo-controlled study, *Lancet* 376:875–885, 2010.
48. Gissi-HF Investigators, Tavazzi L, Maggioni AP, et al: Effect of rosuvastatin in patients with chronic heart failure (the GISSI-HF trial): a randomised, double-blind, placebo-controlled trial, *Lancet* 372:1231–1239, 2008.
49. Dietary supplementation with n-3 polyunsaturated fatty acids and vitamin E after myocardial infarction: results of the GISSI-Prevenzione trial. Gruppo Italiano per lo Studio della Sopravvivenza nell'Infarto miocardico, *Lancet* 354:447–455, 1999.
50. Marchioli R, Marfisi RM, Borrelli G, et al: Efficacy of n-3 polyunsaturated fatty acids according to clinical characteristics of patients with recent myocardial infarction: insights from the GISSI-Prevenzione trial, *J Cardiovasc Med* 8(Suppl 1):S34–S37, 2007.
51. Rauch B, Schiele R, Schneider S, et al: OMEGA, a randomized, placebo-controlled trial to test the effect of highly purified omega-3 fatty acids on top of modern guideline-adjusted therapy after myocardial infarction, *Circulation* 122:2152–2159, 2010.
52. The DIGITALIS Investigation Group: The effect of digoxin on mortality and morbidity in patients with heart failure, *N Engl J Med* 336:525–533, 1997.
53. Bardy GH, Lee KL, Mark DB, et al: for the Sudden Cardiac Death in Heart Failure (SCD-HeFT) Investigators: Amiodarone or an implantable cardioverter-defibrillator for congestive heart failure, *N Engl J Med* 352:225–237, 2005.
54. Moss AJ, Zareba W, Hall WJ, et al: For the Multicenter Automatic Defibrillator Implantation Trial II Investigators: Prophylactic implantation of a defibrillator in patients with myocardial infarction and reduced ejection fraction, *N Engl J Med* 346:877–883, 2002.
55. Kadish A, Dyer A, Daubert JP, et al: for the Defibrillators in Non-Ischemic Cardiomyopathy Treatment Evaluation (DEFINITE) Investigators: *N Engl J Med* 350:2151–2158, 2004.
56. Wittenberg SM, Cook JR, Hall WJ, et al: for the Multicenter Automatic Defibrillator Implantation Trial: Comparison of efficacy of implanted cardioverter-defibrillator in patients with versus without diabetes mellitus, *Am J Cardiol* 96:417–419, 2005.
57. Bristow MR, Saxon LA, Boehmer J, et al: Comparison of Medical Therapy, Pacing, and Defibrillation in Heart Failure (COMPANION) Investigators: Cardiac-resynchronization therapy with or without an implantable defibrillator in advanced chronic heart failure, *N Engl J Med* 350:2140–2150, 2004.
58. Cleland JG, Daubert JC, Erdmann E, et al: Cardiac Resynchronization-Heart Failure (CARE-HF) Study Investigators: The effect of cardiac resynchronization on morbidity and mortality in heart failure, *N Engl J Med* 352:1539–1549, 2005.
59. Moss AJ, Hall WJ, Cannom DS, et al: MADIT-CRT Trial Investigators: Cardiac-resynchronization therapy for the prevention of heart-failure events, *N Engl J Med* 361:1329–1338, 2009.
60. Tang ASL, Wells GA, Talajic M, et al: for the Resynchronization-Defibrillation for Ambulatory Heart Failure Trial (RAFT) Investigators: *N Engl J Med* 363:2385–2395, 2010.
61. Ghali JK, Boehmer J, Feldman AM, et al: Influence of diabetes on cardiac resynchronization therapy with or without defibrillator in patient with advanced heart failure, *J Card Fail* 13:769–773, 2007.
62. Hoppe UC, Freemantle N, Cleland JGF, et al: Effect of cardiac resynchronization on morbidity and mortality of diabetic patients with severe heart failure, *Diabetes Care* 30:722–724, 2007.
63. Martin DT, McNitt S, Nesto RW, et al: Cardiac resynchronization therapy reduces the risk of cardiac events in patients with diabetes enrolled in the multicenter automatic defibrillator implantation trial with cardiac resynchronization therapy (MADIT-CRT), *Circ Heart Fail* 4:332–338, 2011.
64. Jones RH, Velazquez EJ, Michler RE, et al: STICH Hypothesis 2 Investigators. Coronary bypass surgery with or without surgical ventricular reconstruction, *N Engl J Med* 360:1705–1717, 2009.
65. Feldman D, Pamboukian SV, Teuteberg JJ, et al: The 2013 International Society for Heart and Lung Transplantation Guidelines for mechanical circulatory support: executive summary, *J Heart Lung Transplant* 32:157–187, 2013.
66. Mehra MR, Kobashigawa J, Starling R, et al: Listing criteria for heart transplantation: International Society for Heart and Lung Transplantation guidelines for the care of cardiac transplant candidates–200, *Listing J Heart Lung Transplant* 25:1024–1042, 2006.
67. O'Connor CM, Whellan DJ, Lee KL, et al: HF-ACTION Investigators: Efficacy and safety of exercise training in patients with chronic heart failure: HF-ACTION randomized controlled trial, *JAMA* 301:1439–1450, 2009.
68. Effect of intensive blood-glucose control with metformin on complications in overweight patients with type 2 diabetes (UKPDS 34). UK Prospective Diabetes Study (UKPDS) Group, *Lancet* 352:854–865, 1998.
69. Holman RR, Paul SK, Bethel MA, et al: 10-year follow-up of intensive glucose control in type 2 diabetes, *N Engl J Med* 359:1577–1589, 2008.
70. Eurich DT, Weir DL, Majumdar SR, et al: Comparative safety and effectiveness of metformin in patients with diabetes and heart failure: systematic review of observational studies involving 34000 patients, *Circ Heart Fail* 2013 Mar 18, [Epub ahead of print].
71. MacDonald MR, Eurich DT, Majumdar SR, et al: Treatment of type 2 diabetes and outcomes in patients with heart failure: a nested case-control study from the UK. General Practice Research Database, *Diabetes Care* 33:1213–1218, 2010.
72. Eurich DT, Majumdar SR, McAlister FA, et al: Improved clinical outcomes associated with metformin in patients with diabetes and heart failure, *Diabetes Care* 28:2345–2351, 2005.
73. Andersson C, Olesen JB, Hansen PR, et al: Metformin treatment is associated with a low risk of mortality in diabetic patients with heart failure: a retrospective nationwide cohort study, *Diabetologia* 53:2546–2553, 2010.
74. Massoudi FA, Inzucchi SE, Wang Y, et al: Thiazolidinediones, metformin, and outcomes in older patients with diabetes and heart failure: an observational study, *Circulation* 111:583–590, 2005.
75. Eurich DT, Majumdar SR, McAlister FA, et al: Changes in labelling for metformin use in patients with type 2 diabetes and heart failure: documented safety outweighs theoretical risks, *Open Med* 5:e22–e24, 2011.
76. Inzucchi SE, Masoudi FA, McGuire DK, et al: Metformin in heart failure, *Diabetes Care* 30:e129, 2007.
77. Home PD, Pocock SJ, Beck-Nielsen H, et al: RECORD Study Team: Rosiglitazone evaluated for cardiovascular outcomes in oral agent combination therapy for type 2 diabetes (RECORD): a multicentre, randomised, open-label trial, *Lancet* 373:2125–2135, 2009.
78. Komajda M, McMurray JJ, Beck-Nielsen H, et al: Heart failure events with rosiglitazone in type 2 diabetes: data from the RECORD clinical trial, *Eur Heart J* 31:824–831, 2010.
79. Erdman E, Charbonnel B, Wilcox RG, et al: PROactive investigators: Pioglitazone use and heart failure in patients with type 2 diabetes and preexisting cardiovascular disease: data from the PROactive study (PROactive 08), *Diabetes Care* 30:2773–2778, 2007.
80. Dargie HJ, Hildebrandt PR, Riegger GA, et al: A randomized, placebo-controlled trial assessing the effects of rosiglitazone on echocardiographic function and cardiac status in type 2 diabetic patients with New York Heart Association Functional Class I or II Heart Failure, *J Am Coll Cardiol* 49:1696–1704, 2007.
81. Giles TD, Miller AB, Elkayam U, et al: Pioglitazone and heart failure: results from a controlled study in patients with type 2 diabetes mellitus and systolic dysfunction, *J Card Fail* 14:445–452, 2008.
82. Lago RM, Singh PP, Nesto RW: Congestive heart failure and cardiovascular death in patients with prediabetes and type 2 diabetes given thiazolidinediones: a meta-analysis of randomised clinical trials, *Lancet* 370:1129–1136, 2007.
83. ORIGIN Trial Investigators, Gerstein HC, Bosch J, et al: Basal insulin and cardiovascular and other outcomes in dysglycemia, *N Engl J Med* 367:319–328, 2012.
84. Smooke S, Horwich TB, Fonarow GC: Insulin-treated diabetes is associated with a marked increase in mortality in patients with advanced heart failure, *Am Heart J* 149:168–174, 2005.
85. Pocock SJ, Wang D, Pfeffer MA, et al: Predictor of mortality and morbidity in patients with chronic heart failure, *Eur Heart J* 27:65–75, 2006.
86. Khan MA, Deaton C, Rutter MK, et al: Incretins as a novel therapeutic strategy in patients with diabetes and heart failure, *Heart Fail Rev* 18:141–148, 2013.
87. Nathanson D, Ullman B, Lufstrom U, et al: Effects of intravenous exenatide in type 2 diabetic patients with congestive heart failure: a double-blind, randomised controlled clinical trial of efficacy and safety, *Diabetologia* 55:926–935, 2012.
88. Scirica BM, Bhatt DL, Braunwald E, et al: SAVOR-TIMI 53 Steering Committee and Investigators: Saxagliptin and cardiovascular outcomes in patients with type 2 diabetes mellitus, *N Engl J Med* 369:1317–1326, 2013.
89. White WB, Cannon CP, Heller SR, et al: EXAMINE Investigators: Alogliptin after acute coronary syndrome in patients with type 2 diabetes, *N Engl J Med* 369:1327–1335, 2013.
90. Dos Santos L, Salles TA, Arruda-Junior DF, et al: Circulating dipeptidyl peptidase IV activity correlates with cardiac dysfunction in human and experimental heart failure, *Circ Heart Fail* 6:1029–1038, 2013.
91. Lourenço P, Friões F, Silva N, et al: Dipeptidyl peptidase IV and mortality after an acute heart failure episode, *J Cardiovasc Pharmacol* 62:138–142, 2013.
92. Shigeta T, Aoyama M, Bando YK, et al: Dipeptidyl peptidase-4 modulates left ventricular dysfunction in chronic heart failure via angiogenesis-dependent and -independent actions, *Circulation* 126:1838–1851, 2012.
93. Gomez N, Touihri K, Matheeussen V, et al: Dipeptidyl peptidase IV inhibition improves cardiorenal function in overpacing-induced heart failure, *Eur J Heart Fail* 14:14–21, 2012.
94. Takahashi A, Asakura M, Ito S, et al: Dipeptidyl-peptidase IV inhibition improves pathophysiology of heart failure and increases survival rate in pressure-overloaded mice, *Am J Physiol Heart Circ Physiol* 304:H1361–H1369, 2013.
95. Gaziano JM, Cincotta AH, Vinik A, et al: Effect of bromocriptine-QR (a quick-release formulation of bromocriptine mesylate) on major adverse cardiovascular events in type 2 diabetes subjects, *J Am Heart Assoc* 1(5):e002279, 2012. http://dx.doi.org/10.1161/JAHA.112.002279.
96. ADVANCE Collaborative Group, Patel A, MacMahon S, et al: Intensive blood glucose control and vascular outcomes in patients with type 2 diabetes, *N Engl J Med* 358:2560–2572, 2008.
97. Duckwork W, Abraira C, Moritz T, et al: VADT Investigators: Glucose control and vascular complications in veterans with type 2 diabetes, *N Engl J Med* 360:129–139, 2009.
98. Castagno D, Baird-Gunning J, Jhund PS, et al: Intensive glycemic control has no impact on the risk of heart failure in type 2 diabetic patients: evidence from a 37,229 patient meta-analysis, *Am Heart J* 162:938–948, 2011.

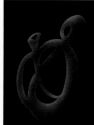

PART VI

OTHER DIABETES-RELATED CARDIOVASCULAR CONSIDERATIONS

27 Peripheral Artery Disease in Diabetes

Neil J. Wimmer and Joshua A. Beckman

Peripheral artery disease (PAD) is generally defined as partial or complete obstruction of one or more arteries affecting the lower extremities and is usually caused by atherosclerosis. Symptoms of PAD include pain with ambulation, resulting from an inadequate blood supply relative to demand in the lower extremities, termed *intermittent claudication*. In severe cases, symptoms occur at rest and tissue ischemia may lead to ulceration or amputation. PAD may also be asymptomatic, but the association of PAD with other comorbid cardiovascular disease often results in an increased risk of mortality. Patients with diabetes are among those most likely to develop PAD and also among those most likely to develop complications resulting from both disease processes.

This chapter provides a framework for the diagnosis and management of patients with PAD, focusing on the overlap and special characteristics of patients with concomitant diabetes.

EPIDEMIOLOGY AND PROGNOSIS OF PERIPHERAL ARTERY DISEASE AND DIABETES—OVERLAPPING EPIDEMICS

The reported prevalence of PAD varies as a function of the population tested, the diagnostic method used, and whether symptoms are included to derive estimates. The ankle-brachial index (ABI) is the most commonly used noninvasive measurement in epidemiologic studies and is described in more detail later. The ABI is the ratio of the ankle to the brachial systolic blood pressure. For intermittent claudication, prevalence estimates range from below 2% to as high as 12%, whereas rates of noninvasively defined disease based on the ABI range from 3% to 33%.[1,2] The prevalence of PAD increases with age, with rates of approximately 4% documented in those 40 years and older compared with rates of 13% to

15% among those 65 years of age and older[3-5] (**Fig. 27-1**). Only a small proportion of those with ABI-defined PAD have claudication, with estimates ranging from approximately 10% to 30%. The prevalence of PAD increases with age[3,6] (**Fig. 27-2**). There is less information about the true incidence of critical limb ischemia or amputation, but estimates suggest that 400 to 450 individuals per million population are affected with ischemia and approximately 112 to 250 individuals per million population require amputation.[6]

Major risk factors for PAD overlap with, but are not identical to, those for coronary artery disease (CAD) and cerebrovascular disease. It is important to note that diabetes, smoking, older age, elevated triglyceride concentrations, and elevated systolic blood pressure are particularly potent risk factors for PAD.[5] Data from the National Health and Nutrition Examination Survey (NHANES) suggest that cigarette smoking and diabetes are the most potent risk factors associated with the development of PAD, with odds ratios for the development of PAD of 4.5 and 2.7, respectively. In the Framingham study, the presence of diabetes increased the risk of intermittent claudication by 3.5-fold in men and 8.6-fold in women.[7] Even in those without frank diabetes, insulin resistance has also been linked to the development of PAD.[8]

The duration and severity of diabetes correlates with the incidence and extent of PAD. In a prospective cohort study, Al-Delaimy and colleagues[9] found a strong association between the duration of diabetes and the risk of developing PAD. The association was particularly strong among men with hypertension or who were current smokers. Adler and colleagues[10] estimated the prevalence of PAD up to 18 years after the diagnosis of diabetes in almost 5000 patients from the United Kingdom Prospective Diabetes Study (UKPDS). They demonstrated a higher prevalence of PAD in those with a longer duration of diabetes. The degree of diabetic glycemic control is an independent risk factor for PAD; with every 1%

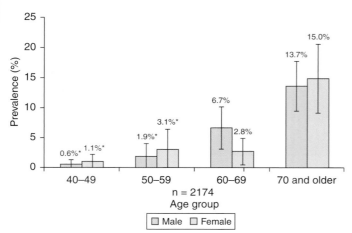

FIGURE 27-1 PAD prevalence and age from the National Health and Nutrition Examination Survey (NHANES).[5] *(Modified from Selvin E, Erlinger TP: Prevalence of and risk factors for peripheral arterial disease in the United States: results from the National Health and Nutrition Examination Survey, 1999-2000, Circulation 110:738-743, 2004.)*

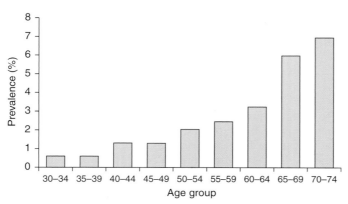

FIGURE 27-2 The prevalence of claudication with age. From TransAtlantic Inter-Society Consensus Document on Management of Peripheral Arterial Disease II (TASC II).[6] *(Modified from Norgren L, Hiatt WR, Dormandy JA, et al: Inter-society Consensus for the Management of Peripheral Arterial Disease [TASC II], Eur J Vasc Endovasc Surg 2007;33[Suppl 1]:S1-S75, 2007.)*

increase in glycosylated hemoglobin (HbA1c), the risk of PAD has been shown to increase by 28%.[11]

Furthermore, patients with diabetes and PAD are more likely to present with an ischemic ulcer or gangrene than patients without diabetes, increasing the risk of lower-extremity amputation.[12] Faglia and colleagues observed a positive trend between PAD severity and amputation rates in patients with diabetes.[13] Individuals with diabetes are approximately 15 times more likely to have an amputation than those without diabetes,[14] and an annual amputation incidence rate of 0.6% has been reported in diabetic patients.[15,16] Patients with diabetes often have extensive and severe PAD and a greater propensity for arterial calcification.[17,18] Involvement of the femoral and popliteal arteries often resembles that of nondiabetics, but distal disease affecting the tibial and peroneal arteries occurs more frequently in diabetics.[12]

CLINICAL PRESENTATION, DIAGNOSIS, AND NATURAL HISTORY OF PERIPHERAL ARTERY DISEASE IN DIABETES

The hallmark features of clinical PAD include intermittent claudication and rest pain. The location of the symptoms

often relates to the site of the most proximal stenosis. In general, buttock, hip, or thigh claudication typically occurs in patients with aortic or iliac stenoses. Calf claudication characterizes femoral or popliteal involvement. Ankle or foot claudication occurs in patients with tibial or peroneal disease. Claudication symptoms should be brought on by exertion and should resolve within minutes after cessation of effort. Leg pain that occurs at rest, such as nocturnal cramping in the calf or thigh, should not be confused with claudication.

Symptoms may occur at rest in patients with critical limb ischemia. Typically, patients complain of paresthesias or pain in the foot or toes of the affected limb. This discomfort worsens with limb elevation and often improves when the limb is lowered, as would be expected because of the increased perfusion pressure to the distal limb by the effect of gravity. The pain can be particularly severe at sites of skin breakdown, and often the skin is exquisitely sensitive to light touch. These symptoms may be absent, however, in diabetic patients with significant peripheral neuropathy, who may have important limb ischemia but experience few symptoms.

A complete cardiovascular physical examination is necessary to detect all the findings of PAD in diabetic patients. Pulse abnormalities and bruits increase the likelihood of PAD.[19] The legs of patients with chronic aortoiliac disease may demonstrate muscular atrophy. Hair loss, thick or brittle toenails, and smooth and shiny skin on the legs can also indicate PAD. Patients with severe limb ischemia often have cool skin and may have petechiae, cyanosis or pallor, dependent rubor, skin fissures, ulceration, or gangrene. Ulcers that result from PAD often have a pale base with irregular borders and usually involve the tips of the toes, the heel of the foot, or other sites that bear chronic pressure (**Fig. 27-3**). Overall, physical examination has a low sensitivity but high specificity for PAD.[20]

The clinical stage of symptomatic PAD can be classified according to the Fontaine or Rutherford scoring systems.[6,21] Fontaine stage I represents those who have PAD but are asymptomatic. Stages IIa and IIb include patients with mild and moderate-to-severe intermittent claudication. Patients with ischemic rest pain are classified as stage III, and those with ulceration or gangrene are stage IV. In the Rutherford classification, asymptomatic patients are classified as category 0. Patients with mild claudication are category 1. Patients with moderate claudication are category 2, and patients with severe claudication are category 3. Patients

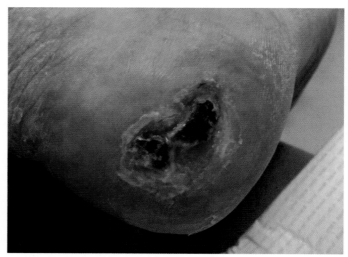

FIGURE 27-3 A typical nonhealing arterial ulcer.

TABLE 27-1 Clinical Classification Schemes for Peripheral Artery Disease

FONTAINE CLASSIFICATION		RUTHERFORD CLASSIFICATION		
Stage	Clinical Description	Grade	Category	Clinical Description
I	Asymptomatic	0	0	Asymptomatic
IIa	Mild claudication	I	1	Mild claudication
IIb	Moderate-to-severe claudication	I I	2 3	Moderate claudication Severe claudication
III	Rest pain	II	4	Rest pain
IV	Ulceration or gangrene	III IV	5 6	Minor tissue loss Ulceration or gangrene

Data from White CJ, Gray WA: Endovascular therapies for peripheral arterial disease: an evidence-based review, *Circulation* 116:2203-2215, 2007.

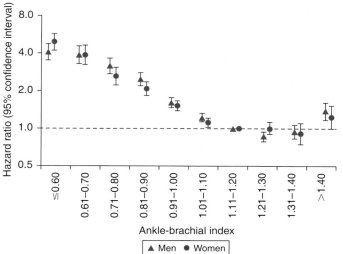

FIGURE 27-4 Ankle-brachial index (ABI) and overall mortality in men and women.[127] *(Modified from Fowkes FG, Murray GD, Butcher I, et al: Ankle brachial index combined with Framingham risk score to predict cardiovascular events and mortality: a meta-analysis, JAMA 300:197-208, 2008.)*

with rest pain are category 4. Patients with minor tissue loss, ulceration, or gangrene are categories 5 and 6 (**Table 27-1**).

The main reasons to diagnose PAD in diabetic individuals are to initiate therapies that decrease the risk of atherothrombotic events, to improve the overall quality of life, and to decrease disability. A diagnosis of PAD indicates the presence of systemic atherosclerosis that confers additional cardiovascular risk to the patient with diabetes, which gives further impetus to aggressively manage vascular risk factors in this high-risk group. Although the physical examination provides important information, additional noninvasive testing is necessary to ensure the diagnosis of PAD. The ABI is a reproducible and reasonably accurate measurement for the detection of PAD. The American Heart Association recently published a consensus scientific statement regarding use of the ABI and suggested standard definitions and interpretation.[22] As mentioned earlier, the ABI is defined as the ratio of the ankle systolic blood pressure divided by the brachial systolic blood pressure. The ABI is normally between 1.00 and 1.40.[22,23] In PAD, the ankle systolic blood pressure is less than the brachial systolic blood pressure, and the ABI is reduced to below 1.00. PAD is defined as an ABI of 0.90 or lower, with values from 0.91 to 1.00 classified as borderline.[22,24] Lower ABI values indicate more severe PAD. Patients with symptoms of leg claudication often have ABIs from 0.5 to 0.8, and patients with critical limb ischemia usually have an ABI below 0.5. The ABI has been shown to correlate inversely with walking distance and walking speed (**Fig. 27-4**). For example, less than 40% of patients with an ABI below 0.4 can complete a 6-minute walking test.[25] One limitation of the ABI in patients with diabetes, however, is that leg blood pressure recordings cannot be reliably interpreted in patients with calcified vessels because these vessels are not reliably compressed during inflation of the blood pressure cuff. Because diabetic patients are more likely than nondiabetics to have arterial calcifications, ABI measurements in certain individuals can be difficult to interpret, and other noninvasive tests, such as a toe-brachial index, should be used to make the diagnosis. The diagnostic measurement of the ABI for the detection of lower-extremity PAD varies according to the population studied, the cutoff threshold, and the comparison gold standard test (invasive angiography or duplex ultrasound). The sensitivity and specificity of the ABI range from 0.17 to 1.0 and from 0.8 to 1.0, respectively.[22] Overall, lower sensitivities are reported in diabetic patients.[26–28]

The American Diabetes Association (ADA) consensus statement recommends that a screening ABI be performed in all diabetic individuals older than 50 years or in anyone with symptoms consistent with PAD.[29] For the general, nondiabetic population, screening ABI testing is recommended at age 65, or at age 50 in individuals with a history of tobacco smoking.[24] In general, PAD is underdiagnosed in the primary care setting.[30] A large-scale PAD screening study demonstrated that only one third of patients with documented PAD had classical claudication symptoms.[20] These data suggest that classic symptoms are inadequate in determining a person's health status with regard to PAD. Particularly in diabetic patients with peripheral neuropathy, ABI screening of asymptomatic individuals represents an important tool in diagnosing PAD and allowing for an appropriately tailored strategy for therapeutic decisions.

Recent data from the National Health and Nutrition Examination Study[31] demonstrate that there are significant treatment gaps, even once patients have been identified as having abnormal ABI measurements. For example, among patients with ABI-documented PAD, statin use was reported in only 30.5% ± 2.5%, angiotensin-converting enzyme (ACE) inhibitor or angiotensin receptor blocker (ARB) use in 24.9% ± 1.9%, and aspirin use in 35.8% ± 2.9%. These numbers correspond to estimates of 5.0 million adults with PAD not taking statins, 5.4 million not taking ACE inhibitors or ARBs, and 4.5 million not taking aspirin. In the same study, these treatment gaps were shown to be associated with elevated mortality rates even after adjustment for other important confounding factors.

In a patient with confirmed PAD for whom further investigation is required, usually at a time when revascularization is considered, there are other modalities available for investigating the extent and nature of the PAD. Segmental pressure and pulse volume recordings are both noninvasive hemodynamic studies that aid in the localization of arterial occlusive disease.[32] Other noninvasive imaging techniques, including magnetic resonance angiography (MRA) and computed tomographic angiography (CTA), or duplex ultrasonography can provide more precise anatomic information for revascularization planning purposes. Conventional, contrast-based angiography can still be useful, particularly when other modalities have left doubts as to the diagnosis.

Overall, patients with PAD have an increased risk of adverse cardiovascular events, as well as impaired quality of life, and an increased risk of limb loss. In addition, patients with PAD and concomitant diabetes are at risk for higher cardiovascular and cerebrovascular event rates than comparable nondiabetics.[29] The combination of PAD and diabetes causes most nontraumatic lower-extremity amputations in the United States.[33] The relative risk for lower-extremity amputation in patients with diabetes was 12.7 (95% confidence interval [CI] 10.9-14.9) compared with 23.5 (95% CI 19.3-29.1) for diabetic patients in the Medicare population.[33]

RISK FACTOR IDENTIFICATION, LIFESTYLE MODIFICATION, AND PHARMACOTHERAPY

Once diabetic individuals with PAD have been identified, the aim of medical management is to aggressively modify cardiovascular risk factors for the prevention of adverse cardiovascular events and to relieve symptoms related to PAD to improve functional status and quality of life. These two goals should be addressed simultaneously in every patient.

Lowering Cardiovascular Morbidity and Mortality

The risk factors for PAD are identical to those for other forms of atherosclerotic vascular disease, and PAD is similarly associated with an increased risk of coronary, cerebrovascular, and renovascular disease. As a result, PAD is considered a coronary heart disease equivalent, elevating it to the highest category of cardiovascular risk.[34] The 2005 American College of Cardiology/American Heart Association (ACC/AHA) practice guidelines (with the 2011 focused update), the 2003 ADA consensus statement, and the 2007 TransAtlantic Inter-Society Consensus (TASC II) document on the management of PAD recommend smoking cessation, lipid-lowering therapy with statins, and the treatment of diabetes and hypertension.[24,29,35,36] Data from a Dutch prospective cohort study of 2420 patients with PAD (ABI 0.90 or lower) support these conclusions and demonstrate that a comprehensive approach to risk factor modification can have additive benefits.[37] In this study, Feringa and colleagues demonstrated that after adjustment for risk factors and propensity scores, statins (hazard ratio [HR] 0.46, 95% CI 0.36-0.58), beta blockers (HR 0.68, 95% CI 0.58-0.80), aspirin (HR 0.72, 95% CI 0.61-0.84), and ACE inhibitors (HR 0.80, 95% CI 0.69-0.94) were significantly associated with a reduced risk of long-term mortality in this cohort. The benefits of these therapies appear additive, and these data support the universal nature of atherosclerotic vascular disease, whether in the form of PAD or elsewhere.

Dyslipidemia

Several cholesterol-lowering trials in patients with dyslipidemia and CAD and/or PAD have evaluated the effects of lipid lowering on PAD. Initial studies, performed before the availability of statins, showed either regression or less progression of femoral atherosclerosis with lipid-lowering therapy.[38–40] The Program on the Surgical Control of the Hyperlipidemias (POSCH) randomized men with previous MI and dyslipidemia to diet therapy or diet therapy plus surgical ileal bypass. At 5 years, those in the surgical group had better control of lipid levels, decreased overall mortality, and decreased mortality from atherosclerotic coronary heart disease.[41]

Studies in the statin era confirm these initial results. For example, in the Heart Protection Study, which randomized 20,536 high-risk participants to 40 mg/day of simvastatin or placebo, a 24% relative risk reduction was observed in first-time cardiovascular events in the patients who received simvastatin. The subgroup of patients with PAD had similar cardiovascular benefits regardless of history of myocardial infarction (MI) or CAD. Even the subgroup population who had low-density lipoprotein cholesterol (LDL-C) levels less than 100 mg/dL at baseline benefited from statin therapy.[42] A post hoc analysis of the Scandinavian Simvastatin Survival Study (4S), which included 4444 patients with angina or previous MI and a baseline total cholesterol level of 212 to 309 mg/dL, found that treatment with 20 to 40 mg of simvastatin per day reduced the incidence of new or worsening claudication by 38% (2.3% versus 3.6% with placebo).[43]

Independent of cholesterol-lowering effects, statin use improves pain-free walking distance and walking speed in patients with PAD and claudication.[44] Two studies randomized patients with claudication to simvastatin 40 mg daily or placebo. Aronow and colleagues reported an improvement in pain-free walking distance of 24% increase at 6 months and of 42% increase at 1 year after initiation of treatment. It is interesting to note that total walking distance and ABI did not improve.[45] In contrast, Mondillo and colleagues reported increases in ABI, total walking distance, and pain-free survival in patients randomized to simvastatin (**Fig. 27-5**).[46] Mohler and colleagues randomized 354 patients with claudication to atorvastatin 10 mg or 80 mg or placebo.[47] Patients receiving atorvastatin had an increased pain-free walking distance, but not total walking distance or ABI. Patients with PAD who take statins have been shown to have less annual decline in lower-extremity performance than those that do not.[48] Overall, the aggregate data suggest that statin use may increase the walking distance until the onset of pain, but statin use does not clearly affect total walking time or change lower-extremity blood flow as measured by ABI.

The current recommendations advocate a goal LDL-C of less than 100 mg/dL for patients with PAD; for very high-risk patients, the goal is an LDL-C below 70 mg/dL. All patients

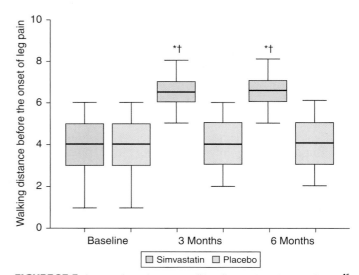

FIGURE 27-5 Simvastatin can improve walking distance in patients with PAD.[46] *(Modified from Mondillo S, Ballo P, Barbati R, et al: Effects of simvastatin on walking performance and symptoms of intermittent claudication in hypercholesterolemic patients with peripheral vascular disease, Am J Med 114:359-364, 2003.)*

with PAD should be treated with statins as first-line lipid-lowering therapy, if tolerable.[24,35]

There is also a role for fibrate therapy in the treatment of PAD. The Fenofibrate Intervention and Event Lowering in Diabetes (FIELD) study randomized 9795 patients aged 50 to 75 years with type 2 diabetes to either fenofibrate 200 mg/day or placebo for 5 years' duration. The risks of first amputation (45 versus 70 events; HR 0.64, 95% CI 0.44-0.94; $P = .02$) and minor amputation events without known large-vessel disease (18 versus 34 events; 0.53, 0.30-0.94; $P = 0.027$) were lower for patients assigned to fenofibrate than for patients assigned to placebo, with no difference between groups in risk of major amputations.[49] A reduction in amputation events has not been similarly shown with statin therapy.

Smoking Cessation

Several nonrandomized studies have shown that patients who successfully quit smoking have decreased rates of PAD progression, critical limb ischemia, amputation, MI, and stroke, and have increased survival.[50,51] Unfortunately, the spontaneous cessation rates without intervention range from 2% to 5% in the United States, despite nearly 75% of smokers expressing a desire to stop. Given the importance of smoking cessation, it is important for health care providers to consistently convey to patients that discontinuation of tobacco products is extremely important to overall survival, well-being, and limb preservation.[52,53] Behavioral interventions can improve cessation rates, but only modestly. Only 5% of patients who receive physician advice, follow-up correspondence, phone calls, and supplementary visits will quit smoking.[54] Randomized trial evidence, however, has demonstrated that a 10-week intervention that results in just a 21.7% smoking cessation rate at 5 years significantly improves survival in patients with chronic lung disease compared with those treated with usual care.[55] Thus, efforts at cessation should be made.

Hennrikus and colleagues have specifically demonstrated that individuals with PAD respond to intensive counseling and education in a randomized trial of 124 patients. These researchers compared an intensive tobacco cessation counseling program with a minimal educational program over 6 months. Study participants assigned to the intensive intervention group were significantly more likely to be abstinent from tobacco at 6-month follow-up: 21.3% versus 6.8% in the minimal intervention group ($P = 0.023$).[56]

Smoking cessation can be aided in many ways, including the use of pharmacotherapy such as short-term nicotine replacement products including gums, long-acting nicotine replacement patches, bupropion, or varenicline. Pharmacologic interventions are more effective than medical advice alone. In controlled studies, the rates of stopping smoking with use of pharmacologic treatment interventions has varied from 17% to 48% at 6 months and from 11% to 34% at 1 year.[57] Bupropion, via a poorly understood mechanism, diminishes the desire for smoking. It is associated with cessation rates of 27% to 35% at 6 months and 23% to 30% at 1 year.[58] Varenicline, a partial agonist selective for the $alpha_4$, $beta_2$ nicotinic acetylcholine receptor, is a newer agent than bupropion. Two large, randomized trials have suggested that varenicline performs better when the two are compared directly. In a study of 1025 smokers where patients were randomized to placebo, sustained-release bupropion, or varenicline, abstinence rates from weeks 9 to 52 were significantly elevated in the two drug arms compared with placebo. Cessation rates were 8.4%, 16.1%, and 21.9% respectively for individuals taking placebo, bupropion, and varenicline.[59] In a second large randomized trial, Jorenby and colleagues found similar abstinence rates in individuals treated with placebo, bupropion, or varenicline.[60]

The U.S. Public Health Service task force smoking cessation guidelines do not recommend any one of the first-line agents over another.[61] Instead, they recommend that patient preference and previous experience with the medications guide the choice of the first-line therapy (nicotine replacement, bupropion, and varenicline). Meta-analyses done for the guideline update addressed the question of whether any drug was more effective than the nicotine patch. In this analysis, there was no statistically significant difference between the patch and other nicotine replacement products or bupropion, but varenicline had a higher efficacy than the nicotine patch (OR 1.6, 95% CI 1.3-2.0). The analysis also compared the nicotine patch with combinations of drugs. The combination of nicotine patch and short-acting nicotine replacement products, used for an extended period of time, was more effective than the patch alone (OR 1.9, 95% CI 1.3-2.7), as was the combination of nicotine patch and sustained-release bupropion (OR 1.3, 95% CI 1.0-1.8).

Until further trials have been performed, varenicline and the combination of long-acting patch plus short-acting nicotine replacement therapies appear to be roughly equivalent first-line choices. Patients treated with varenicline should be monitored for possible adverse neuropsychiatric events.

Despite multiple options for the approach to tobacco cessation in individuals with PAD, there appears to be continued risk in individuals who successfully become abstinent. Data from the Women's Health Study demonstrate that although smoking cessation substantially reduces risk for PAD events in women, there remains an increased occurrence of PAD events in former smokers compared with individuals who never smoked.[62]

Hypertension

In a large number of clinical trials involving thousands of patients, antihypertensive drug therapy has been associated with a 35% to 40% mean reduction in the rate of stroke, a 20% to 25% reduction in MI, more than a 50% reduction in heart failure, and a significant reduction in the development of chronic kidney disease.[63] Although treatment of hypertension has been studied in many contexts, there are limited data available to determine whether treatment of hypertension will prevent the development of claudication or alter the course of PAD itself.

The Treatment of Mild Hypertension Study (TOMHS) showed that drug treatment in addition to nutritional interventions was superior to nutritional interventions alone in preventing the development of intermittent claudication and PAD over an average follow-up of 4.4 years.[64] Reports on the effect of blood pressure lowering on the ability to walk in patients with intermittent claudication are mixed.[65–67] However, these small studies have demonstrated that the ACE inhibitor captopril maintains and may increase walking distance in patients with claudication. Alpha-adrenergic blockers, beta blockers, and calcium channel blockers may adversely affect walking distance, particularly if there is a substantial decrease in systolic blood pressure. In a 6-month crossover trial of 20 hypertensive patients with PAD randomized to atenolol, labetalol, pindolol, captopril, or placebo, only individuals treated with captopril maintained walking distance.[67] This appears to be a class effect, as enalapril and ramipril also seem to improve lower-extremity blood flow in patients with claudication.[68,69]

Antihypertensive therapy should be administered to hypertensive patients with PAD to achieve a goal of less than 140/80 mm Hg to reduce the risk of MI, stroke, heart failure, and cardiovascular death.[69a,69b]

In PAD patients with diabetes, the Appropriate Blood Pressure Control in Diabetes (ABCD) study supports intensive management of hypertension.[70] The ABCD study randomized 480 normotensive patients (baseline diastolic blood pressure of 80 to 89 mm Hg) with type 2 diabetes to either an intensive blood pressure regimen with enalapril or nisoldipine or placebo. Individuals were followed for 5 years. Fifty-three of the patients had PAD as defined by an ABI below 0.90. In patients with PAD, there were 3 cardiovascular events (13.6%) in the intensive treatment group compared with 12 events (38.7%) in patients taking placebo ($P = .046$). After adjustment for multiple cardiovascular risk factors, an inverse relationship between ABI and cardiovascular events was observed with placebo ($P = .009$), but not with intensive treatment ($P = .91$). Thus, with intensive blood pressure control, the risk of an event was not increased, even at the lowest ABI values, and was the same as in patients without PAD. The conclusion from the trial was that intensive blood pressure lowering to a mean of 128/75 mm Hg resulted in a marked reduction in cardiovascular events.

Diabetes Mellitus

To date, no prospective trials have been performed to assess whether improved glycemic control decreases the cardiovascular risk associated with PAD, the walking distance of patients with claudication, or the frequency of amputation. In a retrospective review of the Diabetes Control and Complications Trial of patients with type 1 diabetes mellitus, there was a 22% risk reduction in the development of PAD in the group that received intensive insulin therapy.[79] Epidemiologic studies also support the benefit of tight glycemic control. The prospective Belfast Diet Study of type 2 diabetic patients demonstrated an increasing risk for MI of 1.04 per mmol increase in fasting plasma glucose.[80] In the UK Prospective Diabetes Study of 2693 patients followed for nearly 8 years, patients in the highest tertile of HbA1c had a 1.5-fold greater risk for MI compared with those in the lowest tertile.[81] Although no prospective trial has demonstrated the noncoronary vascular benefits of improved glycemic control, it is nevertheless recommended. The current recommendations based on a joint position statement from the ADA and the European Association for the Study of Diabetes (EASD) advocate a less algorithm-driven treatment plan based on individualized comorbidities than previously articulated, but do not advocate a specific HbA1c goal for treatment.[82] However, the current position document does not specifically mention PAD at all. Previous versions of ADA guidelines recommended that all patients with diabetes and PAD should be aggressively treated to reduce their HbA1c levels to less than 7%.[83]

Further reductions in goal HbA1c levels have been tested in several recent trials.[84–86] Although intensive glycemic control reduced the incidence of microvascular events, there were no significant reductions in macrovascular outcomes between standard and intensive glycemic control. The Action to Control Cardiovascular Risk in Diabetes (ACCORD) trial, for example, randomized 10,251 patients with a history of a cardiovascular event or significant cardiovascular risk to intensive glycemic control (target HbA1c

below 6.0%) or standard glycemic control (target HbA1c 7.0% to 7.9%). Within 12 months of randomization, the intensive glycemic group reached a median HbA1c of 6.4% (from a baseline median of 8.1%) compared with a median HbA1c of 7.5% in the standard glycemic group. However, the glycemic control arm was stopped because of an increased mortality rate in the intensive glycemic control group.[84] At this time, the optimal HbA1c goal for individuals with PAD has not been clearly defined for all patients.

Despite a paucity of clinical trial evidence, meticulous foot care is also recommended for patients with diabetes and PAD to reduce the risk of skin ulceration, necrosis, and subsequent amputation. This includes the use of appropriate footwear to avoid pressure injury, daily inspection and cleansing by the patient, and the use of moisturizing cream to prevent dryness and fissuring. Frequent foot inspection by patients and health care providers is thought to enable early identification of foot lesions and ulcerations and facilitate prompt referral for treatment.[83]

Obesity and Weight Reduction

An association between obesity and PAD has been observed in some studies but not others. For example, in the Framingham cohort of 5209 patients, relative weight was only a weak risk factor for claudication.[7] In contrast, obesity, as determined by a body mass index over 30, was not a risk factor for PAD or intermittent claudication in the Edinburgh Artery Study, Whitehall study, or Lipid Research Clinics study.[87–89] Despite the mixed evidence for a direct relationship between obesity and PAD, obesity may heighten the risk for PAD by increasing the prevalence of other previously established risk factors. For example, in a study of 8688 men followed for 5 years, being overweight was the most significant predictor of who was going to develop type 2 diabetes mellitus.[90] McDermott and colleagues have shown that over 4 years of follow-up, patients with intermittent claudication and a body mass index over 30 kg/m² had significantly more functional decline.[91] Thus it stands to reason that any decrease in weight will decrease the work required for walking and will improve exercise capacity. Therefore, weight reduction is recommended for patients with PAD.

Antiplatelet Therapy

There is substantial evidence that the cardiovascular morbidity and mortality related to PAD in patients with diabetes is related to platelet activity and inflammation. Platelet activity can be modified by the use of antiplatelet agents. The data supporting the use of antiplatelet agents for the prevention of cardiovascular events in patients with PAD in general is mixed, as is described here.

A meta-analysis of approximately 150 prospective controlled trials of antiplatelet therapy (mostly aspirin) has been reported as part of the Antithrombotic Trialists' Collaborative. This analysis combined data from more than 135,000 individuals with evidence of cardiovascular disease, including PAD. Investigators demonstrated a 22% reduction in the odds ratio in the composite primary endpoint of MI, stroke, and vascular death in patients taking antiplatelet therapy compared with controls. When the subset of approximately 9000 patients with claudication was analyzed, the protective effect of antiplatelet therapy was similar.[92] A more recent meta-analysis of 18 prospective trials totaling 5269 patients with PAD found that aspirin therapy compared with placebo was not associated with significant reductions in all-cause or cardiovascular mortality, MI, or major bleeding.[93]

The Aspirin for Asymptomatic Atherosclerosis (AAA) trial enrolled asymptomatic patients with ABI of 0.95 or lower (instead of the standard cutoff value of 0.90 used in the multisociety guidelines) to 100 mg of aspirin daily or placebo. After a mean 8.2-year follow-up there were no differences in the composite number of vascular events, defined as MI, stroke, or coronary revascularization, between groups treated with aspirin or placebo.[94]

Specifically with regard to diabetic patients and PAD, the Prevention of Progression of Arterial Disease and Diabetes (POPADAD), trial enrolled diabetic patients with asymptomatic PAD. This study did not find a beneficial effect of aspirin compared with placebo on a primary endpoint of death from coronary disease, nonfatal MI, nonfatal stroke, or amputation.[95]

Clopidogrel has also been studied in patients with PAD. The Clopidogrel Versus Aspirin in Patients at Risk of Ischaemic Events (CAPRIE) trial compared aspirin versus clopidogrel in patients with recent stroke, recent MI, or established PAD.[96] Patients treated with clopidogrel had an 8.7% relative risk reduction (5.3% versus 5.8%, $P = .043$) in the primary endpoint of stroke, MI, or vascular death compared with those treated with aspirin. In the subset analysis of patients with PAD who were enrolled in the trial, there was a 23.8% relative risk reduction in favor of clopidogrel. The Clopidogrel for High Atherothrombotic Risk and Ischemic Stabilization, Management, and Avoidance (CHARISMA) trial compared the efficacy of dual antiplatelet therapy with clopidogrel plus aspirin versus aspirin alone in patients with established CAD, cerebrovascular disease, or PAD, as well as in patients with multiple atherosclerotic risk factors.[97] Overall, dual antiplatelet therapy produced no significant benefit compared with aspirin alone on the primary endpoint of MI, stroke, or cardiovascular death. Among the 3096 patients with PAD who enrolled, clopidogrel plus aspirin did reduce the rates of MI and hospitalization for ischemic events compared with aspirin alone.[98]

Oral anticoagulation with warfarin has also been studied in patients with PAD. The Warfarin Antiplatelet Vascular Evaluation (WAVE) study evaluated antiplatelet therapy in addition to warfarin compared with antiplatelet therapy alone in patients with PAD.[99] There was no significant improvement with warfarin therapy; however, patients treated with warfarin and antiplatelet agent together had more life-threatening bleeding than those treated with warfarin alone.

Current guidelines recommend that patients with PAD be treated with an antiplatelet drug, such as aspirin or clopidogrel (recommended as a class I recommendation for symptomatic patients and a class II recommendation for asymptomatic patients) to reduce the risk of MI, stroke, or vascular death.[24] Oral anticoagulants are not recommended to reduce cardiovascular events. Newer antiplatelet agents (such as prasugrel or ticagrelor) and nonwarfarin anticoagulants (such as factor Xa inhibitors or direct thrombin inhibitors) have not been rigorously studied in patients with PAD for the prevention of cardiovascular events.

Renin Angiotensin System Antagonism in Peripheral Artery Disease

Although the achievement of goal blood pressure level outweighs the use of a specific class of antihypertensive agents, renin-angiotensin system antagonists should be considered an initial drug class of choice.

Both ACE inhibitors and ARBs have favorable effects on the cardiovascular system beyond their ability to lower blood pressure. Based on the Heart Outcomes Prevention Evaluation (HOPE) study, patients with diabetes or evidence of vascular disease plus one other cardiovascular risk factor who received ramipril had a 22% relative risk reduction of the combined endpoint of stroke, MI, and death compared with patients who received placebo, despite a baseline blood pressure considered at goal for most patients. These outcomes were seen despite a modest overall blood pressure reduction of 3/2 mm Hg.[71] Overall, 17.8% of patients in the placebo group reached the primary study endpoint of MI, stroke, or cardiovascular death. The rate was 22% for the 4051 patients with PAD compared with 14.3% for the 5246 patients without PAD.

In the European Trial on Reduction of Cardiac Events with Perindopril in Patients with Stable Coronary Artery Disease (EUROPA), 12,218 patients with stable CAD were randomly assigned to perindopril or placebo. After a mean follow-up of 4.2 years, cardiovascular events were significantly decreased in patients treated with perindopril. All predefined subgroups, including the 883 patients who had documented PAD, benefited from perindopril.[72] These data concurred with the findings of the HOPE trial. Thus, based on two studies of patients with normal blood pressure at rest and only modest changes in blood pressure with therapy, ACE inhibitors decrease cardiovascular morbidity and mortality more than expected with the observed blood pressure lowering.

Similar to ACE inhibitors, ARBs have documented cardiovascular benefits beyond their antihypertensive properties. In particular, ARBs have been shown to improve endothelial function through decreased vascular inflammation.[73] Patients with high cardiovascular risk, including those with PAD, are likely to benefit from ARBs. ARBs, such as losartan and candesartan, have shown morbidity and mortality benefits either alone or in combination with ACE inhibitors, as demonstrated in the Losartan Intervention for Endpoint Reduction in Hypertension (LIFE) and the Candesartan in Heart Failure: Assessment of Reduction in Mortality and Morbidity (CHARM) studies.[74,75] In the LIFE study, losartan was compared with atenolol in hypertensive patients with electrocardiographic evidence of left ventricular hypertrophy. Overall, losartan significantly lowered the incidence of cardiovascular events, particularly stroke, despite similar decreases in blood pressure. Thus, similar to ACE inhibitors, ARBs should be thought of as having cardiovascular benefits beyond blood pressure reduction. It is interesting to note that in Swedish National Registry data, patients treated with candesartan were less likely to develop PAD compared with patients treated with losartan despite similar blood pressure lowering.[76]

Beta-adrenergic Blockers in Peripheral Artery Disease

The commonly held belief that beta-blocking agents worsen claudication and shorten the amount of exercise required to bring on discomfort in the legs has been well challenged. In a carefully performed meta-analysis of 11 randomized, controlled trials, Radack and Deck demonstrated that beta-adrenergic blocker therapy does not worsen claudication symptoms in people with PAD.[77] Only 1 of 11 studies in this meta-analysis showed that pain-free and maximal treadmill walking distances were decreased by atenolol, labetalol, or pindolol, but not captopril. However, beta blockers should not be considered as first-line agents in the treatment of hypertension and PAD, given the beneficial effects of ACE inhibitors and ARBs already discussed. If there are clear indications for beta-blocker use, such as congestive heart failure, post-MI status, angina pectoris, or arrhythmias or for perioperative cardiovascular protection, then beta blockers can and should be used.[78]

Therapy for the Treatment of Claudication

In addition to modifying risk factors to improve overall cardiovascular morbidity and mortality, there are noninterventional strategies available to treat the mobility limitations caused by symptomatic PAD. Only two medications carry U.S. Food and Drug Administration (FDA) approval for the improvement of walking distance in PAD: pentoxifylline and cilostazol.

Pentoxifylline

Pentoxifylline is a rheologic modifier approved by the FDA for symptomatic relief of claudication. It is thought to act by improving red blood cell and leukocyte flexibility, inhibiting neutrophil activation and adhesion, decreasing fibrinogen concentrations, and reducing blood viscosity, permitting improved muscular perfusion. Studies investigating the efficacy of pentoxifylline have yielded conflicting results. A meta-analysis found that pentoxifylline improved walking distance by 29 meters compared with placebo.[100] The improvement was approximately 50% in the placebo group, whereas pentoxifylline added an additional 30%. The benefit was substantially less, however, than that achieved with a supervised exercise program.[101]

The beneficial response to pentoxifylline is small in most patients, and the overall data are insufficient to support its widespread use in patients with claudication. Pentoxifylline may be considered for patients who cannot take cilostazol, have not responded adequately to an exercise program, and/or are not candidates for revascularization, either with percutaneous or surgical approaches.

Cilostazol

Cilostazol is a phosphodiesterase-3 inhibitor that suppresses platelet aggregation and is a direct arterial dilator.[102] The efficacy of cilostazol has been demonstrated in several studies[103–105] and in a meta-analysis[106] of eight randomized, placebo-controlled trials that included 2702 patients with stable moderate-to-severe claudication. In the meta-analysis, treatment with 100 mg twice daily for 12 to 24 weeks increased maximal and pain-free walking distances by 50% and 67%, respectively. Because cilostazol is a phosphodiesterase inhibitor similar to milrinone, it is contraindicated in patients with symptomatic congestive heart failure or patients with a left ventricular ejection fraction less than 40%.

Cilostazol is more effective than pentoxifylline when compared directly. Superiority was illustrated in a trial of 698 patients randomized to cilostazol, pentoxifylline, or placebo for 24 weeks. The increase in mean walking distance over baseline with pentoxifylline and placebo was the same (30% and 34%, respectively), but the increase with cilostazol was significantly greater (54%) (**Fig. 27-6**).[107] The most common adverse effects with cilostazol are headache, palpitations, and diarrhea. The optimal dose of cilostazol is 100 mg twice daily. The medication should be given on an empty stomach. Because of the inhibitory effects of cilostazol on drug metabolism, the dose should be halved in patients taking medications that inhibit the cytochrome

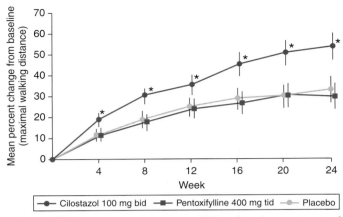

FIGURE 27-6 Cilostazol versus pentoxifylline for the treatment of claudication.[107] (Modified from Dawson DL, Cutler BS, Hiatt WR, et al: A comparison of cilostazol and pentoxifylline for treating intermittent claudication, Am J Med 109:523-530, 2000.)

P-450 isoenzymes CYP3A4 and CYP2C19 (e.g., erythromycin, diltiazem, omeprazole).[108]

Other Pharmacologic Agents

Multiple other agents have been used in the treatment of claudication. Naftidrofuryl, a 5-hydroxytryptamine serotonin receptor inhibitor, has been available in Europe for a number of years. The mechanism of action of this drug is not clear, but it is thought to promote glucose uptake and increase adenosine triphosphate levels. A meta-analysis of four trials showed an increase in the time to initial pain development with treadmill walking over a 3- to 6-month period.[109]

Buflomedil is an alpha-adrenolytic agent available in Europe, but not the United States, that has been used in the treatment of claudication. The Limbs International Medicinal Buflomedil (LIMB) trial evaluated the efficacy and safety of buflomedil in 2078 patients with claudication and an ABI of 0.3 to 0.8, in a randomized, placebo-controlled trial. At a median follow-up of 2.8 years, the rate of a composite endpoint of cardiovascular death, nonfatal MI, nonfatal stroke, symptomatic deterioration in PAD, or leg amputation was significantly lower in the patients who received buflomedil (9.1% versus 12.4%). The benefit was largely driven by a reduction in symptoms of PAD.[110]

Ginkgo biloba has also been studied in the treatment of claudication with some modest success. Ginkgo is thought to act via an antioxidant mechanism that inhibits vascular injury. It is also thought to have some antithrombotic effects. The effect of ginkgo has been reviewed in a meta-analysis that showed that patients receiving ginkgo extract increased pain-free walking by approximately 34 meters, a significant increase compared with placebo.[111]

Many other agents have been tried in the treatment of symptomatic claudication. These include estrogen replacement therapy, chelation therapy with intravenous ethylenediaminetetraacetic acid (EDTA), and vitamin E supplementation. None have been shown to have significant benefit, and none are recommended by current therapy guidelines.

Exercise

Many prospective trials have demonstrated that supervised exercise is an effective method of treating patients with claudication.[112] The magnitude of the effect from a supervised exercise program exceeds that achieved with any of the

TABLE 27-2 Effect of Supervised Exercise from a Meta-analysis of 21 Studies

COMPONENTS OF EXERCISE PROGRAMS	NO. OF STUDIES	CHANGE IN THE DISTANCE TO ONSET OF PAIN, m	P	CHANGE IN THE DISTANCE TO MAXIMAL PAIN, m	P
Exercise Duration					
≤30 min/session	8	143.1±162.8	.039	143.6±418.9	.007
>30 min/session	6	314.2±172.4		652.6±363.9	
Exercise Frequency					
<3 sessions/wk	7	177.8±129.6	.048	249.0±349.5	.045
≥3 sessions/wk	11	270.7±221.4		541.5±253.2	
Length of Program					
<26 wk	10	131.9±158.6	.008	275.1±228.3	.009
≥26 wk	11	345.6±161.7		518.5±409.2	
Claudication Pain End Point Used During Training Sessions					
Onset of pain	15	104.7±91.2	.007	195.5±78.3	.005
Near-maximal pain	6	350.2±246.2		606.8±426.6	
Mode of Exercise					
Walking	6	294.3±289.7	.042	511.9±483.2	.023
Combination of exercises	15	152.1±158.4		286.9±127.4	
Level of Supervision					
Supervised	11	238.3±120.5	.476	448.6±291.7	.518
Combination of home and supervised	8	208.4±198.4		339.8±471.9	

Values for each componant are adjusted means ± standard deviations (SDs) of the change in the distances to onset and to maximal claudication pain after the other five exercise program components were controlled for.
    Data from Gardner AW, Poehlman ET: Exercise rehabilitation programs for the treatment of claudication pain, A meta-analysis, *JAMA* 274:975-980, 1995.

pharmacologic agents available. A meta-analysis of 21 studies by Gardner and Poehlman,[113] which included both randomized and nonrandomized trials, showed that pain-free walking time improved by an average of 180% and maximal walking time by 120% in patients with claudication who underwent supervised exercise training (**Table 27-2**). Furthermore, a meta-analysis from the Cochrane Collaboration that included only randomized, controlled trials showed that exercise improved maximal walking ability by an average of 150% (range 74% to 230%).[114] The most recent randomized, controlled trial of exercise in PAD was the Claudication: Exercise Versus Endoluminal Revascularization (CLEVER) study.[115] Investigators randomized 111 patients with aortoiliac disease to medical therapy, medical therapy plus supervised exercise, or medical therapy plus endovascular revascularization. Patients in the medical therapy plus supervised exercise therapy group were able to increase their peak walking time by 5.8±4.9 minutes compared with 1.2±2.6 minutes for those in the medical therapy alone group. It is interesting to note that the increase in peak walking time was intermediate in the revascularization group, but quality of life as measured by the Peripheral Artery Questionnaire improved most in the revascularization group.

There are several mechanisms by which exercise training may improve claudication, although the available data are not sufficient to render firm conclusions regarding their relative importance. These mechanisms include improved endothelial function via increases in nitric oxide synthase and prostacyclin; reduction of local inflammation; increased exercise pain tolerance; induction of vascular angiogenesis; improved muscle metabolism by favorable effects on muscle carnitine metabolism; and reductions in blood viscosity and red cell aggregation.[116]

Although less well studied, exercise may also improve survival in PAD. This idea was addressed in a prospective, observational study of 225 men with PAD in whom physical activity was measured with a vertical accelerometer. Patients were followed for a mean duration of 57 months, over which time 33% of patients died. Individuals in the highest quartile of accelerometer-measured activity had a significantly lower mortality than those in the lowest quartile (HR 0.29, 95% CI 0.10-0.83).[117]

The current PAD guidelines state that a program of supervised exercise training is recommended as an initial treatment modality for patients with claudication (class I, level of evidence A) and that supervised exercise training should be performed for a minimum of 30 to 45 minutes, in sessions performed at least three times per week for a minimum of 12 weeks (class I, level of evidence A).[24,35]

Exercise programs have several important limitations. First patients must be motivated, which is often difficult when they experience claudication-related pain whenever they walk. Second, the best results occur when patients enroll in a supervised program as with cardiac rehabilitation, ensuring compliance. Unfortunately, there is often a lack of financial reimbursement for supervised programs, and patients instructed by health care providers to exercise on their own do not achieve the same improvement as those in structured programs.[118]

REVASCULARIZATION

Many patients do not experience optimal improvement in symptoms related to PAD from medical therapy or risk factor modification alone. Two general revascularization strategies exist: endovascular interventions and open surgical techniques. As in the coronary circulation, the success of revascularization in the lower extremities depends on many variables including lesion location, lesion length, and the nature of the distal runoff. Diabetes alters the distribution of lower-extremity atherosclerosis so that these patients tend to have severe arterial occlusive disease below the knee in the runoff vessels. As the distal runoff declines, the results of endovascular interventions worsen and the need for surgery increases.

Endovascular Management

In general, endovascular revascularization is more appropriate in patients with relatively focal disease in arteries above the knee.[119] However, short-term success rates for opening long totally occluded vessels and below-the-knee arteries are improving.[120] Thus far, the best results have been seen in aortoiliac vessels, in which 1-year patency rates of 80% to 90% have been demonstrated.[36,121,122] Femoral interventions have 1-year patency rates that vary widely, from approximately 30% to 80%, with diabetes adversely affecting the long-term rates of success.[123–125] However, in diabetic patients with reasonable runoff, patency rates are similar to those in nondiabetics.[126]

Surgical Management

In diabetes, open surgical revascularization tends to have greater durability than endovascular procedures. Bypass to the tibial or pedal vessels with autogenous vein is the most predictable method of improving blood flow to the threatened limb. Surgical bypass with greater saphenous vein is the procedure of choice for patients with diabetes and tibial disease; however, this comes at the price of increased periprocedural cardiovascular morbidity and mortality.[6] The specific operation must take into account the anatomic location of the arterial lesions and the presence of comorbid conditions. The surgical procedure is planned after identification of the arterial obstruction by imaging, ensuring that there is sufficient arterial inflow to and outflow from the graft to maintain patency.

Revascularization is the definitive therapy for the management of patients with chronic limb ischemia, with the aim of healing ischemic ulcers and preventing limb loss. Although most limbs can be revascularized, the lack of target vessel, the unavailability of autogenous vein, or irreversible gangrene means that some cannot. In these patients, amputation is often a better option than prolonged, but failing, medical therapy.

APPROACH TO THE TREATMENT OF DIABETIC PATIENTS WITH PERIPHERAL ARTERY DISEASE

Overall, the approach to treatment of the diabetic patient with PAD is similar to that of other patients with PAD. A schematic of the overall approach is presented in **Figure 27-7**.

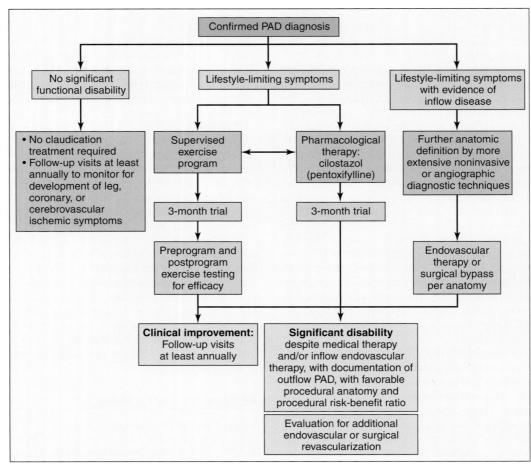

FIGURE 27-7 Treatment algorithm for peripheral artery disease. *(Modified from multi-society guidelines, from Creager and Libby in Braunwald's Heart Disease, Figure 61-17, page 1352).*

SUMMARY AND CONCLUSION

PAD is a common cardiovascular complication in patients with diabetes. The risk of developing PAD is higher in patients with diabetes, and the disease is more severe and progresses more rapidly than in nondiabetic individuals. Moreover, the presence of PAD is an important and potent marker of overall cardiovascular risk. Because the major threat to patients with diabetes and PAD is from cardiovascular events (and not limb-related events), the primary therapeutic goal is to modify atherosclerotic risk factors. Risk factor management includes lifestyle modifications, treatment of associated conditions (tobacco cessation, hypertension, dyslipidemia, diabetes itself), and prevention of ischemic events with antiplatelet therapy. A supervised exercise program, tobacco cessation, and/or cilostazol are the preferred first steps in the management of symptomatic PAD. Revascularization plays an important role in the management of patients for whom risk factor modification and pharmacologic therapy have proven inadequate.

References

1. Kornitzer M, Dramaix M, Sobolski J, et al: Ankle/arm pressure index in asymptomatic middle-aged males: an independent predictor of ten-year coronary heart disease mortality, *Angiology* 46:211–219, 1995.
2. Postiglione A, Cicerano U, Gallotta G, et al: Prevalence of peripheral arterial disease and related risk factors in elderly institutionalized subjects, *Gerontology* 38:330–337, 1992.
3. Criqui MH: Peripheral arterial disease—epidemiological aspects, *Vasc Med* 6:3–7, 2001.
4. Diehm C, Schuster A, Allenberg JR, et al: High prevalence of peripheral arterial disease and co-morbidity in 6880 primary care patients: cross-sectional study, *Atherosclerosis* 172:95–105, 2004.
5. Selvin E, Erlinger TP: Prevalence of and risk factors for peripheral arterial disease in the United States: results from the National Health and Nutrition Examination Survey, 1999–2000, *Circulation* 110:738–743, 2004.
6. Norgren L, Hiatt WR, Dormandy JA, et al: Inter-society consensus for the management of peripheral arterial disease (TASC II), *Eur J Vasc Endovasc Surg* 33(Suppl 1):S1–S75, 2007.
7. Kannel WB, McGee DL: Update on some epidemiologic features of intermittent claudication: the Framingham study, *J Am Geriatr Soc* 33:13–18, 1985.
8. Pande RL, Perlstein TS, Beckman JA, Creager MA: Association of insulin resistance and inflammation with peripheral arterial disease: the National Health and Nutrition Examination Survey, 1999 to 2004, *Circulation* 118:33–41, 2008.
9. Al-Delaimy WK, Merchant AT, Rimm EB, et al: Effect of type 2 diabetes and its duration on the risk of peripheral arterial disease among men, *Am J Med* 116:236–240, 2004.
10. Adler AI, Stevens RJ, Neil A, et al: UKPDS 59: hyperglycemia and other potentially modifiable risk factors for peripheral vascular disease in type 2 diabetes, *Diabetes Care* 25:894–899, 2002.
11. Selvin E, Marinopoulos S, Berkenblit G, et al: Meta-analysis: glycosylated hemoglobin and cardiovascular disease in diabetes mellitus, *Ann Intern Med* 141:421–431, 2004.
12. Jude EB, Oyibo SO, Chalmers N, Boulton AJ: Peripheral arterial disease in diabetic and nondiabetic patients: a comparison of severity and outcome, *Diabetes Care* 24:1433–1437, 2001.
13. Faglia E, Favales F, Quarantiello A, et al: Angiographic evaluation of peripheral arterial occlusive disease and its role as a prognostic determinant for major amputation in diabetic subjects with foot ulcers, *Diabetes Care* 21:625–630, 1998.
14. Bild DE, Selby JV, Sinnock P, et al: Lower-extremity amputation in people with diabetes. Epidemiology and prevention, *Diabetes Care* 12:24–31, 1989.
15. Holzer SE, Camerota A, Martens L, et al: Costs and duration of care for lower extremity ulcers in patients with diabetes, *Clin Ther* 20:169–181, 1998.
16. Gonzalez ER, Oley MA: The management of lower-extremity diabetic ulcers, *Manag Care Interface* 13:80–87, 2000.
17. Marso SP, Hiatt WR: Peripheral arterial disease in patients with diabetes, *J Am Coll Cardiol* 47:921–929, 2006.
18. Aboyans V, Criqui MH, Denenberg JO, et al: Risk factors for progression of peripheral arterial disease in large and small vessels, *Circulation* 113:2623–2629, 2006.
19. Khan NA, Rahim SA, Anand SS, et al: Does the clinical examination predict lower extremity peripheral arterial disease? *JAMA* 295:536–546, 2006.
20. Criqui MH, Fronek A, Klauber MR, et al: The sensitivity, specificity, and predictive value of traditional clinical evaluation of peripheral arterial disease: results from noninvasive testing in a defined population, *Circulation* 71:516–522, 1985.
21. Rutherford RB, Baker JD, Ernst C, et al: Recommended standards for reports dealing with lower extremity ischemia: revised version, *J Vasc Surg* 26:517–538, 1997.
22. Aboyans V, Criqui MH, Abraham P, et al: Measurement and interpretation of the ankle-brachial index: a scientific statement from the American Heart Association, *Circulation* 126:2890–2909, 2012.
23. Hiatt WR: Medical treatment of peripheral arterial disease and claudication, *N Engl J Med* 344:1608–1621, 2001.
24. Rooke TW, Hirsch AT, Misra S, et al: 2011 ACCF/AHA focused update of the guideline for the management of patients with peripheral artery disease (updating the 2005 guideline): a report of the American College of Cardiology Foundation/American Heart Association Task Force on Practice Guidelines, *J Am Coll Cardiol* 58:2020–2045, 2011.
25. McDermott MM, Guralnik JM, Ferrucci L, et al: Physical activity, walking exercise, and calf skeletal muscle characteristics in patients with peripheral arterial disease, *J Vasc Surg* 46:87–93, 2007.
26. Premalatha G, Ravikumar R, Sanjay R, et al: Comparison of colour duplex ultrasound and ankle-brachial pressure index measurements in peripheral vascular disease in type 2 diabetic patients with foot infections, *J Assoc Physicians India* 50:1240–1244, 2002.
27. Alnaeb ME, Crabtree VP, Boutin A, et al: Prospective assessment of lower-extremity peripheral arterial disease in diabetic patients using a novel automated optical device, *Angiology* 58:579–585, 2007.
28. Clairotte C, Retout S, Potier L, et al: Automated ankle-brachial pressure index measurement by clinical staff for peripheral arterial disease diagnosis in nondiabetic and diabetic patients, *Diabetes Care* 32:1231–1236, 2009.
29. Peripheral arterial disease in people with diabetes, *Diabetes Care* 26:3333–3341, 2003.
30. Hirsch AT, Criqui MH, Treat-Jacobson D, et al: Peripheral arterial disease detection, awareness, and treatment in primary care, *JAMA* 286:1317–1324, 2001.
31. Pande RL, Perlstein TS, Beckman JA, Creager MA: Secondary prevention and mortality in peripheral artery disease: National Health and Nutrition Examination Study, 1999 to 2004, *Circulation* 124:17–23, 2011.
32. Mohler ER 3rd: Peripheral arterial disease: identification and implications, *Arch Intern Med* 163:2306–2314, 2003.
33. Diabetes-related amputations of lower extremities in the Medicare population—Minnesota, 1993–1995, *MMWR Morb Mortal Wkly Rep* 47:649–652, 1998.
34. Third report of the National Cholesterol Education Program (NCEP) Expert Panel on Detection, Evaluation, and Treatment of High Blood Cholesterol in Adults (Adult Treatment Panel III) final report, *Circulation* 106:3143–3421, 2002.
35. Hirsch AT, Haskal ZJ, Hertzer NR, et al: ACC/AHA 2005 practice guidelines for the management of patients with peripheral arterial disease (lower extremity, renal, mesenteric, and abdominal aortic): A collaborative report from the american association for vascular surgery/society for vascular surgery, society for cardiovascular angiography and interventions, society for vascular medicine and biology, society of interventional radiology, and the ACC/AHA Task Force on Practice Guidelines (writing committee to develop guidelines for the management of patients with peripheral arterial disease): Endorsed by the American Association of Cardiovascular and Pulmonary Rehabilitation; National Heart, Lung, and Blood Institute; Society for Vascular Nursing; Transatlantic Inter-Society Consensus; and Vascular Disease Foundation, *Circulation* 113:e463–e654, 2006.
36. Norgren L, Hiatt WR, Dormandy JA, et al: Inter-society consensus for the management of peripheral arterial disease (TASC II), *J Vasc Surg* 45(Suppl S):S5–S67, 2007.
37. Feringa HH, van Waning VH, Bax JJ, et al: Cardioprotective medication is associated with improved survival in patients with peripheral arterial disease, *J Am Coll Cardiol* 47:1182–1187, 2006.
38. Barndt R Jr, Blankenhorn DH, Crawford DW, Brooks SH: Regression and progression of early femoral atherosclerosis in treated hyperlipoproteinemic patients, *Ann Intern Med* 86:139–146, 1977.
39. Duffield RG, Lewis B, Miller NE, et al: Treatment of hyperlipidaemia retards progression of symptomatic femoral atherosclerosis. A randomised controlled trial, *Lancet* 2:639–642, 1983.
40. Blankenhorn DH, Azen SP, Crawford DW, et al: Effects of colestipol-niacin therapy on human femoral atherosclerosis, *Circulation* 83:438–447, 1991.
41. Buchwald H, Varco RL, Boen JR, et al: Effective lipid modification by partial ileal bypass reduced long-term coronary heart disease mortality and morbidity: five-year posttrial follow-up report from the POSCH. Program on the Surgical Control of the Hyperlipidemias, *Arch Intern Med* 158:1253–1261, 1998.
42. MRC/BHF heart protection study of cholesterol lowering with simvastatin in 20,536 high-risk individuals: a randomised placebo-controlled trial, *Lancet* 360:7–22, 2002.
43. Pedersen TR, Kjekshus J, Pyoralai K, et al: Effect of simvastatin on ischemic signs and symptoms in the Scandinavian simvastatin survival study (4 s), *Am J Cardiol* 81:333–335, 1998.
44. McDermott MM, Guralnik JM, Greenland P, et al: Statin use and leg functioning in patients with and without lower-extremity peripheral arterial disease, *Circulation* 107:757–761, 2003.
45. Aronow WS, Nayak D, Woodworth S, Ahn C: Effect of simvastatin versus placebo on treadmill exercise time until the onset of intermittent claudication in older patients with peripheral arterial disease at six months and at one year after treatment, *Am J Cardiol* 92:711–712, 2003.
46. Mondillo S, Ballo P, Barbati R, et al: Effects of simvastatin on walking performance and symptoms of intermittent claudication in hypercholesterolemic patients with peripheral vascular disease, *Am J Med* 114:359–364, 2003.
47. Mohler ER 3rd, Hiatt WR, Creager MA: Cholesterol reduction with atorvastatin improves walking distance in patients with peripheral arterial disease, *Circulation* 108:1481–1486, 2003.
48. Giri J, McDermott MM, Greenland P, et al: Statin use and functional decline in patients with and without peripheral arterial disease, *J Am Coll Cardiol* 47:998–1004, 2006.
49. Rajamani K, Colman PG, Li LP, et al: Effect of fenofibrate on amputation events in people with type 2 diabetes mellitus (field study): a prespecified analysis of a randomised controlled trial, *Lancet* 373:1780–1788, 2009.
50. Jonason T, Bergstrom R: Cessation of smoking in patients with intermittent claudication. Effects on the risk of peripheral vascular complications, myocardial infarction and mortality, *Acta Med Scand* 221:253–260, 1987.
51. Quick CR, Cotton LT: The measured effect of stopping smoking on intermittent claudication, *Br J Surg* 69(Suppl):S24–S26, 1982.
52. Hobbs SD, Wilmink AB, Adam DJ, Bradbury AW: Assessment of smoking status in patients with peripheral arterial disease, *J Vasc Surg* 41:451–456, 2005.
53. Hobbs SD, Bradbury AW: Smoking cessation strategies in patients with peripheral arterial disease: an evidence-based approach, *Eur J Vasc Endovasc Surg* 26:341–347, 2003.
54. Law M, Tang JL: An analysis of the effectiveness of interventions intended to help people stop smoking, *Arch Intern Med* 155:1933–1941, 1995.
55. Anthonisen NR, Skeans MA, Wise RA, et al: The effects of a smoking cessation intervention on 14.5-year mortality: a randomized clinical trial, *Ann Intern Med* 142:233–239, 2005.
56. Hennrikus D, Joseph AM, Lando HA, et al: Effectiveness of a smoking cessation program for peripheral artery disease patients: a randomized controlled trial, *J Am Coll Cardiol* 56:2105–2112, 2010.
57. Okuyemi KS, Ahluwalia JS, Harris KJ: Pharmacotherapy of smoking cessation, *Arch Fam Med* 9:270–281, 2000.
58. Dalsgareth OJ, Hansen NC, Soes-Petersen U, et al: A multicenter, randomized, double-blind, placebo-controlled, 6-month trial of bupropion hydrochloride sustained-release tablets as an aid to smoking cessation in hospital employees, *Nicotine Tob Res* 6:55–61, 2004.
59. Gonzales D, Rennard SI, Nides M, et al: Varenicline, an alpha4beta2 nicotinic acetylcholine receptor partial agonist, vs sustained-release bupropion and placebo for smoking cessation: a randomized controlled trial, *JAMA* 296:47–55, 2006.
60. Jorenby DE, Hays JT, Rigotti NA, et al: Efficacy of varenicline, an alpha4beta2 nicotinic acetylcholine receptor partial agonist, vs placebo or sustained-release bupropion for smoking cessation: a randomized controlled trial, *JAMA* 296:56–63, 2006.
61. Fiore MC, Jaen CR: A clinical blueprint to accelerate the elimination of tobacco use, *JAMA* 299:2083–2085, 2008.
62. Conen D, Everett BM, Kurth T, et al: Smoking, smoking status, and risk for symptomatic peripheral artery disease in women: a cohort study, *Ann Intern Med* 154:719–726, 2011.
63. Chobanian AV, Bakris GL, Black HR, et al: The seventh report of the joint national committee on prevention, detection, evaluation, and treatment of high blood pressure: the JNC 7 report, *JAMA* 289:2560–2572, 2003.
64. The treatment of mild hypertension study. A randomized, placebo-controlled trial of a nutritional-hygienic regimen along with various drug monotherapies. The treatment of mild hypertension research group, *Arch Intern Med* 151:1413–1423, 1991.
65. Novo S, Abrignani MG, Pavone G, et al: Effects of captopril and ticlopidine, alone or in combination, in hypertensive patients with intermittent claudication, *Int Angiol* 15:169–174, 1996.
66. Solomon SA, Ramsay LE, Yeo WW, et al: Beta blockade and intermittent claudication: placebo controlled trial of atenolol and nifedipine and their combination, *BMJ* 303:1100–1104, 1991.

67. Roberts DH, Tsao Y, McLoughlin GA, et al: Placebo-controlled comparison of captopril, atenolol, labetalol, and pindolol in hypertension complicated by intermittent claudication, *Lancet* 2:650–653, 1987.
68. Sonecha TN, Nicolaides AN, Kyprianou P, et al: The effect of enalapril on leg muscle blood flow in patients with claudication, *Int Angiol* 9:22–24, 1990.
69. Ahimastos AA, Lawler A, Reid CM, et al: Brief communication: ramipril markedly improves walking ability in patients with peripheral arterial disease: a randomized trial, *Ann Intern Med* 144:660–664, 2006.
69a. Mancia G, Fagard R, Narkiewicz K, et al: 2013 ESH/ESC guidelines for the management of arterial hypertension: the Task Force for the Management of Arterial Hypertension of the European Society of Hypertension (ESH) and of the European Society of Cardiology (ESC), *Eur Heart J* 34:2159–2219, 2013.
69b. James PA, Oparil S, Carter BL, et al: 2014 evidence-based guideline for the management of high blood pressure in adults: report from the panel members appointed to the Eighth Joint National Committee (JNC 8), *JAMA* 311:507–520, 2014.
70. Mehler PS, Coll JR, Estacio R, et al: Intensive blood pressure control reduces the risk of cardiovascular events in patients with peripheral arterial disease and type 2 diabetes, *Circulation* 107:753–756, 2003.
71. Yusuf S, Sleight P, Pogue J, et al: Effects of an angiotensin-converting-enzyme inhibitor, ramipril, on cardiovascular events in high-risk patients. The heart outcomes prevention evaluation study investigators, *N Engl J Med* 342:145–153, 2000.
72. Fox KM: Efficacy of perindopril in reduction of cardiovascular events among patients with stable coronary artery disease: Randomised, double-blind, placebo-controlled, multicentre trial (the EUROPA study), *Lancet* 362:782–788, 2003.
73. Navalkar S, Parthasarathy S, Santanam N, Khan BV: Irbesartan, an angiotensin type 1 receptor inhibitor, regulates markers of inflammation in patients with premature atherosclerosis, *J Am Coll Cardiol* 37:440–444, 2001.
74. Dahlof B, Devereux RB, Kjeldsen SE, et al: Cardiovascular morbidity and mortality in the losartan intervention for endpoint reduction in hypertension study (life): a randomised trial against atenolol, *Lancet* 359:995–1003, 2002.
75. Pfeffer MA, Swedberg K, Granger CB, et al: Effects of candesartan on mortality and morbidity in patients with chronic heart failure: the charm-overall programme, *Lancet* 362:759–766, 2003.
76. Kjeldsen SE, Stålhammar J, Hasvold P, et al: Effects of losartan vs candesartan in reducing cardiovascular events in the primary treatment of hypertension, *J Hum Hypertens* 24:263–273, 2010.
77. Radack K, Deck C: Beta-adrenergic blocker therapy does not worsen intermittent claudication in subjects with peripheral arterial disease. A meta-analysis of randomized controlled trials, *Arch Intern Med* 151:1769–1776, 1991.
78. Olin JW: Hypertension and peripheral arterial disease, *Vasc Med* 10:241–246, 2005.
79. Effect of intensive diabetes management on macrovascular events and risk factors in the diabetes control and complications trial, *Am J Cardiol* 75:894–903, 1995.
80. Hadden DR, Patterson CC, Atkinson AB, et al: Macrovascular disease and hyperglycaemia: 10-year survival analysis in type 2 diabetes mellitus: the Belfast Diet Study, *Diabet Med* 14:663–672, 1997.
81. The effect of intensive treatment of diabetes on the development and progression of long-term complications in insulin-dependent diabetes mellitus. The diabetes control and complications trial research group, *N Engl J Med* 329:977–986, 1993.
82. Inzucchi SE, Bergenstal RM, Buse JB, et al: Management of hyperglycemia in type 2 diabetes: a patient-centered approach: position statement of the American Diabetes Association (ADA) and the European Association for the Study of Diabetes (EASD), *Diabetes Care* 35:1364–1379, 2012.
83. Standards of medical care for patients with diabetes mellitus, *Diabetes Care* 26(Suppl 1): S33–S50, 2003.
84. Gerstein HC, Miller ME, Byington RP, et al: Effects of intensive glucose lowering in type 2 diabetes, *N Engl J Med* 358:2545–2559, 2008.
85. Patel A, MacMahon S, Chalmers J, et al: Intensive blood glucose control and vascular outcomes in patients with type 2 diabetes, *N Engl J Med* 358:2560–2572, 2008.
86. Duckworth W, Abraira C, Moritz T, et al: Glucose control and vascular complications in veterans with type 2 diabetes, *N Engl J Med* 360:129–139, 2009.
87. Fowkes FG, Housley E, Riemersma RA, et al: Smoking, lipids, glucose intolerance, and blood pressure as risk factors for peripheral atherosclerosis compared with ischemic heart disease in the Edinburgh Artery Study, *Am J Epidemiol* 135:331–340, 1992.
88. Smith GD, Shipley MJ, Rose G: Intermittent claudication, heart disease risk factors, and mortality. The Whitehall Study, *Circulation* 82:1925–1931, 1990.
89. Criqui MH, Browner D, Fronek A, et al: Peripheral arterial disease in large vessels is epidemiologically distinct from small vessel disease. An analysis of risk factors, *Am J Epidemiol* 129:1110–1119, 1989.
90. Medalie JH, Papier CM, Goldbourt U, Herman JB: Major factors in the development of diabetes mellitus in 10,000 men, *Arch Intern Med* 135:811–817, 1975.
91. McDermott MM, Criqui MH, Ferrucci L, et al: Obesity, weight change, and functional decline in peripheral arterial disease, *J Vasc Surg* 43:1198–1204, 2006.
92. Antithrombotic Trialists' Collaboration: Collaborative meta-analysis of randomised trials of antiplatelet therapy for prevention of death, myocardial infarction, and stroke in high risk patients, *BMJ* 324:71–86, 2002.
93. Berger JS, Krantz MJ, Kittelson JM, Hiatt WR: Aspirin for the prevention of cardiovascular events in patients with peripheral artery disease: a meta-analysis of randomized trials, *JAMA* 301:1909–1919, 2009.
94. Fowkes FG, Price JF, Stewart MC, et al: Aspirin for prevention of cardiovascular events in a general population screened for a low ankle brachial index: a randomized controlled trial, *JAMA* 303:841–848, 2010.
95. Belch J, MacCuish A, Campbell I, et al: The Prevention of Progression of Arterial Disease and Diabetes (POPADAD) trial: Factorial randomised placebo controlled trial of aspirin and antioxidants in patients with diabetes and asymptomatic peripheral arterial disease, *BMJ* 337: a1840, 2008.
96. A randomised, blinded, trial of Clopidogrel Versus Aspirin in Patients at Risk of Ischaemic Events (CAPRIE). CAPRIE Steering Committee, *Lancet* 348:1329–1339, 1996.
97. Bhatt DL, Fox KA, Hacke W, et al: Clopidogrel and aspirin versus aspirin alone for the prevention of atherothrombotic events, *N Engl J Med* 354:1706–1717, 2006.
98. Cacoub PP, Bhatt DL, Steg PG, et al: Patients with peripheral arterial disease in the charisma trial, *Eur Heart J* 30:192–201, 2009.
99. Anand S, Yusuf S, Xie C, et al: Oral anticoagulant and antiplatelet therapy and peripheral arterial disease, *N Engl J Med* 357:217–227, 2007.
100. Hood SC, Moher D, Barber GG: Management of intermittent claudication with pentoxifylline: meta-analysis of randomized controlled trials, *CMAJ* 155:1053–1059, 1996.
101. Hiatt WR, Regensteiner JG, Hargarten ME, et al: Benefit of exercise conditioning for patients with peripheral arterial disease, *Circulation* 81:602–609, 1990.
102. Reilly MP, Mohler ER 3rd: Cilostazol: treatment of intermittent claudication, *Ann Pharmacother* 35:48–56, 2001.
103. Dawson DL, Cutler BS, Meissner MH, Strandness DE Jr.: Cilostazol has beneficial effects in treatment of intermittent claudication: results from a multicenter, randomized, prospective, double-blind trial, *Circulation* 98:678–686, 1998.
104. Money SR, Herd JA, Isaacsohn JL, et al: Effect of cilostazol on walking distances in patients with intermittent claudication caused by peripheral vascular disease, *J Vasc Surg* 27:267–274, 1998, discussion 274–265.
105. Beebe HG, Dawson DL, Cutler BS, et al: A new pharmacological treatment for intermittent claudication: results of a randomized, multicenter trial, *Arch Intern Med* 159:2041–2050, 1999.
106. Thompson PD, Zimet R, Forbes WP, Zhang P: Meta-analysis of results from eight randomized, placebo-controlled trials on the effect of cilostazol on patients with intermittent claudication, *Am J Cardiol* 90:1314–1319, 2002.
107. Dawson DL, Cutler BS, Hiatt WR, et al: A comparison of cilostazol and pentoxifylline for treating intermittent claudication, *Am J Med* 109:523–530, 2000.
108. Dobesh PP, Stacy ZA, Persson EL: Pharmacologic therapy for intermittent claudication, *Pharmacotherapy* 29:526–553, 2009.
109. Girolami B, Bernardi E, Prins MH, et al: Treatment of intermittent claudication with physical training, smoking cessation, pentoxifylline, or nafronyl: a meta-analysis, *Arch Intern Med* 159:337–345, 1999.
110. Leizorovicz A, Becker F: Oral buflomedil in the prevention of cardiovascular events in patients with peripheral arterial obstructive disease: a randomized, placebo-controlled, 4-year study, *Circulation* 117:816–822, 2008.
111. Pittler MH, Ernst E: Ginkgo biloba extract for the treatment of intermittent claudication: a meta-analysis of randomized trials, *Am J Med* 108:276–281, 2000.
112. Regensteiner JG, Gardner A, Hiatt WR: Exercise testing and exercise rehabilitation for patients with peripheral arterial disease: status in 1997, *Vasc Med* 2:147–155, 1997.
113. Gardner AW, Poehlman ET: Exercise rehabilitation programs for the treatment of claudication pain. A meta-analysis, *JAMA* 274:975–980, 1995.
114. Watson L, Ellis B, Leng GC: Exercise for intermittent claudication, *Cochrane Database Syst Rev*, 2008, CD000990.
115. Murphy TP, Cutlip DE, Regensteiner JG, et al: Supervised exercise versus primary stenting for claudication resulting from aortoiliac peripheral artery disease: six-month outcomes from the Claudication: Exercise Versus Endoluminal Revascularization (CLEVER) study, *Circulation* 125:130–139, 2012.
116. Hamburg NM, Balady GJ: Exercise rehabilitation in peripheral artery disease: functional impact and mechanisms of benefits, *Circulation* 123:87–97, 2011.
117. Garg PK, Tian L, Criqui MH, et al: Physical activity during daily life and mortality in patients with peripheral arterial disease, *Circulation* 114:242–248, 2006.
118. Bendermacher BL, Willigendael EM, Teijink JA, Prins MH: Supervised exercise therapy versus non-supervised exercise therapy for intermittent claudication, *Cochrane Database Syst Rev*, 2006, CD005263.
119. White CJ, Gray WA: Endovascular therapies for peripheral arterial disease: an evidence-based review, *Circulation* 116:2203–2215, 2007.
120. Mahmud E, Cavendish JJ, Salami A: Current treatment of peripheral arterial disease: role of percutaneous interventional therapies, *J Am Coll Cardiol* 50:473–490, 2007.
121. Sullivan TM, Childs MB, Bacharach JM, et al: Percutaneous transluminal angioplasty and primary stenting of the iliac arteries in 288 patients, *J Vasc Surg* 25:829–838, 1997, discussion 838–829.
122. Dormandy JA, Rutherford RB: Management of peripheral arterial disease (PAD). TASC working group. Transatlantic Inter-Society Consensus (TASC), *J Vasc Surg* 31:S1–S296, 2000.
123. Capek P, McLean GK, Berkowitz HD: Femoropopliteal angioplasty. Factors influencing long-term success, *Circulation* 83:I70–I80, 1991.
124. Johnston KW, Rae M, Hogg-Johnston SA, et al: 5-year results of a prospective study of percutaneous transluminal angioplasty, *Ann Surg* 206:403–413, 1987.
125. Zeller T: Current state of endovascular treatment of femoro-popliteal artery disease, *Vasc Med* 12:223–234, 2007.
126. Stokes KR, Strunk HM, Campbell DR, et al: Five-year results of iliac and femoropopliteal angioplasty in diabetic patients, *Radiology* 174:977–982, 1990.
127. Fowkes FG, Murray GD, Butcher I, et al: Ankle brachial index combined with Framingham risk score to predict cardiovascular events and mortality: a meta-analysis, *JAMA* 300:197–208, 2008.

28 Cerebrovascular Disease in Patients with Diabetes

Frank Joachim Erbguth

Stroke—in particular the ischemic subtype—is one of the major vascular manifestations of diabetes, together with coronary heart disease (CHD), peripheral arterial occlusive disease, and diabetic retinopathy. The relationship between hyperglycemia and stroke is bidirectional: on the one hand, diabetic patients exhibit more than a twofold risk of ischemic stroke compared with patients without diabetes (see the later discussion of epidemiology of stroke in diabetes), even after statistical correction for other vascular risk factors. On the other hand, acute stroke can generate acute disturbances of glucose metabolism with poststroke hyperglycemia (PSH) (see the later discussion of PSH), which is associated with an approximate twofold risk of a bad outcome. Treatment of hyperglycemia in patients with diabetes combined with multiple vascular risk factor management can substantially decrease the rate of stroke in primary as well as in secondary prevention. However, diabetes-associated end-organ damage to the brain is not only restricted to neuronal damage by strokes, but also involves chronic and insidious damage of the brain resulting in cognitive decline and dementia. Dementia in patients with diabetes not only results from vascular-mediated neuronal damage manifesting as vascular dementia (VD), but also is caused by an enhancement of neurodegenerative changes in the brain manifesting as Alzheimer disease (AD). In addition, between diabetes and dementia, bidirectional relations are likely: on the one hand, people with diabetes have double the risk of developing dementia by mechanisms that are not yet fully understood; and on the

other hand, the cognitive and behavioral manifestations of dementia such as lack of physical exercise and interference with therapeutic compliance may lead to disturbances of glucose metabolism resulting in lability of glucose control, including an increased frequency of episodes of severe hypoglycemia.

EPIDEMIOLOGY OF STROKE IN DIABETES

Epidemiology of Stroke: General Observations and Time Trends

Stroke is the second most frequent cause of death worldwide and the second leading cause of long-term disability in industrialized countries. The incidence of stroke is considerable across the United States and European countries, with the subtypes of ischemic stroke and transient ischemic attack (TIA) being the most common events (80% to 85%). Stroke incidence in European epidemiologic studies ranges from 114 cases/100,000 persons per year in France for first-ever stroke to 350 cases/100,000 persons per year in Germany for all stroke subtypes. Stroke prevalence estimates range from 1.5% in Italy and 3% in the United Kingdom and United States.[1]

The epidemiologic Oxford Vascular Study[2] analyzed the frequency of three types of vascular events (acute coronary, cerebrovascular, and peripheral) in a population of 91,106 inhabitants in Oxfordshire, United Kingdom, from 2002 to 2005. Cerebrovascular events (618 strokes and 300 TIAs), with a proportion of 45%, were more frequent than coronary

341

vascular events, which affected 42% of the cohort (159 ST-segment elevation myocardial infarctions (STEMIs); 316 non–ST-elevation MIs; 218 unstable angina events; 163 sudden cardiac deaths), and peripheral vascular events, with an incidence of 9% (43 aortic; 53 embolic visceral or limb ischemic events; 92 critical limb ischemic events). Sixty-two deaths remained unclassifiable. The relative incidence of cerebrovascular events compared with coronary events was 1.19 (95% confidence interval [CI] 1.06-1.33) overall, and 1.40 (1.23-1.59) for nonfatal events. Event and incidence rates rose steeply with age in all arterial territories, with 735 (80%) cerebrovascular, 623 (73%) coronary, and 147 (78%) peripheral vascular events in 12,886 (14%) individuals aged 65 years or older; and 503 (54%), 402 (47%), and 105 (56%), respectively, in the 5919 (6%) aged 75 years or older (**Fig. 28-1**). Similar data were shown by French investigators.[3]

A comparison of incidence rates among different subtypes of stroke shows approximately 80% to 85% for ischemic stroke, 10% to 15% for intracerebral hemorrhage, and 5% for subarachnoid hemorrhage. It is not surprising that all studies have demonstrated that the incidence and prevalence of stroke in general increase with age.[1] However, the stroke subtype involving subarachnoid hemorrhage, because of its distinct cause (ruptured aneurysms), does not follow this pattern. The stroke incidence is higher in men than in women of the same age, based on age-adjusted data. Some studies on time trends of stroke epidemiology have indicated that the incidence and the individual personal risk have decreased during the last 20 years.[1]

Stroke mortality rates have been decreasing consistently over time, with recent reports indicating a 29.2% reduction in stroke mortality between 1999 and 2008 in the United States. A German registry found decreased mortality rates from 52.4 deaths per population of 100,000 in 2000 to 32.3 deaths per 100,000 in 2008 in both men and women combined; a greater rate of decline was observed in women.[1] Such increased survival of stroke patients may be linked to advances in preclinical and hospital treatment in acute stroke and in neurorehabilitation.

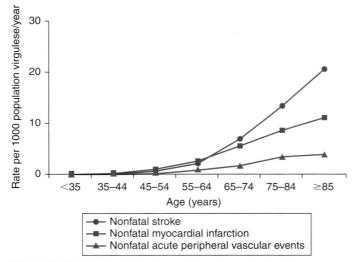

FIGURE 28-1 Age-specific event rates for nonfatal stroke (red line), nonfatal myocardial infarction (blue line), and nonfatal acute peripheral vascular events (green line). (Modified from Rothwell PM, Coull AJ, Silver LE, et al: Population-based study of event-rate, incidence, case fatality, and mortality for all acute vascular events in all arterial territories [Oxford Vascular Study], Lancet 366:1773-1783, 2005.)

In the United Kingdom, an analysis of 32,151 stroke patients within the UK General Practice Research Database[4] revealed that stroke incidence fell significantly by 30% from 1.48/1000 person-years in 1999 to 1.04/1000 person-years in 2008. Fifty-six–day stroke mortality after first stroke was reduced significantly from 21% in 1999 to 12% in 2008. Stroke prevalence, however, increased significantly by 12.5%, from 6.40/1000 in 1999 to 7.20/1000 in 2008. The positive changes in stroke incidence coincided with a marked increase in primary care prescription of primary and secondary cardiovascular preventive medications such as lipid-lowering, antihypertensive, and antithrombotic drugs. Despite these positive findings, the study clearly demonstrated an underuse of oral anticoagulation in patients with atrial fibrillation (AF) at high risk of stroke, and lower use of all preventive treatments in women compared with men.

Diabetes and Other Risk Factors for Stroke

The risk of stroke associated with diabetes has been assessed predominantly in people with type 2 diabetes, because stroke is more common in that population than in the age group typical of persons with type 1 diabetes. Epidemiologic studies identified a twofold to fourfold increase in stroke risk for persons with diabetes.[5] As early as 1988, a population-based study demonstrated diabetes mellitus (DM) as an independent risk factor for stroke; during a follow-up of 3778 persons aged 50 to 79 years over 12 years, diabetes was associated with an increase in risk of 1.8 in men (95% CI 1.0-3.2) and 2.2 in women (95% CI 1.0-4.5).[6] The Nurses' Health Study observed 120,000 women for more than 8 years and found an unadjusted 5.4-fold increase in stroke risk that was associated with diabetes and, after correction for other confounding variables, an adjusted threefold increased stroke risk with diabetes.[7] During the longest observation period of 30 years in the Framingham Heart Study, a 2.5- to 3.6-fold increased risk of stroke in diabetic patients was found.[8] A meta-analysis of 102 prospective studies including 530,083 participants demonstrated a hazard ratio (HR) for ischemic stroke of 2.3 (95% CI 2.0-2.7) for patients with versus without diabetes.[9] A Finnish cohort study with 25,155 men and 26,423 women aged 25 to 74 years showed that diabetes at baseline carried a similar risk for stroke as a prior stroke (PS) at baseline.[10]

The duration of diabetes was independently associated with ischemic stroke risk according to data from the Northern Manhattan Study, adjusting for other risk factors. The observed risk increase associated with diabetes overall was 3% each year, and tripled with diabetes duration of 10 years or longer (**Table 28-1**).[11]

Assuming a population-wide prevalence of diabetes of 10%, these epidemiologic findings indicate a diabetes-attributable risk of stroke of approximately 12%. Hence, one in eight cases of stroke may be attributable to diabetes. Taking into account overall stroke mortality in general and its observed increased risk in diabetes, cerebrovascular disease causes approximately 20% of deaths of diabetic patients.[5]

Comparison of Vascular Risk Factors Between Stroke and Coronary Heart Disease

The case-control study INTERSTROKE[12]—analogous to the INTERHEART study—examined the worldwide burden of stroke and the quantitative impact of known risk factors in different countries, in particular in developing countries.

TABLE 28-1 Duration of Diabetes and Ischemic Stroke Risk

DIABETES DURATION (YEARS)	ADJUSTED HAZARD RATIO (HR)	95% CONFIDENCE INTERVAL (CI)
0-5	1.7	1.1-2.7
5-10	1.8	1.1-3.0
>10	3.2	2.4-4.5

Data from Banerjee C, Moon YP, Paik MC, et al: Duration of diabetes and risk of ischemic stroke: the Northern Manhattan Study. *Stroke* 43:1212-1217, 2012.

TABLE 28-2 Impact of Ten Vascular Risk Factors on Stroke and Myocardial Infarction: Odds Ratios and Percentage of the Population Attributable Risk (PAR)

RISK FACTOR/ BEHAVIOR	ODDS RATIO	PAR (%) FOR STROKE	PAR (%) FOR MYOCARDIAL INFARCTION
1. Arterial hypertension	2.64	34.6	17.9
2. Waist-to-hip ratio	1.65	26.5	20.1
3. Regular physical activity	0.69	28.5	12.2
4. Smoking	2.09	18.9	35,7
5. Diet risk score	1.35	18.8	13.7
6. Diabetes	1.36	5.0	9.9
7. Alcohol intake	1.51	3.8	6.7
8. Psychosocial factors (stress, depression)	1.3	9.8	32.5
9. Cardiac causes	2.38	6.7	—
10. Ratio of apolipoproteins B to A1	1.89	24.9	49.2

Of all fatal strokes worldwide, 85% occur in countries with low to middle income, and the number of strokes worldwide is massively driven by the increase in stroke incidence in developing and newly industrialized countries. Comparing 3000 stroke patients (78% ischemic stroke, 22% hemorrhagic stroke) and 3000 controls, the study extracted the 10 risk factors listed in decreasing order in **Table 28-2** (odds ratios [ORs] and percentage of the population attributable risk [PAR]). For comparison, the corresponding numbers from the INTERHEART study are given in a third column.

Collectively the listed 10 risk factors account for 90% of all strokes, and the first five risk factors—namely, arterial hypertension, smoking, abdominal adiposity, diet habits, and little physical exercise—explain 80% of all strokes. Hypertension was the most important individual epidemiologic risk factor, which tripled the stroke risk, and therefore has a higher relative importance for the risk of stroke than for the risk of CHD. DM as the sixth strongest by PAR% was placed in the middle field, being surrounded by diabetes-related risk factors such as adiposity, lack of physical exercise, and diet habits.

From the mentioned epidemiologic data, an individual stroke risk calculation can be deduced. Kothari and colleagues[13] developed a mathematical model from the United Kingdom Prospective Diabetes Study (UKPDS) data to calculate an individual's risk of stroke within the following 5 years. In this model, for example, a 67-year-old smoker with arterial hypertension, hypercholesterolemia, and diabetes duration of 12 years has a 10.5% risk of stroke within the next 5 years.

It is not surprising that diabetes not only doubles the risk for a first-ever stroke, but in the same manner doubles the risk for a recurrent stroke after a first event.[14,15]

Obviously, there has been a decline in cardiovascular death including stroke in individuals with diabetes; a recent report from the U.S. National Institutes of Health compared 3-year death rates between 1997 and 2004 and found a decline in the cardiovascular disease (CVD) death rate of 40%.[16]

Diabetes as a Stroke Risk Factor IN Younger Patients

Type 1 and type 2 diabetes play an important role as stroke risk factors, particularly in younger and middle-aged patients, because in these age groups other competing stroke risk factors are less prevalent and henceforth contribute less attributable risk than at older ages. According to an observational study in the United States of persons aged 18 to 44 years, diabetes raised the relative stroke risk from 6-fold to 23-fold, depending on gender and race or ethnicity.[17] In general, in patients younger than 60 years, the relative risk (RR) of stroke in those with versus without diabetes is approximately double that of individuals older than 70 years.[9] According to calculations from several studies, diabetes leads to an advanced cerebrovascular aging of approximately 10 to 15 years.

Multiplicative Risk Increase by Additional Vascular Risk Factors

Patients with diabetes almost always have additional vascular risk factors such as arterial hypertension, dyslipoproteinemia, obesity, lack of physical exercise, and nonvalvular AF. These comorbidities not only add to the risk of stroke from diabetes, but multiplicatively affect the risk of stroke. Some studies, for example, found that the combination of diabetes and hypertension was associated with a 5-fold to 10-fold increased risk of stroke, suggesting a synergistic impact on stroke risk.[18]

Stroke Risk in Prediabetes- and Diabetes-Associated Metabolic Risk Configurations (Insulin Resistance, Metabolic Syndrome, Adiposity)

Prediabetes (Impaired Fasting Glucose, Impaired Glucose Tolerance, Hemoglobin A1c)

Not only in diabetes per se, but also in prediabetic states, the risk for cerebrovascular disease is increased, although in general more modestly than with fully established diabetes. Prediabetes is defined as the condition in which glycemic variables are higher than normal but lower than the established diabetes thresholds. Prediabetes is a high-risk state for diabetes development: 5% to 10% of people with prediabetes will convert to diabetes each year.

A prospective study found a significant relationship between levels of fasting plasma glucose (FPG) even below the diabetes threshold and the incidence of stroke in 43,933 asymptomatic nondiabetic men with a mean age of 44 years, who were free of known CVD at baseline.[19] A total of 595 stroke events occurred during 702,928 person-years of follow-up. Age-adjusted fatal, nonfatal, and total stroke event rates per 10,000 person-years for normal FPG (80 to 109 mg/dL), impaired fasting glucose (110 to 125 mg/dL), and undiagnosed diabetes (≥126 mg/dL) are listed in **Table 28-3**. For FPG levels of 110 mg/dL or greater, each 10-unit increment of FPG was associated with a 6% higher risk of total stroke events ($P = .05$).

TABLE 28-3 Stroke Rates per 10,000 Patient-Years in Different Levels of Fasting Plasma Glucose (FPG)

	NORMAL FPG (80-109 g/dL)	IMPAIRED FPG (110-125 mg/dL)	UNDIAGNOSED DIABETES (≥126 mg/dL)	SIGNIFICANCE
Fatal strokes	2.1	3.4	4.0	$P < .002$
Nonfatal strokes	10.3	11.8	18.0	$P < .008$
Total strokes	8.2	9.6	12.4	$P < .008$

Data from Sui X, Lavie CJ, Hooker SP, et al: A prospective study of fasting plasma glucose and risk of stroke in asymptomatic men, *Mayo Clin Proc* 86:1042-1049, 2011.

In another study of 14,000 patients with CHD, a J-shaped association was found between fasting glucose and incident stroke.[20] Stroke events after adjustment were increased in patients with fasting glucose levels of 100 to 109 mg/dL (OR 1.3), 110 to 125 mg/dL (OR 1.6), when compared with levels of 90 to 99 mg/dL. However, patients with very low fasting glucose levels (<80 mg/dL) also exhibited a 1.5-fold increased risk of stroke. The mechanisms underlying this association remain unclear.

In 3127 patients with TIA or minor ischemic stroke in the Dutch TIA Trial,[21] a J-shaped relationship between baseline nonfasting glucose levels and stroke risk was also observed. In patients with impaired glucose tolerance (defined as glucose 7.8 to 11.0 mmol/L), risk of stroke was almost doubled compared with those with normal glucose levels (HR 1.8, 95% CI 1.1-3.0) and almost tripled in diabetic patients (glucose ≥11.1 mmol/L; HR 2.8, 95% CI 1.9-4.1). Patients with low glucose levels (<4.6 mmol/L) had a 50% increased stroke risk (HR 1.5, 95% CI 1.0-2.2) compared with those with normal glucose levels. There was no association between glucose levels and risk of MI or cardiac death. When impaired glucose tolerance was measured by oral glucose tolerance test (OGTT) as in the Japanese Hisayama study,[22] 2-hour values of the OGTT of 11.1 mmol/L were associated with a more-than-doubled risk for stroke (in men, HR 2.71; in women, HR 2.19).

Glycated hemoglobin concentrations are also associated with the risk of stroke even below diabetes thresholds. On analysis of nondiabetic adults participating in the community-based Atherosclerosis Risk in Communities (ARIC) study,[23] HbA1c concentrations—adjusted for potential confounders and for other vascular risk factors—of greater than 6% were associated with two to three times increased risk of stroke. The adjusted HRs for ischemic stroke according to baseline HbA1c are displayed in **Figure 28-2**.

A meta-analysis from 15 prospective cohort studies, which included 760,925 participants, tested the association of stroke risk with prediabetes defined in two ways. Among the eight studies that defined prediabetes as fasting glucose levels ranging from 100 to 125 mg/dL (5.6 to 6.9 mmol/L), which is the current American Diabetes Association (ADA) definition, there was no increase in the risk for stroke after adjustment for established cardiovascular risk factors (1.08; 95% CI 0.94-1.23). In contrast, among the five studies that used the ADA's more stringent 1997 definition of prediabetes (fasting glucose levels ranging from 110 to 125 mg/dL [6.1-6.9 mmol/L]), there was a 21% increased RR after adjustment for established cardiovascular risk factors (1.21; 95% CI 1.02-1.44; $P = .03$), indicating that the extent of the relationship between prediabetes and risk for stroke is a matter of definition of prediabetes.[24]

For those studies that included data on impaired glucose tolerance or combined impaired glucose tolerance and

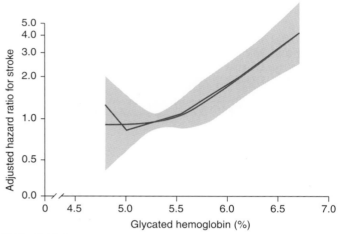

FIGURE 28-2 Adjusted hazard ratios for ischemic stroke according to baseline glycated hemoglobin. *(Modified with permission from Selvin E, Steffes MW, Zhu H, et al: Glycated hemoglobin, diabetes, and cardiovascular risk in nondiabetic adults,* N Engl J Med *362:800-811, 2010.)*

impaired fasting glucose, there was an increased risk for stroke after adjustment for established cardiovascular risk factors (1.26; 95% CI 1.10-1.43; $P < .001$).

Metabolic Risk Configurations (Insulin Resistance, Metabolic Syndrome, Adiposity)

Insulin resistance (IR), a state in which cells fail to respond to the normal actions of insulin, has also been found to be associated with an increased risk of stroke. In the Cardiovascular Health Study,[25] individuals without prevalent diabetes or stroke at baseline were followed for 17 years. Higher IR measured with the Gutt index[26] or 2-hour postload glucose levels was associated with a higher stroke incidence. For calculation of the Gutt index (insulin sensitivity index), plasma glucose and insulin concentrations from fasting (0-min) and 120-minute samples from the OGTT are used. The index is defined as follows:

$$MCR/\log MSI$$

The metabolic clearance rate (MCR) is obtained by $MCR = m/MPG$, where MPG is the mean of the 0- and 120-min glucose values from the OGTT. The mean serum insulin (MSI, mU/L) is the mean insulin concentration obtained from the 0- and 120-min samples of the OGTT.

The glucose uptake rate in peripheral tissues, m (mg/min), is obtained by the following formula:

$$m = [75,000\,\text{mg} + (\text{Glucose}_0 - \text{Glucose}_{120}) \times 0.19 \times \text{BW}]/120\,\text{min}$$

where the term ($0.19 \times$ BW) denotes glucose space, and BW is body weight (kg).

The RR for the lowest quartile versus the highest quartile of the Gutt index was 1.64 (95% CI 1.24-2.16), adjusted for demographics and prevalent cardiovascular and kidney disease. Similarly, the adjusted risk ratio (RR) for the highest quartile versus the lowest quartile of 2-hour glucose was 1.84 (95% CI 1.39-2.42). In contrast, the adjusted RR for the highest quartile versus the lowest quartile of fasting insulin was not significant (1.10; 95% CI 0.84-1.46).

Higher levels of IR are associated with a 10% to 100% increased risk of stroke, depending on the degree of elevation and on the presence of other associated vascular risk factors. The U.S. National Health and Nutrition Examination Survey (NHANES) revealed the homeostatic model assessment of insulin resistance (HOMA-IR; equation: Fasting glucose [mmol/L] × Fasting insulin [mU/L]/22.5) as a measure for insulin resistance[27] to be independently and significantly associated with stroke risk with an OR of 1.06 (95% CI 1.01-1.12) for each HOMA-IR unit, after adjustment for age, history of MI, the presence of hypertension or claudication, activity level, and HbA1c.[28] It seems clear that IR is a risk factor for stroke, but it remains controversial whether insulin concentrations themselves or markers of glucose tolerance convey the highest risk.

The role, and impact of the metabolic syndrome (MetS), a clustering of disturbed glucose and insulin metabolism, obesity, and abdominal fat distribution, dyslipidemia, and hypertension remain controversial. A Finnish population-based cohort study on stroke risk[29] with an average follow-up of 14.3 years revealed for men a 2.41-fold (95% CI 1.12-5.32) increased risk for ischemic stroke associated with MetS, after adjustment for socioeconomic status, smoking, alcohol, and family history of CHD. After additional adjustments the results remained significant.

In the Northern Manhattan Study, 3298 stroke-free individuals were prospectively followed for 6.4 years with a 44% prevalence of MetS, which was associated with a 50% increase in stroke risk after adjustment for sociodemographic and risk factors.[30] The effect of MetS on stroke risk was greater in women (HR 2.0; 95% CI 1.3-3.1) than in men (HR 1.1; 95% CI 0.6-1.9) and among Hispanics (HR 2.0; 95% CI 1.2-3.4) compared with blacks (HR 1.3; 95% CI 0.7-2.3) and whites (HR 1.28; 95% CI 0.6-2.5).

A contrary result was found in a Greek study with a 10-year follow-up,[31] in which MetS per se at baseline or combinations of its components did not predict the development of ischemic stroke in patients with type 2 diabetes. After statistical calculations, only waist circumference (HR 1.006) and age (HR 1.061) were significant predictors for stroke risk. However, habits of food consumption and the influence of the Mediterranean diet in the Greek population were not considered.

Also, in the Stroke Prevention by Aggressive Reduction in Cholesterol Levels (SPARCL) trial,[15] which analyzed the effect of treatment with atorvastatin versus placebo in reducing stroke in patients with a recent stroke or TIA, patients with MetS were not at increased risk for stroke or major cardiovascular events, but more frequently had revascularization procedures (adjusted HR 1.78; 95% CI 1.26-2.5; $P = .001$).

The difference in the results of epidemiologic studies compared with an intervention study such as SPARCL might be a result of the effect of intensive risk factor management for patients enrolled in clinical drug trials. For example, during the SPARCL trial, blood pressure—as a component of MetS—and other risk factors were carefully controlled, and all persons received appropriate antithrombotic treatment, which is usually not reliably the case for those included in epidemiologic studies.

All together, the available data support the consideration of MetS as an independent risk factor for stroke, depending on the metabolic and vascular risk configuration of the affected person on the whole and depending on the definition of MetS. The fact that the incremental stroke risk associated with MetS appears greater than the sum of its components suggests potential biologic interaction among MetS components, generating a risk that is more than additive. According to the type of study and the definition of MetS, its relation to increased risk of stroke is most commonly statistically significant.

The methodologic problems of such association studies with MetS are also obvious, if one notes the variability of the proportion of patients with diabetes included, which ranged from 0% to 100%: the Northern Manhattan Study[30] had a proportion of 17% with diabetes; in the Finnish study[29] no patients with diabetes were included; and the Greek study[31] analyzed a group with 100% prevalence of diabetes. However, all studies similarly analyzed and reported the "independent" contribution of MetS to the risk of stroke.

Obesity in most studies is associated with an increased risk of stroke, whether measured by body mass index (BMI), waist-to-hip ratio, waist-to-height ratio, or waist circumference.[32] Persons with a BMI of 30 kg/m^2 or more have a twofold risk of stroke compared with individuals with a BMI of less than 23 kg/m^2.[33] According to the results of a collaborative analysis of 57 prospective studies with 900,000 individuals, each unit increase in BMI is associated with an increase in the adjusted risk of stroke by approximately 6%. Among adults who are overweight or obese (BMI 25 to 50 kg/m^2), each 5 kg/m^2 increase in BMI is associated with an approximately 40% higher mortality rate from stroke (HR 1.39; 95% CI 1.31-1.48).[34] In the INTERSTROKE study,[12] persons with a waist-to-hip ratio in the highest tertile had a 65% increased risk of stroke (OR 1.65, 99% CI 1.36-1.99) compared with those in the lowest tertile.

However, all measures of adiposity and obesity such as BMI, waist-to-hip ratio, and waist circumference do not consistently improve prediction of stroke risk when added to the most robustly associated stroke risk factors such as arterial hypertension and diabetes. Despite these often discordant observations, excess adiposity remains a major modifiable determinant of these causal risk factors for stroke.

PATHOPHYSIOLOGY AND SUBTYPES OF ISCHEMIC STROKE IN DIABETES

Stroke in diabetes is the clinical culmination of atherosclerotic changes in the extracranial and intracranial large and small arteries associated with hyperglycemia. The proatherogenic effects in diabetes on cerebral blood vessels are not different from effects on coronary arteries and encompass advanced glycation endproducts (AGEs), oxidative stress, endothelial dysfunction, inflammation, and hypercoagulability. In addition, the increased rate of CHD among patients with diabetes causes cardiomyopathy and AF, both of which predispose to cardioembolic stroke. AF is responsible for at least 20% to 30% of ischemic strokes.[35] Recent findings indicate that AF may be relatively common in diabetic patients, with the risk of AF increased by 30% to 40% in individuals with diabetes.[36] The severity of cardioembolic strokes and the resulting disability are greater than with noncardioembolic stroke, and hospital mortality is doubled.

A recent U.S. cohort study comparing 17,372 patients with diabetes with age- and gender-matched patients without

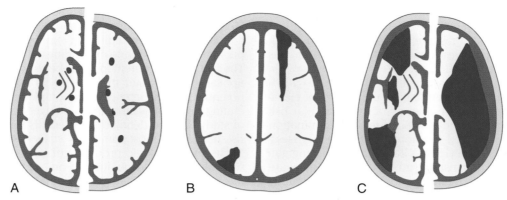

FIGURE 28-3 Diabetes increases the risk for all subtypes of ischemic stroke: **A,** lacunar; **B,** hemodynamic by large artery occlusion; and **C,** cardioembolic.

type 2 diabetes[37] found a significantly higher prevalence of AF among patients with versus without diabetes (3.6 versus 2.5%). Over a mean follow-up of 7.2 ± 2.8 years, diabetic patients without AF at baseline developed AF at an age- and gender-adjusted rate of 9.1 per 1000 person-years (95% CI 8.6-9.7) compared with a rate of 6.6 (95% CI 6.2-7.1) among nondiabetic patients. After full adjustment for other risk factors, diabetes was associated with a 26% increased risk of AF in women (HR 1.26; 95% CI 1.08-1.46), but diabetes was not a statistically significant factor in men (HR 1.09; 0.96-1.24). Diabetes not only is a risk factor for developing AF, but also increases the risk of its systemic and cerebral embolic complications. Depending on other accompanying risk factors, stroke rates in AF can reach almost 20% per year. Diabetes is one of the risk items counting as one point in the six-point $CHADS_2$ score and the nine-point CHA_2DS_2-VASc score, both of which are used to calculate an individual's stroke risk in AF and to inform clinical decision making with regard to antithrombotic therapies.

Because of its impact on cerebrovascular and cardiac systems, diabetes incrementally increases risk for all three subtypes of ischemic stroke: lacunar, large artery occlusive, and thromboembolic. The distribution of these stroke subtypes among patients with diabetes is similar to that in the general population; however, those with diabetes have a greater burden of small-vessel, or lacunar, infarcts, which sometimes are clinically silent.[38] In addition, the proportion of ischemic strokes with infratentorial localization is relatively increased in patients with diabetes (**Fig. 28-3**).

PRIMARY AND SECONDARY PREVENTION OF STROKE IN DIABETES

Glucose Control

In the 1441 patients with type 1 diabetes (aged 13 to 40 years) enrolled in the Diabetes Control and Complications Trial (DCCT) and Epidemiology of Diabetes Interventions and Complications (EDIC) study,[39] intensive glucose management for 6.5 years reduced the risk of cardiovascular composite events (nonfatal MI, stroke, or cardiovascular deaths) significantly by 57% over a mean follow-up period of 17 years, compared with individuals under conventional treatment. However, the absolute numbers of stroke were low, with only one event in the intensive treatment group and five in the conventional treatment group. The target preprandial blood glucose in the intensively treated group was 70 to 120 mg/dL (<180 mg/dL postprandial); the mean HbA1c values were approximately

2% lower than in the conventional treatment group (7.4% versus 9.1%).

In patients with type 2 diabetes in the UKPDS study,[40] intensive treatment with sulfonylureas or insulin did not significantly reduce cardiovascular outcomes compared with conventional diet therapy. However, in the substudy within the UKPDS in which obese patients received metformin as a first-line treatment, the risk of stroke was reduced by 42% compared with the group receiving conventional treatment (3.3 versus 6.2 events per 1000 patient-years).[41]

Three more recent large long-term trials (Action in Diabetes and Vascular Disease: Preterax and Diamicron MR Controlled Evaluation [ADVANCE]; Action to Control Cardiovascular Risk in Diabetes [ACCORD]; Veterans Affairs Diabetes Trial [VADT]) also compared the effects of intensive versus standard treatment in individuals with longstanding type 2 diabetes and a fairly high risk of cardiovascular and cerebrovascular events.[42-44] In the ADVANCE and the VADT studies, no difference in cardiovascular outcomes—including stroke—could be found between the two glucose-lowering strategies. In the ACCORD study the rates of nonfatal stroke were similar in the intervention and control groups.

No beneficial effects of tight glucose management over a mean period of 5 years could be found in a meta-analysis of 34,533 patients with type 2 diabetes (HR 0.96; 95% CI 0.83-1.1).[45] A similar result was communicated in a Cochrane review summarizing the findings from 29,986 patients with type 2 diabetes from 20 randomized trials.[46] The duration of intervention varied from 3 days to 12.5 years. Targeting intensive glycemic control did not reduce the RR of nonfatal stroke (risk ratio 0.96; 95% CI 0.8-1.2).

Taken together, to date, insufficient data are available to prove that intensive and tight glycemic control per se improves occurrence of stroke—in particular in type 2 diabetes. Treatment of patients with a high risk of stroke must balance the risk of recurrent hypoglycemia against the potential advantages of lower targets of HbA1c.

Management of Diabetes Associated Vascular Risk Factors

In the UKPDS, the variables that predicted the 188 incident strokes in DM included duration of diabetes, age, gender, smoking, systolic blood pressure (SBP), dyslipoproteinemia, and the presence of AF. Modifiable risk factors for stroke accompanying diabetes have been targeted for stroke prevention in several randomized controlled trials.

Hypertension

Hypertension has long been recognized as the major modifiable risk factor for stroke. Lowering of blood pressure has a large effect on the risk of stroke. In the UKPDS, better blood pressure control among patients with type 2 diabetes was associated with a 44% reduction in stroke incidence for each 10–mm Hg reduction in mean SBP.[47] In a meta-analysis of 13 trials with 37,736 patients with type 2 diabetes, impaired fasting glucose, or impaired glucose tolerance, more intensive blood pressure control in comparison with standard treatment was associated with a 10% relative reduction in all-cause mortality and a 17% reduction in stroke (OR 0.83; 95% CI 0.73-0.95).[48] The stroke-preventing effect of blood pressure lowering was mainly detected in those trials, in which the target of SBP was 130 to 135 mm Hg. Tighter blood pressure control below the threshold of 130 mm Hg was associated with a significant reduction in stroke, but a 40% increase in serious adverse events, with no benefit for cardiac, renal, and retinal complications.

In the ACCORD trial, a total of 4733 participants with type 2 diabetes were randomly assigned to intensive blood pressure treatment targeting a systolic pressure of less than 120 mm Hg, or standard therapy targeting a systolic pressure of less than 140 mm Hg.[49] After 1 year, a mean SBP of 119.3 mm Hg was achieved in the intensive therapy group and 133.5 mm Hg in the standard therapy group. The annual risk rates of stroke after a mean follow-up of 4.7 years were 0.32% and 0.53% in the two groups, respectively (HR 0.59; 95% CI 0.39-0.89). However, the intensive blood pressure management did not reduce the rate of the composite outcome of fatal and nonfatal major cardiovascular events and led to an increase in adverse events such as syncope and hyperkalemia.

A recent meta-analysis of 11 studies with 42,572 participants compared the effects of tight SBP control (target SBP <130 mm Hg) versus usual SBP control (SBP 130 to 139 mm Hg) on stroke prevention in general[50] and in subgroups. Achieving a tight SBP level was associated with a significant 20% lower stroke risk (RR 0.80; 95% CI 0.70-0.92). The subgroup of patients with cardiovascular risk factors but without established CVD showed substantial reduction of future stroke risk with tight control (RR 0.49; 95% CI 0.34-0.69), but those with established CVD at entry did not experience stroke risk reduction with tight control (RR 0.92; 95% CI 0.83-1.03). Patients with DM at entry showed reduction of future stroke risk with tight control, but those without DM at entry only experienced marginal stroke risk reduction with tight control (RR 0.65, 95% CI 0.48-0.87; versus RR 0.85, 95% CI 0.73-1.00).

Most guidelines for stroke prevention recommend a blood pressure less than 130/80 mm Hg. Reaching these target levels is probably more important than the choice of antihypertensive drug. However, for stroke prevention, beta blockers seem to be inferior to other antihypertensives and, in contrast, calcium channel blockers have been shown to be superior. As a potential explanation for such observed differences in efficacy in stroke prevention by drug classes, different effects on within-individual blood pressure variability across the classes have been proposed, which seems to be an independent risk predictor for stroke (**Fig. 28-4**).[51]

Lipids

In a subgroup of 6000 patients of the Heart Protection Study with diabetes, simvastatin at a daily dose of 40 mg versus

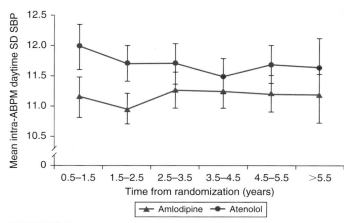

FIGURE 28-4 Lower variability in daytime systolic blood pressure (standard deviation [SD]) of the calcium-channel blocker amlodipine compared with the beta blocker atenolol. A higher blood pressure variability was an independent risk factor for stroke. *(Modified from Rothwell PM, Howard SC, Dolan E, et al: Effects of beta blockers and calcium-channel blockers on within-individual variability in blood pressure and risk of stroke,* Lancet Neurol *9:469-480, 2010.)*

placebo was associated with a 28% (95% CI 8-44) reduction in ischemic stroke, independent of baseline lipid levels.[52] The Collaborative Atorvastatin Diabetes Study (CARDS) found a 48% (95% CI 17-52) reduction in all types of stroke in patients with type 2 diabetes without manifest CVD in the intervention group with 10 mg atorvastatin daily compared with placebo.[53] The Cholesterol Treatment Trialists' Collaboration meta-analysis of 18,686 people with diabetes included 14 placebo-controlled randomized trials of statins.[54] There was a significant 21% (95% CI 7-33) reduction of first stroke, which was similar to the effect observed in the 71,370 patients without diabetes.

For secondary stroke prevention, fewer data are available. The SPARCL trial found that atorvastatin 80 mg daily versus placebo reduced stroke risk in patients with recent stroke or TIA and no known CHD by 16% with a 5-year absolute reduction in stroke risk of 2.2%[55] In the secondary analysis of the SPARCL trial for the subgroup of individuals with type 2 diabetes and MetS, no treatment-by-subgroup interactions were found, indicating a similar stroke preventive effect for the subgroup of patients with diabetes.[55]

Platelet Inhibition

In a meta-analysis on the use of aspirin for primary prevention in persons with diabetes, no significant benefits could be recorded with respect to reduction of serious vascular events, including stroke (RR for stroke 0.83, 95% CI 0.60-1.14).[56] For secondary prevention of stroke, no major studies specifically for individuals with diabetes have been performed. Although a subgroup analysis of the Clopidogrel Versus Aspirin in Patients at Risk of Ischaemic Events (CAPRIE) trial suggested a slightly greater benefit of clopidogrel versus aspirin for patients with diabetes,[57] the meta-analysis of the Antithrombotic Trialists' Collaboration[58] found a similar stroke reduction for both cardiovascular events and ischemic stroke.

Although there is no clear proof for a substantial effect of platelet inhibition on the risk of stroke in primary prevention, antiplatelet agents—mostly aspirin—should be considered for every patient with diabetes identified to be at increased risk of future cerebrovascular complications.

Multifactor Risk Factor Management

The efficacy of multifactorial preventive measures on the risk of stroke in individuals with type 2 diabetes was assessed in three trials.[59–61] No clear benefits specifically for stroke prevention were found in the Euro Heart Survey on Diabetes and the Heart, apart from a general 40% risk reduction in cardiovascular events.[59] Cerebrovascular revascularization procedures, however, were reduced by half. The ADDITION-Europe trial, which focused on early multifactorial treatment after diagnosis of diabetes versus usual care, did not find a different stroke rate between the groups during a mean follow-up of 5.3 years, but the stroke rate was low in both groups with only 1.3% and 1.4%, respectively.[61] A small 17% nonsignificant reduction in the incidence of cardiovascular events and death was observed.

In contrast, a substantial benefit of multifactorial management was found in the Steno-2 trial,[60] in which the 7.8-year multifactorial approach encompassed the use of statins, angiotensin-converting enzyme (ACE) inhibitors, angiotensin II receptor blockers, platelet inhibition, glucose control, and lifestyle modification. At the end of the 13.3 years of follow-up, among 160 high-risk individuals with longstanding type 2 diabetes and microalbuminuria who participated in the study, a reduction in cardiovascular events by 59% (HR 0.41; 95% CI 0.25-0.67] was found. The number of all types of stroke was reduced by 80% (6 versus 30 events) (**Table 28-4**). These findings underscore that multifactorial risk factor management may be the key for a substantial reduction of stroke in diabetes.

Oral Anticoagulation in Atrial Fibrillation in Patients with Diabetes

Twenty percent to 30% of ischemic strokes are caused by cardiac embolism, most commonly from the left atrium and its appendage in nonvalvular AF. Diabetes, together with previous stroke, hypertension, advancing age, congestive heart failure, female gender, and atherosclerosis, is one of the major risk factors for stroke in individuals with AF (see the discussion of pathophysiology and subtypes of ischemic stroke in diabetes) and counts for 1 point in the six-point CHADS$_2$ score and the nine-point CHA$_2$DS$_2$-VASc score, both of which are used for the calculation of an individual´s stroke risk in AF (**Tables 28-5** and **28-6**).

Primary stroke prevention with adjusted-dose warfarin, a vitamin K antagonist (VKA), with a target international normalized ratio (INR) of 2.0 to 3.0, reduces the RR of first-ever stroke in individuals with AF with a moderate vascular risk profile by approximately two thirds compared with placebo (annual stroke risk 1.8% versus 4.6%), without a statistically

TABLE 28-4 Numbers of Events after 13.3 Years with Intensive Versus Conventional Multifactorial Cardiovascular Risk-Modifying Therapy among 160 High-Risk Patients with Diabetes

	INTENSIVE THERAPY (NUMBER OF EVENTS)	CONVENTIONAL THERAPY (NUMBER OF EVENTS)
Death from any cause	24	40
Myocardial infarction	9	35
Stroke	6	30
All cardiovascular events	51	158

TABLE 28-5 Conditions and Points for Calculation of the CHA$_2$DS$_2$-VASc Score (Maximum 9 Points)

C	Congestive heart failure (or left ventricular systolic dysfunction)	1
H	Hypertension: blood pressure consistently above 140/90 mm Hg (or treated hypertension on medication)	1
A$_2$	Age 75 years or older	2
D	Diabetes mellitus	1
S$_2$	Prior stroke or transient ischemic attack or thromboembolism	2
V	Vascular disease (e.g., peripheral artery disease, myocardial infarction, aortic plaque)	1
A	Age 65 to 74 years	1
Sc	Sex category is female	1

TABLE 28-6 Annual Stroke Risk According to CHA$_2$DS$_2$-VASc score

CHA$_2$DS$_2$-VASC SCORE	STROKE RISK %
0	0
1	1.3
2	2.2
3	3.2
4	4.0
5	6.7
6	9.8
7	9.6
8	6.7
9	15.2

Data from Lip GY, Frison L, Halperin JL, et al: Identifying patients at high risk for stroke despite anticoagulation: a comparison of contemporary stroke risk stratification schemes in an anticoagulated atrial fibrillation cohort, *Stroke* 41:2731-2738, 2010.

significant increase in the annual rates of intracranial hemorrhage (0.4% versus 0.2%) or major extracranial bleeding (approximately 2% versus 1%). For secondary stroke prevention, warfarin with a target INR of 2.0 to 3.0 also reduces the risk of recurrent stroke significantly by approximately two thirds compared with placebo (annual stroke risk 3.9% versus 12.3%; HR 0.34, 95% CI 0.20-0.57) and is associated with an annual nonsignificant increase in major bleeding (2.8% versus 0.7%; HR 3.20, 95% CI 0.91-11.3).[62]

Aspirin is not an adequate strategy to replace warfarin and is associated with a nonsignificant reduction in the RR of stroke by approximately 20% compared with placebo (5.2% per year with aspirin versus 6.3% with placebo; RR 0.81, 95% CI 0.65-1.01).[63] For patients with AF and previous ischemic stroke or TIA, aspirin did not show a significant reduction in risk of recurrent stroke compared with placebo (10% per year with aspirin versus 12% with placebo; HR 0.86, 95% CI 0.64-1.15).[64]

Particularly in older patients, aspirin is often prescribed with the assumption that it will cause fewer bleeding complications than warfarin. However, not only is aspirin not efficacious in stroke prevention in AF, but it also causes a similar rate of intracranial bleeding compared with warfarin. The Birmingham Atrial Fibrillation Treatment of the Aged (BAFTA) trial compared warfarin and aspirin in patients aged 75 years or older with a 14% prevalence of diabetes, and demonstrated a twofold increased stroke rate with aspirin versus warfarin without a significant difference in major intracranial or extracranial hemorrhage (1.9% versus 2.0%).[65]

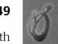

Despite its great efficacy in stroke prevention, oral anticoagulation with VKAs such as warfarin is sometimes poorly managed; register data show that only approximately 50% to 70% of suitable patients receive adequate anticoagulant treatment. And even when treatment is administered, the achieved "time in therapeutic range"—which ensures sufficient stroke protection and a low number of serious bleeding events—is generally poor and does not exceed a proportion of 50% to 60%.[64]

Three newer direct oral anticoagulants (DOACs) have been proven to be successful competitors with warfarin. The direct thrombin inhibitor dabigatran etexilate and the factor Xa inhibitors rivaroxaban and apixaban were shown in large prospective trials to be at least as efficacious and safe as warfarin. The corresponding trials were the Randomized Evaluation of Long-Term Anticoagulation Therapy (RE-LY) trial, in which 23% of the patients had diabetes[66]; the Rivaroxaban Once-Daily Oral Direct Factor Xa Inhibition Compared with Vitamin K Antagonism for Prevention of Stroke and Embolism Trial in Atrial Fibrillation (ROCKET-AF), in which 40% had diabetes[67]; and the Apixaban for the Prevention of Stroke in Subjects with Atrial Fibrillation (ARISTOTLE) trial, in which 20% had diabetes,[68] respectively. These three DOACs so far tested in clinical trials have all shown noninferiority in stroke prevention compared with VKAs, with better safety, consistently limiting the number of intracranial hemorrhages. In the subgroups of patients with diabetes or who otherwise are at high risk for stroke in the three studies, similar results with respect to efficacy and serious bleeding side effects were found, compared with the entire study populations. Rivaroxaban is taken once daily, whereas dabigatran and apixaban have twice-daily dosage regimens. Some drug interactions are evident with the DOACs; patients with severe renal impairment were excluded from the trials, and, in particular, dabigatran has a high renal clearance.

A recent meta-analysis of the mentioned studies analyzing the subgroup of patients with previous stroke or TIA showed that in 14,527 patients, DOACs were associated with a significant reduction of annual stroke or systemic embolism (OR 0.85, 95% CI 0.74-0.99; RR reduction 14%; absolute risk reduction, 0.7%; number needed to treat (NNT) = 134 over 1.8 to 2.0 years) compared with warfarin. DOACs were also associated with a significant reduction in major bleeding compared with warfarin (OR 0.86; 95% CI 0.75-0.99; RR reduction, 13%; absolute risk reduction, 0.8%; NNT = 125), mainly driven by the significant reduction of hemorrhagic stroke (OR 0.44; 95% CI 0.32-0.62; RR reduction 57.9%; absolute risk reduction 0.7% per year; NNT = 139).[69]

The advantages of the DOACs are predictable anticoagulant effects without the need for monitoring coagulation, low propensity for drug interactions, and lower rates of intracranial hemorrhage than with warfarin. Disadvantages might be the short half-life, which in noncompliant patients causes regression to normal coagulation, and until now the absence of specific antidotes. There is a need for standardized tests that accurately measure plasma concentrations and anticoagulant effects. Other disadvantages are possibly higher rates of gastrointestinal hemorrhage and greater expense than with warfarin. With DOACs it is possible that an increasing number of patients with AF who are at risk of stroke—including individuals with diabetes—will be optimally anticoagulated, and consequently the burden of AF-related stroke can be reduced. The guidelines of the European Society of Cardiology of 2012 recommend the DOACs as being broadly preferable to VKA in the vast majority of patients with nonvalvular AF,[70] and a similar recommendation has been provided by the American Heart Association and American Stroke Association.[71]

Carotid Artery Interventions in Diabetes: Carotid Endarterectomy and Carotid Artery Stenting

Carotid artery stenosis is one of the macrovascular complications of diabetes. The presence of an atherosclerotic stenotic lesion in the extracranial internal carotid artery or carotid bulb has been associated with an increased risk of stroke. Randomized trials have shown that carotid endarterectomy (CEA) in appropriately selected patients with carotid stenosis modestly reduces stroke risk compared with patients treated by medical management alone.

However, the risk of stroke in patients undergoing intensive contemporary medical treatment has fallen significantly since the mid-1980s. Recent estimates suggest that the stroke risk in patients undergoing contemporary best medical treatment is overlapping that of patients who have undergone surgery in historical randomized trials, such that the advantages of CEA demonstrated in older trials in such patients are the subject of present controversy.[72,73] According to the guidelines of the American Stroke Association, patients with asymptomatic carotid artery stenosis should receive lifestyle interventions and treatment of all vascular risk factors. Prophylactic CEA performed with less than 3% morbidity and mortality is regarded as useful in highly selected patients with asymptomatic carotid stenosis (minimum 60% by angiography, 70% by validated Doppler ultrasound).

The usefulness of carotid artery stenting (CAS) as an alternative to CEA in asymptomatic patients at high risk for the surgical procedure is uncertain.

For secondary stroke prevention in patients with high-grade internal carotid artery stenosis, CEA has proved its effectiveness, but it has not exclusively been investigated in patients with diabetes. In CEA, both periprocedural and long-term risks are higher in patients with diabetes than without; for example, pooled data[74] from the European Carotid Surgery Trial (ECST)[75] and North American Symptomatic Carotid Endarterectomy Trial (NASCET)[76] found a significant 1.45 periprocedural risk of complications for patients with versus without diabetes (9.7% versus 7.0%; RR 1.45; 95% CI 1.05-2.02).

However, the advantages of the surgical intervention have also been shown in subgroups of patients with diabetes. Three major prospective randomized trials (ECST, NASCET, Veterans Affairs Cooperative Study [VACS])[77] have demonstrated the superiority of CEA plus medical therapy over medical therapy alone for symptomatic patients with an atherosclerotic carotid stenosis greater than 70% (on angiography). The absolute risk reduction with CEA for the subgroup of patients with diabetes was 16% (95% CI 6.0-27.4), higher than for the overall study cohort with absolute reduction of 13.5% (95% CI 9.1-17.9).

Pooled analysis of these trials, including more than 3000 symptomatic patients, found a combined 30-day stroke and death rate of 7.1% in surgically treated patients. There is a controversy for patients with symptomatic stenosis of 50% to 69%. In the NASCET trial of symptomatic patients with a stenosis of 50% to 69%, the 5-year rate of any ipsilateral stroke was 15.7% in patients treated surgically compared with 22.2% in those treated medically. Thus, to prevent one ipsilateral stroke during the 5-year follow-up, 15 patients would have to undergo CEA. The conclusions justify use of CEA only with appropriate case selection when the risk-benefit ratio is favorable for the patient. Patients with a moderate (50% to 69%) stenosis who are at reasonable surgical and anesthetic risk may benefit from an intervention performed by a surgeon with excellent operative skills and a perioperative morbidity and mortality rate of less than 6%.

CAS has emerged as a therapeutic alternative to CEA for treatment of symptomatic extracranial carotid artery occlusive disease; it seems to be advantageous because of its less invasive nature, decreased patient discomfort, and a shorter recuperation period.

However, two randomized trials, the French EVA-3S (Endarterectomy Versus Angioplasty in Patients with Symptomatic Severe Carotid Stenosis)[78] and European SPACE (Stent-Supported Percutaneous Angioplasty of the Carotid Artery Versus Endarterectomy)[79] trials, had to be stopped prematurely for reasons of safety and futility because of a higher 30-day stroke and death rate in the CAS group. In the EVA-3S trial, for example, the 30-day combined stroke and death rate for CAS was 9.6% compared with 3.9% for CEA, with an RR of 2.5 for any stroke or death for CAS compared with CEA. Both trials have been criticized for possible inadequate and nonuniform operator experience, which may have had a negative impact on CAS performance and associated clinical outcomes.

The most recent Carotid Revascularization Endarterectomy Versus Stent Trial[80] (CREST), in which 30% of patients had diabetes, found no significant difference in the composite primary outcome (30-day rate of stroke, death, MI, and 4-year ipsilateral stroke) in patients treated with CAS compared with CEA (7.2% with CAS versus 6.8% with CEA; HR with stenting, 1.11; 95% CI 0.81-1.51). In symptomatic patients, the 4-year rate of stroke or death was nonsignificantly different—8% with CAS compared with 6.4% with CEA. In symptomatic patients, the rate of any periprocedural stroke or postprocedural ipsilateral stroke was significantly higher in the CAS group than in the CEA group (5.5% versus 3.2%). However, in symptomatic patients the rate of MI was significantly higher in the CEA group (2.3% versus 1.0%). For the entire study population, a significant qualitative interaction between age and treatment efficacy was found: for patients older than 70 years, CAS showed greater efficacy, whereas for patients younger than 70 years, CEA results were superior (**Table 28-7**).

In the long-term observation of the CREST study, rates of restenosis or occlusion after CAS or CEA at 2 years showed no significant difference, with 6.0% of patients who had undergone CAS versus 6.3% of those who had undergone CEA developing restenosis or occlusion (HR 0.90, 95% CI 0.63-1.29). Diabetes was the strongest independent predictor of restenosis or occlusion after both procedures, with a 2.31-fold (95% CI 1.61-3.31) increased risk.

Based on these data, the guidelines of the American Stroke Association[81] recommend CEA for patients with recent TIA or ischemic stroke within the past 6 months and ipsilateral severe (70% to 99%) carotid artery stenosis, if the perioperative morbidity and mortality risk is estimated to be below 6%. For a lower degree of stenosis (50% to 69%), CEA is recommended depending on patient-specific factors, such as age, gender, and comorbidities, if the perioperative morbidity and mortality risk is estimated to be below 6%. In patients with stenosis with a degree greater than 50%, no indication for carotid revascularization exists. If surgical revascularization is performed, it should be within 2 weeks after the stroke or TIA. CAS is indicated as an alternative to CEA for symptomatic patients at average or low risk of complications associated with endovascular intervention when the diameter of the lumen of the internal carotid artery is reduced by more than 70% on noninvasive imaging or by more than 50% on catheter angiography. In patients with symptomatic severe stenosis (>70%) in whom the stenosis is difficult to access surgically, when medical conditions are present that greatly increase the risk for surgery, or when other specific circumstances exist, such as radiation-induced stenosis or restenosis after CEA, CAS may be considered. CAS in the these settings is held to be reasonable when performed by operators with established periprocedural morbidity and mortality rates of 4% to 6%.

Mechanical Revascularization of Severe Intracranial Arterial Stenosis

Patients with a recent cerebrovascular event and severe stenosis (70% to 99%) of major intracranial arteries are at high annual risk of approximately 23% for recurrent stroke in the territory of the stenotic artery, despite treatment with aspirin and standard management of vascular risk factors. As a promising prevention strategy, percutaneous transluminal angioplasty and stenting (PTAS) was suggested. The self-expanding Wingspan stent was approved by the Food and Drug Administration (FDA) for use in patients with atherosclerotic intracranial arterial stenosis. Despite the mechanically attractive and therefore feasible way of revascularization, PTAS was not proved to be useful when compared with aggressive medical management of such intracranial stenosis. The Stenting and Aggressive Medical Management for Preventing Recurrent Stroke in Intracranial Stenosis (SAMMPRIS) trial[82] tried to overcome this uncertainty, but the enrollment was halted after 451 randomized patients because of the high risk of stroke or death within 30 days of enrollment in the PTAS arm relative to the medical arm. Of the participants, 46% had type 2 diabetes. The 30-day rate of stroke or death was 14.7% in the PTAS group (nonfatal stroke, 12.5%; fatal stroke, 2.2%) almost threefold higher than in the medically managed group with 5.8% (nonfatal stroke, 5.3%; non–stroke-related death, 0.4%). Beyond 30 days, stroke in the same brain territory occurred in 13 patients in each group. An analysis of

TABLE 28-7 Endpoint Events According to Treatment Group in the CREST Trial

	PERIPROCEDURAL PERIOD			FOUR-YEAR STUDY PERIOD (INCLUDING PERIPROCEDURAL PERIOD)		
	CAS	CEA	HR for CAS versus CEA (95% CI)	CAS	CEA	HR for CAS versus CEA (95% CI)
Death	0.7%	0.3%	2.25 (0.69-7.30)	11.3	12.6	1.12 (0.83-1.51)
Any Stroke	4.1%	2.3%	1.79 (1.14-2.82)	10.2	7.9	1.40 (1.04-1.89)

patient and procedural factors that may have been associated with periprocedural cerebrovascular events in the trial found that diabetes was one of the major factors that were significantly associated with ischemic events, with an OR of 4.5 (95% CI 1.3-16.1) associated with diabetes. Based on this study, in severe intracranial stenosis, the following composition of aggressive medical management is recommended: aspirin at a dose of 325 mg/day; clopidogrel at a dose of 75 mg/day for the first 90 days after the incident event; management of the primary risk factors such as elevated SBP and elevated low-density lipoprotein (LDL) cholesterol levels; and management of secondary risk factors (diabetes, elevated non–high-density lipoprotein (non-HDL) cholesterol levels, smoking, excess weight, and insufficient exercise) with the help of a lifestyle modification program. The corresponding targets of intervention were SBP of less than 140 mm Hg (<130 mm Hg in patients with diabetes), and an LDL cholesterol level of less than 70 mg/dl. Thus, stenting in intracranial stenosis cannot be recommended at this time.

HYPOGLYCEMIA AND STROKE

The brain is directly and rapidly affected by a critical decrease in blood glucose because its metabolism relies exclusively on glucose supply. In this context, repeated episodes of severe hypoglycemia are thought to contribute to the development of cognitive decline and dementia, because of their cumulative neurotoxic effect (see the later discussion of diabetes as a vascular risk factor for cognitive impairment and dementia).

However, hypoglycemia may also cause adverse cerebrovascular events. Acute hypoglycemia provokes profound physiologic changes affecting the cardiovascular system and several hematologic parameters, as a consequence of sympathoadrenal activation and counter-regulatory hormonal secretion. Many of these responses have an important role in protecting the brain from neuroglycopenia, through altering regional blood flow and promoting metabolic changes that will restore blood glucose to normal. Some of these effects are potentially pathophysiologic, and in people with diabetes who have not yet developed endothelial dysfunction, they may have an adverse impact on a vasculature that is already damaged. The acute hemodynamic and hematologic changes may increase the risk of localized tissue ischemia, and major vascular events can certainly be precipitated by acute hypoglycemia. These include myocardial and cerebral ischemia, and occasionally infarction. The possible mechanisms underlying these hypoglycemia-induced cerebrovascular effects include hemorrheologic changes, white cell activation, vasoconstriction, and the release of inflammatory mediators and cytokines. Therefore it is suggested that acute and repeated hypoglycemia could aggravate cerebrovascular complications associated with diabetes by enhancing atherosclerotic vascular and proembolic changes.[83]

DIABETES AND ACUTE STROKE—POSTSTROKE HYPERGLYCEMIA

Epidemiology and Definition of Poststroke Hyperglycemia

If one analyzes the patient characteristics in acute stroke studies, approximately one fifth of patients have diabetes. The prevalence of DM ranges from 10.6% (MAST-E study)

to 24.4% (SAINT-II study,; CLASS] study). In the large study of systemic thrombolysis in acute ischemic stroke, ECASS-3), the prevalence of diabetes was 15.7%.[84] Other epidemiologic data suggest the prevalence of diabetes to be 10% to 20% among patient populations with acute stroke, not accounting for a number of undiagnosed cases of diabetes that also must be assumed.

Poststroke hyperglycemia occurs not only in the acute stroke phase in patients with preexisting DM, but also in patients without a prior diagnosis of diabetes. PSH can occur in all subtypes of strokes. The frequency found in various studies depends on the following:

1 The definition of the threshold of hyperglycemia (fasting glucose from 6.0 mmol/L to 7.8 mmol/L)
2 The definition of the duration of the acute poststroke period (12 to 96 hours)
3 The frequency of blood glucose testing (single test on admission versus repeated single tests versus continuous glucose monitoring)
4 The nutritional status of patients (no nutrition versus parenteral nutrition versus intravenous nutrition)

With a glucose limit value of 7.0 mmol/L, the frequency of PSH is approximately 40% to 50%,[85,86] at least twice as high as the diabetes prevalence in stroke patients. In a study with continuous glucose monitoring, Allport and colleagues were able to demonstrate that PSH can have a dynamic progression. After an initial peak, blood glucose levels were lower approximately 14 to 16 hours later; this was followed by a second hyperglycemic peak 48 to 69 hours later.[85] More recent studies,[87,88] however, could not show this "two-peak" dynamic. Various patterns were shown with respect to latency and duration of PSH, namely "initial" or "delayed" PSH peaks as well as permanent hyperglycemia. The PSH pattern distribution varied significantly between patients with and without diabetes; whereas patients with diabetes more frequently had permanent hyperglycemia, patients without diabetes more frequently had initial PSH peaks (**Table 28-8**).[88] Only 15% of patients with diabetes but 70% of those without diabetes showed a permanent normoglycemic state within 24 hours poststroke.

This possible variability of PSH over time explains that frequencies and patterns of PSH in various studies depend on the respective times of glucose measures. This makes it difficult to interpret and compare different studies.

Causes of Poststroke Hyperglycemia

If one takes the previously described prevalence rates, half of PSH patients have a preexisting disturbance of glucose

TABLE 28-8 Distribution of Patients With and Without Diabetes in the Four Progression Patterns of Poststroke Hyperglycemia

	DIABETES (n=161) N (%)	NO DIABETES (n=587) N (%)
Initial hyperglycemia	21 (13%)	79 (13%)
Hyperglycemia after 24 hours	16 (10%)	54 (9%)
Persistent hyperglycemia	100 (62%)	46 (8%)
Persistent normoglycemia	24 (15%)	408 (70%)

Data from Yong M, Kaste M: Dynamic of hyperglycemia as a predictor of stroke outcome in the ECASS-II trial, *Stroke* 39:2749-2755, 2008.

metabolism such as diabetes or prediabetes. In non-preexisting diabetes, a postulated cause of PSH is a neuro-metabolic "stress hyperglycemia" with the activation of the hypothalamus-pituitary-adrenal (HPA) axis with the release of cortisol and adrenaline and subsequent glycolysis and gluconeogenesis.[89] However, this theory may be too global and simplified. There are contradictory endocrinologic findings in reference to the "stress postulates" because some studies could not prove the claimed stress metabolism.[90]

Neurotoxicity in Poststroke Hyperglycemia

The findings with regard to neuronal damage mechanisms of PSH are mainly the result of experimental studies performed on animals and a few patient examinations with functional cerebral imaging. These have shown that there is not one singular damage mechanism, but rather there are a coaction and an interaction of various "neurotoxic" effects. **Table 28-9** summarizes the potential direct and indirect mechanisms of neuronal damage by hyperglycemia during the acute phase of ischemic stroke.[91–93]

Poststroke Hyperglycemia as a Global Negative Outcome Predictor

In animal models, the extent of hyperglycemia in acute cerebral ischemia determined the size of cerebral lesions and mortality. In patient studies, the negative prognostic impact of hyperglycemia was identified after adjustment for other variables such as age, severity, and extent of the stroke.[94] A meta-analysis based on 32 clinical trials[95] found a relative 93% increase for the in-hospital or 30-day mortality rates in patients with PSH on admission (unadjusted OR 1.93; 95% CI 1.15-3.24). It is interesting to note that the negative effect of PSH in clinical studies was lower in patients with diabetes, with a nonsignificant unadjusted OR for in-hospital or 30-day

mortality of 1.3 (95% CI 0.49-3.43), compared with those without diabetes, with an OR of 3.07 (95% CI 2.5-3.79). Despite the large heterogeneity of the studies that were part of this meta-analysis, even after subgroup analyses the negative predictive value of PSH in patients without prevalent diabetes remained stable with an increased risk of 41% for an unfavorable clinical outcome in a relatively homogeneous group of patients with cerebral ischemia (OR 1.41; CI 1.16-1.73). Even more recent studies, such as one conducted at the Mayo Clinic,[96] found that glucose levels of more than 7.2 mmol/L led to a significantly more severe clinical progression of the stroke and was associated with a risk of mortality that was 2.3 times higher. Even in this study, the PSH in patients without diabetes had a significantly greater negative effect than in those with diabetes; the increase in mortality associated with PSH was 3.4-fold in nondiabetic patients, compared with 1.6-fold in patients with diabetes. The data from the Gruppo Italiano di Farmacoepidemiologia nell'Anziano (GIFA) register for strokes allowed extraction of PSH as a significant negative predictor for hospital mortality, with a significant OR of 1.066 (95% CI 1.028-1.104). With regard to the cognitive prognosis, PSH proved to be non-negative predictive, which was confirmed by another study that dealt exclusively with this question; however, the case number of 113 is low.[97]

In general, the negative implications of PSH have not been studied specifically with regard to the various types of strokes. However, there are indications that PSH does not necessarily have an unfavorable effect in small lacunar infarctions or even could be favorable in terms of prognosis. The analysis of the patient population participating in the studies with the neuroprotectant lubeluzole (LUB-INT-9 and LUB-INT-5])[98] showed that glucose levels in excess of 8 mmol/L within 6 hours after the stroke event coincided with larger infarctions with an expected lower functional outcome (OR 0.60; 95% CI 0.41-0.88), whereas in lacunar ischemia the chance for a good functional outcome was almost three times better (OR 2.70; 95% CI 1.01-7.13). However, this positive correlation turned negative with higher glucose levels (>12 mmol/L) (**Fig. 28-5**).

The prospective Spanish multicenter observational study Glycaemia in Acute Stroke (GLIAS)[99] examined the question concerning a critical predictive threshold value of PSH in 476 acute stroke patients with mean glucose levels of 7.6 ± 3.2 mmol/L and demonstrated a statistically calculated predictive cut-off value of 8.6 mmol/L, both initially as well as within the first 48 hours, which differentially predicted between a good and a bad outcome after 3 months. After multivariable statistical adjustment, any hyperglycemia above this limit value was associated with a risk of unfavorable progression that was 2.7 times higher (95% CI 1.42-5.24) and a mortality risk that was 3.8 times higher (95% CI 1.79-8.10). There were no differences between those with and without prevalent diabetes. This correlation could be demonstrated not only in larger but also in smaller infarctions. Finally, the presently available evidence is contradictory in terms of the significance of isolated increased glucose levels compared with continuous increases.

TABLE 28-9 Hyperglycemic Damage Mechanisms in Acute Ischemic Stroke

Parenchyma toxicity (anaerobic/glucose metabolism)	Acidosis Lactate accumulation Increase of the NMDA receptor–dependent cellular calcium flux Inflammation Increased formation of free radicals Increased expression of matrix metalloproteinase 9 (MMP-9)
Vascular damage and perfusion defect	Endothelial dysfunction Reduced vessel reactivity Inflammation Prothrombotic state—for example, activation of plasminogen activator inhibitor 1 (PAI-1) Reduced NO production
Impairment of the blood-brain barrier	Edema formation Increased rate of hemorrhage
Noncerebral effects	Immune system Shift in fluid balance Disruption in peripheral perfusion
Consequences of the insulin deficit	Increased formation of free fatty acids with prothrombotic effect and reduction in vessel reactivity

MMP-9 = Matrix metalloproteinase 9; NMDA = N-methyl-D-aspartate; PAI-1 = plasminogen activator inhibitor 1.

Influence of Diabetes on Acute Stroke Treatments

Diabetes and PSH have been linked to a lower efficacy of intravenous thrombolysis with alteplase in ischemic stroke

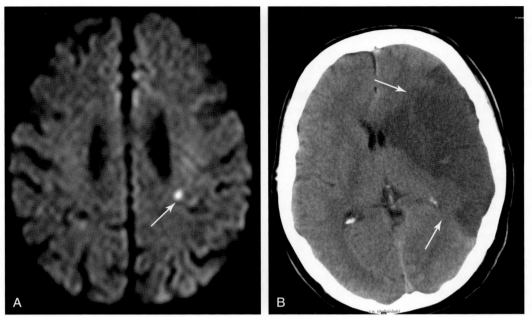

FIGURE 28-5 In small lacunar infarctions (**A,** white dot in the diffusion-weighted magnetic resonance imaging scan; white arrow), poststroke hyperglycemia has a less negative effect on functional outcome than in large territorial infarctions (**B,** large, dark gray infarction demarcation between the two white arrows in the computed tomography scan).

patients, resulting from both lower rates of recanalization and increased rates of complicating symptomatic intracerebral hemorrhage (SICH).[100,101]

In a multivariable analysis of 16,049 patients from the SITS-ISTR (Stroke Registry) of thrombolysis patients,[102] increasing blood glucose levels were independently, linearly, and significantly associated with a higher mortality and disability, and an increased risk of SICH. In particular, blood glucose from 181 to 200 mg/dL were associated with a threefold increased risk levels of SICH compared with the reference level of normoglycemia. The trends of associations between blood glucose and outcomes were similar in patients with diabetes (17% of the cohort) or without such history, except for mortality and SICH, in which the association was not statistically significant in patients with diabetes (mortality $P=.23$; SICH $P=.06$).

In Europe, patients with PS and concomitant DM were excluded from treatment with the approval of systemic intravenous thrombolysis with alteplase. Because of the uncertainty of its benefit-risk ratio in patients with diabetes, thrombolysis is often withheld in many such patients. An analysis of 29,500 patients from SITS-ISTR[103] compared with nonthrombolysed controls from the Virtual International Stroke Trials Archive (VISTA) registry, including 18.5% with diabetes, found a significant 45% better functional outcome (measured by the change in distribution of the modified Rankin Scale score 0 to 6) in the thrombolysed patients compared with controls among the subset of patients with diabetes (adjusted OR for a better outcome = 1.45 [95% CI 1.30-1.62]). This degree of benefit is comparable to the outcome relationship between thrombolysis and control groups among patients without diabetes (OR for a better outcome with thrombolysis = 1.53; 95% CI 1.42-1.63). Hence, outcomes with thrombolysis are better than controls among patients with diabetes, indicating no statistical justification for the exclusion of patients with diabetes who are otherwise eligible from receiving thrombolytic therapy in acute ischemic stroke.

Glucose-Lowering Treatment of Poststroke Hyperglycemia
Feasibility of Glycemic Control in Poststroke Hyperglycemia

There is no consensus regarding the best type of glycemic control, the best method for achieving it, and the necessary monitoring in the setting of acute stroke. The mentioned fluctuating course of PSH includes the risk of induced hypoglycemia when strict control is attempted. The type of insulin delivery has differed in reported studies; for example, whereas intravenous glucose-insulin-potassium (GIK) infusions were administered in the intervention study Glucose Insulin in Stroke Trial (GIST-UK),[104] other studies used staggered perfusion rates of insulin in NaCl 0.9% strictly applied according to the measured glucose levels, or they used 5% glucose or insulin in individual intravenous bolus dosages. One study from Glasgow involving 13 patients[105] showed the basic feasibility of a strict decrease in increased values by approximately 1 to 2 mmol/L with only one observed hypoglycemic event. There was no correlation between the better control of glycemia and any clinical success; however, the number of patients was clearly too low to address such a question. In the THIS) study,[95] which compared 46 diabetic patients with a glucose level of more than 8.3 mmol/L treated for 72 hours with an aggressive intravenous insulin infusion (N=31; glucose target value <7.2 mmol/L) with conventional glycemia control with use of subcutaneous insulin (N=15; glucose target value <11.1 mmol/L), the achieved mean glucose levels were significantly lower in the group undergoing targeting of strict control (7.4 mmol/L) than in the group treated subcutaneously (10.5 mmol/L). However, 11 patients (35%) became hypoglycemic in the aggressively treated group, and four of them (13%) were symptomatic; no hypoglycemia occurred in the group of patients undergoing conventional glycemia control (N=15). In addition, the number of patients did not allow evaluation of any clinical low effects on the prognosis in this group, as well. A more recent study[106] concluded that the control of glycemia with various regimens was difficult to achieve, particularly postprandial regimens because of discontinuous nutrition. This demonstrated that it is basically possible to lower the blood glucose levels to a normal range with aggressive intravenous insulin therapy during the first 24 to 72 hours after an ischemic infarction; however, the consequence is a not-insignificant number of hypoglycemia events. Although no lasting negative clinical consequences of hypoglycemia were evident, it seems imperative to monitor glucose levels closely.

Does Tight Glycemic Control Improve Outcome in Poststroke Hyperglycemia?

The previous recommendations to lower increased glucose levels during the acute phase of a stroke follow the plausible speculation that control of a clearly negative predictive risk factor should lead to an improvement in the clinical prognosis. However, until 2007 there were insufficient data from large prospective randomized studies with clinical endpoints to confirm this assumption. This gap was at least in part closed by the GIST-UK study,[104] which could not prove a positive endpoint effect of a target value–oriented glycemic control strategy and the results of which lead to large controversies regarding the practical consequences concluded from the data. In the active treatment group (GIK infusion) a mean blood glucose of 0.57 mmol/L was achieved, compared with patients treated with only physiologic saline solution; however, there were no differences between the groups in the primary or secondary endpoints. It is interesting that even in the NaCl infusion group, the blood glucose levels decreased significantly, which may correspond to the spontaneous progression of PSH (**Fig. 28-6**). In addition, the intervention arm showed significantly lower SBP values—on average 9 mm Hg lower.

First responses to the study questioned the efficacy of global control of glycemia. However, a number of limitations and methodologic problems of the GIST-UK trial warrant consideration. In 2005, it was discontinued after 7 years of recruitment after only 933 patients were included instead of the planned 2355 patients, which undermined the statistical power of the trial. In addition, the intervention was relatively delayed in its initiation and the glucose control achieved was not very pronounced—only 0.57 mmol/L lower in a population with initially moderate PSH. In addition, the unintended

lowering of the blood pressure in the active treatment arm could have a negative effect on the endpoints. Therefore the results are unable to contradict the general target of an ambitious glycemic control including the avoidance of hypoglycemia.

The controversies of glycemic control in acute stroke are similar to those ongoing in the context of management of surgical and medical intensive care patients. If the clear results of a 34% reduction in mortality by tight glycemic control in the single-center study from University of Leuven[107] initially led to propagation of the use of such intensive glucose management, then newer results, in which the tight glycemic control with an achieved target value of 4.5 to 6.0 mmol/L[108] proved disadvantageous, have cast doubt on the value of tight glycemic control. However, for the treatment of acute strokes, the results of the GIST study cannot mean that lowering the glucose level in a patient who has sustained an acute stroke is discredited globally as superfluous. In connection with this, a trend toward such laissez-faire behavior can already be observed. The GLIAS results[99] allow speculation that there is a U-shaped curve of correlation between the prognosis and the blood glucose level. Accordingly both hypoglycemic and near-hypoglycemic values would be just as negatively predictive as significantly hyperglycemic values, and the best prognosis would be within the moderately hyperglycemic and normoglycemic ranges. If the hypothesis for such a correlation were to be tested prospectively, it remains plausible that lowering glucose levels from the moderately hyperglycemic to the hypoglycemic range would have a negative effect, whereas interventions to lower hyperglycemia to less-severe hyperglycemia or to normoglycemia could have a favorable effect on clinical outcomes. It is probable that the effectiveness of glycemic control is decisively dependent on the quality of glucose monitoring and the avoidance of hypoglycemia.

The guideline recommendations in Europe versus the United States differ in details, however, they both agree in a defensive manner to such a plausible assumption. The European Stroke Organisation (ESO) recommends lowering the glucose level with insulin if the values exceed 10 mmol/L (180 mg/dL), whereas the American Stroke Association prefers an intervention if the values exceed 140 mg/dL (approximately 7.8 mmol/L). The problem with these recommendations is that although they suggest an

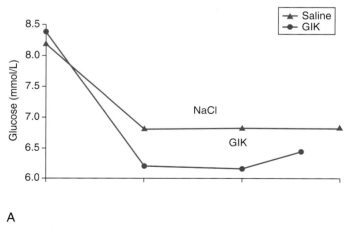

A

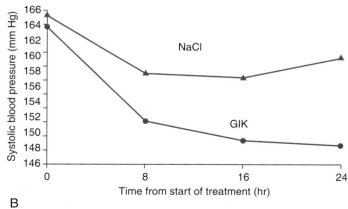

B

FIGURE 28-6 Mean glucose levels **(A)** and systolic blood pressure values **(B)** initially and 8, 16, and 24 hours later in both study arms of the GIST-UK study. GIK = Glucose-potassium-insulin infusion. *(Modified from Gray CS, Hildreth AJ, Sandercock PA, et al: Glucose-potassium-insulin infusions in the management of post-stroke hyperglycaemia: the UK Glucose Insulin in Stroke Trial (GIST-UK). Modified from Lancet Neurol 6:397-406, 2007.)*

upper intervention limit for initiation of the intervention and advocate avoidance of hypoglycemia, neither guideline suggests a target glucose range. Now, it could be assumed that the recommended intervention thresholds are too high and the success of the intervention depends decisively on the avoidance of hypoglycemia; however, the data from clinical studies is insufficient to affirm such an approach.

DIABETES AS A VASCULAR RISK FACTOR FOR COGNITIVE IMPAIRMENT AND DEMENTIA

Because type 2 diabetes doubles the risk of stroke, and stroke alone causes cognitive impairment by strategic cognition-relevant brain lesions in approximately 20% of patients, a statistical and clinical association between diabetes and cognitive impairment is expected. However, brains of patients with diabetes, in addition to having the obvious cerebrovascular pathology, may also be affected by neurodegenerative cerebral pathology, leading to dementia. Although the influence of diabetes on cognitive function has been suggested since the 1930s and a large number of studies have been done in this area since then, no consensus has emerged regarding the role of diabetes in the development of dementia or whether optimal blood glucose control yields a protective effect. In general, the association between type 2 diabetes and dementia seems to be stronger for VD than for AD, but these observations are inconsistent.

Definition and Epidemiology

Type 2 diabetes disproportionally affects older adults in whom dementia is also a common condition. Large population-based studies examining people at an older age (>70 years) demonstrate that patients with type 2 diabetes are overrepresented among individuals with dementia. Dementia is one of the most devastating diseases of late life; approximately 4.6 million new cases of dementia are estimated to occur worldwide every year, and the prevalence of dementia is expected to quadruple by the year 2050 in the United States.

AD is the most common form of dementia, accounting for approximately 80% of all cases, followed by VD. So-called "mixed dementia" describes a combination of clinical and radiologic features of AD and VD. The proportion of these major types of dementia depends on criteria used for the differentiation, which vary widely. Diabetes has been linked not only to the full picture of dementia, but also to more subtle forms of cognitive impairment below the threshold of dementia, defined by neuropsychological testing. People with mild cognitive impairment are at increased risk of developing dementia, although the conversion rates reported range from 1% to 25% or more per year.[109] The determination of cognitive deficits and the diagnosis of the type of dementia are also not always easy. Thus the boundaries among cognitive deficit, early dementia, and more severe stages of dementia are sometimes difficult to discern.

DM is associated with cognitive dysfunction and has been related to accelerated cognitive decline in older adults, development of mild cognitive impairment, and increased risk of dementia, including both AD and VD (**Fig. 28-7**).

The association between DM and risk of mild cognitive impairment and dementia is robust, and diabetes also seems to increase the risk of progression from such impairment to dementia.

Clinical Studies

Cognitive decline in nondemented patients with diabetes has been studied in several cross-sectional case-control studies. Most of them show worse cognitive performance in patients across age groups between 50 and 80 years with type 2 diabetes compared with age-, gender-, and education-matched controls with regard to different cognitive features such as verbal memory, information processing speed, perception, visuoconstruction, language attention, and executive functioning.[110] Cross-sectional population-based

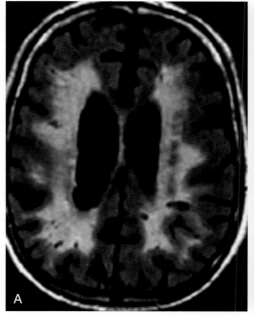
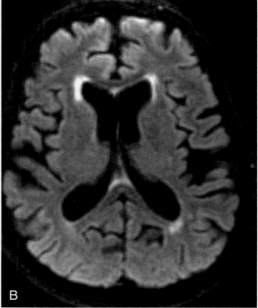

FIGURE 28-7 Magnetic resonance imaging scans of patients with diabetes-related types of dementia. **A,** A patient with vascular dementia with extensive white matter lesion and lacunar infarctions *(black holes)*. **B,** A patient with only small white matter lesions but pronounced brain atrophy.

cohort studies such as ARIC[111] and the Framingham study[112] reported findings similar to those of most of the case-control studies. There seems to be a 1.5-fold increased risk for patients with type 2 diabetes for development of mild cognitive impairment.[113] Not all studies, however, observed significant differences in cognitive performance between patients with diabetes and controls despite elaborate cognitive testing and relatively large sample sizes.[114]

Some large longitudinal studies that examined the impact of diabetes on cognitive function reported cognitive decline over an average period of 5 years that exceeded the effects of normal aging by a factor of 1.5 to 2.17.[115] However, in most studies only a limited number of cognitive test results were affected and the absolute magnitudes of the observed differences were small and clearly distinct from the rate of decline that is typical for pathologic conditions such as AD. Other studies did not observe accelerated cognitive decline in patients with type 2 diabetes.[115] Taken together, the findings of these studies show relatively subtle decrements in cognitive functioning, which slowly progress over time.

However, according to the results of a systematic review of a large number of studies, type 2 diabetes is a risk factor for cognitive impairment crossing the threshold to dementia.[116,117] Type 2 diabetes is associated with a twofold to fourfold increased risk of VD and a 1.5- to 2-fold increased risk of AD. However, in studies, differentiation between the dementia subtypes of VD and AD is difficult, especially when it is based only on a clinical diagnosis. Moreover, many patients may be affected by both vascular and neurodegenerative pathology.[118] On the basis of these numbers, 6% to 8% of all cases of late-life dementia would be attributable to type 2 diabetes. Patients with type 2 diabetes were overrepresented by a factor 1.5 to 2 in subgroups of older individuals (age 65 years and older) with severe cognitive deficits.[113]

In some longitudinal studies, a longer diabetes duration and higher HbA1c levels were predictors for a faster development of cognitive decline.[113,116]

As with the relationship between prediabetic metabolic abnormalities and stroke, cognitive decrements have also been found in prediabetic stages and its vascular risk escorts such as hyperinsulinemia, impaired glucose tolerance, and MetS. They are all associated with an approximately 1.5- to 2-fold increased risk of development of cognitive impairment or dementia.[113,117,119]

Similarly, as with the relationship between diabetes and stroke, additional vascular risk factors and predispositions that are associated with type 2 diabetes (e.g., hypertension, dyslipoproteinemia, depression, stroke, genetics, demographic and lifestyle characteristics) may modulate or mediate cognitive functioning. One longitudinal study, for example, found that cognitive functioning in patients with type 2 diabetes was related to long-term exposure to hypertension, even in prediabetic stages.[120] In a group of middle-aged patients with diabetes, dyslipidemia was associated with worse declarative memory performance.[121] Many of these diabetes-associated risk factors are interrelated, and it therefore remains difficult to assess the exclusive impact of diabetes differentiated from the other risk factors on cognition.

Genetic predisposition might contribute to the association among type 2 diabetes, cognitive decrements, and dementia. The most widely examined risk factor is the apolipoprotein E (apo E) ε4 allele, an important risk factor for CVD and late-onset AD in the general population. Some studies have shown interaction effects between type 2 diabetes and the apo E ε4 allele, further aggravating the diabetes-associated risk of cognitive decline and dementia,[113] whereas others could not confirm such an interaction.[122] Another genetic relationship between type 2 diabetes and AD may be mediated by the insulin-degrading enzyme, which degrades both insulin and amyloid beta, the main component of amyloid plaques and pathologic hallmark of AD. Variations in the insulin-degrading enzyme gene were associated with an increased risk of type 2 diabetes and AD.[123] It is interesting to note that these associations were only observed in individuals who do not carry the apo E ε4 allele.

Brain Imaging Studies

Brain imaging studies have been used to analyze vascular lesions including infarcts, white matter hyperintensities (WMHs) and microbleeds, and cerebral atrophy as possible structural correlates of impaired cognition in type 2 diabetes. According to the increased risk of stroke in diabetes, it is not surprising that population-based studies found a 1.5- to 2-fold higher prevalence and incidence of lacunar infarcts associated with diabetes.[124] The relationship between type 2 diabetes and WMHs is less clear. Several large population-based studies did not observe a significant association between diabetes and WMHs,[125] whereas others observed a modest increase in WMH severity and accelerated WMH progression in patients with type 2 diabetes through use of elaborate WMH scaling and volumetry.[113,116] Some studies identified microbleeds on T2-weighted magnetic resonance imaging (MRI) scans, a marker of cerebrovascular disease, to be more prevalent in patients with type 2 diabetes.[126]

Modest degrees of global and focal cerebral atrophy in patients with diabetes have been reported from cross-sectional studies. Findings of atrophy in specific brain regions such as the frontal or medial temporal lobe, including the hippocampus and amygdala—a typical pattern in AD—suggest a possible association between type 2 diabetes and neurodegenerative brain changes and dementia.[124]

Autopsy Studies

In line with the findings from imaging studies, autopsy studies in patients with diabetes have revealed an approximately 2.5-fold increased risk for cortical and subcortical cerebral infarctions and Alzheimer pathology.[116] Diabetes was also associated with changes in the cerebral microvasculature, including amyloid angiopathy and capillary basement thickening. In contrast, no link has been demonstrated between type 2 diabetes and the severity of Alzheimer-typical amyloid plaques and neurofibrillary tangles.[127,128] Some studies have even reported a reverse association, with a decreased amount of Alzheimer pathology in patients with diabetes.[129] In the Honolulu-Asia Aging Study, no relationship between type 2 diabetes per se and the amount of plaques and tangles was observed; however, there was an interaction between type 2 diabetes and the presence of the apo E ε4 allele, showing that patients with type 2 diabetes who carried the apo E ε4 allele had a higher number of plaques and tangles than nondiabetic apo E ε4 carriers.[130] Thus, the current evidence from autopsy studies does not confirm a direct link between diabetes and Alzheimer pathology, but several possible interactions. Just as much, it is possible that diabetes-associated vascular pathology may lower the threshold at which Alzheimer-type pathology becomes clinically manifest.

Prevention and Treatment of Diabetes-Related Dementia

There is no evidence that approved medical treatments used in the treatment of AD such as cholinesterase inhibitors or N-methyl-D-aspartate (NMDA) receptor antagonists have a deviant effect on patients with versus without diabetes. However, the beneficial effects of antidementive medications are limited.

As yet, there is also no evidence-based disease-modifying treatment for diabetes-related cognitive decrements. However, there are some hints that modest cognitive decrements in patients with type 2 diabetes are partially reversible with improvement of glycemic control,[131] although some studies found no such effect.[132]

The recently published ACCORD-MIND study, a nested substudy of the ACCORD trial comprising 2977 trial participants, followed various outcome parameters of brain function and structure. The Digit Symbol Substitution Test (DSST) score was used as a neuropsychological measure at baseline and at 20 and 40 months, and total brain volume (TBV) was assessed as a brain structure outcome measure with MRI at baseline and 40 months in a subset of participants.[133] The investigators found no significant treatment difference after 40 months in the mean DSST score between the groups randomized to more intensive versus standard glucose control. The intensive treatment group, however, had a significantly greater mean TBV than the standard treatment group (4.62 cm^3, 95% CI 2.0-7.3). The authors concluded that, in conjunction with the nonsignificant effects of more intensive glycemic control on other ACCORD outcomes and with the increased mortality in participants in the intensive treatment group, the findings of the study do not support the use of intensive therapy to reduce the adverse effects of diabetes on the brain in patients with similar characteristics to those of the study participants.

A current analysis sought to determine whether poor glucose control was related to worse cognitive performance in 3069 elderly individuals aged 70 to 79 years within a follow-up period of 10 years. There was a link between cognition and HbA1c levels, and the authors concluded that poor glucose control among those with diabetes is associated with worse cognitive function and greater decline, although the study was not a prospective interventional study.[83]

Multifactorial vascular risk factor intervention (hypertension, dyslipidemia, hyperglycemia, tobacco smoking) was found to slow cognitive decline in patients with preexisting AD in an observational study.[134]

Insulin therapy in patients with diabetes may also be effective in slowing cognitive decline in patients with preexisting AD. The investigators[135] compared oral glucose-lowering drugs alone versus a combination of oral drugs with insulin in 104 patients with mild-to-moderate AD and type 2 diabetes for a follow-up period of 12 months. Cognitive function, assessed by the Mini Mental State Examination (MMSE) worsened significantly from baseline by 56.5% in the oral therapy alone group compared with 23.2% in patients in the oral plus insulin group. Also, measurements with the scored Clinical Global Impression (CGI) survey instrument showed a significant worsening for all domains after 12 months in the oral medication group but not in the oral-insulin group. The two groups were matched for body mass index, serum lipids, triglycerides, apo E ε4 allele, and smoking status. After adjustment for imbalance in ischemic heart disease and hypertension, each with higher baseline prevalence in the oral-insulin group, the results remained significant.

A possible relationship between glucose-lowering drug treatment and dementia was detected with metformin treatment. One study in cellular models showed that metformin increases the production of amyloid beta through upregulation of beta-secretase,[136] and the authors raised the concern that metformin could increase the risk of AD. However, the findings of this study require replication, and the relevance of its findings to humans has not been demonstrated. Of note, clinical data published to date have been discordant, with some studies suggesting increased dementia among metformin users[137] and others finding the opposite.[138] The effect of metformin on cognition will be assessed in the ongoing phase II trial (NCT00620191) testing whether metformin can decrease cognitive decline and dementia in overweight persons aged 55 to 90 years with mild cognitive impairment.

One example of other approaches that have been examined with regard to impact on dementia is physical activity, which in observational studies assessing associations with light and moderate exercise was associated with better cognitive function in patients with type 2 diabetes.[139]

A surprising result was found in a French study of patients with AD with a mean age of 77 years, of whom those with type 2 diabetes showed a significantly lower rate of cognitive decline than did individuals without diabetes.[131] Causes for this paradox may include confounding factors such as a survival bias related to diabetes, but also different nutrition habits of cognitively impaired patients.

The Role of Hypoglycemia on Cognitive Impairment and Dementia

Assessing the role of hypoglycemia on cognitive disorders in patients with diabetes is complex, because the influence of hyperglycemia in the course of the diabetic metabolic disorder itself, its duration, and its vascular and degenerative complications interact to a great extent.

In type 1 diabetes, a meta-analysis[140] and results from DCCT and EDIC[141,142] did not provide evidence for an association between the occurrence of more hypoglycemic episodes in the intensive treatment group (**Table 28-10**) and impaired cognition in young adult patients.

In type 2 diabetes, two longitudinal studies examined the relationship between severe hypoglycemic events and cognitive decline. Data from the large diabetes registry of the Kaiser-Permanente Northern California Diabetes Registry showed a dose-response relationship between the number of severe hypoglycemic episodes and the risk of development of dementia up to 17 years after the events.[143]

In contrast, the Fremantle diabetes study[144] found no evidence that severe hypoglycemia contributes to cognitive decline in older patients with type 2 diabetes, but suggested a reverse direction of causality: People with dementia were at increased risk of further severe hypoglycemic episodes over the subsequent 5 years of follow-up. Thus, a bidirectional relationship between diabetes-associated hypoglycemia episodes and cognitive disturbances may be considered. Differential

OTHER DIABETES-RELATED CARDIOVASCULAR CONSIDERATIONS

VI

TABLE 28-10 Number of Hypoglycemic Episodes During the Three Periods of the DCCT/EDIC Study

EPISODES	DCCT (6.5 YEARS)		EDIC FOLLOW-UP (12 YEARS)		18 YEARS FOLLOW-UP	
	Intensive treatment (N=588)	Conventional treatment (N=556)	Intensive treatment (N=588)	Conventional treatment (N=556)	Intensive treatment (N=588)	Conventional treatment (N=556)
0	364	445	465	424	326	365
1-5	190	104	119	127	212	175
>5	34	7	4	4	50	16

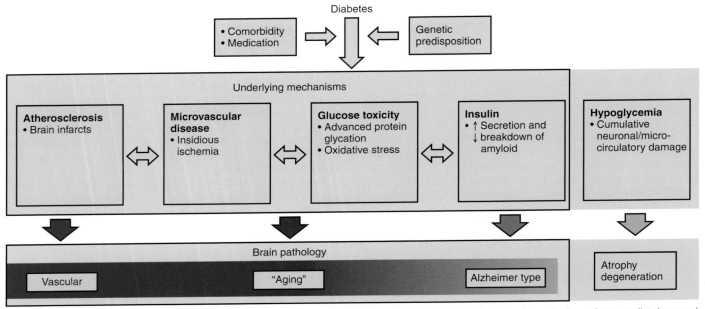

FIGURE 28-8 Proposed pathophysiologic interaction between diabetes and advanced brain aging or dementia including vascular mechanisms, glucose-mediated neuronal toxicity, interference with Alzheimer-typical cerebral amyloid deposition, and cerebral damage by episodes of hypoglycemia. *(Modified from Biessels GJ, Staekenborg S, Brunner E, et al: Risk of dementia in diabetes mellitus: a systematic review,* Lancet Neurol 5:64-74, 2006.)

vulnerability of the brain to hypoglycemia in young and older patient populations may be another reason for the observed discrepancy in between type 1 and type 2 diabetes.[114,116]

Vascular and Degenerative Mechanisms in Diabetes-Related Dementia

Mechanisms through which type 2 diabetes may adversely affect cognitive function include vascular disturbances, glucose toxicity, hypoglycemic episodes, and disturbances of cerebral insulin signaling.[116] Diabetes could interact with the dementia process by accelerating the pathologic processes underlying AD, for example, through disturbances of amyloid metabolism or through vascular (co)morbidity.[145] An alternative explanation is that diabetes affects the reserve capacity of the brain, possibly through the same mechanisms that cause the subtle cognitive decrements, and thereby reduces the threshold for the neurodegenerative dementia process to become clinically manifest. As one potential noncerebrovascular mechanism in the relationship between diabetes and dementia, peripheral hyperinsulinemia with impaired cerebral insulin signaling leading to a type of "cerebral IR" affecting amyloid-beta clearance in the brain has been suggested.[146] Another potential noncerebrovascular mechanism is elevation of AGEs in patients with type 2 diabetes, resulting in upregulation of the AGE receptor (RAGE), which may interfere with AD-related lipid metabolism in the brain.[113] Based on the proposed relationship between

impaired insulin signaling in the brain and dementia, intranasal administration of insulin has been studied as a potential treatment for AD, with promising initial results.[147]

A summary of the discussed relationships between diabetes and dementia is shown in **Figure 28-8**.

SUMMARY

Patients with diabetes have a twofold to fourfold risk of ischemic stroke compared with patients without diabetes. This increased risk encompasses all four subtypes: ischemic, lacunar, large artery occlusive, and thromboembolic strokes. Comorbid vascular risk factors in patients with diabetes not only add to the stroke risk from diabetes, but multiplicatively affect this risk. The risk for cerebrovascular disease is already increased in prediabetic states

Interventional studies that focused exclusively on glucose control in patients with diabetes could not demonstrate a reduction in stroke rates. However, approaches using multifactorial risk factor management—including intensive glucose control—have shown a significant reduction in stroke rates. These findings underscore that multifactorial risk factor management may be the key for a substantial reduction of stroke incidence in patients with diabetes.

Acute stroke can generate acute disturbances of glucose metabolism with PSH, which is associated with an approximately twofold risk of an unfavorable outcome. Tight hyperglycemia management in acute stroke has not yet proven to be beneficial, because in prospective studies its potential beneficial effect has been negatively compensated by high rates of hypoglycemic episodes.

In addition to increasing the risk of stroke, diabetes similarly leads to chronic and insidious damage of the brain, resulting in cognitive decline and dementia. Dementia in patients with diabetes results not only from cerebrovascular-mediated neuronal damage, but also from neurodegenerative processes manifesting as AD.

There are hints regarding a bidirectional relationship between diabetes and dementia. On the one hand, people with diabetes have double the risk of developing dementia; on the other hand, cognitive and behavioral manifestations of dementia lead to disturbances in glucose metabolism.

References

1. Zhang Y, Chapman AM, Plested M, et al: The incidence, prevalence, and mortality of stroke in France, Germany, Italy, Spain, the UK, and the US: a literature review. *Stroke Res Treat* 12:ID 436125, doi:10.1155/2012/436125. Epub
2. Rothwell PM, Coull AJ, Silver LE, et al: Population-based study of event-rate, incidence, case fatality, and mortality for all acute vascular events in all arterial territories (Oxford Vascular Study), *Lancet* 366:1773–1783, 2005.
3. Gentil A, Bejot Y, Lorgis L, et al: Comparative epidemiology of stroke and acute myocardial infarction: the Dijon Vascular project (Diva), *J Neurol Neurosurg Psychiatry* 80:1006–1011, 2009.
4. Lee S, Shafe ACE, Cowie MR: UK stroke incidence, mortality and cardiovascular risk management 1999e2008: time-trend analysis from the General Practice Research Database, *BMJ Open* 1:e000269, http://dx.doi.org/10.1136/bmjopen-2011-000269 2011.
5. Luitse MJ, Biessels GJ, Rutten GE, et al: Diabetes, hyperglycaemia, and acute ischaemic stroke, *Lancet Neurol* 11:261–271, 2012.
6. Barrett-Connor E, Khaw KT: Diabetes mellitus: an independent risk factor for stroke? *Am J Epidemiol* 128:116–123, 1988.
7. Manson JE, Colditz GA, Stampfer MJ, et al: A prospective study of maturity-onset diabetes mellitus and risk of coronary heart disease and stroke in women, *Arch Intern Med* 151:1141–1147, 1991.
8. Kannel WB, McGee DL: Diabetes and cardiovascular disease. The Framingham study, *JAMA* 241:2035–2038, 1979.
9. The Emerging Risk Factors Collaboration: Diabetes mellitus, fasting blood glucose concentration, and risk of vascular disease: a collaborative meta-analysis of 102 prospective studies, *Lancet* 375:2215–2222, 2010.
10. Hu G, Jousilahti P, Sarti C, et al: The effect of diabetes and stroke at baseline and during follow-up on stroke mortality, *Diabetologia* 49:2309–2316, 2006.
11. Banerjee C, Moon YP, Paik MC, et al: Duration of diabetes and risk of ischemic stroke: the Northern Manhattan Study, *Stroke* 43:1212–1217, 2012.
12. O'Donnell MJ, Xavier D, Liu L, et al: Risk factors for ischaemic and intracerebral haemorrhagic stroke in 22 countries (the INTERSTROKE study): a case-control study, *Lancet* 376:112–123, 2010.
13. Kothari V, Stevens RJ, Adler AI, et al: UKPDS 60: risk of stroke in type 2 diabetes estimated by the UK Prospective Diabetes Study risk engine, *Stroke* 33:1776–1781, 2002.
14. Hankey GJ, Jamrozik K, Broadhurst RJ, et al: Long-term risk of first recurrent stroke in the Perth Community Stroke Study, *Stroke* 29:2491–2500, 1998.
15. Callahan A, Amarenco P, Goldstein LB, et al: Risk of stroke and cardiovascular events after ischemic stroke or transient ischemic attack in patients with type 2 diabetes or metabolic syndrome: secondary analysis of the Stroke Prevention by Aggressive Reduction in Cholesterol Levels (SPARCL) trial, *Arch Neurol* 68:1245–1251, 2011.
16. Gregg EW, Cheng YJ, Saydah S, et al: Trends in death rates among U.S. adults with and without diabetes between 1997 and 2006: findings from the National Health Interview Survey, *Diabetes Care* 35:1252–1257, 2012.
17. Rohr J, Kittner S, Feeser B, et al: Traditional risk factors and ischemic stroke in young adults: the Baltimore-Washington Cooperative Young Stroke Study, *Arch Neurol* 53:603–607, 1996.
18. Hu G, Sart C, Jousilahti P, et al: The impact of history of hypertension and type 2 diabetes at baseline on the incidence of stroke and stroke mortality, *Stroke* 21:18–25, 2005.
19. Sui X, Lavie CJ, Hooker SP, et al: A prospective study of fasting plasma glucose and risk of stroke in asymptomatic men, *Mayo Clin Proc* 86:1042–1049, 2011.
20. Tanne D, Koren-Morag N, Goldbourt U: Fasting plasma glucose and risk of incident ischemic stroke or transient ischemic attacks: a prospective cohort study, *Stroke* 35:2351–2355, 2004.
21. Vermeer SE, Sandee W, Algra A, et al: Dutch TIA Trial Study Group: Impaired glucose tolerance increases stroke risk in nondiabetic patients with transient ischemic attack or minor ischemic stroke, *Stroke* 37:1413–1417, 2006.
22. Doi Y, Ninomiya T, Hata J, et al: Impact of glucose tolerance status on development of ischemic stroke and coronary heart disease in a general Japanese population: the Hisayama study, *Stroke* 41:203–209, 2010.
23. Selvin E, Steffes MW, Zhu H, et al: Glycated hemoglobin, diabetes, and cardiovascular risk in nondiabetic adults, *N Engl J Med* 362:800–811, 2010.
24. Lee M, Saver JL, Hong KS, et al: Effect of pre-diabetes on future risk of stroke: meta-analysis, *BMJ* 344:e3564, http://dx.doi.org/10.1136/bmj.e3564 2012 Review.
25. Thacker EL, Psaty BM, McKnight B, et al: Fasting and post-glucose load measures of insulin resistance and risk of ischemic stroke in older adults, *Stroke* 42:3347–3351, 2011.
26. Gutt M, Davis CL, Spitzer SB, et al: Validation of the insulin sensitivity index (ISI(0,120)): comparison with other measures, *Diabetes Res Clin Pract* 47:177–184, 2000.
27. Rudenski AS, Matthews DR, Levy JC, et al: Understanding insulin resistance: both glucose resistance and insulin resistance are required to model human diabetes, *Metabolism* 40:908–917, 1991.
28. Bravata DM, Wells CK, Kernan WN, et al: Association between impaired insulin sensitivity and stroke, *Neuroepidemiology* 25:69–74, 2005.
29. Wang J, Ruotsalainen S, Moilanen L, et al: The metabolic syndrome predicts incident stroke: a 14-year follow-up study in elderly people in Finland, *Stroke* 39:1078–1083, 2008.
30. Boden-Albala B, Sacco RL, Lee HS, et al: Metabolic syndrome and ischemic stroke risk: Northern Manhattan Study, *Stroke* 39:30–35, 2008.
31. Protopsaltis I, et al: Metabolic syndrome and its components as predictors of ischemic stroke in type 2 diabetic patients, *Stroke* 39:1036–1038, 2008.
32. Hankey GJ: Nutrition and the risk of stroke, *Lancet Neurol* 11:66–81, 2012.
33. Kurth T, Gaziano JM, Berger K, et al: Body mass index and the risk of stroke in men, *Arch Intern Med* 162:2557–2562, 2002.
34. Whitlock G, Lewington S, Sherliker P, et al: Body-mass index and cause-specific mortality in 900,000 adults: collaborative analyses of 57 prospective studies, *Lancet* 373:1083–1096, 2009.
35. Lip GY, Tse HF, Lane DA: Atrial fibrillation, *Lancet* 379:648–661, 2012.
36. Huxley RR, Filion KB, Konety S, et al: Meta-analysis of cohort and case-control studies of type 2 diabetes mellitus and risk of atrial fibrillation, *Am J Cardiol* 108:56–62, 2011.
37. Nichols GA, et al: Independent contribution of diabetes to increased prevalence and incidence of atrial fibrillation, *Diabetes Care* 32:1851–1856, 2009.
38. Cui R, Iso H, Yamagishi K, et al: Diabetes mellitus and risk of stroke and its subtypes among Japanese: the Japan public health center study, *Stroke* 42:2611–2614, 2011.
39. Nathan DM, Cleary PA, Backlund JY, et al: Diabetes Control and Complications Trial/Epidemiology of Diabetes Interventions and Complications (DCCT/EDIC) Study Research Group: Intensive diabetes treatment and cardiovascular disease in patients with type 1 diabetes, *N Engl J Med* 353:2643–2653, 2005.
40. UKPDS-study group: Intensive blood-glucose control with sulphonylureas or insulin compared with conventional treatment and risk of complications in patients with type 2 diabetes (UKPDS 33). UK Prospective Diabetes Study (UKPDS) Group, *Lancet* 352:837–853, 1998.
41. Effect of intensive blood-glucose control with metformin on complications in overweight patients with type 2 diabetes (UKPDS 34). UK Prospective Diabetes Study (UKPDS) Group, *Lancet* 352:854–865, 1998.
42. Action to Control Cardiovascular Risk in Diabetes Study Group: Effects of intensive glucose lowering in type 2 diabetes, *N Engl J Med* 358:2545–2559, 2008.
43. ADVANCE Collaborative Group: Intensive blood glucose control and vascular outcomes in patients with type 2 diabetes, *N Engl J Med* 358:2560–2572, 2008.
44. Duckworth W, Abraira C, Moritz T, et al: VADT Investigators: Glucose control and vascular complications in veterans with type 2 diabetes, *N Engl J Med* 360:129–139, 2009.
45. Boussageon R, Bejan-Angoulvant T, Saadatian-Elahi M, et al: Effect of intensive glucose lowering treatment on all cause mortality, cardiovascular death, and microvascular events in type 2 diabetes: meta-analysis of randomised controlled trials, *BMJ* 343:d4169, 2011 Jul 26.
46. Hemmingsen B, Lund SS, Gluud C, et al: Targeting intensive glycaemic control versus targeting conventional glycaemic control for type 2 diabetes mellitus, *Cochrane Database Syst Rev* (6): http://dx.doi.org/10.1002/14651858, 2011 Jun 15. CD008143.
47. UKPDS: Tight blood pressure control and risk of macrovascular and microvascular complications in type 2 diabetes: UKPDS 38. UK Prospective Diabetes Study Group, *BMJ* 317:703–713, 1998.
48. Bangalore S, Kumar S, Lobach I, et al: Blood pressure targets in subjects with type 2 diabetes mellitus/impaired fasting glucose: observations from traditional and Bayesian random-effects meta-analyses of randomized trials, *Circulation* 123:2799–2810, 2011.
49. ACCORD Study Group: Effects of intensive blood-pressure control in type 2 diabetes mellitus, *N Engl J Med* 362:1575–1585, 2010.
50. Lee M, Saver JL, Hong KS, et al: Does achieving an intensive versus usual blood pressure level prevent stroke? *Ann Neurol* 71:133–140, 2012.
51. Rothwell PM, Howard SC, Dolan E, et al: Effects of beta blockers and calcium-channel blockers on within-individual variability in blood pressure and risk of stroke, *Lancet Neurol* 9:469–480, 2010.
52. Collins R, Armitage J, Parish S, et al: MRC/BHF Heart Protection Study of cholesterol-lowering with simvastatin in 5963 people with diabetes: a randomised placebo-controlled trial, *Lancet* 361:2005–2016, 2003.
53. Colhoun HM, Betteridge DJ, Durrington PN, et al: primary prevention of cardiovascular disease with atorvastatin in type 2 diabetes in the Collaborative Atorvastatin Diabetes Study (CARDS): multicentre randomised placebo-controlled trial, *Lancet* 364:685–696, 2004.
54. Kearney PM, Blackwell L, Collins R, et al: Cholesterol Treatment Trialists' (CTT) Collaborators: Efficacy of cholesterol-lowering therapy in 18 686 people with diabetes in 14 randomised trials of statins: a meta-analysis, *Lancet* 371:117–125, 2008.
55. Amarenco P, Bogousslavsky J, Callahan A 3rd, : Stroke Prevention by Aggressive Reduction in Cholesterol Levels (SPARCL) Investigators: High-dose atorvastatin after stroke or transient ischemic attack, *N Engl J Med* 355:549–559, 2006.
56. De Berardis G, Sacco M, Strippoli GF, et al: Aspirin for primary prevention of cardiovascular events in people with diabetes: meta-analysis of randomized controlled trials, *BMJ* 339:b4531, 2009 6.
57. Bhatt DL, Marso SP, Hirsch AT, et al: Amplified benefit of clopidogrel versus aspirin in patients with diabetes mellitus, *Am J Cardiol* 90:625–628, 2002.
58. Antithrombotic Trialists' Collaboration: Collaborative meta-analysis of randomized trials of antiplatelet therapy for prevention of death, myocardial infarction, and stroke in high risk patients, *BMJ* 324:71–86, 2002.
59. Anselmino M, Malmberg K, Öhrvik J, et al: Evidence-based medication and revascularization: powerful tools in the management of patients with diabetes and coronary artery disease: a report from the Euro Heart Survey on diabetes and the heart, *Eur J Cardiovasc Prev Rehabil* 15:216–223, 2008.
60. Gaede P, Lund-Andersen H, Parving H-H, et al: Effect of a multifactorial intervention on mortality in type 2 diabetes, *N Engl J Med* 358:580–591, 2008.
61. Griffin SJ, Borch-Johnsen K, Davies MJ, et al: Effect of early intensive multifactorial therapy on 5-year cardiovascular outcomes in individuals with type 2 diabetes detected by screening (ADDITION-Europe): a cluster-randomised trial, *Lancet* 378:156–167, 2011.
62. Alberts MJ, Eikelboom JW, Hankey GJ: Antithrombotic therapy for stroke prevention in non-valvular atrial fibrillation, *Lancet Neurol* 11:1066–1081, 2012.
63. Koudstaal PJ: Antiplatelet therapy for preventing stroke in patients with nonrheumatic atrial fibrillation and a history of stroke or transient ischemic attacks, *Cochrane Database Syst Rev* 2:2000 CD000186.
64. EAFT (European Atrial Fibrillation Trial) Study Group: Secondary prevention in non-rheumatic atrial fibrillation after transient ischaemic attack or minor stroke, *Lancet* 342:1255–1262, 1993.
65. Mant J, Hobbs FDR, Fletcher K, et al: Warfarin versus aspirin for stroke prevention in an elderly community population with atrial fibrillation (the Birmingham Atrial Fibrillation Treatment of the Aged Study, BAFTA): a randomised controlled trial, *Lancet* 370:493–503, 2007.
66. Connolly SJ, Ezekowitz MD, Yusuf S, et al: Dabigatran versus warfarin in patients with atrial fibrillation, *N Engl J Med* 361:1139–1151, 2009.
67. Patel MR, Mahaffey KW, Garg J, et al: Rivaroxaban versus warfarin in nonvalvular atrial fibrillation, *N Engl J Med* 365:883–891, 2011.
68. Granger CB, Alexander JH, McMurray JJV, et al: Apixaban versus warfarin in patients with atrial fibrillation, *N Engl J Med* 365:981–992, 2011.
69. Ntaios G, Papavasileiou V, Diener HC, et al: Nonvitamin-k-antagonist oral anticoagulants in patients with atrial fibrillation and previous stroke or transient ischemic attack: a systematic review and meta-analysis of randomized controlled trials, *Stroke* 43:3298–3304, 2012.
70. Camm AJ, Lip GY, De Caterina R, et al: 2012 focused update of the ESC Guidelines for the management of atrial fibrillation: an update of the 2010 ESC Guidelines for the management of atrial fibrillation. Developed with the special contribution of the European Heart Rhythm Association, *Eur Heart J* 33:2719–2747, 2012.
71. Furie KL, Goldstein LB, Albers GW, et al: Oral antithrombotic agents for the prevention of stroke in nonvalvular atrial fibrillation. A science advisory for healthcare professionals from the American Heart Association/American Stroke Association, *Stroke* 43:3442–3453, 2012.

72. Abbott AL: Medical (nonsurgical) intervention alone is now best for prevention of stroke associated with asymptomatic severe carotid stenosis: results of a systematic review and analysis, *Stroke* 40:e573–e583, 2009.
73. Marquardt L, Geraghty OC, Mehta Z, et al: Low risk of ipsilateral stroke in patients with asymptomatic carotid stenosis on best medical treatment: a prospective, population-based study, *Stroke* 41:e11–e17, 2010.
74. Rothwell PM, Eliasziw M, Gutnikov SA, et al: Endarterectomy for symptomatic carotid stenosis in relation to clinical subgroups and timing of surgery, *Lancet* 363:915–924, 2004.
75. ECST Collaborative Group: Randomised trial of endarterectomy for recently symptomatic carotid stenosis: final results of the MRC European Carotid Surgery Trial (ECST), *Lancet* 351:1379–1387, 1998.
76. North American Symptomatic Carotid Endarterectomy Trial Collaborators: Beneficial effect of carotid endarterectomy in symptomatic patients with high-grade carotid stenosis, *N Engl J Med* 325:445–453, 1991.
77. Hobson RW 2nd, Weiss DG, Fields WS, et al: Efficacy of carotid endarterectomy for asymptomatic carotid stenosis. The Veterans Affairs Cooperative Study Group, *N Engl J Med* 328:221–227, 1993.
78. Mas JL, Chatellier G, Beyssen B, et al: Endarterectomy versus stenting in patients with symptomatic severe carotid stenosis, *N Engl J Med* 355:1660–1671, 2006.
79. Ringleb PA, Allenberg J, Bruckmann H, et al: 30 day results from the SPACE trial of stent-protected angioplasty versus carotid endarterectomy in symptomatic patients: a randomised non-inferiority trial, *Lancet* 368:1239–1247, 2006.
80. Brott TG, Hobson RW II, Howard G, et al: Crest investigators: Stenting versus endarterectomy for treatment of carotid-artery stenosis, *N Engl J Med* 363:11–23, 2006.
81. Furie KL, Kasner SE, Adams RJ, et al: Guidelines for the prevention of stroke in patients with stroke or transient ischemic attack: a guideline for healthcare professionals from the American Heart Association / American Stroke Association, *Stroke* 42:227–276, 2011.
82. Chimowitz MI, Lynn MJ, Derdeyn CP, et al: Stenting versus aggressive medical therapy for intracranial arterial stenosis, *N Engl J Med* 365:993–1003, 2011.
83. Wright RJ, Frier BM: Vascular disease and diabetes: is hypoglycaemia an aggravating factor? *Diabetes Metab Res Rev* 24:353–363, 2008.
84. Hacke W, Kaste M, Bluhmki E, et al: Thrombolysis with alteplase 3 to 4.5 hours after acute ischemic stroke, *N Engl J Med* 359:1317–1329, 2009.
85. Allport L, Baird T, Butcher K, et al: Frequency and temporal profile of post stroke hyperglycaemia using continuous glucose monitoring, *Diabetes Care* 29:1839–1844, 2006.
86. Scott JF, Robinson GM, French JM, et al: Prevalence of admission hyperglycaemia across clinical subtypes of acute stroke, *Lancet* 353:376–377, 1999.
87. Wong AA, Schluter PJ, Henderson RD, et al: Natural history of blood glucose within the first 48 hours after ischemic stroke, *Neurology* 70:1036–1041, 2008.
88. Yong M, Kaste M: Dynamic of hyperglycemia as a predictor of stroke outcome in the ECASS-II trial, *Stroke* 39:2749–2755, 2008.
89. O'Neill PA, Davies I, Fullerton KJ, et al: Stress hormone and blood glucose response following acute stroke in the elderly, *Stroke* 22:842–847, 1991.
90. van Kooten F, Hoogerbrugge N, Naarding P, et al: Hyperglycaemia in the acute phase of stroke is not caused by stress, *Stroke* 24:1129–1132, 1993.
91. Garg R, Chaudhuri A, Munschauer F, et al: Hyperglycaemia, insulin and acute ischaemic stroke, *Stroke* 37:267–273, 2006.
92. Gilmore RM, Stead LG: The role of hyperglycemia in acute ischemic stroke, *Neurocrit Care* 5:153–158, 2006.
93. Quinn TJ, Lees KR: Hyperglycaemia in acute stroke–to treat or not to treat, *Cerebrovasc Dis* 27(Suppl 1):148–155, 2009.
94. Weir CJ, Murray GD, Dyker AG, et al: Is hyperglycaemia an independent predictor of poor outcome after acute stroke? Results of a long term follow up study, *BMJ* 314:1303–1306, 1997.
95. Capes SE, Hunt D, Malmberg K, et al: Stress hyperglycemia and prognosis of stroke in nondiabetic and diabetic patients: a systematic overview, *Stroke* 32:2426–2432, 2001.
96. Stead LG, Gilmore RM, Bellolio MF, et al: Hyperglycemia as an independent predictor of worse outcome in non-diabetic patients presenting with acute ischemic stroke, *Neurocrit Care* 10:181–186, 2009.
97. Kruyt ND, Nys GM, van der Worp HB, et al: Hyperglycemia and cognitive outcome after ischemic stroke, *J Neurol Sci* 270:141–147, 2008.
98. Uyttenboogaart M, Koch MW, Stewart RE, et al: Moderate hyperglycaemia is associated with favourable outcome in acute lacunar stroke, *Brain* 130:1626–1630, 2007.
99. Fuentes B, Castillo J, San José B, et al: The prognostic value of capillary glucose levels in acute stroke. The GLycemia in Acute Stroke (GLIAS) study, *Stroke* 40:562–568, 2009.
100. Bruno A, Levnie SR, Frankel MR, et al: for the NINDS rt-PA stroke study group: Admission glucose level and clinical outcomes in the NINDS rt-PA stroke trial, *Neurology* 59:669–674, 2002.
101. Ribo M, Molina C, Montaner J, et al: Acute hyperglycemia state is associated with lower tPA-induced recanalization rates in stroke patients, *Stroke* 36:1705–1709, 2005.
102. Ahmed N, Davalos A, Eriksson N, et al: for the SITS Investigators: Association of admission blood glucose and outcome in patients treated with intravenous thrombolysis: results from the Safe Implementation of Treatments in Stroke International Stroke Thrombolysis Register (SITS-ISTR), *Arch Neurol* 67:1123–1130, 2010.
103. Mishra NK, Davis SM, Kaste M, et al: Comparison of outcomes following thrombolytic therapy among patients with prior stroke and diabetes in the Virtual International Stroke Trials Archive (VISTA), *Diabetes Care* 33:2531–2537, 2010.
104. Gray CS, Hildreth AJ, Sandercock PA, et al: Glucose-potassium-insulin infusions in the management of post-stroke hyperglycaemia: the UK Glucose Insulin in Stroke Trial (GIST-UK), *Lancet Neurol* 6:397–406, 2007.
105. Walters MR, Weir CJ, Lees K: A randomised, controlled pilot study to investigate the potential benefit of intervention with insulin in hyperglycaemic acute ischaemic stroke patients, *Cerebrovasc Dis* 22:116–122, 2006.
106. Vriesendorp TM, Roos YB, Kruyt ND, et al: Efficacy and safety of two 5 day insulin dosing regimens to achieve strict glycaemic control in patients with acute ischaemic stroke, *J Neurol Neurosurg Psychiatry* 80:1040–1043, 2009.
107. Van den Berghe G, Wouters P, Weekers F, et al: Intensive insulin therapy in the critically ill patient, *N Engl J Med* 345:1359–1367, 2001.
108. NICE-SUGAR Study Investigators, Finfer S, Chittock DR, Su SY, et al: Intensive versus conventional glucose control in critically ill patients, *N Engl J Med* 360:1283–1297, 2009.
109. Velayudhan LV, Poppe M, Archer N, et al: Risk of developing dementia in people with diabetes and mild cognitive impairment, *Br J Psychiatry* 196:36–40, 2010.
110. Reijmer YD, van den Berg E, Ruis C, et al: Cognitive dysfunction in patients with type 2 diabetes, *Diabetes Metab Res Rev* 26:507–519, 2010.
111. Cerhan JR, Folsom AR, Mortimer JA, et al: Correlates of cognitive function in middle-aged adults, *Gerontology* 44:95–105, 1998.
112. Elias PK, Elias MF, D'Agostino RB, et al: NIDDM and blood pressure as risk factors for poor cognitive performance. The Framingham Study, *Diabetes Care* 20:1388–1395, 1997.
113. Luchsinger JA, Reitz C, Patel B, et al: Relation of diabetes to mild cognitive impairment, *Arch Neurol* 64:570–575, 2007.
114. Luchsinger JA: Diabetes, related conditions, and dementia, *J Neurol Sci* 299:35–38, 2010.
115. van den Berg E, Reijmer YD, de Bresser J, et al: A 4 year follow-up study of cognitive functioning in patients with type 2 diabetes mellitus, *Diabetologia* 53:58–65, 2010.
116. Biessels GJ, Staekenborg S, Brunner E, et al: Risk of dementia in diabetes mellitus: a systematic review, *Lancet Neurol* 5:64–74, 2006.
117. Biessels GJ: Hypoglycemia and dementia in type 2 diabetes: chick or egg? *Nat Rev Endocrinol* 5:532–534, 2009.
118. Jellinger KA, Attems J: Prevalence of dementia disorders in the oldest-old: an autopsy study, *Acta Neuropathol* 119:421–433, 2010.
119. Yaffe K, Blackwell T, Kanaya AM, et al: Diabetes, impaired fasting glucose, and development of cognitive impairment in older women, *Neurology* 63:658–663, 2004.
120. van den Berg E, Dekker JM, Nijpels G, et al: Blood pressure levels in pre-diabetic stages are associated with worse cognitive functioning in patients with type 2 diabetes, *Diabetes Metab Res Rev* 25:657–664, 2009.
121. Bruehl H, Wolf OT, Sweat V, et al: Modifiers of cognitive function and brain structure in middleaged and elderly individuals with type 2 diabetes mellitus, *Brain Res* 1280:186–194, 2009.
122. Kanaya AM, Barrett-Connor E, Gildengorin G, et al: Change in cognitive function by glucose tolerance status in older adults: a 4-year prospective study of the Rancho Bernardo study cohort, *Arch Intern Med* 164:1327–1333, 2004.
123. Edland SD: Insulin-degrading enzyme, apolipoprotein E, and Alzheimer's disease, *J Mol Neurosci* 23:213–217, 2004.
124. van Harten B, de Leeuw FE, Weinstein HC, et al: Brain imaging in patients with diabetes: a systematic review, *Diabetes Care* 29:2539–2548, 2006.
125. Schmidt R, Launer LJ, Nilsson LG, et al: CASCADE Consortium: Magnetic resonance imaging of the brain in diabetes: the Cardiovascular Determinants of Dementia (CASCADE) Study, *Diabetes* 53:687–692, 2004.
126. Cordonnier C, Al-Shahi SR, Wardlaw J: Spontaneous brain microbleeds: systematic review, subgroup analyses and standards for study design and reporting, *Brain* 130: 1988–2003, 2007.
127. Alafuzoff I, Aho L, Helisalmi S, et al: ß-Amyloid deposition in brains of subjects with diabetes, *Neuropathol Appl Neurobiol* 35:60–68, 2009.
128. Arvanitakis Z, Schneider JA, Wilson RS, et al: Diabetes is related to cerebral infarction but not to AD pathology in older persons, *Neurology* 67:1960–1965, 2006.
129. Schnaider Beeri M, Silverman JM, Davis KL, et al: Type 2 diabetes is negatively associated with Alzheimer's disease neuropathology, *J Gerontol A Biol Sci Med Sci* 60:471–475, 2005.
130. Peila R, Rodriguez BL, Launer LJ: Type 2 diabetes, APOE gene, and the risk for dementia and related pathologies: the Honolulu-Asia Aging Study, *Diabetes* 51:1256–1262, 2002.
131. Ryan CM, Freed MI, Rood JA, et al: Improving metabolic control leads to better working memory in adults with type 2 diabetes, *Diabetes Care* 29:345–351, 2006.
132. Mussell M, Hewer W, Kulzer B, et al: Effects of improved glycaemic control maintained for 3 months on cognitive function in patients with Type 2 diabetes, *Diabet Med* 21: 1253–1256, 2004.
133. Launer LJ, Miller ME, Williamson JD, et al: Effects of intensive glucose lowering on brain structure and function in people with type 2 diabetes (ACCORD MIND): a randomised open-label substudy, *Lancet Neurol* 10:969–977, 2011.
134. Deschaintre Y, Richard F, Leys D, et al: Treatment of vascular risk factors is associated with slower decline in Alzheimer disease, *Neurology* 73:674–680, 2009.
135. Plastino M, Fava A, Pirritano D, et al: Effects of insulinic therapy on cognitive impairment in patients with Alzheimer disease and diabetes mellitus type-2, *J Neurol Sci* 288:112–116, 2010.
136. Chen Y, Zhou K, Wang R, et al: Antidiabetic drug metformin (GlucophageR) increases biogenesis of Alzheimer's amyloid peptides via up-regulating BACE1 transcription, *Proc Natl Acad Sci* 106:3907–3912, 2009.
137. Imfeld P, Bodmer M, Jick SS, et al: Metformin, other antidiabetic drugs, and risk of Alzheimer's disease: a population-based case-control study, *J Am Geriatr Soc* 60:916–921, 2012.
138. Hsu CC, Wahlqvist ML, Lee MS, et al: Incidence of dementia is increased in type 2 diabetes and reduced by the use of sulfonylureas and metformin, *J Alzheimers Dis* 24:485–493, 2011.
139. Colberg SR, Somma CT, Sechrist SR: Physical activity participation may offset some of the negative impact of diabetes on cognitive function, *J Am Med Dir Assoc* 9:434–438, 2008.
140. Brands AMA, Biessels GJ, De Haan EHF, et al: The effects of Type 1 diabetes on cognitive performance: a meta-analysis, *Diabetes Care* 28:726–735, 2005.
141. Austin EJ, Deary IJ: Effects of repeated hypoglycemia on cognitive function: a psychometrically validated reanalysis of the Diabetes Control and Complications Trial data, *Diabetes Care* 22:1273–1277, 1999.
142. The Diabetes Control and Complications Trial Research Group: Long-term effect of diabetes and its treatment on cognitive function, *N Engl J Med* 356:1842–1852, 2007.
143. Whitmer RA, Karter AJ, Yaffe K, et al: Hypoglycemic episodes and risk of dementia in older patients with type 2 diabetes mellitus, *JAMA* 301:1565–1572, 2009.
144. Bruce DG, Davis WA, Casey GP, et al: Severe hypoglycaemia and cognitive impairment in older patients with diabetes: the Fremantle Diabetes Study, *Diabetologia* 52:1808–1815, 2009.
145. Messier C, Gagnon M: Cognitive decline associated with dementia and type 2 diabetes: the interplay of risk factors, *Diabetologia* 52:2471–2474, 2009.
146. Craft S: Insulin resistance and Alzheimer's disease pathogenesis: potential mechanisms and implications for treatment, *Curr Alzheimer Res* 4:147–152, 2007.
147. Craft S, Baker LD, Montine TJ, et al: Intranasal insulin therapy for Alzheimer disease and amnestic mild cognitive impairment: a pilot clinical trial, *Arch Neurol* 69:29–38, 2012.

29 Cardiovascular Autonomic Neuropathy

Paul Valensi

Cardiovascular autonomic neuropathy (CAN) is defined as the impairment of autonomic control of the cardiovascular system in the setting of diabetes after exclusion of other causes. CAN is usually detected at a subclinical stage by means of several cardiovascular autonomic reflex tests and may affect patients with type 1 or type 2 diabetes mellitus (T1DM or T2DM). Poor glycemic control is a major determinant of this complication. CAN predicts a higher mortality and may induce significant cardiovascular changes in diabetic patients.

PATHOPHYSIOLOGY OF VAGOSYMPATHETIC IMBALANCE

The relationships between cardiac autonomic dysfunction and insulin resistance are complex. Each of them may aggravate the other (**Fig. 29-1**). Moreover, vagosympathetic imbalance may induce hemodynamic changes.

Role of Vagosympathetic Impairment in Insulin Resistance

Obesity is a major determinant of CAN in T2DM patients. Data suggest that cardiac autonomic dysfunction may occur in obese individuals before diabetes. In obese patients, cardiac vagal tests more often show impairment in those with the metabolic syndrome, and the impairment is more commensurate with the severity of perturbations of the components of the syndrome. In individuals with the metabolic syndrome, increased activity of the sympathetic nervous system was found to be associated with several of the components of the metabolic syndrome, including elevated blood pressure (BP).[1] However, whether this disorder contributes to the development of the metabolic syndrome or is a consequence of it remains still a matter of debate. Because cardiac autonomic dysfunction may occur in individuals with only one or two metabolic abnormalities without

insulin resistance, cardiac autonomic dysfunction is suggested to precede insulin resistance in the metabolic syndrome.[2] This hypothesis is strongly supported by a recent demonstration that the progression to T2DM is associated with increased central sympathetic drive, blunted sympathetic responsiveness, and altered norepinephrine disposition.[3] Indeed, vagal depression and sympathetic predominance might contribute to insulin resistance and depression of insulin secretion. Several findings support this hypothesis. In obese normotensive patients, central fat distribution is associated with higher sympathetic activity.[4] Glucose usage has been found to correlate negatively with the low frequency–to–high frequency ratio (LF/HF) on spectral analysis of heart rate (HR) variations, which means that glucose usage was reduced when sympathetic activity was relatively higher.[5] We reported that in obese patients with vagal cardiac impairment, insulin levels correlated negatively with glucose oxidation rate (indirect calorimetry), suggesting a more severe insulin resistance that may again result from sympathetic overactivity.[6]

Effects of Insulin and Glucagon-like Peptide 1 on Autonomic Activity

Hyperinsulinemia subsequent to insulin resistance may also modulate autonomic activity and induce changes in hemodynamic parameters.[7] Insulin may increase HR slightly, as shown during hyperinsulinemic euglycemic clamps in healthy individuals.[8,9] HR elevation results from both vagal depression[8,9] and cardiac sympathetic activation as indicated by increased muscle sympathetic nerve activity (MSNA),[9,10] plasma catecholamines,[11] and in some studies[8] LF/HF ratio (an index for relative sympathetic predominance). Sympathoexcitatory effects of insulin result from a central nervous action and possibly from baroreflex activation secondary to insulin-induced peripheral vasodilation. However, during insulin clamp the shift in the cardiac

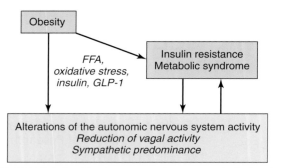

FIGURE 29-1 Relationships between cardiac autonomic dysfunction and obesity and insulin resistance. FFA = Free fatty acids; GLP-1 = glucagon-like peptide 1.

autonomic activity toward sympathetic predominance was reported to be lower in obese than in lean individuals[12] and in insulin-resistant patients,[13] suggesting that chronic hyperinsulinemia may prevent further enhancement of cardiac sympathetic tone during an acute rise in insulin.

In addition, recent data suggest that the incretin hormone glucagon-like peptide 1 (GLP-1) may also play a role in this context. Regarding the effects of GLP-1 on autonomic activity, both the acute and chronic administration of central long-lasting GLP-1 receptor agonist exendin-4 was shown to reduce HF and LF powers of HR variations and to inhibit neurotransmission to cardiac vagal neurons.[14] GLP-1, administered peripherally or centrally, also increases sympathetic activity in rats.[15] Further studies on the effects of GLP-1 on autonomic activity need to be performed in diabetic and obese patients to determine the role of GLP-1 in these populations.

Thus, insulin and GLP-1 are able to induce vagal depression and sympathetic activation (see **Fig. 29-1**). Both hormones may potentially affect BP with effects that might differ depending on the presence of hypertension, cardiac autonomic impairment, and endothelium function.

Vagosympathetic Imbalance and Hemodynamic Changes

Sympathetic activity was found to be greater and baroreflex sensitivity more severely impaired in individuals with obesity and hypertension than in those with either obesity or hypertension alone[16] and similarly for individuals with the metabolic syndrome and hypertension,[17] suggesting that sympathetic overactivity may contribute to hypertension. Vagal impairment and/or sympathetic overactivity may also contribute to resting sinus tachycardia.

At advanced stages of diabetic CAN sympathetic activity is depressed, which may induce orthostatic hypotension (OH).[18] Postprandial hypotension may also occur as a result of meal-induced splanchnic vasodilation while sympathetic response is blunted (**Fig. 29-2**).

EPIDEMIOLOGICAL DATA

Prevalence and Correlates of Cardiovascular Autonomic Neuropathy

In clinical studies including both T1DM and T2DM patients, the prevalence of confirmed CAN (defined by at least two abnormal cardiovascular autonomic reflex test [CART] results) was approximately 20%.[19,20] However, prevalence rates increased with age and diabetes duration (up to 35% in T1DM and 65% in T2DM patients with longstanding diabetes). Glycemic control and the presence of microvascular complications (polyneuropathy, retinopathy, nephropathy) are other correlates of CAN.[19–21] A contributing role of several cardiovascular risk factors (high BP or hypertension, smoking, dyslipidemia, overweight or obesity in T2DM, large waist circumference, high insulin levels in T2DM, and cardiovascular disease) has also been reported. The influence of overweight and obesity is supported by the high prevalence of impaired cardiac vagal activity in nondiabetic obese patients[22] and the finding of an inverse correlation between HR variability and body weight in the general population.[23] This suggests that cardiac autonomic dysfunction precedes the onset of T2DM and might play a role in metabolic disorders.

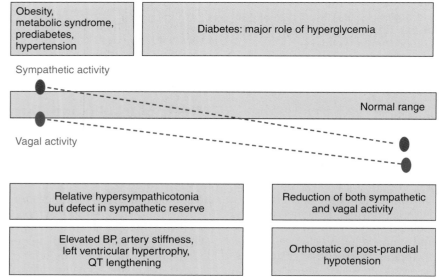

FIGURE 29-2 Changes in vagal and sympathetic activity in the diabetes continuum. BP = Blood pressure.

Cardiovascular Autonomic Neuropathy as a Predictor of Cardiovascular Morbidity and Mortality

CAN is a risk marker for all-cause and cardiac mortality, stroke, coronary events, silent myocardial ischemia (SMI), heart failure, arrhythmia, sudden death, and nephropathy progression.[24] A meta-analysis of 15 longitudinal studies, which included 2900 patients followed for 1 to 16 years, showed that the diagnosis of CAN based on at least two abnormal CART results determined a relative risk of mortality of 3.45 (95% confidence interval 2.66-4.47; $P<0.001$).[25] Subsequent studies including the Action to Control Cardiovascular Risk in Diabetes (ACCORD) trial[26] confirmed the independent predictive value of CAN for all-cause and cardiovascular mortality (still predictive after adjustment for cardiovascular risk factors). The presence of OH, a clinical manifestation of severe CAN, impaired the prognosis and was associated with a higher mortality risk than the increase in risk associated with vagal cardiac test abnormalities.[25] Prolongation of the QT interval corrected for HR (QTc), which may result from CAN, is also an independent predictor of all-cause and cardiovascular mortality.[27]

CARDIOVASCULAR DISORDERS ASSOCIATED WITH CARDIOVASCULAR AUTONOMIC NEUROPATHY

Several disorders associated with subclinical CAN and subsequent to sympathetic predominance may account for the increase in cardiovascular events (**Fig. 29-3**).

Silent Myocardial Ischemia

SMI may be detected by stress ECG or by stress myocardial scintigraphy or echocardiography. In a meta-analysis of 12 studies including 1468 diabetic patients, SMI was present in 20% of those with CAN compared with 10% of those without CAN, with a prevalence rate ratio of 1.96.[28] The Detection of Ischemia in Asymptomatic Diabetics (DIAD) trial, which assessed the role of routine screening for ischemia using nuclear stress testing compared with usual care, showed that in 1123 T2DM patients an abnormal Valsalva maneuver was the strongest determinant of SMI.[29] The lowest quartile of HR response in the lying-to-standing test was associated with an adjusted hazard ratio of 4.33 for cardiac death or nonfatal myocardial infarction over a mean follow-up of 4.8 years.[30] In addition, we reported that CAN enhances the cardiac risk associated with SMI.[31] Thus, CAN testing may be considered a main component of a diabetes-specific risk pattern to identify high-risk patients in whom screening for SMI is more

effective,[32] although the efficacy of such a strategy awaits confirmation in a controlled clinical trial.

Hypertension

A defect in vagal activity might contribute to hypertension through a relative sympathetic override. This is supported by a study in rats with ventromedial hypothalamic obesity that exhibited a marked bradycardia and only a mild increase in BP. In these rats heart vagal tone was increased, and adrenal medulla secretion was enhanced probably as a result of hyperinsulinemia. In addition, increased vagal activity was observed, and cardiac responsiveness to beta-agonist stimulation was also increased.[33] This suggests that high vagal activity may be protective against hypertension associated with obesity. In patients with T1DM or T2DM we showed that the prevalence of hypertension increased with CAN severity, which supports the role of CAN contributing to hypertension in diabetic patients.[34] Furthermore, a large majority of the patients with macrovascular complications, retinopathy, or nephropathy exhibited the CAN-plus-hypertension profile, which is consistent with a deleterious effect of CAN on vascular hemodynamics and structure, additive to the effects of hypertension.[34] Similarly, we recently found a relationship between the severity of cardiac autonomic dysfunction and the prevalence of hypertension in nondiabetic obese patients (unpublished data).

Left Ventricular Dysfunction

CAN has been reported to be associated with left ventricular systolic and particularly diastolic dysfunction.[35,36] However, it is difficult to evaluate the independent role of CAN in these disorders and in chronic heart failure, because interstitial myocardial fibrosis and microangiopathic or metabolic changes may also contribute to diabetic myocardial disease and left ventricular dysfunction.

QT Interval Prolongation

QTc prolongation may result from imbalance in cardiac sympathetic innervation but also from metabolic and electrolytic myocardial changes, left ventricular hypertrophy, coronary artery disease, and genetic factors. In a meta-analysis of 17 studies including 4584 diabetic patients, QTc prolongation (corrected QT for HR >441 milliseconds) was a specific (86%) but insensitive (28%) index of CAN.[37] Using 24-hour electrocardiographic recordings, we showed that the day-night modulation of the QT/RR-interval relationship was altered in CAN patients free of coronary artery disease or left ventricular dysfunction or hypertrophy, with a reversed day-night pattern and an increased nocturnal QT-HR dependence.[38]

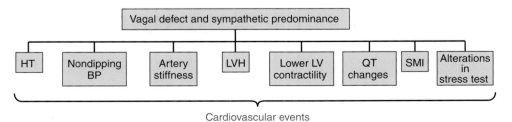

FIGURE 29-3 **Cardiovascular disorders induced by CAN.** BP = Blood pressure; HT = hypertension; LV = left ventricular; LVH = left ventricular hypertrophy; SMI = silent myocardial infarction.

In T1DM patients, prolonged QTc has been reported to occur frequently during overnight hypoglycemia and to be associated with cardiac rate and rhythm disturbances. Reversible QTc prolongation may be induced by hyperglycemia and by acute hypoglycemia in both healthy and diabetic patients. These findings support an arrhythmic basis for the "dead in bed" syndrome and possibly a provocative role in cardiovascular events of hypoglycemia-induced sympathetic activation.[39] Thus, the presence of CAN may identify diabetic patients more susceptible to the deleterious effects of hypoglycemia, in particular among those with a coronary artery disease. CAN testing may also serve to inform the choice of glycemic control targets according to the patient's risk profile and to balance the advantage of aggressive glucose-lowering treatment versus its risk. Moreover, QTc measurement may be used for cardiovascular risk stratification.[24]

Abnormal Circadian Blood Pressure Pattern

An abnormal circadian BP pattern on ambulatory blood pressure monitoring (ABPM) is associated with CAN. Normal circadian BP changes are characterized by lower levels during the night than during the day. Nondipping and reverse dipping, defined as attenuation or loss of BP and nocturnal fall, respectively, may result from CAN. Several studies linked nondipping to changes in the circadian variation of sympathovagal activity, consisting of a diminished increase in vagal activity and sympathetic predominance during the night.[40,41] Nondipping or reverse dipping was associated with left ventricle hypertrophy[42] and was found to predict the progression of nephropathy independently of 24-hour BP level. Thus ABPM may be useful in patients with CAN to detect disturbance of normal circadian BP variability, to determine risk stratification for cardiovascular mortality and nephropathy progression, and to adjust antihypertensive treatment.

Exercise Intolerance

In diabetic patients with cardiac autonomic neuropathy, exercise capacity and the HR, BP, and cardiac stroke volume responses to exercise are found to be diminished, with a further decrease in exercise capacity and BP response in patients with both vagal neuropathy and OH. The severity of CAN correlates inversely with maximal HR increase during exercise, suggesting CAN contribution to altered exercise tolerance.[43] We also found an impairment of HR recovery after exercise in diabetic patients with CAN but free of SMI. CAN testing offers a useful tool to identify patients with potentially poor exercise performance and to prevent adverse outcomes when patients are introduced to exercise training programs.[24] Thus, CAN testing may be considered before a stress exercise test and also before initiation of a program of vigorous physical activity.[24]

Arterial Stiffness

Using spectral analysis we showed in obese and diabetic hypertensive patients that the low-frequency peak of systolic BP variations in the standing position, which reflects sympathetic activity, correlated significantly with pulse pressure measured in the lying position, suggesting that an increase in arterial stiffness is associated with a higher sympathetic activity.[44] In the Pittsburgh Epidemiology of Diabetes Complications study, CAN function was evaluated in a childhood-onset T1DM population and was associated with increased arterial stiffness measured 18 years later.[45] Some experimental data support the role of a possible protective effect of vagal activity and an aggravating role of sympathetic predominance in arterial stiffness.[46]

DETECTION OF SUBCLINICAL CARDIOVASCULAR AUTONOMIC NEUROPATHY

Detection in Clinical Practice
Standard Tests
Subclinical CAN is a frequent condition that is usually documented with CARTs, the gold standard for clinical autonomic testing. These tests consist of analysis of HR response to deep breathing, lying to standing, and Valsalva maneuver (HR tests), and BP response to standing.[24] HR variations during these tests are indices mainly of parasympathetic function, whereas the presence of OH indicates a sympathetic defect (**Table 29-1**). Knowledge of age-related normal ranges of HR test results is mandatory for accurate analysis of the results (**Fig. 29-4**). These tests are noninvasive, safe, clinically relevant, easy to perform, sensitive, specific, reproducible, and standardized.[24] However, in the absence of data on the potential risk of retinal complications, avoiding the Valsalva maneuver in patients with proliferative retinopathy may be appropriate.[24]

CARTs need to be performed with avoidance of confounding factors. Patients should be requested to avoid strenuous physical exercise in the 24 hours preceding the tests and caffeinated beverages, smoking, and alcohol at least 2 hours before the tests. Testing should be performed at fasting or at least 2 hours after a light meal, and in insulin-treated patients at least 2 hours after short-acting insulin administration, and not during hypoglycemia or marked hyperglycemia. In addition, test results should be interpreted with caution in patients with chronic obstructive pulmonary disease, respiratory failure, obstructive sleep apnea syndrome, or cardiac diseases, in particular heart failure. An appropriate washout of interfering drugs, particularly diuretics, sympatholytic agents, and psychoactive drugs should be considered, and if this is not feasible, then results should be interpreted cautiously.

CARTs need to be performed in a standardized way, with HR variations during the tests being analyzed with use of a

TABLE 29-1 Tests to Detect Subclinical Cardiovascular Autonomic Neuropathy in Clinical Practice or in Clinical Research

SETTING	TESTS
Standard tests in clinical practice	Analysis of HR variations during: • Deep breathing • Lying to standing • Valsalva Assess postural hypotension
In clinical research	• Cardiac vagal baroreflex sensitivity • Frequency domain measures of HR and BP variations • Measurement of muscle or skin sympathetic nerve activity • Plasma catecholamines • Heart sympathetic imaging

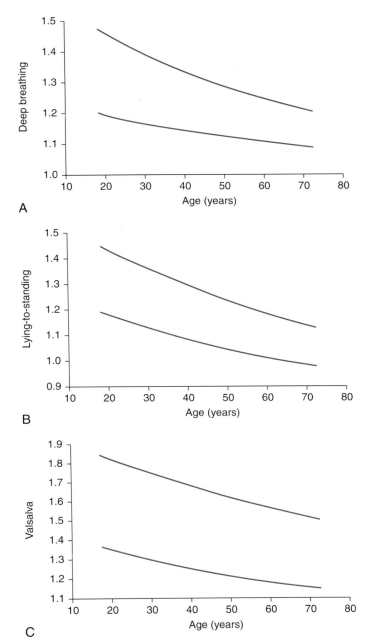

FIGURE 29-4 Influence of age on autonomic HR test results. Correlations (blue line) between RR ratio during the three CAN function tests—**A,** deep breathing; **B,** lying to standing; and **C,** Valsalva—with age in healthy individuals. Results obtained in one patient need to be located on the figures. Results are abnormal if below the 5th percentile line (red line). *(Modified from Valensi P: Comment rechercher une neuropathie autonome cardiaque? In: Coeur et Diabète, Frison Roche Ed, Paris, 1999.)*

simple cardiograph or an electrocardiographic computer system. Briefly, the deep-breathing test consists of six deep respiratory cycles in one minute in the recumbent position; the result is expressed as the mean value for the ratio of maximal RR (interval between two consecutive R waves on the electrocardiogram [ECG]) during breathing out to minimal RR during breathing in at each respiratory cycle. For the lying-to-standing test, the patient is asked to remain lying for 1 minute and then to stand up quickly; the result is expressed as the ratio of the longest RR interval (approximately the 30th beat after standing up) to the shortest RR interval (approximately the 15th beat). The Valsalva test is carried out with the patient seated. He or she is asked to

exhale a deep breath to maintain 40 mm Hg pressure for 15 seconds; the Valsalva ratio is calculated by the longest RR interval after breathing out divided by the shortest RR interval while breathing out. OH is defined as a reduction of systolic BP of at least 20 mm Hg or diastolic BP of at least 10 mm Hg within 3 minutes of standing, and a systolic fall in BP of 30 mm Hg in hypertensive patients.[24]

Cardiovascular Autonomic Neuropathy Staging
A definite diagnosis of CAN and CAN staging require more than one HR test and the measurement of BP response to standing. One abnormal cardiovagal test result identifies the condition of possible or early CAN, to be confirmed over time; at least two abnormal cardiovagal test results among the three HR tests are required for a definite or confirmed diagnosis of CAN. The presence of OH in addition to HR test abnormalities identifies severe or advanced CAN (**Fig. 29-5**).[18,24]

Evaluation of Vagosympathetic Activity in Clinical Research
More sophisticated approaches to evaluate CAN may be used in clinical research, including frequency domain measures of HR and BP variations, baroreflex sensitivity, muscle or skin sympathetic nerve activity, plasma catecholamines, and heart sympathetic imaging (see **Table 29-1**).[18,47]
- Frequency-domain indexes can be obtained by spectral analysis of HR variations applied on short (5- to 7-minute) and longer (24-hour) ECG recordings. HF spectral power provides a measure of parasympathetic modulation, whereas LF power evaluates both sympathetic and parasympathetic modulation. The LF power of BP variations provides a measure of sympathetic modulation.
- Cardiac vagal baroreflex sensitivity can be assessed by analysis of HR and BP response to pharmacologic or spontaneous BP perturbations.
- Sympathetic outflow can be measured directly via microelectrodes inserted into a fascicle of a distal sympathetic nerve to the skin or muscle, at rest and in response to various physiologic perturbations.
- Whole-body sympathetic activity is assessed by measuring plasma concentrations of noradrenaline and adrenaline.
- Cardiac sympathetic innervation may be analyzed through scintigraphic studies performed with radiolabelled noradrenaline analogues (iodine-123 [^{123}I]–metaiodobenzylguanidine [MIBG] or carbon-11 [^{11}C]–hydroxyephedrine [HED]).

CLINICAL CONTEXT

Diagnosing Cardiovascular Autonomic Neuropathy in Symptomatic Patients
Symptomatic manifestations of CAN include resting sinus tachycardia, OH, postprandial hypotension, and poor exercise tolerance.

Patients may report palpitations, and tachycardia may be repetitively observed. Emerging evidence on the prognostic value of resting HR has led to the advice in the current hypertension guidelines to measure HR in clinical practice[48] and to use it for cardiovascular risk stratification and as a therapeutic target in high-risk patients.[24]

OH may result from advanced CAN and other factors including drugs and hypovolemia. OH may induce orthostatic symptoms including dizziness, blurred vision, fainting, or pain in the neck or shoulder when standing, and may

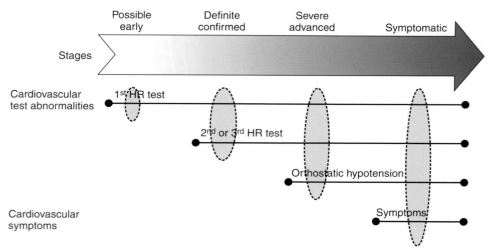

FIGURE 29-5 Staging cardiac autonomic neuropathy (CAN). *(Modified from Spallone V, Ziegler D, Freeman R, et al: on behalf of the Toronto Consensus Panel on Diabetic Neuropathy: Cardiovascular autonomic neuropathy in diabetes: clinical impact, assessment, diagnosis, and management, Diabetes Metab Res Rev, 2011 [Epub ahead of print].)*

induce falls in older adults. Symptoms may be disabling and are often a barrier to an effective antihypertensive treatment.

Postprandial hypotension may induce dizziness and fainting. After excluding any concomitant hypoglycemia, postprandial hypotension may be confirmed by self-measured BP or 24-hour BP monitoring.

The potential cause of CAN in these manifestations or in nondipping or reverse dipping or QT interval prolongation should be confirmed by CARTs.

Screening Asymptomatic Patients

In October 2009 in Toronto (Canada), expert panels were convened to provide updates on the diabetic neuropathies. They suggested screening for CAN at the diagnosis of T2DM and 5 years after the diagnosis of T1DM, particularly in patients at greater risk of CAN because of a history of poor glycemic control, cardiovascular risk factors, diabetic peripheral neuropathy, and macroangiopathic and microangiopathic diabetic complications.[18]

MANAGEMENT OF CARDIOVASCULAR AUTONOMIC NEUROPATHY

Role of Glycemic Control

The Diabetes Control and Complications Trial (DCCT) was a multicenter, randomized, clinical study designed to determine whether an intensive treatment regimen directed at maintaining blood glucose concentrations as close to normal as possible would affect the appearance or progression of early vascular complications in patients with T1DM. This study showed that intensive insulin treatment reduced the incidence of CAN by 53% compared with conventional therapy. In the Epidemiology of Diabetes Interventions and Complications (EDIC) study, a prospective observational follow-up of the DCCT cohort, CAN prevalence and incidence at the 13th to 14th year after DCCT closeout remained significantly lower in the former intensive than in the former conventional group (**Table 29-2**).[49] In the Steno-2 study, which included 160 T2DM patients with microalbuminuria, an

TABLE 29-2 Management of Cardiovascular Autonomic Neuropathy

Role of glycemic control	Prevents CAN and its aggravation in patients with T1DM. Avoid hypoglycemia in patients with CAN.
Management of tachycardia	Cardioselective beta blockers can be used to treat resting tachycardia associated with CAN.
Management of OH	Identify other causes of OH—in particular, volume depletion. Avoid drugs exacerbating postural symptoms. Educate patients regarding behavioral strategies, increased fluid and salt intake if not contraindicated. Use elastic garment over the legs and abdomen. If symptoms persist, consider a pharmacologic treatment, weighing its potential risks against its possible benefit.

intensive multifactorial cardiovascular risk intervention based on tight glucose regulation and the use of renin-angiotensin system blockers, aspirin, and lipid-lowering agents reduced the progression or the development of CAN compared with the conventional-therapy group.[50]

However, the achievement of tight glycemic control is associated with an increased risk of hypoglycemic events. Through sympathetic activation hypoglycemia may elevate BP, lengthen QT interval with higher risk of arrhythmia, increase cardiac load, and reduce coronary reserve.[39] These effects might be greater in the patients with vagal depression and relative hypersympathicotonia with potential amplification in those treated with insulin (**Fig. 29-6**). Hypoglycemia may also have some delayed deleterious effects on the autonomic nervous system function and affect the responses to future hypoglycemic episodes. Indeed, it has been shown in healthy individuals that a 2-hour hypoglycemic clamp at 2.8 mmol/L depresses sympathetic reactivity measured 16 hours later.[51] Such a prolonged depression of sympathetic reactivity after a hypoglycemic episode may contribute to future hypoglycemia and to the lack of perception of recurrent hypoglycemia. This concept of autonomic failure associated with repeated hypoglycemia is supported by the reversal of

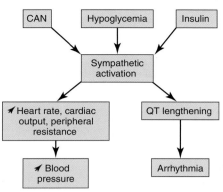

FIGURE 29-6 Cardiovascular changes during hypoglycemic episodes. Potential additional effects of cardiac autonomic neuropathy (CAN) and insulin treatment.

hypoglycemia unawareness and the improvement of the epinephrine response to hypoglycemia after scrupulous avoidance of hypoglycemia for 2 to 3 weeks.[52] Altogether these data should lead to prevention of hypoglycemia in patients with CAN—in particular, those with coronary artery disease.

Management of Tachycardia and Orthostatic Hypotension

An increase in HR variability has been described in diabetic patients taking angiotensin-converting enzyme (ACE) inhibitors, angiotensin II type 1 receptor blockers, cardioselective beta blockers without intrinsic sympathomimetic activity, digoxin, and verapamil. Cardioselective beta blockers can be used to treat resting tachycardia associated with CAN.

In patients with OH, the first steps are to identify other causes of OH—for example, volume depletion—and avoid drugs that exacerbate postural symptoms, such as psychotropic drugs, diuretics, and alpha-adrenoreceptor antagonists; to educate patients regarding behavioral strategies (e.g., gradual staged movements with postural change, head-up bed position during sleep) and increased fluid and salt intake if not contraindicated; and to prescribe the use of elastic garments over the legs and abdomen. If symptoms persist, a pharmacologic treatment should be considered, weighing its potential risks against its possible benefit (balance between the increase in standing BP and the avoidance of marked supine hypertension). The peripheral selective alpha$_1$-adrenergic agonist midodrine is a first-line drug. Fludrocortisone, erythropoietin (in particular in patients with anemia associated with severe CAN), and acarbose (useful in attenuating postprandial hypotension) are other possible treatments (see **Table 29-2**).

In conclusion, CAN assessment is relevant in clinical practice for diagnosis of asymptomatic forms of CAN, to confirm the cause of CAN in patients with resting tachycardia and orthostatic hypotension, and to explain symptoms (e.g., gastrointestinal or urinary symptoms) suggestive of diabetic autonomic dysfunction. CAN contributes to the increase in cardiovascular risk in patients with diabetes. The detection of CAN may help tailor therapeutic strategies and exercise programs. It may help in the individualized treatment of OH, tachycardia, and nondipping and nocturnal

hypertension. In the presence of CAN, drugs with adverse autonomic consequences should be avoided, and drugs with the potential to prolong QT interval should be excluded where possible. CAN assessment is also relevant for tailoring glycemic targets of antidiabetic therapy.

References

1. Licht CM, Vreeburg SA, van Reedt Dortland AK, et al: Increased sympathetic and decreased parasympathetic activity rather than changes in hypothalamic-pituitary-adrenal axis activity is associated with metabolic abnormalities, *J Clin Endocrinol Metab* 95:2458, 2010.
2. Chang CJ, Yang YC, Lu FH, et al: Altered cardiac autonomic function may precede insulin resistance in metabolic syndrome, *Am J Med* 123:432, 2010.
3. Straznicky NE, Grima MT, Sari CI, et al: Neuroadrenergic dysfunction along the diabetes continuum: a comparative study in obese metabolic syndrome subjects, *Diabetes* 61:2506, 2012.
4. Grassi G, Dell'Oro R, Facchini A, et al: Effect of central and peripheral body fat distribution on sympathetic and baroreflex function in obese normotensives, *J Hypertens* 22:2363, 2004.
5. Lindmark S, Lönn L, Wiklund U, et al: Dysregulation of the autonomic nervous system can be a link between visceral adiposity and insulin resistance, *Obes Res* 13:717–728, 2005.
6. Valensi P, Lormeau B, Dabbech M, et al: Glucose-induced thermogenesis, inhibition of lipid oxidation rate and autonomic dysfunction in non-diabetic obese women, *Int J Obes Relat Metab Disord* 22:494, 1998.
7. Valensi P, Chiheb S, Fysekidis M: Insulin- and Glucagon-Like Peptide-1-induced changes in heart rate and vagosympathetic activity: why they matter? *Diabetologia* 56:1196, 2013.
8. Bellavere F, Cacciatori V, Moghetti P, et al: Acute effect of insulin on autonomic regulation of the cardiovascular system: a study by heart rate spectral analysis, *Diabet Med* 13:709, 1996.
9. Van De Borne P, Hausberg M, Hoffman RP, et al: Hyperinsulinemia produces cardiac vagal withdrawal and nonuniform sympathetic activation in normal subjects, *Am J Physiol* 276:178, 1999.
10. Vollenweider L, Tappy L, Owlya R, et al: Insulin-induced sympathetic activation and vasodilation in skeletal muscle. Effects of insulin resistance in lean subjects, *Diabetes* 44:641, 1995.
11. Rowe JW, Young JB, Minaker KL, et al: Effect of insulin and glucose infusions on sympathetic nervous system activity in normal man, *Diabetes* 30:219, 1981.
12. Paolisso G, Manzella D, Tagliamonte MR, et al: Effects of different insulin infusion rates on heart rate variability in lean and obese subjects, *Metabolism* 48:755, 1999.
13. Paolisso G, Manzella D, Rizzo MR, et al: Effects of insulin on the cardiac autonomic nervous system in insulin-resistant states, *Clin Sci (Lond)* 98:129, 2000.
14. Griffioen KJ, Wan R, Okun E, et al: GLP-1 receptor stimulation depresses heart rate variability and inhibits neurotransmission to cardiac vagal neurons, *Cardiovasc Res* 89:72, 2011.
15. Yamamoto H, Lee CE, Marcus JN, et al: Glucagon-like peptide-1 receptor stimulation increases blood pressure and heart rate and activates autonomic regulatory neurons, *J Clin Invest* 110:43, 2002.
16. Grassi G, Seravalle G, Dell'Oro R, et al: Adrenergic and reflex abnormalities in obesity-related hypertension, *Hypertension* 36:538, 2000.
17. Grassi G, Dell'Oro R, Quarti-Trevano F, et al: Neuroadrenergic and reflex abnormalities in patients with metabolic syndrome, *Diabetologia* 48:1359, 2005.
18. Tesfaye S, Boulton AJ, Dyck PJ, et al: Toronto Diabetic Neuropathy Expert Group: Diabetic neuropathies: update on definitions, diagnostic criteria, estimation of severity, and treatments, *Diabetes Care* 33:2285, 2010.
19. Valensi P, Pariès J, Attali JR: French Group for Research and Study of Diabetic Neuropathy: Cardiac autonomic neuropathy in diabetic patients: influence of diabetes duration, obesity, and microangiopathic complications-the French multicenter study, *Metabolism* 52:815, 2003.
20. Witte DR, Tesfaye S, Chaturvedi N, et al: EURODIAB Prospective Complications Study Group: Risk factors for cardiac autonomic neuropathy in type 1 diabetes mellitus, *Diabetologia* 48:164, 2005.
21. Ziegler D, Gries FA, Mühlen H, et al: the DiaCAN Multicenter Study Group: Prevalence and clinical correlates of cardiovascular autonomic and peripheral diabetic neuropathy in patients attending diabetes centers, *Diabete Metab* 19:143, 1993.
22. Valensi P, Thi BN, Lormeau B, et al: Cardiac autonomic function in obese patients, *Int J Obes Relat Metab Disord* 19:113, 1995.
23. Valensi P, Extramiana F, Lange C, et al: DESIR Study Group: Influence of blood glucose on heart rate and cardiac autonomic function. The DESIR study, *Diabet Med* 28:440, 2011.
24. Spallone V, Ziegler D, Freeman R, et al: on behalf of the Toronto Consensus Panel on Diabetic Neuropathy: Cardiovascular autonomic neuropathy in diabetes: clinical impact, assessment, diagnosis, and management, *Diabetes Metab Res Rev* 2011 [Epub ahead of print].
25. Maser RE, Mitchell BD, Vinik AI, et al: The association between cardiovascular autonomic neuropathy and mortality in individuals with diabetes: a meta-analysis, *Diabetes Care* 26:1895, 2003.
26. Pop-Busui R, Evans GW, Gerstein HC, et al: Action to Control Cardiovascular Risk in Diabetes Study Group: Effects of cardiac autonomic dysfunction on mortality risk in the Action to Control Cardiovascular Risk in Diabetes (ACCORD) trial, *Diabetes Care* 33:1578, 2010.
27. Ziegler D, Zentai CP, Perz S, et al: KORA Study Group: Prediction of mortality using measures of cardiac autonomic dysfunction in the diabetic and nondiabetic population: the MONICA/KORA Augsburg Cohort Study, *Diabetes Care* 31:556, 2008.
28. Vinik AI, Maser RE, Mitchell BD, et al: Diabetic autonomic neuropathy, *Diabetes Care* 26:1553, 2003.
29. Wackers FJ, Young LH, Inzucchi SE, Detection of Ischemia in Asymptomatic Diabetics Investigators: Detection of silent myocardial ischemia in asymptomatic diabetic subjects: the DIAD study, *Diabetes Care* 27:1954, 2004.
30. Young LH, Wackers FJ, Chyun DA, et al: DIAD Investigators: Cardiac outcomes after screening for asymptomatic coronary artery disease in patients with type 2 diabetes: the DIAD study: a randomized controlled trial, *JAMA* 301:1547, 2009.
31. Valensi P, Sachs RN, Harfouche B, et al: Predictive value of cardiac autonomic neuropathy in diabetic patients with or without silent myocardial ischemia, *Diabetes Care* 24:339, 2001.
32. Valensi P, Cosson E: It is not yet the time to stop screening diabetic patients for silent myocardial ischaemia, *Diabetes Metab* 36:91, 2010.
33. Valensi P, Doaré L, Perret G, et al: Cardiovascular vagosympathetic activity in rats with ventromedial hypothalamic obesity, *Obes Res* 11:54, 2003.
34. Ayad F, Belhadj M, Pariès J, et al: Association between cardiac autonomic neuropathy and hypertension and its potential influence on diabetic complications, *Diabet Med* 27:804, 2010.
35. Dinh W, Füth R, Lankisch M, et al: Cardiovascular autonomic neuropathy contributes to left ventricular diastolic dysfunction in subjects with type 2 diabetes and impaired glucose tolerance undergoing coronary angiography, *Diabet Med* 28:311, 2011.
36. Zola B, Kahn JK, Juni JE, et al: Abnormal cardiac function in diabetic patients with autonomic neuropathy in the absence of ischemic heart disease, *J Clin Endocrinol Metab* 63:208, 1986.
37. Whitsel EA, Boyko EJ, Siscovick DS: Reassessing the role of QTc in the diagnosis of autonomic failure among patients with diabetes, *Diabetes Care* 23:241, 2000.
38. Valensi P, Johnson NB, Maison-Blanche P, et al: Influence of cardiac autonomic neuropathy on heart rate dependence of ventricular repolarization in diabetic patients, *Diabetes Care* 25:918, 2002.

39. Desouza CV, Bolli GB, Fonseca V: Hypoglycemia, diabetes, and cardiovascular events, *Diabetes Care* 33:1389, 2010.

40. Spallone V, Bernardi L, Ricordi L, et al: Relationship between the circadian rhythms of blood pressure and sympathovagal balance in diabetic autonomic neuropathy, *Diabetes* 42:1745, 1993.

41. Spallone V, Maiello MR, Morganti R, et al: Usefulness of ambulatory blood pressure monitoring in predicting the presence of autonomic neuropathy in type 1 diabetic patients, *J Hum Hypertens* 21:381, 2007.

42. Vinik AI, Ziegler D: Diabetic cardiovascular autonomic neuropathy, *Circulation* 115:387, 2007.

43. Hilsted J: Pathophysiology in diabetic autonomic neuropathy: cardiovascular, hormonal, and metabolic studies, *Diabetes* 31:730, 1982.

44. Brahimi M, Dabire H, Platon P, et al: Arterial rigidity and cardiovascular vagosympathetic activity in normotensive and hypertensive obese patients and type 2 diabetes, *Arch Mal Coeur* 94:944, 2001.

45. Prince CT, Secrest AM, Mackey RH, et al: Cardiovascular autonomic neuropathy, HDL cholesterol, and smoking correlate with arterial stiffness markers determined 18 years later in type 1 diabetes, *Diabetes Care* 33:652, 2010.

46. Cosson E, Valensi P, Laude D, et al: Arterial stiffness and the autonomic nervous system during the development of Zucker diabetic fatty rats, *Diabetes Metab* 35:364, 2009.

47. Bernardi L, Spallone V, Stevens M, et al: on behalf of the Toronto Consensus Panel on Diabetic Neuropathy: Investigation methods for cardiac autonomic function in human research studies, *Diabetes Metab Res Rev* 2011 [Epub ahead of print].

48. Mancia G, De Backer G, Dominiczak A, et al: European Society of Hypertension, European Society of Cardiology: 2007 ESH-ESC guidelines for the management of arterial hypertension: the task force for the management of arterial hypertension of the European Society of Hypertension (ESH) and of the European Society of Cardiology (ESC), *Blood Press* 16:135, 2007.

49. Pop-Busui R, Low PA, Waberski BH, et al: DCCT/EDIC Research Group: Effects of prior intensive insulin therapy on cardiac autonomic nervous system function in type 1 diabetes mellitus: the Diabetes Control and Complications Trial/Epidemiology of Diabetes Interventions and Complications study (DCCT/EDIC), *Circulation* 119:2886, 2009.

50. Gaede P, Lund-Andersen H, Parving HH, et al: Effect of a multifactorial intervention on mortality in type 2 diabetes, *N Engl J Med* 358:580, 2008.

51. Adler GK, Bonyhay I, Failing H, et al: Antecedent hypoglycemia impairs autonomic cardiovascular function: implications for rigorous glycemic control, *Diabetes* 58:360, 2009.

52. Cryer PE: The barrier of hypoglycemia in diabetes, *Diabetes* 57:3169, 2008.

30 Disparities in Diabetes Risk, Cardiovascular Consequences, and Care

Women, Ethnic Minorities, and the Elderly

Cheryl P. Lynch, Kelly J. Hunt, and Leonard E. Egede

DISPARITIES IN DIABETES RISK

Type 2 diabetes is a growing problem that closely parallels the obesity epidemic and places a severe burden on health care resources in the United States (see also **Chapter 1**). Diabetes currently affects 25.8 million Americans, 8.3% of the United States population, approximately 95% of whom have type 2 diabetes.[1,2] The lifetime risk of developing type 2 diabetes for individuals born in 2000 in the United States was estimated to be 32.8% in men and 38.5% in women.[3] Diabetes affects all age, sex, ethnic, and racial groups, but disproportionately affects minority populations, with African Americans and Hispanics having a twofold to threefold increased risk of developing diabetes relative to whites.[2,4] Projections indicate that over half of Hispanic women (i.e., 52.5%), almost half of African American women (i.e., 49.0%), and almost one out of every three white women (i.e., 31.2%) will develop diabetes in their lifetime.[3] Projections are slightly lower in men but remain high, with 45.5% of Hispanic men, 40.2% of African American men, and 26.7% of white men projected to develop diabetes during their lifetime.[3]

As the prevalence of diabetes increases, individuals are diagnosed at earlier ages, resulting in greater duration and comorbidity burden and earlier mortality.[3] In African Americans, diabetes diagnosed at age 50 implies living with diabetes for over a quarter of one's life (i.e., average duration, 18.1 years; 10.1 years of life lost), and diagnosis at 30 implies living with diabetes for almost half one's life (i.e., average duration, 28.2 years; 17.1 years of life lost).[3] In Hispanics and whites, diagnosis at age 30 similarly implies living with diabetes for over half one's life (i.e., average duration, 37.7 and 35.3 years, respectively; 14.8 and 13.2 years of life lost, respectively).[3]

From 1980 through 2011, based on information from the National Health Interview Survey (NHIS),[5,6] the prevalence of people with self-reported diagnosed diabetes increased by 167% (from 0.6% to 1.6%) for those aged 0 to 44 years, 118% (from 5.5% to 12.0%) for those aged 45 to 64 years, 140% (9.1% to 21.8%) for those aged 65 to 74 years, and 125% (8.9% to 20.0%) for those aged 75 years and older (**Fig. 30-1**). In general, throughout the time period, the percentage of people with diagnosed diabetes increased among all age groups. In 2011 the percentage of diagnosed diabetes among people aged 65 to 74 (21.8%) was more than 13 times that of people younger than 45 years (1.6%). The NHIS is a health survey of the civilian, noninstitutionalized household population of the United States and has been conducted continuously since 1957 by the National Center for Health Statistics (NCHS), Centers for Disease Control and Prevention (CDC).[5,6] In 2011, 63% of the adult incident cases (i.e., cases diagnosed within the previous year) of diabetes were diagnosed in patients between the ages of 40 and 64 years.[6] About 16% were diagnosed in individuals younger than age 40, and approximately 21% were diagnosed in individuals age 65 or older (**Fig. 30-2**).[6,7]

From 1980 to 1998, the age-adjusted prevalence of self-reported diagnosed diabetes for men and women was similar. However, in 1999 the percentage for men began to increase at a faster rate than the percentage for women. From 1980 to 2011, the age-adjusted percentage of diagnosed diabetes increased from 2.7% to 6.9% for men and from 2.9% to 5.9% for women (**Fig. 30-3**).

Using data from the NHIS, the incidence of diagnosed diabetes in the United States was estimated from 1997 to 2011 and during this time period the age-adjusted incidence of diagnosed diabetes increased among all racial and ethnic groups and was higher in African Americans and Hispanics than in whites. The age-adjusted incidence of diagnosed diabetes was 12.4/1000 in African Americans, 11.1/1000 in Hispanics, and 7.0/1000 in whites (**Fig. 30-4**).

DISPARITIES IN CARDIOVASCULAR CONSEQUENCES

Diabetes Comorbidities in Racial and Ethnic Minorities

Diabetes is the seventh leading cause of death in the United States. Previous studies report up to a threefold increase in mortality risk associated with diabetes.[8-13] In the Framingham Heart Study, which included white men and women living in Framingham from 1950 through 1975, the age- and sex-adjusted hazard ratio (HR) associated with diabetes

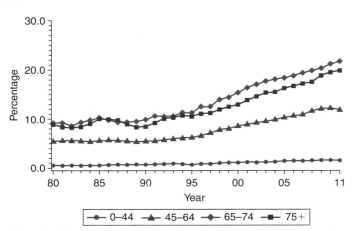

FIGURE 30-1 Percentage of civilian, noninstitutionalized population with diagnosed diabetes, by age, United States, 1980-2011. *(Centers for Disease Control and Prevention (CDC), National Center for Chronic Disease Prevention and Health Promotion, Division of Diabetes Translation. Percentage of civilian, noninstitutionalized population with self-reported physician diagnosed diabetes, by age, United States, 1980-2011. Data from the National Health Interview Survey, National Center for Health Statistics, Division of Health Interview Statistics. Available at: http://www.cdc.gov/diabetes/statistics/prev/national/figbyage.htm. Accessed on 5/11/2014.)*

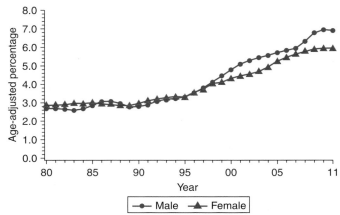

FIGURE 30-3 Age-adjusted percentage of civilian, noninstitutionalized population with diagnosed diabetes, by sex, United States, 1980-2010. *(Centers for Disease Control and Prevention (CDC), National Center for Chronic Disease Prevention and Health Promotion, Division of Diabetes Translation. Age-adjusted percentage of civilian, noninstitutionalized population with diagnosed diabetes, by sex, United States, 1980-2011. Data from the National Health Interview Survey, National Center for Health Statistics, Division of Health Interview Statistics. Available at: http://www.cdc.gov/diabetes/statistics/prev/national/figbysex.htm. Accessed on 5/11/2014.)*

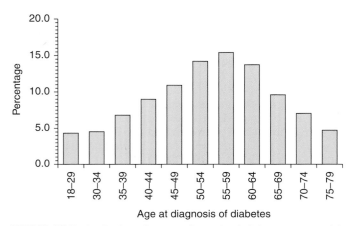

FIGURE 30-2 Distribution of age at diagnosis of diabetes among adult incident cases in patients aged 18 to 79 years, United States, 2008. *(Centers for Disease Control and Prevention (CDC), National Center for Chronic Disease Prevention and Health Promotion, Division of Diabetes Translation. Distribution of age at diagnosis of diabetes among adult incident cases in patients aged 18 to 79 years, United States, 2011. Data from the National Health Interview Survey, National Center for Health Statistics, Division of Health Interview Statistics. Available at: http://www.cdc.gov/diabetes/statistics/age/fig1.htm. Accessed on 5/11/2014.)*

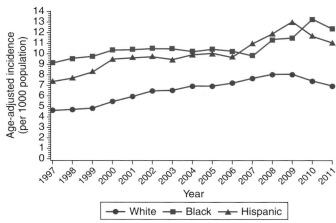

FIGURE 30-4 Age-adjusted incidence of self-reported diagnosed diabetes per 1000 population aged 18 to 79 years, by race or ethnicity, United States, 1997-2010. *(Centers for Disease Control and Prevention (CDC), National Center for Chronic Disease Prevention and Health Promotion, Division of Diabetes Translation. Age-adjusted incidence of self-reported diagnosed diabetes per 1000 population aged 18 to 79 years, by race or ethnicity, United States, 1997-2011. Data from the National Health Interview Survey, National Center for Health Statistics, Division of Health Interview Statistics. Available at: http://www.cdc.gov/diabetes/statistics/incidence/fig6.htm. Accessed on 5/11/2014.)*

for all-cause mortality was 2.44 (95% confidence interval [CI] 1.99-2.98), whereas the respective HR for the time period 1976 to 2001 was 1.95 (95% CI 1.63-2.33).[12] The age- and sex-adjusted HR for diabetes in non-Hispanic whites in the San Antonio Heart Study, a cohort study of non-Hispanic whites and Mexican Americans living in San Antonio, Texas, is 1.88 (95% CI 1.28-2.77) and is comparable to results from the second time period of the Framingham Heart Study.[14] In contrast, in U.S.-born Mexican Americans in the San Antonio Heart Study, there was a threefold increased risk of mortality associated with diabetes.[14] Unexpectedly, in the San Antonio Heart Study, adjusting for cardiovascular risk factors altered associations only slightly, indicating that the increased mortality risk associated with diabetes in U.S.-born Mexican Americans is independent of cardiovascular risk factors at least to the extent that they were adjusted for.

In the United States, diabetes is a major cause of heart disease and stroke as well as the leading cause of kidney failure, nontraumatic lower-limb amputations, and development of blindness in adults (see also **Chapters 7, 11, 27,** and **28**). The incidence of coronary disease is twofold to fivefold higher in those with diabetes relative to those without diabetes[9,15–19]; the risk of renal failure is twofold higher, the risk of blindness is 20-fold higher, and the risk of lower-extremity amputation is 40-fold higher in those with diabetes relative to those without diabetes.[20,21] At the Veterans Health Administration (VHA), diabetes accounts for approximately 50% of cerebrovascular events, 40% of patients with end-stage renal disease receiving dialysis, and over 70% of amputations.[22]

Relative to whites, African Americans with diabetes are at higher risk of complications typically related to hypertension including end stage renal disease, lower-extremity amputation, blindness, and stroke. This is not surprising, given that it is well established that hypertension is more common and less well controlled in African Americans than whites.[23–25] In studies conducted using the Third National Health and Nutrition Examination Survey (NHANES III), the presence of any diabetic retinopathy lesion was 46% higher in African Americans than in whites, with African Americans also more likely to have moderate or severe retinopathy when compared with whites.[26] End-stage renal disease is a growing problem in the United States, with diabetes accounting for approximately 45% of new patients requiring renal replacement therapy and the incidence of end-stage renal disease increasing more than 80% between 1993 and 2003.[27] Disparities in end-stage renal disease are vast, with incidence rates of 976/million in African Americans and 277/million in whites in 2009, a 3.5-fold higher incidence in African Americans than whites.[27,28] Between 1980 and 2008, the age-adjusted incidence of treatment (i.e., dialysis or transplant) for end-stage renal disease in individuals with diabetes varied by race and gender groups (**Fig. 30-5**).[29] Among individuals with diabetes, the incidence of end-stage renal disease was highest in African American men and lowest in white women. In whites and African Americans with diabetes, the incidence of end-stage renal disease increased in the 1980s, but started to decrease in the 1990s.[29] This can be explained by the increasing incidence of end-stage renal disease in the U.S. population because, although in recent years a lower percentage of individuals with diabetes have developed incident end-stage renal disease, the total number of individuals with diabetes and end-stage renal disease continues to increase. In a study conducted within the Veterans Administration, in which differences in socioeconomic status (SES) and access to care are limited, African Americans with diabetes were also more likely to have nephropathy and end-stage renal disease than whites with diabetes after adjustment for age, sex, and economic status.[31]

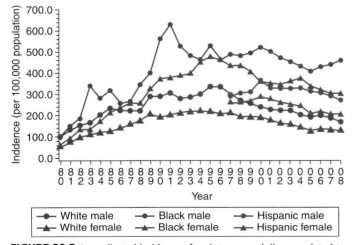

FIGURE 30-5 Age-adjusted incidence of end-stage renal disease related to diabetes mellitus (ESRD-DM) per 100,000 diabetic population, by race, ethnicity, and sex, United States, 1980-2008. *(Centers for Disease Control and Prevention (CDC), National Center for Chronic Disease Prevention and Health Promotion, Division of Diabetes Translation. Age-adjusted incidence of end-stage renal disease related to diabetes mellitus (ESRD-DM) per 100,000 diabetic population, by race, ethnicity, and sex, United States, 1980-2008. Data from the United States Renal Data System funded by National Institutes of Health; National Health Interview Survey, National Center for Health Statistics. Available at: http://www.cdc.gov/diabetes/statistics/esrd/fig5.htm. Accessed on 11/14/2013.)*

Similar to end-stage renal disease, the incidence and prevalence of lower-extremity amputation is higher in African Americans with diabetes than in whites with diabetes. Using age-adjusted hospital discharge rates for nontraumatic lower-extremity amputation, in whites the rates declined from 6.2/1000 individuals with diabetes in 1988 to 2.3/1000 individuals with diabetes in 2009.[32] During the same time period, rates also declined in African Americans, from 6.7/1000 to 4.5/1000 individuals with diabetes, but remained almost twice as high when compared with whites in 2009. In a study conducted within the Veteran Administration, African Americans with diabetes were more likely to undergo a lower-extremity amputation than whites with diabetes.[33]

In contrast to microvascular disease, macrovascular complications, including myocardial infarction and cardiovascular mortality, which are typically related to dyslipidemia, seem to have similar or even lower rates in African Americans with diabetes than whites with diabetes.[34] The similar or even lower rates of heart disease in African Americans may be a result of their distinct but favorable lipid profiles when compared with whites.[35–37]

Relative to whites, Mexican Americans with diabetes are at higher risk of microvascular as well as macrovascular disease.[13,38] In NHANES III, the presence of any diabetic retinopathy lesion was 84% higher in Mexican Americans than whites, with Mexican Americans also more likely to have moderate or severe retinopathy when compared with whites.[26] Rates of end-stage renal disease are also higher in Hispanics than whites.[29,30] In 1997, when the United States Renal Data System began collecting information on ethnicity, the age-adjusted incidences of end-stage renal disease were 293.2/100,000 men and 264.1/100,000 women with diabetes (see **Fig. 30-5**).[29,30] In 2008, rates had declined to 271.8/100,000 men and 205.8/100,000 women with diabetes. However, in contrast to African Americans, Mexican Americans with diabetes also appear to have increased risk of macrovascular disease relative to whites, although there remains some controversy.[29,30] In a study of 827 diabetic San Antonio Heart Study participants, age- and sex-adjusted HRs indicated that U.S.-born Mexican Americans with diabetes had a 70% greater risk of all-cause mortality and a 60% greater risk of cardiovascular mortality than non-Hispanic whites with diabetes.[13] In the San Luis Valley Diabetes Study, of nondiabetic participants, Mexican Americans and whites were at equal risk of incident coronary heart disease (CHD), whereas of diabetic participants, whites were at a higher risk than Mexican Americans of incident CHD.[39] In contrast, a community-based surveillance project, the Corpus Christi Heart Project, reported a higher incidence of hospitalized CHD among Mexican Americans than whites,[40] a higher CHD fatality rate among Mexican Americans than non-Hispanic whites,[41,42] and higher community-wide CHD mortality (both in and out of hospital) in Mexican Americans than non-Hispanic whites.[43]

Factors potentially associated with racial or ethnic differences in comorbidity burden include biologic differences in diabetes severity triggered by genetic or environmental factors as well as differences in health care access, treatment practices, and ongoing prevention efforts. Unfortunately, available markers of biologic differences in disease severity including medication use, insulin use, fasting glucose levels, and duration of clinically recognized diabetes are intrinsically tied to health care use and treatment. Increased access to care and disease awareness likely result in a shorter time to recognition and treatment of disease, a higher prevalence of recognized diabetes, a lower prevalence of unrecognized diabetes, and improved outcomes. Duration of diagnosed and duration of undiagnosed diabetes (i.e., time to recognition and treatment) may also be affecting severity and outcomes differently across populations.

Diabetes Comorbidities in Women

A large number of studies and at least three meta-analyses have examined whether diabetes reduces the sex difference in CHD mortality.[44–46] Reports from two of the three meta-analyses indicate that the impact of diabetes on the risk of CHD death is greater in women than in men and that standard cardiovascular disease (CVD) risk factors do not fully account for the sex difference,[44,46] whereas the third meta-analysis found that elevated levels of the standard CVD risk factors (i.e., age, hypertension, total cholesterol, and smoking) are responsible for the excess relative risk of CHD mortality in women with diabetes versus men with diabetes.[45] Sex-specific elevations in CVD risk factors (established or novel), sex-specific interactions among CVD risk factors, or sex-specific increased substrate susceptibility may all operate to reduce the sex difference in CHD mortality among individuals with diabetes. If differences in CVD risk factor levels (established or novel) account for all or part of the attenuation of the CHD mortality sex difference in individuals with diabetes, then relative to men, women with diabetes must have higher CVD risk factor levels. This could be explained if diabetes had a more adverse effect on CVD risk factor levels (established or novel) in women than in men, or if diabetes and CVD shared a common antecedent that affected men and women differently. Elevated CVD risk factors in prediabetic individuals,[47–51] elevated CVD risk before a clinical diagnosis of diabetes in the Nurses' Health Study,[48] and elevated carotid artery intima-media thickness in prediabetic individuals in the Mexico City study[52] each suggest an atherogenic state before the onset of clinical diabetes that is consistent with a common cause underlying diabetes and CVD. Furthermore, the metabolic syndrome, recognized as a cluster of CVD risk factors that frequently coincides with insulin resistance and hyperglycemia,[53,54] may be an early manifestation of the common cause underlying diabetes and CHD.

Obesity, specifically increased central adiposity, affects men and women differently and is distributed differently between men and women with and without diabetes. In the Strong Heart Study, differences in waist-to-hip ratio and waist circumference between diabetic and nondiabetic individuals were greater in women than men.[55] Studies also indicate that adverse lipoprotein changes associated with diabetes affect women and men differently.[56–62] In the San Antonio Heart Study, diabetes in Mexican American women was associated with a greater increase in low-density lipoprotein cholesterol (LDL-C) and a greater decrease in high-density lipoprotein cholesterol (HDL-C) levels than in Mexican American men.[61] Adverse lipoprotein changes reported in other studies include greater decreases in HDL-C, apolipoprotein (apo) A-I, and LDL particle size and greater increases in LDL-C and apo B in diabetic women than in diabetic men.[56–62] These lipoprotein changes may be one explanation for the reduced sex difference in CHD mortality among individuals with diabetes.

Disparities in Access to Care

Disparity in access to care is a central issue often directly affected by patients, providers, and the health care system. Access to health care is defined by the Institute of Medicine as having "the timely use of personal health services to achieve the best health outcomes".[63] It requires entry into the health care system, receipt of needed services at health care sites, and development of a relationship of mutual communication and trust with providers who meet the needs of individual patients. The trend of disparities in access to care factors is presented annually by the Agency for Healthcare Research and Quality (AHRQ) in the National Healthcare Disparities report[64] demonstrating issues with basic health care services. An approach to addressing issues in access to cardiovascular care was introduced by an ad hoc task force of the American College of Cardiology in the early 1990s, which reported and provided recommendations in a series of conference reports that presented the current state of care and recommendations for change or improvement (1992 and 1993). This work culminated in a formal policy statement on access to cardiovascular care[65] that supported the "development of an organized system of health care for the underserved," access to "a basic set of essential, clinically appropriate cardiovascular services," and research to explain "differences in utilization of health care procedures in certain populations." Such efforts stimulated a multitude of studies to report on underlying issues regarding differences in the prevention and management of cardiovascular health and use and quality of cardiovascular services. However, studies examining trends in access to cardiovascular care are limited, and even fewer studies attempt to explain disparities in access to cardiovascular care. No formal reporting method exists to reveal the trends in disparities in access to cardiovascular care, particularly in high-risk groups such as patients with preexisting CVD, diabetes, hypertension, hyperlipidemia, and chronic kidney disease.

Despite understanding that access to care is a major barrier to the receipt and use of care services, and that disparities exist with regard to race and ethnicity, SES, provider behavior and practice, and organizational factors, many of the existing disparities remain unexplained.[66] Data from the National Healthcare Disparities Report[64] indicate that there has been no change in disparities between rates of health insurance coverage for ethnic minorities versus non-Hispanic whites (<70% vs. 83%), except in African Americans, for whom insurance coverage is now at 81%. It will be interesting to see how the Affordable Care Act impacts disparities in health and health care with expansion of insurance coverage and reduction in cost-sharing for preventive services. One recent study suggests that the most important contributing factors to the growing disparities between Hispanics and whites are health insurance, education, and income differences.[67] Such disparities in access-related factors are further amplified with loss of employment and periods of uninsurance across all population subgroups. Currently, access to care specific to cardiovascular health is largely limited by racial or ethnic and socioeconomic differences for heart disease and hypertension, congestive heart failure, diabetes, and cardiac procedures.[68]

Pincus and colleagues summarized several studies demonstrating persistent and widened disparities in health according to SES as evidence for the limitations in access to care.[69] For example, in the United States, lack of a high school diploma was a greater risk factor than biologic factors for development of many diseases, an association only partly explained by age, ethnicity, sex or smoking status. One study of 17,530 employed London civil servants with universal access to the National Health Service showed that job classification, as a measure of SES, was a better predictor of cardiovascular death over 7 years than cholesterol level, blood pressure, and smoking combined. Disparities in health according to SES widened between 1970 and 1980 in the United States and in the United Kingdom, despite universal access. Finally, level of formal education predicted cardiovascular mortality better than random assignment to active drug or placebo over 3 years in a clinical trial that provided optimal access to care.[69] Although Canada has universal health coverage, a study that examined the relationship between access to care and 1-year mortality among patients hospitalized with acute myocardial infarction in the Ontario Myocardial Infarction Database showed that Ontario residents living in lower-income areas had reduced access to invasive procedures and higher mortality rates compared with residents of wealthier neighborhoods.[70]

In the United States, the U.S. Department of Veterans Affairs (VA) health care system is a universal access system for military veterans, yet several studies have clearly demonstrated disparities in cardiovascular prevention and management among veterans with diabetes.[71–74] One study showed that African American veterans with diabetes were 0.72 times less likely to receive lipid-lowering medications than their white counterparts[71] and less likely (40.9% versus 56.9%, respectively) to meet guideline-specific goals for LDL-C (<100 mg/dL).[75] A large cohort study examining control of hyperglycemia among insulin-treated veterans with type 2 diabetes showed poorer glycemic control and less intensive insulin treatment in African Americans compared with whites.[72] However, no differences in control of other CVD risk factors were found. Similar ethnic differences in glycemic control[76] and in blood pressure control[77] over time have been demonstrated in longitudinal studies. One longitudinal study of multiple cardiovascular risk factor control among ethnic minority veterans with diabetes showed that non-Hispanic blacks had a twofold risk of poor control and Hispanics had a 48% higher likelihood of poor control compared with non-Hispanic whites.[78] Such disparities in a health care system that provides a universal level of benefit for its members may reflect differences in treatment intensity, provider behaviors (prescribing patterns), and/or patient behaviors (medication adherence) or preferences.[72]

The collective evidence from these studies strongly suggests that equal access to care does not necessarily translate into equity in clinical outcomes. True equity is achieved when there is equity in access, usage, and outcomes.[79] A number of factors can influence access to cardiovascular services, such as geographic distance, economic barriers, and cultural variables.[80] Access can be further conceptualized to include overall access, contact access, and appointment access.[81] However, access is tightly linked with SES. In addition, SES is often correlated with race and ethnicity through key environmental variables that affect CVD outcomes, such as stress from residence in crime-prone communities, substandard housing, exposure to toxic waste sites, density of fast-food restaurants, limited transportation, and limited educational opportunities. Therefore, studies on disparities in access to care for CVD risk and outcomes need to account for SES.

Sex Disparities in Access to Care

Data on cardiovascular health in women continue to demonstrate that CVD remains a leading cause of death, although CVD-related mortality rates have been declining over time.[82] Sex differences have also been demonstrated in clinical outcomes for CVD. A cross-sectional analysis of 44,893 patients with type 2 diabetes (51% women) showed that women with CVD were less likely to have control of important modifiable risk factors (systolic blood pressure [SBP], LDL-C, and hemoglobin A1c [HbA1c]) and less likely to receive intensive lipid-lowering treatment.[83] Similarly, women without CVD were less likely than men to have lipids controlled, with no differences in SBP or HbA1c control. Such treatment differences can well be attributed to different access to or use of care. A meta-analysis identified 37 studies of type 2 diabetes and fatal CHD among a total of 447,064 patients. Whereas CHD fatality rates were higher in patients with diabetes than in those without (5.4% versus 1.6%), the overall summary relative risk for fatal CHD in patients with diabetes compared with no diabetes was significantly greater among women (3.50, 95% CI 2.70-4.53) than it was among men (2.06, 95% CI 1.81-2.34). This excess CHD risk was attributed to patient and provider factors, with more adverse CVD risk profiles among women with diabetes and possible disparities in treatment that favor men.[84] Excess CHD risk in women has also been attributed to different treatment of CVD risk factors. Studies demonstrate a heavier burden of traditional risk factors and a greater effect of blood pressure and atherogenic dyslipidemia in women with diabetes.[85] Studies have also found greater prescribing of statins (45% versus 35%)[86] and lipid-lowering therapy to achieve recommended LDL-C levels[87] in men compared with women with diabetes.

Studies have shown that women with CVD are screened and treated less aggressively than men and are less likely to undergo cardiac procedures. From a national sample of commercial health plans, women with diabetes had a 19% lower odds (95% CI 0.76-0.86) and women with a history of CVD had a 28% lower odds (0.64-0.82) of achieving the LDL-C goal of below 100 mg/dL. However, women performed better than men with blood pressure control (Odds ratio [OR] 1.12; 95% CI 1.02-1.21). Despite similar access to care, sex disparities were shown in the management and outcomes of CVD among this cohort of privately insured patients. Overall, poor performance in LDL control was seen in both men and women. This suggests that less intensive treatment of cholesterol occurred in the cohort of women.[88] Therefore the differences in patterns of care demonstrate the need for interventions tailored to address sex disparities.

Although awareness among women of their risk for CVD has improved, disparities in knowledge persist.[89] It is particularly alarming when data suggest that only 57% of women will seek emergency care for symptoms suggestive of a heart attack.[89] The lack of priority in addressing cardiovascular health is supported by findings that middle-aged women with diabetes or cardiovascular conditions were more likely to report delays in care (85% to 111% higher adjusted odds among diabetes patients, 56% to 84% higher adjusted odds among cardiovascular patients; all $P < 0.01$) than men.[90]

Ethnic Disparities in Access to Care

The latest CDC report[82] indicates that non-Hispanic blacks continue to have the highest age-adjusted prevalence rates of diagnosed diabetes (12.6%) among all racial and ethnic groups, and Puerto Ricans had the absolute highest rate (13.8%) among all Hispanics. From 1997 to 2011, the age-adjusted percentage of people with diabetes aged 35 years and older reporting heart disease or stroke was lowest among Hispanics compared with whites or African Americans. In a systematic review of studies on cardiovascular health disparities, most were descriptive in nature with the vast majority of evidence being presented for African American populations.[91] Disparities in access to care can include different provider practice patterns, lack of availability of insurance, and membership in restrictive health plans, as well as other factors that can differently affect the care of certain patient groups.[92] For example, disparities may occur among racial-ethnic groups as a result of observed patient characteristics (e.g., income, language fluency, and health status) and unobserved heterogeneity (e.g., discrimination, attitudes, and cultural differences even among individuals within the same racial-ethnic group).[92,93] To dampen the impact of such issues, recently implemented ACA provisions broaden access to health care services and will increase workforce diversity as a means of improving observed disparities. In summary, a range of system-related and patient-related factors can contribute to racial and ethnic disparities in access to care.

The higher risk of fatal CHD among blacks compared with whites was associated with CVD risk factor burden.[94] When other risk factors are held constant, ethnic minority individuals are at higher risk of CVD mortality at younger ages than non-Hispanic whites.[95] In a study of low-income patients with diabetes, all-cause mortality risk was higher for both African Americans with diabetes (HR 1.84; 95% CI 1.71-1.99) and whites with diabetes (HR 1.80; 95% CI 1.58-2.04) versus those without diabetes. However, among those with diabetes, mortality was lower among African Americans than whites (HR 0.78; 95% CI 0.69-0.87). Mortality risk increased with duration of diabetes, with insulin therapy, and with a history of CVD, hypertension, and stroke. Despite a lower baseline prevalence of CVD, the HRs associated with these multiple risk factors tended to be similar by sex and race with the exception of a higher impact of prevalent CVD on mortality among African Americans. With similarly low SES and access to health care, strong and generally similar predictors of mortality were identified for African Americans and whites with diabetes, with African Americans at a moderately but significantly lower mortality risk.[96]

Whether factors related to health care access can further explain racial disparities in CVD have not been thoroughly examined. The Health, Aging, and Body Composition (Health ABC) Study is a longitudinal study of 3075 well-functioning older adults aged 70 to 79. One Health ABC study examined racial and health care (i.e., health insurance and access to care) associations with CVD indicators (i.e., hypertension, low ankle-arm index, and left ventricular hypertrophy) and found that older African Americans had significantly worse health care compared with white adults. Overall, health care only slightly reduced the significant association between African American ethnicity and risk for CVD, whereas race remained strongly associated with CVD after adjustment for demographics, SES, body mass index, and comorbidity.[97] However, this study may have been limited in demonstrating significant differences, given that all participants had Medicare and access to a regular source of care and that selection bias may have excluded a sicker cohort of individuals. Although studies continue to describe disparities in CVD outcomes and examine underlying reasons for these associations, research on disparities in access to and quality of cardiovascular care, patient- and provider-level characteristics, and the interaction among these factors is needed to provide a more comprehensive understanding of disparities in CVD outcomes.

Studies that address cardiovascular health disparities and access to cardiovascular care in Hispanic, Asian, and Native American populations with diabetes are relatively scarce. In more recent studies among U.S. Hispanic adults of diverse backgrounds, a sizeable proportion of men and women had adverse major risk factors. The prevalence of adverse CVD risk profiles was higher among participants with Puerto Rican background, lower SES, and higher levels of acculturation.[98] In a cross-sectional survey of 211 Latinos (predominantly Puerto Ricans) with type 2 diabetes, higher food insecurity score was a risk factor for experiencing enabling factor (OR 1.46; 95% CI 1.17-1.82), medication access (OR 1.26; 95 CI% 1.06-1.50), and forgetfulness (OR 1.22; 95 CI% 1.04-1.43) barriers.[99] Higher diabetes management self-efficacy was protective against all barriers. Evidence for CVD risk with early-stage disease demonstrates that cardiovascular risk estimates from prehypertension have ranged from no increased cardiovascular mortality, after adjustment for the presence of any CVD risk factor, in NHANES[100] to an 80% increase in CVD risk with prehypertension to a 270% increase with coexisting prehypertension and diabetes among American Indians in the Strong Heart Study.[101]

Age-Related Disparities in Access to Care

Both the quality and quantity of access to health care may be associated with better health through health insurance.[102] Therefore in older adults, Medicare coverage among those who are 65 years of age and older may improve access and outcomes. However, whereas traditional Medicare insurance afforded older adults near universal coverage, current Medicare packages provide more variable access to health care that is dependent on the purchase of supplemental insurance coverage through Medicare or private companies and selection of a regular source of health care. Invariably, access to cardiovascular care is affected by the level of reimbursement for packaged health care services, such as that offered by managed care plans, for older adults. This is supported by findings from a study comparing equity of care according to the Healthcare Effectiveness Data and Information Set (HEDIS) between the VA and Medicare Advantage (a for-profit managed care plan), showing that the VA outperformed Medicare Advantage health plans on widely used clinical performance indicators for diabetes and cardiovascular care among enrollees aged 65 years or older.[103] Further research is needed to understand the role of health care access in racial and ethnic disparities in heart disease among older adults.

Older adults represent a population that can have increased difficulty with access to care. The aging population is faced with multiple coexisting chronic conditions, called multimorbidity. More than 50% of older adults have three or more chronic diseases.[104,105] Despite their eligibility for Medicare at age 65 many of them exist on fixed incomes. Independently living elderly in a lower income bracket creates a barrier for paying premiums for supplemental insurance, affording the copays for multiple primary and specialty care visits, obtaining durable medical equipment, and bearing the burden of medication costs particularly when Medicare Part D (for prescription coverage) reaches the gap where less coverage is provided. This type of "disparity of aging" prompted development of models of comprehensive care for the elderly that demonstrate improved access to and quality of care[106] such as the Geriatric Resources for Assessment and Care of Elders (GRACE) model, Guided Care, and the Program of All-inclusive Care for the Elderly (PACE).

When examining the pattern of multimorbidity hypertension and diabetes are amongst common clusters of comorbid conditions in the elderly.[107–109] Using diabetes as an example of the burden of health disparities, recent estimates show that diabetes is most prevalent among older adults (65 years and older) at nearly 27%.[110] While several demographic changes are occurring in the US population, one of the most impactful is the proportion of older adults projected to account for a larger segment of the population by year 2050. If current increases in the incidence rate of diabetes continues among adults 65 years of age and older (see **Fig. 30-1**), diabetes cases can be expected to affect one in every two older adults.[111] With the recent implementation of Patient Protection and Affordable Care Act (PPACA) initiatives that address elimination of cost sharing for preventive services and reduced cost sharing for prescription drug benefit, greater availability and access to alternative models of care for the elderly is a distinct possibility. Consequently, health care disparities can be alleviated partly through more efficient and effective complex care that improve health outcomes, functional status, and quality of life among the elderly.

IDENTIFICATION, SCREENING, AND PREVENTION IN HIGH-RISK GROUPS: PRE-DIABETES

Diabetes has an asymptomatic preclinical phase; hence, in the absence of routine screening a significant proportion of individuals with diabetes remain undiagnosed. In a publication using NHANES data from 2005 and 2006, based on fasting plasma glucose as well as 2-hour plasma glucose from an oral glucose tolerance test, it was estimated that in the U.S. adult population aged 20 years or older, the prevalence of undiagnosed diabetes was 5.1%.[112] This translates to a prevalence of undiagnosed diabetes among those with diabetes of 39.7%.[112] Using the American Diabetes Association recently endorsed HbA1c cut point of 6.5% or greater as diagnostic of diabetes, estimates for undiagnosed diabetes were slightly lower at 2.1% in 1988 to 1994, 1.6% in 1999 to 2002, and 1.8% in 2003 to 2006 in the U.S. adult population aged 20 years or older.[113] These values translated to a prevalence of undiagnosed diabetes among those with diabetes of 28.9% in 1988 to 1994, of 20.6% in 1999 to 2002, and of 21.5% in 2003 to 2006.[64] Hence, with fasting and 2-hour plasma glucose used to diagnose diabetes in 2005 and 2006, roughly two fifths of all cases of diabetes were undiagnosed in the U.S. adult population aged 20 years or older.[112] When HbA1c was used to diagnose diabetes in 2003 to 2006, roughly one fifth of all cases of diabetes were undiagnosed.[113]

Expanding the time period to a 10-year window from 1999 through 2008 and defining diabetes based on HbA1c of 6.5%

or greater, based on NHANES data in adults aged 20 years or older, the overall prevalence of undiagnosed diabetes was 1.5% (95% CI 1.2-1.8) in whites, 3.1% (95% CI 2.6-3.5) in African Americans, and 2.7% (95% CI 2.1-3.3) in Mexican Americans, whereas the prevalence of diagnosed diabetes was 6.7% (95% CI 6.0-7.3) in whites, 11.3% (95% CI 10.3-12.3) in African Americans, and 7.6% (95% CI 6.8-8.4) in Mexican Americans.[65] Hence, undiagnosed diabetes accounted for 18.5% (95% CI 15.4-21.5), 21.3% (95% CI 18.1-24.6), and 26.0% (95% CI 21.5-30.4) of diabetes in whites, African Americans, and Mexican Americans, respectively.[114] The prevalence of undiagnosed diabetes in the general population increases with age, is higher in men than in women, and is higher in African Americans and Mexican Americans than in whites.[2,112–115]

Based on NHANES data in adults aged 20 years or older from 1999 through 2008, in individuals with undiagnosed diabetes, Mexican Americans were the youngest at 49.1 years, followed by African Americans at 56.5 years and whites at 60.7 years.[114] Mexican Americans and whites were more likely to be male than female—57.5% and 62.4% male, respectively—whereas only 38.1% of African Americans were male.[114] Mexican and African Americans were less likely to have graduated from high school and were more likely to have a low household income than whites.[114] In this study the authors report that in a population representative of individuals in the United States with undiagnosed diabetes, cardiometabolic risk factor levels were high across racial and ethnic groups, but African and Mexican Americans had poorer cardiometabolic risk factor control than whites.[114]

In a recent retrospective cohort study conducted among 1456 African American and 2624 white veterans with recently diagnosed diabetes who were receiving consistent primary care at VHA facilities, the authors reported that at the time of diagnosis of diabetes and at the time of initiation of glucose-lowering medication, glucose and HbA1c levels were higher in African Americans than in whites.[116] Specifically, at the time of diabetes diagnosis, average HbA1c levels were 7.8% in African Americans, but only 7.1% in whites (with similar results for glucose: 154 versus 148 mg/dL). At the time of initiation of glucose-lowering medication, average HbA1c levels were 8.5% in African Americans, but only 7.8% in whites (with similar results for glucose: 176 versus 169 mg/dL).[116]

Several studies have examined chronic complications of diabetes and the economic cost before the onset of clinical diabetes. Studies of chronic complications of diabetes indicate that cardiovascular risk factor levels,[47,49–51,117] atherosclerosis (as measured by carotid artery intima-media thickness),[52] microalbuminuria,[117,118] and cardiovascular events[48] are elevated before the clinical recognition of diabetes. Similarly, economic studies indicate that cost is elevated before the onset of clinical disease.[119,120] The few studies completed in individuals with unrecognized diabetes indicate elevated levels of chronic complications of diabetes, including elevated levels of nephropathy and peripheral neuropathy[121] as well as elevated estimated cardiovascular risk relative to those without diabetes.[122] Finally, in 2007 in the United States, the economic cost of undiagnosed diabetes was estimated to be $18 billion dollars, or $2864 per person with undiagnosed diabetes.[123,124] This estimate includes $11 billion in medical costs and $7 billion in indirect costs.[123,124]

Type 2 diabetes is an incurable relentless, progressive disease with significant associated complications and increased mortality risk, and recent studies demonstrate that even tight control of hyperglycemia in individuals with type 2 diabetes does not reduce associated complications and mortality.[125-127] The Veterans Affairs Diabetes Trial (VADT) is one of a series of recent clinical trials demonstrating that tight control of hyperglycemia does not reduce the risk of cardiovascular events or microvascular complications in individuals with poorly controlled longstanding diabetes.[125] In contrast, earlier studies of individuals with newly diagnosed diabetes had the opposite outcome. Results from the Diabetes Control and Complications Trial indicate that retinopathy and long-term incidence of CVD are lowered by tight control of hyperglycemia in individuals with early-stage type 1 diabetes.[128,129] Moreover, in the United Kingdom Prospective Diabetes Study (UKPDS), which enrolled individuals with newly diagnosed type 2 diabetes, HbA1c levels were a strong predictor of both microvascular and macrovascular complications.[130] Moreover, the early termination of the Look AHEAD (Action for Health in Diabetes) trial because of null results provides further evidence that prevention of diabetes comorbidities must occur before diabetes onset.[131] Look AHEAD tested whether a lifestyle intervention resulting in weight loss would reduce cardiovascular events in overweight and obese people with type 2 diabetes.

Based on the negative results of these recent trials that demonstrate the difficulty in preventing comorbidities once diabetes is clinically manifest, focus is shifting to identifying individuals at high risk for the disease as evidenced by clinical guidelines that present specific cutoffs for HgbA1c (5.7 to 6.4%) to diagnose pre-diabetes (ADA 2008[132]) and development of treatment guidelines by endocrine societies (ACE/AACE 2008[133]). The term *prediabetes* refers to individuals with impaired fasting glucose (IFG) or impaired glucose tolerance (IGT) who do not yet meet the criteria for diabetes (see also **Chapter 4**). With use of HbA1c levels of 6.0 to less than 6.5% in NHANES 2003 to 2006, the prevalence of prediabetes in adults 20 years of age and older was estimated to be 3.1% in whites, 6.7% in African Americans, and 2.8% in Mexican Americans.[113] The prevalence of prediabetes is similar in men and women, 3.5% and 3.4%, respectively.[113] When the population was limited to adults 65 years of age and older, the prevalence of prediabetes increased substantially to 7.7% in whites, 13.2% in African Americans, and 8.3% in Mexican Americans.[113] Hence, the prevalence of prediabetes reflects the prevalence of diabetes in the population.

ACKNOWLEDGMENTS

Dr. Egede is supported by grant #K24 DK093699 from the National Institute for Diabetes and Digestive and Kidney Diseases.

This study was supported by resources from the Charleston Veteran's Affairs Research Enhancement Award Program (grant #REA 08-261) funded by the VHA Health Services Research and Development (HSR&D) program. The funding agency did not participate in the design and conduct of the study; collection, management, analysis, and interpretation of the data; and preparation, review, or approval of the manuscript.

The manuscript represents the views of the authors and not those of NIH, the VA or HSR&D.

Disclosure: None of the authors disclosed any financial or other conflicts of interest.

References

1. Centers for Disease Control and Prevention (CDC): *National diabetes fact sheet: national estimates and general information on diabetes and prediabetes in the United States, 2011,* Atlanta, GA, 2011, U.S. Department of Health and Human Services, Centers for Disease Control and Prevention. Available at: http://www.cdc.gov/diabetes/pubs/pdf/ndfs_2011.pdf.
2. Cowie C: Prevalence of diabetes and impaired fasting glucose in adults in the U.S. population: National Health And Nutrition Examination Survey 1999–2002, *Diabetes Care* 29(6):1263–1268, 2006.
3. Narayan KM, Boyle JP, Thompson TJ, et al: Lifetime risk for diabetes mellitus in the United States, *JAMA* 290(14):1884–1890, 2003.
4. Mokdad A: Diabetes trends in the U.S.: 1990–1998, (see comment) *Diabetes Care* 23 (9):1278–1283, 2000.
5. Massey JT, Moore TF, Parsons VL, et al: Design and estimation for the National Health Interview Survey, 1985–1994. Hyattsville, MD: National Center for Health Statistics, *Vital Health Stat* 2(110) 1989.
6. Botman SL, Moore TF, Moriarity CL, et al: Design and estimation for the national Health Interview Survey, 1995–2004. National Center for Health Statistics, *Vital Health Stat* 2(130)2000.
7. 2007–2009 National Health Interview Survey (NHIS): *Diabetes Data & Trends,* 2012, National Center for Health Statistics, Centers for Disease Control and Prevention (CDC).
8. Gregg EW, Gu Q, Cheng YJ, et al: Mortality trends in men and women with diabetes, 1971 to 2000, *Ann Intern Med* 147(3):149–155, 2007.
9. Kannel WB, McGee DL: Diabetes and cardiovascular disease. The Framingham study, *JAMA* 241 (19):2035–2038, 1979.
10. Preis SR, Hwang SJ, Coady S, et al: Trends in all-cause and cardiovascular disease mortality among women and men with and without diabetes mellitus in the Framingham Heart Study, 1950 to 2005, *Circulation* 119(13):1728–1735, 2009.
11. Burke J: Rapid rise in the incidence of type 2 diabetes from 1987 to 1996: results from the San Antonio Heart Study, *Arch Intern Med* 159(13):1450–1456, 1999.
12. Fox CS, Coady S, Sorlie PD, et al: Trends in cardiovascular complications of diabetes, *JAMA* 292 (20):2495–2499, 2004.
13. Hunt KJ, Williams K, Resendez RG, et al: All-cause and cardiovascular mortality among diabetic participants in the San Antonio Heart Study: evidence against the "Hispanic Paradox", *Diabetes Care* 25(9):1557–1563, 2002.
14. Hunt KJ, Gonzalez ME, Lopez R, et al: Diabetes is more lethal in Mexicans and Mexican-Americans compared to non-Hispanic whites, *Ann Epidemiol* 21(12):899–906, 2011.
15. Laditka SB, Mastanduno MP, Laditka JN: Health care use of individuals with diabetes in an employer-based insurance population, *Arch Intern Med* 161(10):1301–1308, 2001.
16. Ford ES, DeStefano F: Risk factors for mortality from all causes and from coronary heart disease among persons with diabetes. Findings from the National Health and Nutrition Examination Survey I Epidemiologic Follow-up Study, *Am J Epidemiol* 133(12):1220–1230, 1991.
17. Manson JE, Colditz GA, Stampfer MJ, et al: A prospective study of maturity-onset diabetes mellitus and risk of coronary heart disease and stroke in women, *Arch Intern Med* 151 (6):1141–1147, 1991.
18. Sasaki A, Uehara M, Horiuchi N, et al: A long-term follow-up study of Japanese diabetic patients: mortality and causes of death, *Diabetologia* 25(4):309–312, 1983.
19. Wilson PW, Cupples LA, Kannel WB: Is hyperglycemia associated with cardiovascular disease? The Framingham Study, *Am Heart J* 121(2 Pt 1):586–590, 1991.
20. Nathan DM: Long-term complications of diabetes mellitus, *N Engl J Med* 328(23):1676–1685, 1993.
21. Reiber GE, Pecoraro RE, Koepsell TD: Risk factors for amputation in patients with diabetes mellitus. A case-control study, *Ann Intern Med* 117(2):97–105, 1992.
22. Management of Diabetes Mellitus Update Working Group: *VA/DoD clinical practice guideline for the management of diabetes mellitus. Version 4.0,* Washington, DC, 2010, Veterans Health Administration and Department of Defense. Available at: http://www.healthquality.va.gov/guidelines/CD/diabetes/AboutDM.asp.
23. Egan BM, Zhao Y, Axon RN: US trends in prevalence, awareness, treatment, and control of hypertension, 1988–2008, *JAMA* 303(20):2043–2050, 2010.
24. Guo F, He D, Zhang W, et al: Trends in prevalence, awareness, management, and control of hypertension among United States adults, 1999 to 2010, *J Am Coll Cardiol* 60(7):599–606, 2012.
25. Shuaib FM, Durant RW, Parmar G, et al: Awareness, treatment and control of hypertension, diabetes and hyperlipidemia and area-level mortality regions in the Reasons for Geographic and Racial Differences in Stroke (REGARDS) study, *J Health Care Poor Underserved* 23 (2):903–921, 2012.
26. Harris MI, Klein R, Cowie CC, et al: Is the risk of diabetic retinopathy greater in non-Hispanic African Americans and Mexican Americans than in non-Hispanic whites with type 2 diabetes? A U.S. population study, *Diabetes Care* 21(8):1230–1235, 1998.
27. US Renal Data System: *USRDS 2011 annual data report: atlas of chronic kidney disease and end-stage renal disease in the United Sates,* Bethesda, MD, 2011, National Institutes of Health, National Institute of Diabetes and Digestive Kidney Diseases.
28. Tareen N, Zadshir A, Martins D, et al: Chronic kidney disease in African American and Mexican American populations, *Kidney Int Suppl* 97:S137–S140, 2005.
29. Centers for Disease Control and Prevention (CDC), National Center for Chronic Disease Prevention and Health Promotion, Division of Diabetes Translation: *Age-adjusted incidence of end-stage renal disease related to diabetes mellitus (ESRD-DM) per 100,000 diabetic population, by race, ethnicity, and sex, United States, 1980–2008.* Data from the United States Renal Data System funded by National Institutes of Health; National Health Interview Survey, National Center for Health Statistics. Available at: http://www.cdc.gov/diabetes/statistics/esrd/fig5.htm. Accessed November 14, 2013.
30. U.S. Renal Data System: *USRDS 2013 annual data report: atlas of chronic kidney disease and end-stage renal disease in the United States,* Bethesda, MD, 2013, National Institutes of Health, National Institute of Diabetes and Digestive and Kidney Diseases. Available at: http://www.usrds.org/adr.aspx. Accessed May 07, 2014.
31. Young BA, Maynard C, Boyko EJ: Racial differences in diabetic nephropathy, cardiovascular disease, and mortality in a national population of veterans, *Diabetes Care* 26(8):2392–2399, 2003.
32. Centers for Disease Control and Prevention (CDC), National Center for Chronic Disease Prevention and Health Promotion, Division of Diabetes Translation: *Age-adjusted hospital discharge rates for nontraumatic lower extremity amputation per 1,000 diabetic population, by Race, United States, 1988–2009.* Data from the National Health Interview Survey, National Center for Health Statistics, Division of Health Interview Statistics. Available at: http://www.cdc.gov/diabetes/statistics/lea/fig6.htm. Accessed May 11, 2014.
33. Young BA, Maynard C, Reiber G, et al: Effects of ethnicity and nephropathy on lower-extremity amputation risk among diabetic veterans, *Diabetes Care* 26(2):495–501, 2003.

34. Lowe LP, Liu K, Greenland P, et al: Diabetes, asymptomatic hyperglycemia, and 22-year mortality in black and white men. The Chicago Heart Association Detection Project in Industry Study, *Diabetes Care* 20(2):163–169, 1997.
35. Otten MW Jr., Teutsch SM, Williamson DF, et al: The effect of known risk factors on the excess mortality of black adults in the United States, *JAMA* 263(6):845–850, 1990.
36. Metcalf PA, Sharrett AR, Folsom AR, et al: African American-white differences in lipids, lipoproteins, and apolipoproteins, by educational attainment, among middle-aged adults: the Atherosclerosis Risk in Communities Study, *Am J Epidemiol* 148(8):750–760, 1998.
37. Haffner SM, D'Agostino R Jr., Goff D, et al: LDL size in African Americans, Hispanics, and non-Hispanic whites: the insulin resistance atherosclerosis study, *Arterioscler Thromb Vasc Biol* 19 (9):2234–2240, 1999.
38. Haffner SM, Mitchell BD, Pugh JA, et al: Proteinuria in Mexican Americans and non-Hispanic whites with NIDDM, *Diabetes Care* 12(8):530–536, 1989.
39. Rewers M, Shetterly SM, Hoag S, et al: Is the risk of coronary heart disease lower in Hispanics than in non-Hispanic whites? The San Luis Valley Diabetes Study, *Ethn Dis* 3 (1):44–54, 1993.
40. Goff DC, Nichaman MZ, Chan W, et al: Greater incidence of hospitalized myocardial infarction among Mexican Americans than non-Hispanic whites. The Corpus Christi Heart Project, 1988–1992, *Circulation* 95(6):1433–1440, 1997.
41. Goff DC Jr., Varas C, Ramsey DJ, et al: Mortality after hospitalization for myocardial infarction among Mexican Americans and non-Hispanic whites: the Corpus Christi Heart Project, *Ethn Dis* 3(1):55–63, 1993.
42. Goff DC Jr., Ramsey DJ, Labarthe DR, et al: Greater case-fatality after myocardial infarction among Mexican Americans and women than among non-Hispanic whites and men. The Corpus Christi Heart Project, *Am J Epidemiol* 139(5):474–483, 1994.
43. Pandey DK, Labarthe DR, Goff DC, et al: Community-wide coronary heart disease mortality in Mexican Americans equals or exceeds that in non-Hispanic whites: the Corpus Christi Heart Project, *Am J Med* 110(2):81–87, 2001.
44. Lee WL, Cheung AM, Cape D, et al: Impact of diabetes on coronary artery disease in women and men: a meta-analysis of prospective studies, *Diabetes Care* 23(7):962–968, 2000.
45. Kanaya AM, Grady D, Barrett-Connor E: Explaining the sex difference in coronary heart disease mortality among patients with type 2 diabetes mellitus: a meta-analysis, *Arch Intern Med* 162 (15):1737–1745, 2002.
46. Orchard TJ: The impact of sex and general risk factors on the occurrence of atherosclerotic vascular disease in non-insulin-dependent diabetes mellitus, *Ann Med* 28(4):323–333, 1996.
47. Fagot-Campagna A, Narayan KM, Hanson RL, et al: Plasma lipoproteins and incidence of non-insulin-dependent diabetes mellitus in Pima Indians: protective effect of HDL cholesterol in women, *Atherosclerosis* 128(1):113–119, 1997.
48. Hu FB, Stampfer MJ, Haffner SM, et al: Elevated risk of cardiovascular disease prior to clinical diagnosis of type 2 diabetes, *Diabetes Care* 25(7):1129–1134, 2002.
49. McPhillips JB, Barrett-Connor E, Wingard DL: Cardiovascular disease risk factors prior to the diagnosis of impaired glucose tolerance and non-insulin-dependent diabetes mellitus in a community of older adults, *Am J Epidemiol* 131(3):443–453, 1990.
50. Medalie JH, Papier CM, Goldbourt U, et al: Major factors in the development of diabetes mellitus in 10,000 men, *Arch Intern Med* 135(6):811–817, 1975.
51. Mykkanen L, Kuusisto J, Pyorala K, et al: Cardiovascular disease risk factors as predictors of type 2 (non-insulin-dependent) diabetes mellitus in elderly subjects, *Diabetologia* 36 (6):553–559, 1993.
52. Hunt KJ, Williams K, Rivera D, et al: Elevated carotid artery intima-media thickness levels in individuals who subsequently develop type 2 diabetes, *Arterioscler Thromb Vasc Biol* 23 (10):1845–1850, 2003.
53. The metabolic syndrome and total and cardiovascular disease mortality in middle-aged men, *JAMA* 288(21):2709–2716, 2002.
54. Laaksonen DE, Lakka HM, Niskanen LK, et al: Metabolic syndrome and development of diabetes mellitus: application and validation of recently suggested definitions of the metabolic syndrome in a prospective cohort study, *Am J Epidemiol* 156(11):1070–1077, 2002.
55. Howard BV, Cowan LD, Go O, et al: Adverse effects of diabetes on multiple cardiovascular disease risk factors in women. The Strong Heart Study, *Diabetes Care* 21(8): 1258–1265, 1998.
56. Assmann G, Schulte H: Relation of high-density lipoprotein cholesterol and triglycerides to incidence of atherosclerotic coronary artery disease (the PROCAM experience). Prospective Cardiovascular Munster study, *Am J Cardiol* 70(7):733–737, 1992.
57. Cowie CC, Howard BV, Harris MI: Serum lipoproteins in African Americans and whites with non-insulin-dependent diabetes in the US population, *Circulation* 90(3):1185–1193, 1994.
58. Evans RW, Orchard TJ: Oxidized lipids in insulin-dependent diabetes mellitus: a sex-diabetes interaction? *Metabolism* 43(9):1196–1200, 1994.
59. Howard BV, Knowler WC, Vasquez B, et al: Plasma and lipoprotein cholesterol and triglyceride in the Pima Indian population. Comparison of diabetics and nondiabetics, *Arteriosclerosis* 4(5):462–471, 1984.
60. Orchard TJ: Dyslipoproteinemia and diabetes, *Endocrinol Metab Clin North Am* 19(2):361–380, 1990.
61. Stern MP, Rosenthal M, Haffner SM, et al: Sex difference in the effects of sociocultural status on diabetes and cardiovascular risk factors in Mexican Americans. The San Antonio Heart Study, *Am J Epidemiol* 120(6):834–851, 1984.
62. Walden CE, Knopp RH, Wahl PW, et al: Sex differences in the effect of diabetes mellitus on lipoprotein triglyceride and cholesterol concentrations, *N Engl J Med* 311 (15):953–959, 1984.
63. Institute of Medicine (IOM), Committee on Monitoring Access to Personal Health Care Services: *Access to health care in America*, Washington, DC, 1993, National Academy Press.
64. *2011 National healthcare quality and disparities reports*. Rockville, MD, March 2012, Agency for Healthcare Research and Quality. Available at: http://www.ahrq.gov/research/findings/nhqrdr/nhqrdr11/qrdr11.html. Accessed May 11, 2014.
65. Access to cardiovascular care. ACC policy statement. American College of Cardiology, *J Am Coll Cardiol* 21(1):276–278, 1993.
66. Zuvekas SH, Taliaferro GS: Pathways to access: health insurance, the health care delivery system, and racial/ethnic disparities, 1996–1999, *Health Aff (Millwood)* 22(2):139–153, 2003.
67. Mahmoudi E, Jensen GA: Diverging racial and ethnic disparities in access to physician care: comparing 2000 and 2007, *Med Care* 50(4):327–334, Apr 2012.
68. Mayberry RM, Mili F, Ofili E: Racial and ethnic differences in access to medical care, *Med Care Res Rev* 57(Suppl 1):108–145, 2000.
69. Pincus T, Esther R, DeWalt DA, et al: Social conditions and self-management are more powerful determinants of health than access to care, *Ann Intern Med* 129(5):406–411, 1998.
70. Alter DA, Naylor CD, Austin P, et al: Effects of socioeconomic status on access to invasive cardiac procedures and on mortality after acute myocardial infarction, *N Engl J Med* 341(18):1359–1367, Oct 1999.
71. Safford M, Eaton L, Hawley G, et al: Disparities in use of lipid-lowering medications among people with type 2 diabetes mellitus, *Arch Intern Med* 163(8):922–928, Apr 2003.
72. Wendel CS, Shah JH, Duckworth WC, et al: Racial and ethnic disparities in the control of cardiovascular disease risk factors in Southwest American veterans with type 2 diabetes: the Diabetes Outcomes in Veterans Study, *BMC Health Serv Res* 6:58, 2006.
73. Trivedi AN, Grebla RC, Wright SM, et al: Despite improved quality of care in the Veterans Affairs health system, racial disparity persists for important clinical outcomes, *Health Aff (Millwood)* 30 (4):707–715, Apr 2011.
74. Vimalananda VG, Miller DR, Palnati M, et al: Gender disparities in lipid-lowering therapy among veterans with diabetes, *Womens Health Issues* 21(4 Suppl):S176–S181, 2011.
75. Williams ML, Morris MT, Ahmad U, et al: Racial differences in compliance with NCEP-II recommendations for secondary prevention at a Veterans Affairs medical center, *Ethn Dis* 12(1):S1-58-62, 2002.
76. Egede LE, Mueller M, Echols CL, et al: Longitudinal differences in glycemic control by race/ethnicity among veterans with type 2 diabetes, *Med Care* 48(6):527–533, 2010.
77. Axon RN, Gebregziabher M, Echols C, et al: Racial and ethnic differences in longitudinal blood pressure control in veterans with type 2 diabetes mellitus, *J Gen Intern Med* 26(11):1278–1283, Nov 2011.
78. Egede LE, Gebregziabher M, Lynch CP, et al: Longitudinal ethnic differences in multiple cardiovascular risk factor control in a cohort of US adults with diabetes, *Diabetes Res Clin Pract* 94 (3):385–394, 2011.
79. Oliver A, Mossialos E: Equity of access to health care: outlining the foundations for action, *J Epidemiol Community Health* 58(8):655–658, 2004.
80. Ngana J: Measuring inequity of a health system: a systems perspective - systematic analytical mapping approach. Paper presented at. In *Annual meeting of the international society for systems sciences, Waterloo, ON, Canada*, 2010.
81. Hall A, Lemak C, Steingraber H, et al: Expanding the definition of access: it isn't just about health insurance, *J Health Care Poor Underserved* 19:625–637, 2008.
82. Centers for Disease Control and Prevention: *National diabetes fact sheet: national estimates and general information on diabetes and prediabetes in the United States, 2011*, Atlanta, GA, 2011, U.S. Department of Health and Human Services, Centers for Disease Control and Prevention.
83. Gouni-Berthold I, Berthold HK, Mantzoros CS, et al: Sex disparities in the treatment and control of cardiovascular risk factors in type 2 diabetes, *Diabetes Care* 31(7):1389–1391, Jul 2008.
84. Huxley R, Barzi F, Woodward M: Excess risk of fatal coronary heart disease associated with diabetes in men and women: meta-analysis of 37 prospective cohort studies, *BMJ* 332(7533):73–78, Jan 2006.
85. Juutilainen A, Kortelainen S, Lehto S, et al: Gender difference in the impact of type 2 diabetes on coronary heart disease risk, *Diabetes Care* 27(12):2898–2904, 2004.
86. Tonstad S, Furu K, Rosvold EO, et al: Determinants of control of high blood pressure. The Oslo Health Study 2000-2001, *Blood Press* 13(6):343–349, 2004.
87. Wexler DJ, Grant RW, Meigs JB, et al: Sex disparities in treatment of cardiac risk factors in patients with type 2 diabetes, *Diabetes Care* 28(3):514–520, Mar 2005.
88. Chou AF, Scholle SH, Weisman CS, et al: Gender disparities in the quality of cardiovascular disease care in private managed care plans, *Womens Health Issues* 17(3):120–130, 2007.
89. Mosca L, Mochari-Greenberger H, Dolor RJ, et al: Twelve-year follow-up of American women's awareness of cardiovascular disease risk and barriers to heart health, *Circ Cardiovasc Qual Outcomes* 3(2):120–127, Mar 2010.
90. Ng JH, Kaftarian SJ, Tilson WM, et al: Self-reported delays in receipt of health care among women with diabetes and cardiovascular conditions, *Womens Health Issues* 20(5):316–322, Sep 2010.
91. Davis AM, Vinci LM, Okwuosa TM, et al: Cardiovascular health disparities: a systematic review of health care interventions, *Med Care Res Rev* 64(5 Suppl):29S–100S, 2007.
92. McGuire T, Alegria M, Cook B, et al: Implementing the Institute of Medicine definition of disparities: an application to mental care, *Health Research and Educational Trust* 41(5):1979–2005, 2006.
93. Bustamante A, Fang H, Rizzo J, et al: Understanding observed and unobserved health care access and utilization disparities among U.S. Latino adults, *Med Care Res Rev* 66(5):561–577, 2009.
94. Safford MM, Brown TM, Muntner PM, et al: Association of race and sex with risk of incident acute coronary heart disease events, *JAMA* 308(17):1768–1774, Nov 2012.
95. Hurley LP, Dickinson LM, Estacio RO, et al: Prediction of cardiovascular death in racial/ethnic minorities using Framingham risk factors, *Circ Cardiovasc Qual Outcomes* 3(2):181–187, Mar 2010.
96. Conway BN, May ME, Blot WJ: Mortality among low-income African Americans and whites with diabetes, *Diabetes Care* 35(11):2293–2299, Nov 2012.
97. Rooks RN, Simonsick EM, Klesges LM, et al: Racial disparities in health care access and cardiovascular disease indicators in Black and White older adults in the Health ABC Study, *J Aging Health* 20(6):599–614, Sep 2008.
98. Daviglus ML, Talavera GA, Avilés-Santa ML, et al: Prevalence of major cardiovascular risk factors and cardiovascular diseases among Hispanic/Latino individuals of diverse backgrounds in the United States, *JAMA* 308(17):1775–1784, Nov 2012.
99. Kollannoor-Samuel G, Vega-López S, Chhabra J, et al: Food insecurity and low self-efficacy are associated with health care access barriers among Puerto-Ricans with type 2 diabetes, *J Immigr Minor Health* 14(4):552–562, Aug 2012.
100. Mainous AG, Everett CJ, Liszka H, et al: Prehypertension and mortality in a nationally representative cohort, *Am J Cardiol* 94(12):1496–1500, Dec 2004.
101. Zhang Y, Lee ET, Devereux RB, et al: Prehypertension, diabetes, and cardiovascular disease risk in a population-based sample: the Strong Heart Study, *Hypertension* 47(3):410–414, Mar 2006.
102. Brown VY, Hartung BR: Managed care at the crossroads: can managed care organizations survive government regulation? *Ann Health Law* 7:25–72, 1998.
103. Trivedi AN, Grebla RC: Quality and equity of care in the veterans affairs health-care system and in medicare advantage health plans, *Med Care* 49(6):560–568, Jun 2011.
104. Anderson G: *Chronic care: making the case for ongoing care.* Princeton, NJ, 2010, Robert Wood Johnson Foundation. [on-line]. Available at: http://www.rwjf.org/files/research/50968chronic.care.chartbook.pdf. Accessed May 05, 2014.
105. Marengoni A, Angleman S, Melis R, et al: Aging with multimorbidity: a systematic review of the literature, *Ageing Res Rev* 10(4):430–439, 2011.
106. Boult C, Wieland GD: Comprehensive primary care for older patients with multiple chronic conditions: "Nobody rushes you through", *JAMA* 304:1936–1943, 2010.
107. Marengoni A, Rizzuto D, Wang HX, Winblad B, Fratiglioni L: Patterns of chronic multimorbidity in the elderly population, *J Am Geriatr Soc* 57(2):225–230, 2009.
108. Schafer I, von Leitner EC, Schon G, et al: Multimorbidity patterns in the elderly: a new approach of disease clustering identifies complex interrelations between chronic conditions, *PLoS One* 5 (12):e15941, 2010.
109. Formiga F, Ferrer A, Sanz H, Marengoni A, Alburquerque J, Pujol R: Patterns of comorbidity and multimorbidity in the oldest old: the Octabaix study, *Euro J of Int Med* 24(1):40–44, 2013.
110. Boyle JP, Thompson TJ, Gregg EW, Barker LE, Williamson DF: Projection of the year 2050 burden of diabetes in the US adult population: dynamic modeling of incidence, mortality, and prediabetes prevalence, *Popul Health Metr* 8:29, 2010.
111. Quiñones A, O'Neil M, Saha S, et al: *Interventions to reduce racial and ethnic disparities,* VA-ESP Project #05-225, 2011.
112. Cowie CC, Rust KF, Ford ES, et al: Full accounting of diabetes and pre-diabetes in the U.S. population in 1988–1994 and 2005–2006, *Diabetes Care* 32(2):287–294, 2009.
113. Cowie CC, Rust KF, Byrd-Holt DD, et al: Prevalence of diabetes and high risk for diabetes using A1C criteria in the U.S. population in 1988–2006, *Diabetes Care* 33(3):562–568, 2010.
114. Hunt KJ, Gebregziabher M, Egede LE: Racial and ethnic differences in cardio-metabolic risk in individuals with undiagnosed diabetes: National Health and Nutrition Examination Survey 1999–2008, *J Gen Intern Med* 27(8):893–900, 2012.

115. Harris MI, Flegal KM, Cowie CC, et al: Prevalence of diabetes, impaired fasting glucose, and impaired glucose tolerance in U.S. adults. The Third National Health and Nutrition Examination Survey, 1988–1994, *Diabetes Care* 21(4):518–524, 1998.
116. Twombly JG, Long Q, Zhu M, et al: Diabetes care in black and white veterans in the southeastern U.S, *Diabetes Care* 33(5):958–963, 2010.
117. Haffner SM, Mykkanen L, Festa A, et al: Insulin-resistant prediabetic subjects have more atherogenic risk factors than insulin-sensitive prediabetic subjects: implications for preventing coronary heart disease during the prediabetic state, *Circulation* 101(9):975–980, 2000.
118. Mykkanen L, Haffner SM, Kuusisto J, et al: Microalbuminuria precedes the development of NIDDM, *Diabetes* 43(4):552–557, 1994.
119. Nichols GA, Arondekar B, Herman WH: Medical care costs one year after identification of hyperglycemia below the threshold for diabetes, *Med Care* 46(3):287–292, 2008.
120. Nichols GA, Brown JB: Higher medical care costs accompany impaired fasting glucose, *Diabetes Care* 28(9):2223–2229, 2005.
121. Koopman RJ, Mainous AG 3rd, Liszka HA, et al: Evidence of nephropathy and peripheral neuropathy in US adults with undiagnosed diabetes, *Ann Fam Med* 4(5):427–432, 2006.
122. Borg R, Vistisen D, Witte DR, et al: Comparing risk profiles of individuals diagnosed with diabetes by OGTT and HbA1c The Danish Inter99 study, *Diabet Med* 27(8):906–910, 2010.
123. Dall TM, Zhang Y, Chen YJ, et al: The economic burden of diabetes, *Health Aff* 29(2):1–7, 2010.
124. Zhang Y, Dall TM, Mann SE, et al: The economic costs of undiagnosed diabetes, *Popul Health Manag* 12(2):95–101, 2009.
125. Duckworth W, Abraira C, Moritz T, et al: Glucose control and vascular complications in veterans with type 2 diabetes, *N Engl J Med* 360(2):129–139, 2009.
126. Gerstein HC, Miller ME, Byington RP, et al: Effects of intensive glucose lowering in type 2 diabetes, *N Engl J Med* 358(24):2545–2559, 2008.
127. Patel A, MacMahon S, Chalmers J, et al: Intensive blood glucose control and vascular outcomes in patients with type 2 diabetes, *N Engl J Med* 358(24):2560–2572, 2008.
128. Retinopathy and nephropathy in patients with type 1 diabetes four years after a trial of intensive therapy. The Diabetes Control and Complications Trial/Epidemiology of Diabetes Interventions and Complications Research Group, *N Engl J Med* 342(6):381–389, 2000.
129. Nathan DM, Cleary PA, Backlund JY, et al: Intensive diabetes treatment and cardiovascular disease in patients with type 1 diabetes, *N Engl J Med* 353(25):2643–2653, 2005.
130. Stratton IM, Adler AI, Neil HA, et al: Association of glycaemia with macrovascular and microvascular complications of type 2 diabetes (UKPDS 35): prospective observational study, *BMJ* 321(7258):405–412, 2000.
131. National Institutes of Health: *Weight loss does not lower heart disease risk from type 2 diabetes.* [Released 10/19/2012]; Available from: http://www.nih.gov/news/health/oct2012/niddk-19.htm. Accessed November 19, 2013.
132. American Diabetes Association: Standards of medical care in diabetes — 2008, *Diabetes Care* 31 (Suppl 1):S12–S54, 2008.
133. Consensus statement on the diagnosis and management of pre-diabetes in the continuum of hyperglycemia, *American College of Endocrinology and American Association of Clinical Endocrinologists*, July 23, 2008.

31 The Quality Chasm
Diabetes Mellitus

Jason S. Fish

Over the past several decades there has been much interest in refining the definition of quality of health care, moving the definition beyond an individual's perception of quality. A pivotal article by Avedis Donabedian in 1988 introduced the concept that quality of care can and should be measurable and that there will be multiple dimensions to identifying high-quality care depending on the perspective from which one is looking.[1] A provider may view quality in one way, a patient in another, and a payer in yet another. Furthermore, Donabedian introduced the idea that quality may be related not only to individuals delivering care but also to the systems in which care is delivered. Quality is likely influenced by structural attributes of the system or the processes of care used within the systems to deliver care.[1] Thus, quality becomes much broader than a health care provider's performance; it involves defining and measuring the structures and processes used by these providers and the systems delivering care. Shortly after this pivotal article, the U.S. Institute of Medicine (IOM) put forth a definition of quality of health care that encompassed Donabedian's conceptual model by stating that quality can be defined by how well health care itself aims at increasing the health outcomes for individuals and populations based on some set of agreed-on standards of care.[2]

With this broader definition of quality, the IOM examined the quality of health care in the United States; the culmination of this examination was the publication of two pivotal reports in 2000 and 2001 entitled "To Err Is Human: Building a Safer Health System"[3] and "Crossing the Quality Chasm: A New Health System for the 21st Century."[2] Coupled together, these reports raised significant concerns regarding the state of quality of care delivered by the U.S. health care system. In the second publication, the IOM cited an overwhelming amount of research illustrating the serious variation in quality of care across the nation across multiple settings (hospital, emergency, and ambulatory) and types of care delivered (acute, chronic, and emergent).[2] More specifically, the Quality Chasm report outlined how the U.S. health care system struggled with an overwhelming amount of overuse and underuse of services and errors in health care practice.[2]

After publication of these IOM reports, McGlynn and colleagues published results from an observational study corroborating the IOM observations, which identified that across 12 metropolitan areas involving 490 quality metrics for 30 acute and chronic conditions and preventative services, adults receiving care in the United States were only 54.9% likely to receive all of the evidence-based, recommended care.[4] Further analysis revealed that the variation occurred across all studied settings (hospital, emergency room, and outpatient) and types of care (acute, chronic, and preventative), with no single disease or specific clinical setting driving the low proportional use of guideline-recommended care.[4]

The Quality Chasm report[2] concluded, using Donabedian's quality framework of structure and process as related to outcome, that the United States health care system's struggle with achieving its expected or desired health outcomes is due to four key issues: increasing complexity of science and technology; increased prevalence of chronic conditions; poorly organized delivery systems; and constraints on exploiting the revolution in information technology.[2] In addition, the IOM put forth six specific aims for improvement to obtain comprehensive, consistent health care delivery.[2] The first aim is to optimize safety, focusing on avoiding injury or harm to patients in the context of health care delivery, including diagnostic evaluations, treatments, and the settings in which these are delivered. The second aim is to improve effectiveness, providing health care interventions based on evidence-based knowledge when possible. The third aim is to evolve toward more patient-centered health care delivery, offering care that is respectful of and responsive to individual patient preferences, needs, and values throughout the breadth of clinical decisions. The fourth aim is to improve timeliness of medical evaluation and treatment, reducing delays that are potentially harmful. The fifth aim is to improve efficiency, focusing on eliminating unnecessary processes to reduce cost, time, or use of resources. The last aim is to increase the equitable delivery of health care, providing care across populations with minimization of disparities based on individual patient characteristics, such as race and ethnicity, sex and other personal characteristics.[2]

ASSESSING THE QUALITY OF CARE FOR DIABETES

After publication of the IOM reports on health care quality, significant efforts to systematically improve the quality of health care delivery in the United States were undertaken. Given the increase in diabetes prevalence and the staggering associated health care costs (see also **Chapter 1**), the quality of diabetes care has been a key area of focus to reduce the morbidity and mortality resulting from diabetic macrovascular and microvascular disease complications. To best characterize the quality of care for patients with diabetes, evidence-based metrics of assessment are needed. These metrics should be accurate, reliable, and valid with regard to associations with important patient-experienced clinical outcomes to determine the present level of quality of health care delivery and to prospectively analyze progress.[5] Furthermore, with valid and widely accepted measurements, there can also be accountability regarding achievement of objectives by patient, provider, or health care system.[5]

For diabetes, there are several different measurements endorsed by various professional organizations and societies for determining the quality of health care delivery (**Fig. 31-1**).[6] These measurements include traditional process measurements (e.g., measuring hemoglobin A1c [HbA1c]) and control process measurements (e.g., controlling HbA1c), sometimes called *intermediate outcomes*. It is important to note that none of the measures have been validated as surrogates for clinical outcomes such as retinopathy, end-stage renal disease, or cardiovascular disease, although some have been shown to be associated with potentially lowering the risk of development of these clinical outcomes.[7-10]

QUALITY-OF-CARE MEASURES

During the last decade, there have been several quality improvement projects aimed at improving quality of diabetes care through focusing first on process measurements such as measurement of HbA1c, blood pressure, and low-density lipoprotein (LDL) cholesterol (LDL-C) or screening for retinopathy or neuropathy. Multiple small randomized clinical trials were able to demonstrate the improvement of these diabetes process measures[6]; unfortunately, with additional research, improving these process measures has not consistently translated into improvements in the control of HbA1c, blood pressure, and LDL-C nor in improvements in relevant, patient-experienced diabetes clinical outcomes. In addition, when efforts were successful in improving control measures, control generally faded over time, particularly when feedback ceased.[6]

Focusing on control process measures of quality care improves achievement of therapeutic targets; yet, there is an increasing recognition that many factors outside the traditional health care system influence a person's health and thus the clinical relevance of these measures.[5,6] Provider actions, patient behaviors, comorbid conditions, medication safety, and cost have all been implicated to influence these measures and the achievement of therapeutic targets.[6] What has also complicated interpretation of research analyzing such control markers is the need for targets to be individualized for patients, taking into account patient comorbidities, life expectancy, and risk of therapy side effects.[6] Yet, setting thresholds too aggressively to define high-quality care for control measures may cause harm for some patients, and setting thresholds too liberally may lead to limited accountability or identifiable opportunities for improvement.[6,11-13]

IMPORTANCE OF THE HEALTH CARE PROVIDER-PATIENT INTERFACE IN ACHIEVEMENT OF HIGH-QUALITY CARE

Another area of focus as outlined in the IOM Quality Chasm report[2] is that patient-centeredness is an important aspect of improving quality, taking into account patient preferences.[2] Patients may choose goals or may decline care, and there may be patient characteristics that require amendment of metric goals or foregoing of the metrics altogether.[6] Other approaches have used the comparative analyses of composite scores (diabetes overall control scores), weighted measures (control of HbA1c assigned more points than measurement of HbA1c), and risk-based measures (adjusting for comorbidities affecting diabetes outcomes). However, these approaches have not been proven to improve diabetes outcomes more than the standard approach, and the complexity involved in implementation and measurement, including patient preferences, limits their widespread use.

A promising evolution of diabetes quality measurements is toward clinical action measures for which the assessment of

Process Measures	Control Process Measure / Intermediate Outcomes	Outcomes
HbA1c, % tested in last 12 months	Good blood glucose control (HbA1c < 8%)	Stroke/CVA
BMI, % tested in last 12 months	Poor blood glucose control (HbA1c > 9)	Amputation
Blood pressure, % tested in last 12 months	BMI ≥ 30 kg/m² (obese)	Heart disease
Lipids, % tested in last 12 months	Blood pressure (below 140/80 mm Hg)	Renal disease
Eye exam, % examined in last 12-24 months	Lipids, percentage of those tested with total cholesterol <190 mg/dl	Severe vision loss/retinopathy
Foot exam, % examined in the last 12 months	Lipids, LDL cholesterol < 100 mg/dl	
Microalbuminuria, % tests in the last 12 months		

FIGURE 31-1 Diabetes quality measures. BMI = Body mass index; CVA = cerebrovascular accident; HbA1c = hemoglobin A1c; LDL = low-density lipoprotein.

quality is based on meeting one of four goals: (1) threshold met; (2) appropriate clinical action taken (e.g., starting or increasing the dose of an appropriate medication); (3) longitudinal assessment with resolution without intervention; or (4) identification of an exception such as a contraindication to further therapy intensification (e.g., a very low diastolic blood pressure) or maximal therapy already in use despite risk factor level without achievement of therapeutic target.[6] With continued improvement of electronic health records (EHRs), clinical action measures may prove an important way in which to measure quality, capturing provider action, patient preferences or attributes, and long-term effect.

SURVEY OF CURRENT QUALITY OF DIABETES CARE IN THE UNITED STATES

The main process measures for quality of diabetes care are (at least) annual measurement of HbA1c, lipids, blood pressure, and body mass index (BMI), and preventative measures including annual flu vaccine, testing for nephropathy,

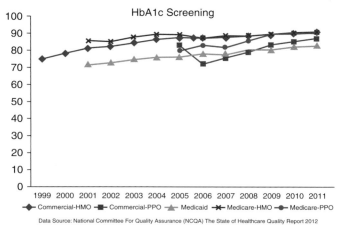

FIGURE 31-2 **Rates of HbA1c testing among US adults with diabetes 1999-2011, stratified by type of health care coverage.** *(Data from the National Committee For Quality Assurance (NCQA) The State of Healthcare Quality Report 2012. Available at: http://www.ncqa.org./Portals/0/SOHC-web1.pdf.)*

eye examination, and foot examination. The proportion of diabetes patients undergoing annual testing of HbA1c has been relatively stable over the past decade with a slight trend upward, in the high 80% range for most payers (**Fig. 31-2**).[14]

In 2010, the National Diabetes Surveillance System published self-reported data on several process measures (**Fig. 31-3**).[15] According to self-reports, 68.5% of patients had HbA1c measured at least twice per year, 62.8% received an annual eye examination, and 67.5% underwent an annual foot examination.[15] As discussed earlier, the past decade involved much effort toward improving process measures as evidenced by the relatively high percentage of patients undergoing HbA1c and LDL-C testing, blood pressure measurement, and nephropathy screening.

In examining control process measures of quality care, metrics associated more closely with outcomes, the United States national data for diabetes present some positive observations and some areas for improvement. The main control process measures are good glucose control (as reflected by HbA1c below 8%) as contrasted with poor glucose control (as defined as HbA1c above 9%); good blood pressure control (defined as blood pressure below 130/80 mm Hg); and good LDL-C control (defined as LDL-C below 100 mg/dL). In 2011, good HbA1c control (below 8%) averaged around 60% across multiple payers, ranging from 48% to 65% (**Fig. 31-4**).[14]

INCENTIVIZATION OR PAY FOR PERFORMANCE

Several major pay-for-performance (P4P) initiatives have reported their results for patients with diabetes. Unfortunately, the effect on quality from these initiatives remains controversial. Many studies indicate that improvements in measurements can be achieved; however, studies also indicate two important points: (1) once the financial incentive is removed, quality declines; and (2) once the quality targets are achieved, little improvement occurs afterward.[6] The largest P4P initiative, also cited as the most aggressive, is the U.K. Health System Quality and Outcomes Framework,

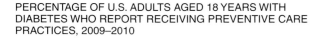
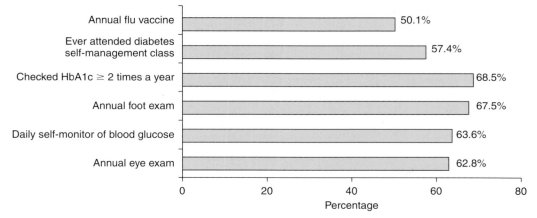

PERCENTAGE OF U.S. ADULTS AGED 18 YEARS WITH DIABETES WHO REPORT RECEIVING PREVENTIVE CARE PRACTICES, 2009–2010

Data were age adjusted. See Technical Notes for more details.

FIGURE 31-3 **Self-reported preventative care for patients with diabetes, 2009 and 2010.** *(Modified from National Diabetes Surveillance System, Behavioral Risk Factor Surveillance System data.)*

GOOD HbA1c CONTROL (HbA1c < 8.0%)

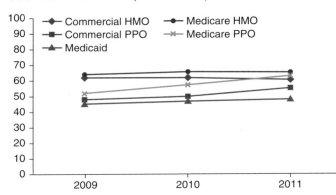

FIGURE 31-4 **Proportion of United States patients with diabetes achieving good glucose control 2009-2011.** HMO = Health maintenance organization; PPO = preferred provider organization. *(Modified from National Committee For Quality Assurance [NCQA]: The State of Healthcare Quality Report 2012.)*

introduced in 2004 as part of the General Medical Services contract. In this system, control of glucose improved dramatically with the program for many years. However, rates of quality for nonincentivized measures declined, and there was little improvement beyond the targeted glycemic goals.[6] In the United States, Kaiser Permanente is another system that has initiated diabetes performance measures aligned with financial incentives. Diabetes eye examinations and retinopathy screening were the focus of these measures. After initiation of the surveillance program, screening rates increased from 85% to 88%.[6] However, when the financial incentive was removed, the rates fell to below 80% (worse than baseline). More concerning are the findings of a cluster-randomized trial done using EHR-based diabetes clinical decision support to improve glucose and blood pressure control through the use of real-time feedback and incentives. In the trial, once the incentives and feedback ceased, even though the clinical decision support remained,

the results of the quality measures decreased.[6] Despite these unintended consequences and difficulty with sustainability, these types of incentives continue to develop, including value-based reimbursements. Time will tell how effective they are or how they will need to be used to maintain the success and improvements sought.

EFFORTS TO IMPROVE CONTROL MEASURES

There have been many other initiatives focused on improvement of control measures for patients with diabetes; unfortunately, many of these efforts have failed. First, efforts to improve patient adherence have been evaluated in several studies.[16–19] Although there were many different methods used, such as diabetes education, home aides, or nurse-led training, only a small effect was seen in improving some control measures.[16,17] These efforts tended to be more associated with improvement in processes of care,[18] consistent with prior observations that treatment intensification has a greater influence on achievement of control measures than does targeting improved patient adherence.[19] Specifically, efforts aimed at improving treatment intensification have shown some short-term improvements in control measures and may be a source of future focus.[10,20,21] One area that has consistently produced improved achievement of control measures is group-based training for self-management strategies. Several studies have demonstrated improved HbA1c, diabetes knowledge, systolic blood pressure, and BMI and a reduction in the need for medications with such group-based intervention programs.[22]

Recently, a promising new model was introduced aiming to help identify more accurately the measurements needed to improve outcomes with accountability tied to the measures (**Fig. 31-5**).[5,23] The model emphasizes areas of control and the primary drivers that affect health outcomes. In this model, health care (high control) accounts for 20% of control of improving health; health behaviors (shared between health care and patient) account for 30%; and socioeconomic and

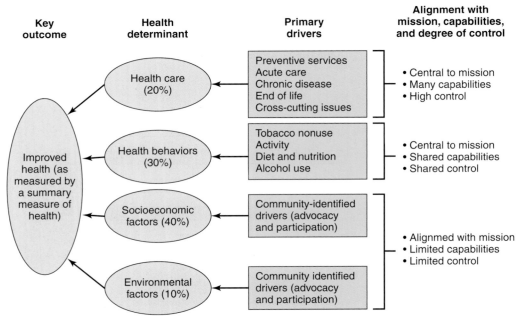

FIGURE 31-5 Framework of the drivers of health determinants.

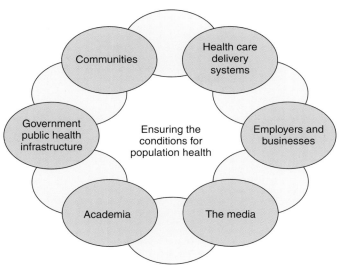

FIGURE 31-6 **The intersectoral public health system.** Ensuring population health.

Within the figure:
- Communities
- Health care delivery systems
- Government public health infrastructure
- Ensuring the conditions for population health
- Employers and businesses
- Academia
- The media

environmental factors accounting for the remaining 50%. With this model, more relevant quality measurements with realistic accountability can be developed.

SUMMARY

In summary, the IOM reports identifying the quality chasm a decade ago remain relevant for contemporary patients with diabetes. Overall, the quality of health care remains inconsistent, with continued variation across the nation, fragmented care lacking coordination, and a remarkable level of investment with little improvement in overall health outcomes.[5] Physicians practicing within engaged health systems, focused on improving processes, are continuing to struggle to translate these process improvements into better patient outcomes.

As illustrated in **Figure 31-6**, health is not defined simply by what happens when patients engage the health care system. There are many key stakeholders that need to be engaged, with health care systems playing a vital part.[24,25] If the health care system is to improve the health of patients with diabetes, given the overwhelming rates of diabetes and all of the sequelae associated with diabetes including health-related costs, then new models of care are going to be needed to improve these outcomes, holding accountable those responsible for each part as well as continuing to improve on diabetes quality measurements.

References

1. Donabedian A: The quality of care. How can it be assessed? *JAMA* 260(12):1743–1748, 1988.
2. Institute of Medicine (IOM): *Crossing the quality chasm: a new health system for the 21st century,* Washington DC, 2001, National Academies Press.
3. Kohn LT, Corrigan J, Donaldson MS: *To err is human: building a safer health system,* Washington, DC, 2000, National Academy Press.
4. McGlynn EA, Asch SM, Adams J, et al: The quality of health care delivered to adults in the United States, *N Engl J Med* 348:2635–2645, 2003.
5. Institute of Medicine (IOM): *Core measurement needs for better care, better health, and lower costs: counting what counts: workshop summary,* Washington, DC, 2013, The National Academies Press.
6. O'Connor P, Bodkin N, Fradkin J, et al: Diabetes performance measures: current status and future directions, *Diabetes Care* 34:1651–1659, July 2011.
7. Sidorenkov G, Voorham J, de Zeeuw D, et al: Do treatment quality indicators predict cardiovascular outcomes in patients with diabetes? *PLoS One* 8(10):e78821, 2013.
8. Sidorenkov G, Haaijer-Ruskamp FM, de Zeeuw D, et al: Relation between quality-of-care indicators for diabetes and patient outcomes: a systematic literature review, *Med Care Res Rev* 68:263–289, June 2011.
9. McEwen LN, Bilik D, Johnson SL, et al: Predictors and impact of intensification of antihyperglycemic therapy in type 2 diabetes: translating research into action for diabetes (TRIAD), *Diabetes Care* 32(6):971–976, 2009.
10. Sidorenkov G, Voorham J, de Zeeuw D, et al: Treatment quality indicators predict short-term outcomes in patients with diabetes: a prospective cohort study using the GIANTT database, *BMJ Qual Saf* 22:339–347, 2013.
11. Inzucchi SE, Bergenstal RM, Buse JB, et al: Management of hyperglycemia in type 2 diabetes: a patient-centered approach: position statement of the American Diabetes Association (ADA) and the European Association for the Study of Diabetes (EASD), *Diabetes Care* 35(6):1364–1379, 2012.
12. Ryden L, Grant PJ, Anker SD, et al: ESC guidelines on diabetes, pre-diabetes, and cardiovascular diseases developed in collaboration with the EASD: the Task Force on diabetes, pre-diabetes, and cardiovascular diseases of the European Society of Cardiology (ESC) and developed in collaboration with the European Association for the Study of Diabetes (EASD), *Eur Heart J* 34(39):3035–3087, 2013.
13. 2014 ADA Standards of Care for Diabetes in Diabetes Care.
14. National Committee for Quality Assurance (NCQA): *The state of healthcare quality 2012.* www.ncqa.org/Directories/HealthPlans/StateofHealthCareQuality.aspx. Last Accessed 9/2/2013.
15. Centers for Disease Control and Prevention: *Diabetes report card 2012,* Atlanta, GA, 2012, Centers for Disease Control and Prevention, U.S. Department of Health and Human Services.
16. Vermeire EIJJ, Wens J, Van Royen P, et al: Interventions for improving adherence to treatment recommendations in people with type 2 diabetes mellitus, *Cochrane Database Syst Rev* (2):2005, CD003638.
17. Loveman E, Royle P, Waugh N: Specialist nurses in diabetes mellitus, *Cochrane Database Syst Rev* (2):2003, CD003286.
18. Mangione CM, Gerzoff RB, Williamson DF, et al: TRIAD Study Group: The association between quality of care and the intensity of diabetes disease management programs, *Ann Intern Med* 145(2):107–116, 2006.
19. Schmittdiel JA, Uratsu CS, Karter AJ, et al: Why don't diabetes patients achieve recommended risk factor targets? Poor adherence versus lack of treatment intensification, *J Gen Intern Med* 23:588–594, 2008.
20. Renders CM, Valk GD, Griffin SJ, et al: Interventions to improve the management of diabetes mellitus in primary care, outpatient and community settings, *Cochrane Database Syst Rev* (4):2000, CD001481.
21. O'Connor PJ, Sperl-Hillen JM, Rush WA, et al: Impact of electronic health record clinical decision support on diabetes care: a randomized trial, *Ann Fam Med* 9(1):12–21, 2011.
22. Deakin TA, McShane CE, Cade JE, et al: Group based training for self-management strategies in people with type 2 diabetes mellitus, *Cochrane Database Syst Rev* (2):2005, CD003417.
23. Isham GJ: *HealthPartners' approach to assessing opportunities to improve community health: a perspective of a consumer governed, not-for-profit healthcare financing and delivery system,* 2012. http://www.iom.edu/~/media/Files/Activity%20Files/Quality/VSRT/Core%20Metrics%20Workshop/Presentations/Isham.pdf, Accessed September 5, 2013.
24. Institute of Medicine (IOM): *Primary care and public health: exploring integration to improve population health,* Washington, DC, 2012, National Academies Press.
25. Institute of Medicine (IOM): *The future of the public's health in the 21st century,* Washington, DC, 2002, National Academies Press.

Index

Note: Page numbers followed by *b* indicate boxes, *f* indicate figures and *t* indicate tables.

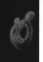